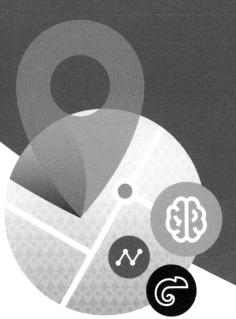

10th EDITION

CONTEMPORARY NURSING
Issues, Trends, & Management

Barbara Cherry, DNSc, MBA, RN, NEA-BC
Professor Emerita
Texas Tech University Health Sciences Center
School of Nursing
Lubbock, Texas

Susan R. Jacob, PhD, MS, RN
Professor Emerita
The University of Tennessee Health Science Center
College of Nursing
Memphis, Tennessee

ELSEVIER

Elsevier
3251 Riverport Lane
St. Louis, Missouri 63043

Notice

Practitioners and researchers must always rely on their own experience and knowledge in evaluating
and using any information, methods, compounds or experiments described herein. Because of rapid
advances in the medical sciences, in particular, independent verification of diagnoses and drug dosages
should be made. To the fullest extent of the law, no responsibility is assumed by Elsevier, authors, editors
or contributors for any injury and/or damage to persons or property as a matter of products liability,
negligence or otherwise, or from any use or operation of any methods, products, instructions, or ideas
contained in the material herein.

Previous editions copyrighted 2023, 2019, 2017, 2014, 2011, 2008, 2005, 2002, 1999.

Content Strategist: Sandra Clark
Senior Content Development Manager: Lisa P. Newton
Publishing Services Manager: Deepthi Unni
Project Manager: Thoufiq Mohammed
Design Direction: Margaret Reid

Printed in India

Last digit is the print number: 9 8 7 6 5 4 3 2 1

Working together
to grow libraries in
developing countries

www.elsevier.com • www.bookaid.org

This book is dedicated to all student nurses whose curiosity and enthusiasm for nursing will provide strong leadership for the profession far into the future, and to all practicing nurses who face serious challenges in the workplace but reap great rewards for providing high-quality health care for individuals, families, and communities.

Being a Nurse Means ...

You will never be bored,
You will always be frustrated,
You will be surrounded by challenges,
So much to do and so little time.
You will carry immense responsibility
And very little authority.
You will step into people's lives,
And you will make a difference.
Some will bless you.
Some will curse you.
You will see people at their worst,
And at their best.
You will never cease to be amazed at people's capacity
For love, courage, and endurance.
You will see life begin
And end.
You will experience resounding triumphs
And devastating failures.
You will cry a lot.
You will laugh a lot.
You will know what it is to be human
And to be humane.

Melodie Chenevert, RN

CONTRIBUTORS

Cindy Acton, DNP, RN, NEA-BC
Associate Professor
School of Nursing
Texas Tech University Health Sciences Center
Amarillo, Texas

Trina Barrett, DNP, RN, CNE, CCRN-K
Assistant Professor
College of Nursing
University of Tennessee Health Science Center
Memphis, Tennessee

Katie Boston-Leary, PhD, MBA, MHA, RN, NEA-BC
Director
Nursing Programs
American Nurses Association
Silver Spring, Maryland

Barbara Cherry, DNSc, MBA, RN, NEA-BC
Professor Emerita
Texas Tech University Health Sciences Center
School of Nursing
Lubbock, Texas

Charlotte Eliopoulos, PhD, MPH, ND, RN
Consultant, Educator, Author of Nursing
Glen Arm, Maryland

Stephanie H. Hoelscher, DNP, RN-BC, CPHIMS, CHISP, FHIMSS
Professor
School of Nursing
Texas Tech University Health Sciences Center
Lubbock, Texas

Susan R. Jacob, PhD, MS, RN
Professor Emerita
The University of Tennessee Health Science Center
College of Nursing
Memphis, Tennessee

Rebecca R. Keck, DNP, RN, NEA-BC
Senior Associate Dean: Faculty Affairs, Professor
Department of Faculty Affairs
Vanderbilt University School of Nursing
Nashville, Tennessee

Patricia R. Keene, DNP, ACNP-BC, ACHPN
Nurse Practitioner
Baptist Reynold's Hospice House
Collierville, Tennessee

Laura Mahlmeister, PhD, RN
President
Nursing Quality and Patient Safety
Mahlmeister & Associates
Belmont, California

Leslie Moro, DNP, APRN, FNP-BC
Assistant Professor
School of Nursing
University of Tennessee at Chattanooga
Chattanooga, Tennessee

Carole R. Myers, PhD, RN, FAAN
Professor Emerita
College of Nursing
University of Tennessee
Knoxville, Tennessee

Tommie L. Norris, DNS, RN
Dean
Benjamin Leon School of Nursing
Miami Dade College
Miami, Florida

Keevia Y. Porter, DNP, APRN, NP-C, PMHNP-BC
Assistant Professor
Dr. Susan L. Davis, RN & Richard J. Henley College of
    Nursing
Sacred Heart University
Fairfield, Connecticut

Anna Marie Sallee, PhD, RN, CCRN-K
ATI Educator, NCLEX Specialist
Department of Nursing
Ascend Learning
Lubbock, Texas

Carla D. Sanderson, PhD, RN, FAAN
Provost
Department of Academics
Chamberlain University
Chicago, Illinois
Provost Emerita
Union University
Jackson, Tennessee

Terri Stewart, MSN, RN
Instructor
College of Nursing
University of Tennessee Health Science Center
Memphis, Tennessee

Elizabeth E. Weiner, PhD, RN-BC, FACMI, FAAN
Senior Associate Dean of Informatics, Emerita
Professor in the School of Nursing, Emerita
Vanderbilt University School of Nursing
Nashville, Tennessee

ANCILLARY WRITERS

Charla K. Hollin, RN, BSN
Allied Health Division Chair
University of Arkansas Rich Mountain
Mena, Arkansas
TEACH for Nurses, PowerPoint Slides

Linda Turchin, RN, MSN, CNE
Professor Emeritus of Nursing
Fairmont State University
School of Nursing
Fairmont, West Virginia
*Test Bank; Student Review Questions;
Student Resource: Next-Generation NCLEX®
    (NGN)-Style Case Study*

REVIEWERS

Lori Sullivan, DNP, MSN, RN
Program Chair/Professor of Nursing
Finlandia University
Hancock, Michigan

Alison S. Knox, RN, MSN
Nursing Faculty
List, MSN, BSN Pitt Community College
Greenville, North Carolina

Eleonor Pusey-Reid, DNP, RN, MEd
Associate Professor
MGH Institute of Health Professions
Boston, Massachusetts

Linda J. Hassler, DNP, RN, GCNS-BC, FGNLA
Assistant Professor
Rutgers University, School of Nursing
Newark, New Jersey

Angela M. Vogel MSN-ED, RN
Assistant Director of Nursing/Assistant Professor
San Bernardino Valley College
San Bernardino, California

Elizabeth A. Thomas, MSN-CNL, RN, CCRN, CEN
Assistant Professor of Nursing
Roane State Community College–Knoxville Campus
Harriman, Tennessee

PREFACE

As we begin 2024 we see that nurses are being challenged like no other time in our history to continue their critically important work of caring for patients, populations, and communities, as well as leading and managing health care settings. The nursing profession is currently confronting serious nursing shortages as a result of an increasing demand for health care, an aging population requiring more care, advanced use of technology in health care requiring nurses' expertise, and an avalanche of nurses who retired or left the profession following the COVID-19 pandemic. Fortunately nursing education has pushed forward with new advancements to educate greater numbers of nurses with an increased emphasis on technology integration, online learning, and simulation-based training. Nurse leaders are also focusing on mental health concerns among nurses with efforts to provide better support systems and resources to address burnout and stress and promote mental well-being for nurses. In another positive movement the nursing profession has recognized the need to advance diversity, equity, and inclusion in the nursing profession and efforts are under way to increase diversity among nursing students and professionals to better reflect the diverse patient populations that we serve. Nurses are also leading the way to optimize the role of nurses in health care delivery to ensure they are supported to practice at the highest level of their education and training. Today, more than ever, nurses have proven their value to society in the multitude of roles in which they function, including caring for critically ill patients, educating the next generation of nurses, promoting the health and wellness of individuals and populations, leading interprofessional teams, and creating healthy work environments and efficient processes of care. Nurses must continue to use their considerable influence, knowledge, and clinical judgment to address the ongoing issues facing the US health care system.

This book will provide the foundational knowledge nurses need to competently address complex issues such as patient safety and quality care, health care reform and the uninsured population, nursing workforce challenges, advancing technology, changing legal and ethical concerns, care at the end of life, evolving nursing education trends, rising health care costs, and working within a multicultural and multigenerational society. The book will also provide students with strategies to prepare for Next-Gen NCLEX-RN examination.

WHO WILL BENEFIT FROM THIS BOOK?

The tenth edition of *Contemporary Nursing: Issues, Trends, & Management* is an excellent resource to help nursing students and practicing nurses understand the complex issues they are facing and use clinical judgment to implement strategies from the direct patient care level to the national legislative arena that can significantly improve patient care, population health, the health care system, and the nursing profession. The book provides many examples of using the Clinical Judgment Model to master nursing practice; it also provides several Next Generation NCLEX (NGN) questions and case studies to help nursing students understand and master the new type of testing they will experience when they face the NGN licensure examination.

ORGANIZATION

Unit 1: The Development of Nursing

The book opens with a presentation about the exciting evolution of nursing, its very visible public image, and its core foundations, which include nursing education, licensure and certification, nursing theory, and nursing research and evidence-based practice. These opening chapters provide the reader with a solid background for understanding and studying current and future trends.

Unit 2: Current Issues in Health Care

This unit provides a comprehensive overview of the most current trends and issues occurring today in nursing and health care, including health care financing and economics, legal and ethical issues, cultural and social issues, complementary and alternative healing, workplace issues and nursing workforce challenges, collective bargaining and unions, technology in the clinical setting, end-of-life care, and emergency preparedness. Students, faculty, and seasoned nurses will be challenged to critically examine each of these significant issues that are shaping the practice of professional nursing and the health care delivery system.

Unit 3: Leadership and Management in Nursing

This unit offers a foundation of knowledge in nursing leadership and management, with a focus on the basic skills that are necessary for all nurses, regardless of the setting or position in which they work, to function effectively in the professional nursing role. Chapters examine the foundation of leadership and management, budgeting basics, effective communication, delegation and supervision, staffing and nursing care delivery models, quality improvement and patient safety, and health policy and politics. The updated content in this unit provides the most current information available related to nursing leadership and management and will serve as both a valuable educational tool for students and a useful resource for practicing nurses.

Unit 4: Career Management

The final unit prepares the student to embark on a career in nursing. Making the transition from student to professional, using the clinical judgment model, managing time, understanding career opportunities, finding a good match between the nurse and the employer, and passing the Next GEN NCLEX-RN® examination are all presented with practical, useful advice that will serve as an excellent resource for both students and novice nurses as they build their careers in professional nursing.

LEARNING AIDS

Each chapter in the tenth edition contains the same features that made the previous editions so successful:

- A **Professional/Ethical Issue** is included in every chapter as an interesting, real-life dilemma that will test the reader's ability to think critically and apply ethical and professional standards to address issues or concerns the reader may face in their nursing practice.
- Real-life **Vignettes** and **Questions to Consider** at the beginning of each chapter, which pique the reader's interest in the chapter content and stimulate critical thinking, are provided.
- Also included are **Key Terms**, which contain clear and concise definitions of terms critical to enhance

readers' understanding of the topics and expand their vocabulary related to health care issues.

- Integrated **Learning Outcomes** provide instructors and students with a clear understanding of what behaviors can be expected after a study of the chapter is completed.
- The **Chapter Overview** is an overall perspective and guide to the chapter content.
- **Clinical Judgment and Next-Generation NCLEX® Examination Style Questions** are included in some chapters as appropriate, to guide students to apply the Clinical Judgment Model to decision-making in practice.
- A **Summary** at the end of each chapter offers a wrap-up based on the questions at the beginning of the chapter and helps students focus on points to remember.
- **References** related to chapter content help students explore further the issues that were covered.

NEW TO THIS EDITION

Every chapter in the tenth edition has been updated to include the most current and relevant information available. New and expanded content in this edition includes:

- New chapter summaries that close the loop from the opening questions at the beginning of the chapter to the summary of key chapter content
- Expanded content on creating joy and engagement in the workplace
- Expanded content on bullying and incivility
- Most current data available on the nursing shortage and retention strategies
- Virtual nursing as a new model of care
- New team-based care models that have evolved as a result of the pandemic
- Undated information on current health information technology laws and initiatives
- Health-related wearable technologies including sensors, biosensors, and remote monitoring
- Artificial intelligence, machine learning, and virtual-, augmented-, and mixed-reality technologies
- Mobile technologies and mHealth
- Updated patient safety goals and nursing quality indicators
- AHRQ's 2023 Report on *Making Healthcare Safer*
- New section on the role of professional nurses in quality improvement based on the AACN 2021 Essentials
- Becoming resilient and practicing mindfulness
- New section on clinically focused time-management strategies

- Rethinking health by reducing disparities to achieve health equity
- Strengthening nursing capacity, expertise, and leadership
- Transforming the delivery of health care services
- Current legal cases involving nurses
- Cultural humility. health disparities, and social determinants of health
- Health equity
- Updated standards of cultural competence
- Healthy People 2030
- Future of Nursing 2020–2030
- Updated statistics on the nursing workforce
- Expanded examples of real-world ethical dilemmas and applications
- The *Nurses Bill of Rights* introduced by the American Nurses Association (ANA) in 2022
- Expanded content on whistleblower protection and ANA's position statement
- Future opportunities for registered nurse (RN) employment
- New section on diversity, equity, inclusion, belonging, and justice and *The National Commission to Address Racism in Nursing*
- Translational research
- Comprehensive overview of the Next-Generation NCLEX-RN examination and strategies to prapare for the exam.
- Case studies using the Clinical Judgment Model and Next-Generation NCLEX® Examination–Style Questions on the following topics:
  - Advanced directives
  - Nurses role in reducing health care costs
  - Delegation and supervision
  - Making assignments
  - Violence in the workplace
  - Bullying in the workplace
  - Quality improvement
  - Health policy to address social determinants of health
  - Time management
  - Developing leadership skills
  - Conflict resolution

TEACHING AND LEARNING RESOURCES

For Instructors

Instructor Resources on Evolve, available at http://evolve.elsevier.com/Cherry/, provide a wealth of material to help you make your nursing instruction a success. In addition to all of the Student Resources the following are provided for faculty:

- **TEACH for Nurses Lesson Plans**, based on textbook chapter Learning Outcomes, serve as ready-made, modifiable lesson plans and a complete road map to link all parts of the educational package. These concise and straightforward lesson plans can be modified or combined to meet your particular scheduling and teaching needs.
- **PowerPoint Presentations** are organized by chapter, with more than 1000 slides for in-class lectures. These are detailed and include customizable text and image lecture slides to enhance learning in the classroom or in Web-based course modules. If you share them with students, they can use the note feature to help them with your lectures.
- The **Test Bank** has more than 500 test items, complete with the correct answer, rationale, cognitive level of each question, corresponding step of the nursing process, appropriate NCLEX format, and text page reference(s).
- **CLINICAL JUDGMENT AND NEXT-GENERATION NCLEX® EXAMINATION-STYLE QUESTIONS** in the textbook for *Contemporary Nursing: Issues, Trends, & Management.*
- **Additional CLINICAL JUDGMENT AND NEXT-GENERATION NCLEX® EXAMINATION- STYLE CASE STUDIES** for Issues and Trends in Nursing.
- **Image Collection** includes all the images from the book.

For Students

Student Resources on Evolve, available at http://evolve.elsevier.com/Cherry/, provide a wealth of valuable learning resources. The Evolve Resources page near the front of the book gives login instructions and a description of each resource.

- **Answer key for CLINICAL JUDGMENT AND NEXT-GENERATION NCLEX® EXAMINATION-STYLE Case Studies** in the textbook for *Contemporary Nursing: Issues, Trends, & Management.*
- **Résumé Builder** offers templates and samples of résumés and cover letters.
- **Case Studies** provide detailed case studies covering the major content in the chapters.
- **Additional CLINICAL JUDGMENT AND NEXT-GENERATION NCLEX® EXAMINATION- STYLE Case Studies** for Issues and Trends in Nursing.
- **Review Questions** assist in preparing for the NCLEX® examination.

Barbara Cherry, DNSc, MBA, RN, NEA-BC, received her diploma in nursing from Methodist Hospital School of Nursing, her BSN from West Texas A&M University, her MBA from Texas Tech University, her MSN from Texas Tech University Health Sciences Center, and her Doctor of Nursing Science from the University of Tennessee Health Science Center. Dr. Cherry's clinical background is in critical care, medical-surgical, and nephrology nursing. Her research was focused on the long-term care nursing workforce and technology. She has more than 25 years of clinical and nursing leadership experience followed by more than 20 years as a nurse educator and academic administrator. She is a professor teaching leadership, nursing administration, and finance at Texas Tech University Health Sciences Center School of Nursing in Lubbock, Texas.

Susan R. Jacob, PhD, MS, RN, received her BSN from West Virginia University, her MS from San Jose State University, and her PhD from the University of Tennessee, Memphis. Her extensive experience as a clinician, educator, and researcher has been focused in the community health arena, specifically home health and hospice. She has been an educator for 40 years and has taught at both the undergraduate and graduate levels. Dr. Jacob's research has addressed the grief experience of older adults and RNs working on the frontlines during the pandemic. She is Professor Emerita in the College of Nursing at the University of Tennessee, Health Science Center, Memphis, Tennessee.

ACKNOWLEDGMENTS

Our contributors deserve our most sincere thanks for their high-quality, timely work that demonstrates genuine expertise and professionalism. Their contributions have made this book a truly first-rate text that will be invaluable to nursing students and faculty and will serve as an outstanding resource for practicing nurses. We extend a special thanks to our reviewers, who gave us helpful suggestions and insights as we developed the 10th edition.

We would like to express our grateful appreciation to the Elsevier staff—Sandra Clark, Senior Content Strategist; Lisa Newton, Senior Content Development Manager; and Thoufiq Mohammed, Project Manager—for their very capable and professional support, guidance, and calm reassurance.

Our deepest appreciation goes to the most important people in our lives—our husbands, Mike and Dick, our families, and our friends. Their enduring support and extreme patience have allowed us to accomplish what sometimes seemed to be the impossible.

CONTENTS

1

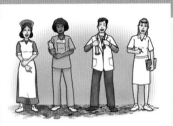

Building on a strong foundation for a bright future.

The Evolution of Professional Nursing

Susan R. Jacob, PhD, MS, RN

(e) Additional resources are available online at: http://evolve.elsevier.com/Cherry/

LEARNING OUTCOMES

After studying this chapter, the reader will be able to:
1. Summarize health practices throughout the course of history.
2. Analyze the effect of historic, political, social, and economic events on the development of nursing.
3. Describe the evolution of professional challenges experienced by nurses of diverse ethnic, racial, and educational backgrounds.

KEY TERMS

Florence Nightingale (1820–1910) She is considered the founder of organized, professional nursing. She is best known for her contributions to the reforms in the British Army Medical Corps, improved sanitation in India, improved public health in Great Britain, use of statistics to document health outcomes, and the development of organized training for nurses.

Professional nurse A specially trained professional who addresses the humanistic and holistic needs of patients, families, and environments and provides responses to patterns and/or needs of patients, families, and communities to actual and potential health problems. The professional nurse has diverse roles, such as health care provider, client advocate, educator, care coordinator, primary care practitioner, and change agent (Katz et al., 2009).

We thank Shiphrah A. Williams-Evans, PhD, APRN, BC, for her contribution to this chapter in the fourth edition.

PROFESSIONAL/ETHICAL ISSUE

Gretchen Ornish graduated from nursing school last year and became active in the local nurses association. She volunteered for the program planning committee because her friend, Beth Aaron, was also on the committee. The committee decided to plan a program for Nurses Week that would highlight pioneers in nursing. Beth agreed to pull a list of famous nurses together for the committee. When the committee met to start planning the program, Beth presented her list, which included Florence Nightingale, Clara Barton, Dorothea Dix, Lillian Wald, Mary Breckenridge, and many others. When Gretchen realized that all of the nurses on Beth's list were White, she suggested that Beth add names of nurses such as Harriet Tubman, Sojourner Truth, Mary Mahoney, Beverly Malone, and Elizabeth Carnegie. Beth was very reluctant to add other nurses to the list she had already developed, saying that there would not be enough time to feature more nurses than those on the list. She also stated that the names she had come up with were widely known and, in her opinion, the most significant. Gretchen was very disappointed because she remembered so many Black nurses of distinction and felt that they should be honored as well. She feared that the program planning committee would be criticized for overlooking some very important Black nursing leaders. Gretchen did not want to be part of providing what might be considered a biased program. She voiced her concerns to Beth and the committee, stating that she felt it would be so much better if a more diverse group of nursing pioneers was highlighted. In spite of Gretchen's concerns, Beth persuaded the committee to proceed with planning the program to include the list of nursing pioneers she presented.

What are some strategies that Gretchen might use to persuade Beth and the committee to present a more diverse group of nursing pioneers at the Nurses Week program?

VIGNETTE

My mother and grandmother, who are both nurses, were very excited when I decided to pursue nursing as a career. They love to talk about their experiences in nursing school in the 1970s and 1990s. They shared with me what they were taught about Florence Nightingale, who began the work of organized nursing. My class on the evolution of nursing covers much of the same history that my mother and grandmother were taught in their nursing programs. However, since the time when they received their education, nursing has evolved into a profession that is focused on meeting the complex needs of the diverse people it serves and preparing providers who can think critically to meet those needs. Nursing education today involves interprofessional experiences and the use of technologies such as vSim for Nursing and Shadow Health, which were unheard of in their day. Although my grandmother, mother, and I have a lot in common when it comes to our desire to help individuals achieve optimal health outcomes, our nursing education and career opportunities are vastly different.

Questions to Consider While Reading This Chapter

1. What were the challenges faced by nurses historically?
2. How has access to care and managed care affected professional nursing practice?
3. What are the challenges facing nurses in the 21st century?

CHAPTER OVERVIEW

Throughout the pages of recorded history, nursing has been integrated into every facet of life. A legacy of human caring was initiated when, according to the book of Exodus, two midwives, Shiphrah and Puah, rescued the baby Moses and hid him to save his life. This legacy of caring has progressed throughout the years, responding to psychological, social, environmental, and physiologic needs of society. Nurses of the past and present have struggled for recognition as knowledgeable professionals. The evolution of this struggle is reflected in political, cultural, environmental, and economic events that have sculpted our nation and world history (Catalano, 2015).

Traditionally, society recognized men as healers. Women challenged the status quo and transformed nursing from a mystical phenomenon to a respected profession (Catalano, 2015). Florence Nightingale played a major role in bringing about changes in nursing. Using the concept of role modeling, she and other nursing leaders demonstrated the value of their worth through their work in fighting for the cause of health and healing. During the 20th century, nurses made tremendous advancements in the areas of education, practice, research, and technology. Nursing as a science progressed through education, clinical practice, development of theory, and rigorous research. Today's nurses continue to be challenged to expand their roles and explore new areas of practice and leadership. This chapter provides a brief glimpse of health care practices and nursing care in the prehistoric period and early civilization; it then describes the evolution of professional nursing practice. Box 1.1 summarizes some of the important events in the evolution of nursing.

BOX 1.1   Important Events in the Evolution of Nursing

1751—The Pennsylvania Hospital is the first hospital established in America.

1798—The US Marine Hospital Service comes into being by an act of Congress on July 16. It is renamed the US Public Health Service in 1912.

1840—Two Black women, Mary Williams and Frances Rose, who founded Nursing Sisters of the Holy Cross, are listed as nurses in the City of Baltimore Directory.

1851—Florence Nightingale (1820–1910) attends Kaiserswerth to train as a nurse.

1854—During the Crimean War, Florence Nightingale transforms the image of nursing.

1861—The outbreak of the Civil War causes Black women to volunteer as nurses. Among these women are Harriet Tubman, Sojourner Truth, and Susie King Taylor.

1872—Another school of nursing opens in the United States: The New England Hospital for Women and Children in Boston, Massachusetts.

1873—Linda Richards is responsible for designing a written patient record and physician's order system—the first in a hospital.

1879—Mary Mahoney, the first trained Black nurse, graduates from the New England Hospital for Women and Children in Boston, Massachusetts.

1881—The American Red Cross is established by Clara Barton.

1886—The Visiting Nurse Association (VNA) is started in Philadelphia, Pennsylvania; Spelman College, Atlanta, Georgia, establishes the first diploma-granting nursing program for African Americans.

1893—Lillian Wald and Mary Brewster establish the Henry Street Visiting Nurse Service in New York.

1896—The Nurses' Associated Alumnae of the United States and Canada is established.

1898—Namahyoke Curtis, an untrained Black nurse, is assigned by the War Department as a contract nurse in the Spanish–American War.

1899—The International Council of Nurses (ICN) is founded.

1900—The first issue of the *American Journal of Nursing* is published.

1901—The Army Nurse Corps is established under the Army Reorganization Act.

1902—School nursing is established in New York City by Linda Rogers.

1903—The first nurse practice acts are passed, and North Carolina is the first state to implement registration of nurses.

1908—The National Association of Colored Graduate Nurses is founded; it is dissolved in 1951.

1909—Ludie Andrews sues the Georgia State Board of Nurse Examiners to secure Black nurses the right to take the state board examination and become licensed; she wins in 1920.

1911—The American Nurses Association (ANA) is established.

1912—The US Public Health Service and the National League for Nursing (NLN) are established.

1918—Eighteen Black nurses are admitted to the Army Nurse Corps after the armistice ending World War I is signed.

1919—*Public Health Nursing* is written by Mary S. Gardner. A public health nursing program is started at the University of Michigan.

1921—The Sheppard–Towner Act is passed providing federal aid for maternal and child health care.

1922—Sigma Theta Tau is founded (becomes the International Honor Society of Nursing in 1985).

1923—The Goldmark Report criticizes the inadequacies of hospital-based nursing schools and recommends increased educational standards.

1924—The US Indian Bureau Nursing Service is founded by Elinor Gregg.

1925—The Frontier Nursing Service is founded by Mary Breckenridge.

1935—The Social Security Act is passed.

1937—Federal appropriations for cancer, venereal diseases, tuberculosis, and mental health begin.

1939—World War II begins.

1943—The US Army establishes a quota of 56 Black nurses for admission to the Army Nurse Corps. The Nurse Training Act is passed.

1943—An amendment to the Nurse Training Act is passed that bars racial bias.

1945—The US Navy drops the color bar and admits four Black nurses.

1946—Nurses are classified as professionals by the US Civil Service Commission. The Hospital Survey and Construction Act (Hill–Burton) is passed.

1948—The Brown Report discusses the future of nursing.

1948—Estelle Osborne is the first Black nurse elected to the board of the ANA. The ANA votes individual membership to all Black nurses excluded from any state association.

1949—M. Elizabeth Carnegie is the first Black nurse to be elected to the board of a state association (Florida).

1950—The Code for Professional Nurses is published by the ANA.

1952—National nursing organizations are reorganized from six to two: ANA and NLN.

Continued

BOX 1.1   Important Events in the Evolution of Nursing—cont'd

1954—The Supreme Court decision in Brown v. Board of Education asserts that "separate educational facilities are inherently unequal."

1965—The Social Security Amendment includes Medicare and Medicaid.

1971—The National Black Nurses Association is organized.

1973—The ANA forms the American Academy of Nursing.

1974—Luther Christman helps establish the National Male Nurse Association, which becomes the American Assembly for Men in Nursing in 1981.

1978—Barbara Nichols is the first Black nurse elected president of the ANA. M. Elizabeth Carnegie, a Black nurse, is elected president of the American Academy of Nursing.

1979—Brigadier General Hazel Johnson Brown is the first Black chief of the Army Nurse Corps.

1983—The American Academy of Nursing (AAN) Task Force on Nursing Practice in Hospitals identifies work environment characteristics known to this day as the "Forces of Magnetism."

1985—Vernice Ferguson, a Black nurse, is elected president of Sigma Theta Tau International.

1986—The Association of Black Nursing Faculty is founded by Dr. Sally Tucker Allen.

1990—Congress proclaims March 10 as Harriet Tubman Day in the United States, honoring her as a brave Black freedom fighter and nurse during the Civil War.

1990—The Bloodborne Pathogen Standard is established by the Occupational Safety and Health Administration (OSHA).

1991—*Healthy People 2000* is published.

1993—The National Center for Nursing Research is upgraded to the National Institute of Nursing Research within the National Institutes of Health.

1994—NCLEX-RN, a computerized nurse-licensing examination, is introduced.

1996—The Commission on Collegiate Nursing Education is established as an agency devoted exclusively to the accreditation of baccalaureate and graduate-degree nursing programs.

1999—Beverly Malone, the second Black president of the ANA, is named Deputy Assistant Secretary for Health, Department of Health and Human Services, Office of Public Health and Science.

1999—The Institute of Medicine (IOM) releases its landmark report: *To Err Is Human: Building a Safer Health System*.

2000—M. Elizabeth Carnegie is inducted into the ANA Hall of Fame. The American Nurses Credentialing Center gives its first psychiatric mental health nurse practitioner examination. *Healthy People 2010* is published.

2001—Beverly Malone is appointed General Secretary, Royal College of Nursing, London. The Health Care Financing Administration (HCFA) becomes the Centers for Medicare & Medicaid Services (CMS).

2002—Johnson & Johnson Health Care Systems Inc. launches The Future of Nursing, a national publicity campaign to address the nursing shortage.

2002—To address the nursing shortage, the Nurse Reinvestment Act is signed into law by President George W. Bush.

2002—Significant funding is obtained for geriatric nursing initiatives.

2003—The American Nurses Foundation launches an "Investment in Nursing" campaign to deal with the nursing shortage.

2003—The IOM report *Keeping Patients Safe: Transforming the Work Environment of Nurses* is released.

2003—The AACN White Paper on the Role of the Clinical Nurse Leader is published.

2005—The CCNE decides that only programs that offer practice doctoral degrees with the Doctor of Nursing Practice (DNP) title will be eligible for CCNE accreditation.

2005—The NLN offers and certifies the first national certification for nurse educators; the initials CNE may be placed behind the names of those certified.

2006—The AACN approves essentials of doctoral education for advanced nursing practice (DNP).

2007—The Commission on Nurse Certification, an autonomous arm of the AACN, begins certifying clinical nurse leaders (CNLs).

2007—American Nurses Credentialing Center acquires the Texas Nurses Association's Nurse Friendly Program and renames it Pathway to Excellence.

2008—The Commission on Collegiate Nursing Education begins accrediting DNP programs.

2010—*Healthy People 2020* is launched by the Department of Health and Human Services.

2010—The Patient Protection and Affordable Care Act (Public Law 111–152) is passed.

2010—The Health Care and Education Affordability Reconciliation Act is passed.

2011—The IOM report *The Future of Nursing: Leading Change, Advancing Health* is released.

2016—*Advancing Healthcare Transformation: A New Era for Academic Nursing*, commissioned by the American Association of Colleges of Nursing (AACN) is released.

2017—The American Nurses Association Enterprise (ANAE) launches Healthy Nurse Healthy Nation.

BOX 1.1   **Important Events in the Evolution of Nursing—cont'd**

2020—*Healthy People 2030* is launched by the Department of Health and Human Services.

2020—COVID-19 Pandemic

2021—The National Commission to Address Racism in Nursing (the Commission) is established. The Commission examines the issue of racism within nursing nationwide, focusing on the impact on nurses, patients, communities, and health care systems to motivate all nurses to confront individual and systemic racism.

2021—The American Association of Colleges of Nursing publishes *The Essentials: Core competencies for professional nursing education.*

2022—The American Association of Colleges of Nursing selected 10 Nursing schools to pilot Learning Strategies to Build Leadership and Resilience Skills in New Nurses.

2023—The National Council of State Boards of Nursing (NCSBN) launched the Next Generation NCLEX (NGN) Exam.

From AACN, 2006; Carnegie, 1995; Deloughery, 1998; Donahue, 1999; Kalisch and Kalisch, 1995; IOM, 2003, 2011.

Prehistoric Period

Nursing in the prehistoric period was delineated by health practices that were strongly guided by beliefs of magic, religion, and superstition. Individuals who were ill were considered to be cursed by evil spirits and evil gods that entered the human body and caused suffering and death if not cast out. These beliefs dictated the behavior of primitive people, who sought to scare away the evil gods and spirits. Members of tribes participated in rituals, wore masks, and engaged in demonstrative dances to rid the sick of demonic possession of the body. Sacrifices and offerings, sometimes including human sacrifices, were made to rid the body of evil gods, demons, and spirits. Many tribes used special herbs, roots, and vegetables to cast out the "curse" of illness.

EARLY CIVILIZATION

Egypt

Ancient Egyptians are noted for their accomplishments in health care at an early period in civilization. They were the first to use the concept of suture in repairing wounds. They also were the first to be recorded as developing community planning that resulted in a decrease in public health problems. One of the main early public health problems was the spread of disease through contaminated water sources. Specific laws on cleanliness, food use and preservation, drinking, exercise, and sexual relations were developed. Health behaviors were usually carried out to accommodate the gods (Catalano, 2015). A pharmacopoeia that classified more than 700 drugs was written to assist in the care and management of disease (Ellis & Hartley, 2012). As in the case of Shiphrah and Puah, the midwives who saved baby Moses, nurses were used by kings and other aristocrats to deliver babies and care for the young, older adults, and those who were sick.

Palestine

From 1400 to 1200 BC, the Hebrews migrated from the Arabian Desert and gradually settled in Palestine, where they became an agricultural society. Under the leadership of Moses, the Hebrews developed a system of laws called the Mosaic Code. This code, one of the first organized methods of disease control and prevention, contained public health laws that dictated personal, family, and public hygiene. For instance, laws were written to prohibit the eating of animals that were dead longer than 3 days and to isolate individuals who were thought to have communicable diseases. Hebrew priests took on the role of health inspectors (Ellis & Hartley, 2012).

Greece

From 1500 to 100 BC, Greek philosophers sought to understand man and his relationship with the gods, nature, and other men. They believed that the gods and goddesses of Greek mythology controlled health and illness. Temples built to honor Aesculapius, the god of medicine, were designated to care for the sick. Aesculapius carried a staff that was intertwined with serpents or snakes, representing wisdom and immortality. This staff is thought to be the model of today's medical caduceus. Hippocrates (460–362 BC), considered the "Father of Medicine," paved the way in establishing scientific knowledge in medicine. Hippocrates was the first to attribute disease to natural causes rather than super-natural causes and curses of the gods. His teachings also emphasized the patient-centered approach and use of the scientific method for solving problems (Catalano, 2015).

India

Dating from 3000 to 1500 BC, the earliest cultures of India were Hindu. The sacred book of Brahmanism (also known as Hinduism), the Vedas, was used to guide health care practices. The Vedas, considered by some to be the oldest written material, emphasized hygiene and prevention of sickness and described major and minor surgical procedures. The Indian practice of surgery was very well developed. The importance of prenatal care to mother and infant was also well understood. Public hospitals were constructed from 274 to 236 BC and were staffed by male nurses with qualifications and duties similar to those of the 20th-century practical nurse (Ellis & Hartley, 2012).

China

The teachings of the Chinese scholar Confucius (551–479 BC) had a powerful effect on the customs and practices of the people of ancient China. Confucius taught a moral philosophy that addressed one's obligation to society. Central to his teachings were service to the community and the value of the family as a unit. However, women were considered inferior to men.

The early Chinese also placed great value on solving life's problems. Their belief about health and illness was based on the yin and yang philosophy. The yin represented the feminine forces, which were considered negative and passive. The yang represented the masculine forces, which were positive and active. The Chinese believed that an imbalance between these two forces would result in illness, whereas balance between the yin and yang represented good health (Ellis & Hartley, 2012). The ancient Chinese used a variety of treatments believed to promote health and harmony, including acupuncture, hydrotherapy, and massage (Giger & Davidhizar, 2008).

Rome

The Roman Empire (27 BC–476 AD), a military dictatorship, adapted medical practices from the countries they conquered and the physicians they enslaved. At the end of the Dark Ages, there was a series of holy wars, including the Crusades. The first military hospital in Europe was established in Rome to care for the injured. Military nursing orders that were made up exclusively of men were also developed. They were very well organized and dedicated, and they wore suits of armor for protection, with the emblem of a red cross (Catalano, 2015; Walton et al., 1994). The Romans practiced advanced hygiene and sanitation and emphasized bathing (Ellis & Hartley, 2012).

THE MIDDLE AGES

The Middle Ages (476–1450) followed the demise of the Roman Empire (Walton et al., 1994). Women began using herbs and new methods of healing, whereas men continued to use purging, leeching, and mercury. This period also saw the Roman Catholic Church become a central figure in the organization and management of health care. Most of the changes in health care were based on the Church's emphasis on charity and the sanctity of human life. Wives of emperors, and other women considered to be noble, became nurses. These women devoted themselves to caring for the sick, often carrying baskets of food and medicine as they journeyed from house to house (Bahr & Johnson, 1997). Widows and unmarried women became nuns and deaconesses. Two deaconesses, Dorcas and Phoebe, had been mentioned in the Bible as outstanding for the care they provided to the sick (Freedman, 1995).

During the Middle Ages, physicians spent most of their time translating medical essays and provided little actual medical care. Poorly trained barbers, who lacked any formal medical education, performed surgery and medical treatments that were considered "bloody" or "messy." Nurses also provided some medical care, although in most hospitals and monasteries, female nurses who were not midwives were forbidden to witness childbirth, help with gynecologic examinations, or even diaper male infants (Kalisch & Kalisch, 1986). During the Crusades, which lasted for almost 200 years (from 1096 to 1291), military nursing orders, known as Templars and Hospitalers, were founded. Monks and Christian knights provided nursing care and defended the hospitals during battle, wearing suits of armor under their religious habits. The habits were distinguished by the Maltese cross to identify the monks and knights as Christian warriors. The same cross was used years later on a badge designed for the first school of nursing and became a forerunner for the design of nursing pins (Buckway & Sowerby, 2023).

THE RENAISSANCE AND THE REFORMATION PERIOD

Following the Middle Ages came the Renaissance and the Reformation, also known as the rebirth of Europe (the 14th to 16th centuries). Major advancements were made in pharmacology, chemistry, and medical knowledge, including anatomy, physiology, and surgery. During the Renaissance, new emphasis was given to medical education, but nursing education was practically nonexistent.

The Reformation, which began in Germany in 1517, was a religious movement that resulted in a dissention between Roman Catholics and Protestants. During this period, religious facilities that provided health care closed. Women were encouraged toward charitable services, but their main duties included bearing and caring for children in their homes. Furthermore, hospital work was no longer appealing to women of high economic status, and the individuals who worked as nurses in hospitals were often female prisoners, prostitutes, and alcoholics. Nursing was no longer the respected profession it had once been. This period is referred to as the "Dark Ages" of nursing (Buckway & Sowerby, 2023).

During the 16th and 17th centuries, famine, plague, filth, and crime ravaged Europe. King Henry VII eliminated the organized monastic relief programs that aided the orphans, poor, and other displaced people. Out of great concern for social welfare, several nursing groups, such as the Order of the Visitation of St. Mary, the Daughters of Charity of St. Vincent de Paul, and the Sisters of Charity, were organized to give time, service, and money to the poor and sick. The Sisters of Charity recruited intelligent young women for training in nursing, developed educational programs, and cared for abandoned children (Buckway & Sowerby, 2023).

THE COLONIAL AMERICAN PERIOD

The first hospital and the first medical school in North America were founded in Mexico—the Hospital of the Immaculate Conception in Mexico City and the medical school at the University of Mexico. During this time in the American colonies, individuals with infectious diseases were isolated in almshouses or "pesthouses" (Ellis & Hartley, 2012). Procedures such as purgatives and bleeding were widely used, leading to shortened life expectancy. Plagues such as scarlet fever, dysentery, and smallpox caused thousands of deaths. Benjamin Franklin, who was outspoken regarding the care of the sick, insisted that a hospital be built in the colonies. He believed that the community should be responsible for the management and treatment of those who were ill. Through his efforts, the first hospital, called the Pennsylvania Hospital, was built in the United States in Philadelphia, in 1751 (Buckway & Sowerby, 2023).

FLORENCE NIGHTINGALE

Florence Nightingale was born in Florence, Italy, on May 12, 1820. Her family was wealthy, well traveled, and well educated. Nightingale was an intelligent, talented, and attractive woman. From an early age, she demonstrated a deep concern for the poor and suffering. At 25 years of age, she became interested in training as a nurse. However, her family was strongly opposed to this choice and preferred that she marry and take her place in society (Joel, 2006). In 1851, her parents finally permitted her to pursue training as a nurse. At 31 years of age, Nightingale attended a 3-month nursing training program at the Institution of Deaconesses at Kaiserswerth, Germany. As her knowledge of hospitals and nursing grew, she began training nurses in London (Buckway & Sowerby, 2023). The outbreak of the Crimean War marked a turning point in Nightingale's career. In October 1854, Sidney Herbert, British Secretary of War and an old friend of the Nightingale family, wrote to Nightingale and asked her to lead a group of nurses to the Crimea to work at one of the military hospitals under government authority and expense. Nightingale accepted his offer and assembled 38 nurses who were sisters and nuns from various Catholic and Anglican orders (Buckway & Sowerby, 2023).

Nightingale and her team were assigned to the Barracks Hospital at Scutari. When Nightingale arrived, she found deplorable conditions. Between 3000 and 4000 sick and wounded men were packed into the hospital, which was originally designed to accommodate 1700 patients. There were no beds, blankets, food, or medicine. Many of the wounded soldiers had been placed on the floor, where lice, maggots, vermin, rodents, and blood covered their bodies. There were no candles or lanterns. All medical care had to be rendered during the light of day (Buckway & Sowerby, 2023).

Despite the distressing conditions at the Barracks Hospital, the army physicians and surgeons at first refused Nightingale's assistance. However, within a week and faced with scurvy, starvation, dysentery, and the eruption of more fighting, the physicians, in desperation, called her to help. Nightingale immediately purchased medical supplies, food, linens, and hospital equipment, using her own money and that of the Times Relief Fund. Within 10 days, she had set up a kitchen for special diets and had rented a house that she converted into a laundry (Gill, 2004; Small, 2002). The wives of soldiers were hired to manage and operate the laundry service. She assigned soldiers to make repairs and clean up the building. Just weeks later, she initiated social services, reading classes, and even coffeehouses where soldiers could enjoy music and recreation (Nies & McEwen, 2022).

Nightingale worked long, hard hours to care for these soldiers. She spent up to 20 hours each day caring for wounds, comforting soldiers, assisting in surgery, directing staff, and keeping records. Nightingale introduced principles of infection control, a system for transcribing physicians' orders, and a procedure to maintain patient records.

Nightingale is credited with using public health principles and statistical methods to advocate for improved health conditions for British soldiers. Through carefully recorded statistics, Nightingale was able to document that the soldiers' death rate decreased from 42% to 2% as a result of health care reforms that emphasized sanitary conditions. Because of her remarkable work in using statistics to demonstrate cause and effect and improve the health of British soldiers, Nightingale is recognized for her contributions to nursing research (Nies & McEwen, 2022).

Nightingale also demonstrated the power of political activism to effect health care reform by writing letters of criticism accompanied by constructive recommendations to British army leaders. Nightingale's ability to overthrow the British army's management method, which had allowed the deplorable conditions to exist in the army hospitals, was considered one of her greatest achievements (Nies & McEwen, 2022).

After her return from the Crimea, Nightingale experienced ongoing health problems. Early writers suggest that she retreated to her bedroom for the next 43 years

and continued her involvement in health care from her secluded apartment. More recent research, however, indicates a more active involvement (Buckway & Sowerby, 2023).

Florence Nightingale's work, from the Crimean War to the establishment of formal nursing education programs, was a catapult for the reorganization and advancement of professional nursing. Nightingale wrote extensively about hospitals, sanitation, health, and health statistics (creating the first pie chart), and nursing education. Among her most popular books is *Notes on Nursing*, published in 1859.

In 1860, Nightingale established the first nursing school in England, St. Thomas' Hospital of London. By 1873, graduates of Nightingale's nurse training program in England migrated to the United States, where they became supervisors in the first of the hospital-based (diploma) nursing schools: Massachusetts General Hospital in Boston, Bellevue Hospital in New York, and the New Haven Hospital in Connecticut.

Until her death in August 1910, Nightingale demonstrated the powerful effect that well-educated, creative, skilled, and competent individuals have in the provision of health care. She is honored as the founder of professional nursing (Buckway & Sowerby, 2023). Nightingale had the means to support her work and the stamina to drive forward in her belief concerning health care. Even though Louis Pasteur's germ theory was not widely known and was very controversial at the time, her theory of environmental cleanliness is still applicable today.

NURSING IN THE UNITED STATES

The Civil War Period

During the US Civil War, or the War Between the States (1861 to 1865), health care conditions in the United States were similar to those encountered by Nightingale. Numerous epidemics plagued the country, including syphilis, gonorrhea, malaria, smallpox, and typhoid (Nelson, 2001; Oermann, 1997).

The Civil War was initiated by the attack on Fort Sumter, South Carolina, April 17, 1861. At the time, there were no nurses formally trained to care for the sick. However, thousands of men and women from the South and North volunteered to care for the wounded. Hospitals were set up in the field, and transports were put in place to carry the wounded to hospitals (Carnegie, 1995).

Secretary of War Simon Cameron appointed a schoolteacher named Dorothea Dix to organize military hospitals and provide medical supplies to the Union Army soldiers. Dix received no official status and no salary for this position.

Women providing nursing care during the Civil War worked under very primitive conditions. Maintaining sanitary conditions was an overwhelming challenge and often not possible. More than 6 million patients were admitted to hospitals. Approximately 500,000 surgical procedures were performed. Unfortunately, there were only about 2000 individuals who served as nurses, far fewer than the number needed to provide adequate care (Fitzpatrick, 1997; Kalisch & Kalisch, 1995). According to records kept at three hospitals, 181 male and female Black nurses served between July 16, 1863, and June 14, 1864. White nurses were paid $12 per month; Black nurses received $10 per month (Carnegie, 1995).

Three Black nurses made particularly important contributions to nursing efforts during the Civil War: Harriet Tubman cared for the sick as a nurse in the Sea Islands off the coast of South Carolina and was later known as the "conductor of the Underground Railroad." It is also reported that she was the first woman to lead American troops into battle (Carnegie, 1995). In 1990 Congress proclaimed March 10 as Harriet Tubman Day in the United States, honoring her as a brave Black Freedom Fighter and nurse during the Civil War. Sojourner Truth, known for her abolitionist and nursing efforts, was an advocate of clean and sanitary conditions for patients. She insisted that these conditions were needed for patients to heal. Susie King Taylor, although hired to work in the laundry, served as a nurse because of the growing number of wounded who needed care. Having learned to read and write, which was against the law for Black people at the time, she also taught many of her comrades in Company E to read and write (Carnegie, 1995).

Many other volunteer nurses made important contributions during the Civil War: Clara Barton served on the front line during the Civil War and operated a war relief program to provide supplies to the battlefields and hospitals. Barton also set up a postwar service to find missing soldiers and is credited with founding the American Red Cross (Nies & McEwen, 2022). Louisa May Alcott, who served as a nurse for 6 weeks until stopped by ill health, authored detailed accounts of the experiences encountered by nurses during the war for a newspaper publication titled *Hospital Sketches* (Kalisch & Kalisch, 1995, 2003).

When the Civil War ended, the number of nurse training schools increased. The war had proven the need for more nurses to be formally trained. These early nursing programs offered little or no classroom education, and on-the-job training occurred in the hospital wards. The students learned routine patient care duties, worked long hours 6 days a week, and were used as supplemental hospital staff. After graduation, most of the nurses practiced as private duty nurses or hospital staff (Lindeman & McAthie, 1990). The first nursing textbook, titled *Hand-Nursing for Family and General Use*, was published in 1878 by a committee of nurses and physicians associated with Connecticut Training School at New Haven Hospital (Buckway & Sowerby, 2023).

During the 1890s, the nationwide establishment of hospitals and nursing schools for Black people gained momentum as Black musicians, educators, and community leaders became alarmed at the high rates of morbidity and mortality among Black Americans. Because of segregation and discrimination, African Americans had to establish their own health care institutions to provide Black patients with access to quality health care and to provide Black men and women with opportunities to enter the nursing profession. However, in 1886, John D. Rockefeller, a White philanthropist, funded the establishment of the first school of nursing for Black women at the Atlanta Baptist Seminary—now known as Spelman College (Buckway & Sowerby, 2023) (Box 1.2).

1900 TO WORLD WAR I

In the 1900s, states began to require nurses to become registered before entering practice. By 1910, most states had upgraded education requirements to high school, upgraded training, and required registration before practice (Buckway & Sowerby 2023). The Army and Navy Nurse Corps were created in 1901 and 1908, respectively, and an estimated 30,000 nurses served in World War I (Buckway & Sowerby, 2023). In 1908 the National Association of Colored Graduate Nurses was founded. In 1920 Ludie Andrews won her lawsuit with the Georgia State Board of Nurse Examiners to secure Black nurses the right to take the state board examination and become licensed.

BOX 1.2 Duties of the Hospital Floor Nurse in 1887

In addition to caring for your 60 patients, each nurse will follow these regulations:

1. Daily sweep and mop the floors of your ward; dust the patient's furniture and windowsill.
2. Maintain an even temperature on your ward by bringing in a scuttle of coal for the day's business.
3. Light is important to observe the patient's condition; therefore, each day fill kerosene lamps, clean chimneys, and trim wicks. Wash the windows once a week.
4. The nurse's notes are important in aiding the physician's work. Make your pens carefully; you may whittle nibs to your individual taste.
5. Each nurse on day duty will report every day at 7 AM and will leave at 8 PM except on Sabbath, on which day you will be off from 12 PM to 2 PM.
6. Graduate nurses in good standing with the director of nurses will be given an evening off each week if she regularly attends church.
7. Each nurse should lay aside from each payday a good sum of her earnings for her benefits during her declining years so that she will not become a burden. For example, if you earn $20 a month, you should set aside $10.
8. Any nurse who smokes, uses liquor in any form, gets her hair done at a beauty shop, or frequents dance halls will have given the director of nurses good reason to suspect her worth, intentions, and integrity.
9. The nurse who performs her labors, serves her patients and physicians faithfully and without fault for a period of 5 years will be given an increase by the hospital administration of 5 cents per day, providing there are no hospital debts that are outstanding.

Lillian Wald, a pioneer in public health nursing, is best known for the development and establishment of the first viable practice for public health nurses. The main location for this practice was the Henry Street Settlement House, located in the Lower East Side of New York City. Its purpose was to provide well-baby care, health education, disease prevention, and treatment of patients with minor illnesses. The nursing practice based at the Henry Street Settlement House formed the basis of public health nursing for the entire country. Instead of relying on patients to visit the clinic, public health nurses made their way to the various tenements located around Henry Street (Nies & McEwen, 2022).

Wald also developed the first nursing service for occupational health. She believed that prevention of disease among workers would improve productivity and was able to persuade the Metropolitan Life Insurance Company that her ideas had merit. As a result, nursing agencies, such as those in place at the Henry Street Settlement House, provided skilled nursing services to employees. Another innovation that emerged from this program was the sliding-fee scale, by which patients were billed according to their income or their ability to pay. In 1911, Wald chaired a committee formed by members of the Associated Alumnae of Training Schools for Nurses, later to become the American Nurses Association (ANA), and the Society of Superintendents of Training Schools for Nurses, the precursor of the National League for Nursing (NLN). The purpose of the committee was to develop standards for nursing services performed outside the hospital environment. The committee determined that a new organization was necessary to meet the needs of community health nurses. The result of the committee's recommendation was the formation of the National Organization for Public Health Nursing, whose goals were to establish educational and practice standards for community health nursing (Stanhope & Lancaster, 2024).

The ANA and the NLN are still leading nursing organizations today. The ANA has focused primarily on professional aspects of nursing, and the NLN was the only accrediting body for nursing schools until 1996, when the Commission on Collegiate Nursing Education (CCNE), an autonomous arm of the American Association of Colleges of Nursing (AACN), was established as an agency devoted exclusively to the accreditation of baccalaureate and graduate degree nursing programs (Buckway & Sowerby, 2023).

In 2013, the National League for Nursing Accreditation Commission (NLNAC) changed its name and is now the Accreditation Commission for Education in Nursing (ACEN). This organization accredits practical, diploma, baccalaureate, and graduate degree nursing programs.

World War I and the 1920s

During the early 1900s, the world was rapidly changing and moving toward global conflict. Germany was arming, and the rest of Europe was trying to ignore the threat. "Prosperous" was the word used to describe the US economy. Women were granted the right to vote and were moving into the workforce on a regular basis.

Advancements in medical care and public health were being made. The primary site for medical care moved from the home to the hospital, and surgical and diagnostic techniques were improved. Pneumonia management was the focus of scientific study. Insulin was discovered in 1922, and in 1928 Alexander Fleming discovered the precursor of penicillin, which would eventually be used to successfully treat patients with pneumonia and other infections (Kalisch & Kalisch, 1995) (Box 1.3).

Environmental conditions improved, and the serious epidemics of the previous century became nonexistent. Lillian Wald, in *The House on Henry Street*, linked poor environmental and social conditions to prevalent illnesses and poverty and used this information to lead the fight for better sanitation and housing conditions (Nies & McEwen, 2022).

With the outbreak of World War I in 1914, nurses were desperately needed to care for the soldiers who were injured or who suffered from the many illnesses resulting from trench warfare (Nies & McEwen, 2022). The war offered nurses a chance to advance into new fields of specialization. For example, nurse anesthetists made their first appearance as part of the surgical teams at the front lines. More than 20,000 US-trained nurses served in World War I (Oermann, 1997). Eighteen Black nurses were admitted to the Army Nurse Corps after the Armistice was signed ending World War I, and by 1943 the Army Nurse Corps had established a quota of 56 Black nurses.

BOX 1.3 Qualities of Good Nurses During Post–World War II

1. Tidy and loyal to the hospital and its personnel
2. Compliant with the orders of the physicians and directives of nursing management
3. Always busy
4. If census was low, fold laundry, clean shelves, prepare supplies to be sterilized
5. Ability to get work done no matter how many patients assigned

From Martell, L.K. (1999). Maternity care during the post–World War II baby boom: The experience of general duty nurses, *Western Journal of Nursing Research, 21*(3), 387–404.

Because many nurses volunteered to provide services during the war, the community health nursing movement in the United States stalled. However, the American Red Cross, founded by Clara Barton in 1882, assisted in efforts to continue public health nursing. The Red Cross nurses originally focused on members of rural communities who were not able to access health care services. As the war continued, however, the Red Cross nurses also moved into urban areas to provide health care services (Stanhope & Lancaster, 2024).

During World War I, the US Public Health Service, founded in 1798 to provide health care services to merchant seamen, was charged with the responsibility to provide health services at military posts located within the United States. A nurse, who was "loaned" by the National Organization for Public Health Nursing, established nursing services at US military outposts. The responsibilities of the US Public Health Service continued to grow; eventually it was composed of physicians, nurses, and other allied health professionals who provided indigent care and practiced in community health programs (Stanhope & Lancaster, 2024).

Further changes were in store for nursing during World War I. In 1918, the Vassar Camp School for Nurses was established. Its purpose was to provide an intensive 2-year nurses' training program for college graduates. Graduates of the program were given an army reserve commission and would be activated during times of war to meet increased nursing needs. Sponsored by the American Red Cross and the Council of National Defense, the school graduated 435 nurses. The Vassar Camp School for Nurses was a short-lived enterprise. After the peace treaty was signed in 1919, the program was permanently disbanded (Snodgrass, 2004; Stanhope & Lancaster, 2024).

In 1921, the federal government recognized the need to improve the health of women and children and passed the Sheppard-Towner Act, one of the first pieces of federal legislation to provide funds to assist in the care of special populations (Nies & McEwen, 2022). This funding provided public health nurses with resources to promote the health and well-being of women, infants, and children.

Following these improvements, the Frontier Nursing Service (FNS) was established in 1925 by Mary Breckenridge of Kentucky. Born into a wealthy family, Breckenridge learned the value of providing care to others from her grandmother. Breckenridge began her career at St. Luke's Hospital School of Nursing in New York. After serving as a nurse during World War I, she returned to Columbia University to learn more about community health nursing. Armed with her new knowledge and a passion to assist disadvantaged women and children, Breckenridge returned to Kentucky and the rural Appalachian Mountains (Stanhope & Lancaster, 2024).

Breckenridge believed that the rural mountain area of Kentucky, cut off from many modern conveniences, was an excellent place to prove the value of community health nursing. She established the FNS in a five-room cabin in Hyden, Kentucky. After serious obstacles such as no water supply or sewage disposal were overcome, six other nursing outposts were constructed in the rural mountains from 1927 to 1930. The FNS based its hospital in Hyden and eventually attracted physicians and nurses to provide medical, dental, surgical, nursing, and midwifery services to the rural poor. Financial support for the FNS ranged from fees for labor and supplies to funds raised through annual family dues to donations and fundraising efforts. Nurses working for the FNS traveled a 700-square-mile area, often on horseback, to provide services to approximately 10,000 patients (Stanhope & Lancaster, 2024).

Breckenridge established an important health care service for rural Kentucky communities. Equally important was her documentation of the results of community health nursing in rural communities. Breckenridge followed the advice of a consulting physician and collected mortality data on the communities before nursing services actually were started. The results were startling; mortality was significantly reduced, and the need for the nursing services was clearly documented. Breckenridge proved that even in appalling environmental conditions without heat, electricity, or running water, nursing services could make a substantial positive impact on the health of the community (Stanhope & Lancaster, 2024). The FNS is still in operation today and provides vital service to the rural communities of Kentucky.

The Great Depression (1930 to 1940)

The US economy prospered during World War I and well into the 1920s. However, after the stock market crash in October 1929, economic prosperity quickly dissipated. Millions of men and women became unemployed. Before the Depression, many people had private duty nurses. However, during the Depression, many nurses found themselves unemployed because most families could no longer afford private duty nurses.

Franklin D. Roosevelt, elected president of the United States in 1932, faced a country in shambles. He responded with several innovative and necessary interventions and ushered in the first major social legislation enacted in US history. Titled the "New Deal," the legislation had several social components that affected the provision of medical care and other services for indigent people across the country (Karger & Stoesz, 2005).

The piece of legislation that had the greatest effect on health care in the United States was the Social Security Act of 1935, which set the precedent for the passage of the Medicare and Medicaid acts in 1965. The main purposes of the 1935 Social Security Act were to provide (1) a national old-age insurance system, (2) federal grants to states for maternal and child welfare services, (3) vocational rehabilitation services for the handicapped, (4) medical care for crippled children and blind people, (5) a plan to strengthen public health services, and (6) a federal–state unemployment system (Karger & Stoesz, 2005).

The passage of the 1935 Social Security Act provided avenues for nursing care, and nursing jobs were created. With funds from the Social Security Act, public health nursing became the major source of health care for dependent mothers and children, the blind, and crippled children. Nurses found employment as public health nurses for county or state health departments (Stanhope & Lancaster, 2024). Hospital job opportunities also were created for nurses, and the hospital became the usual employment setting for graduate nurses.

World War II (1940 to 1945)

The United States officially entered World War II after the bombing of Pearl Harbor in December 1941. At that time, the nursing divisions of all of the military branches had inadequate numbers of nurses. Congress passed legislation to provide needed funds to expand nursing education. In 1943 an amendment to the Nurse Training Act was passed to bar racial bias. A committee of six national nursing organizations, called the National Nursing Council, received $1 million to accomplish the needed expansion. The US Public Health Service became the administrator of the funds, further strengthening the tie between the US Public Health Service and nursing (Stanhope & Lancaster, 2024).

The war was considered a global conflict, and nursing became an essential part of the military advance.

Nurses were required to function under combat conditions and had to adapt nursing care to meet the challenges of different climates, facilities, and supplies. As a result of their service during World War II, nurses finally were recognized as an integral part of the military and attained the ranks of officers in the army and navy. Colonel Julie O. Flikke was the first army nurse to be promoted to colonel in the US Army and served as Superintendent of the Army Nurse Corps from 1937 to 1942 (Deloughery, 1998; Robinson & Perry, 2001).

Post–World War II Period (1945 to 1950)

The period after World War II was a time of prosperity for the average American. The GI Bill enabled returning veterans to complete their interrupted education. The unemployment rate dropped to an all-time low in the United States. In an effort to provide more areas of employment for the returning men, the federal government mounted a massive campaign to encourage women to return to the more traditional roles of wife and mother. Consequently, numerous women in all professions, including nursing, chose to return to marriage and childrearing rather than continue employment outside the home.

After World War II the Soviet Union began invading and taking over Eastern European countries. With support from China, the North Koreans made a grab for South Korea, resulting in the Korean War. Again, nurses volunteered for the armed services to provide care to patients near the battlefields in Korea. This time they worked in mobile army surgical hospitals, better known as MASH units, where medical and surgical techniques were further refined.

The two decades after World War II saw the emergence of nursing as a true profession. National standards for nursing education were established by the National Nursing Accrediting Service. By 1950, all state boards were participating in the test pool; they continue to do so today. Nursing continued to improve the quality and quantity of educational programs as the number of nursing baccalaureate programs increased and associate degree programs developed in community or junior colleges (Buckway & Sowerby, 2023) (see Box 1.1).

The end of World War II and the early 1950s marked the beginning of significant federal intervention in health care. The Nurse Training Act of 1943 was the first instance of federal funding being used to support nurse training. The passage of the Hill-Burton Act, or the Hospital Survey and Construction Act of 1946, marked the largest commitment of federal dollars to health care in the country's history. The purpose of the act was to provide funding to construct hospitals and to assist states in planning for other health care facilities based on the needs of the communities. Nearly 40% of the hospitals constructed in the late 1940s and the early 1950s were built with Hill-Burton funds. The hospital construction boom created by the Hill-Burton Act led to an increased demand for professional nurses to provide care in hospitals (Nies & McEwen, 2022) (see Box 1.3).

It was also in the early 1950s that the National Association of Colored Graduate Nurses (NACGN) went out of existence. This was the organization that had fought for integration of the Black nurse into the ANA. From 1916 to 1948, Black nurses in the South were barred from membership in the ANA because of segregation laws in the Southern states. In the 1940s, the NACGN began to wage an all-out war against discrimination by the Southern constituents of the ANA. The NACGN chose as its central issue the route to membership in ANA. This issue was raised by the NACGN on the floor at every national convention of the ANA, and it evoked strong opposition from the Southern state constituents. Speaking from the floor of the House of Delegates at the 1946 convention in Atlantic City, a White nurse from Georgia referred to Black nurses as "our darkies." Immediately a motion was passed to strike the reference from the record. However, this comment caused an uproar, and the Black nurses who were barred from membership in the Southern states started the wheels turning to bypass the states and join ANA directly. This arrangement, known as *individual membership*, was put into effect in 1948. With the establishment of individual membership, Black nurses in the South could bypass their states and become members of the ANA. This type of individual membership continued until all barriers had been dropped in the early 1960s (Carnegie, 1995). Estelle Osborne was the first Black nurse elected to the Board of the ANA. In 1949 M. Elizabeth Carnegie was the first Black nurse to be elected to a Board of a state association.

Nursing in the 1960s

Federal legislation enacted during the 1960s had a major and lasting effect on nursing and health care. The Community Mental Health Centers Act of 1963 provided funds for the construction of community outpatient mental health centers; opportunities for mental health nursing were expanded when funds to staff these centers were appropriated in 1965 with the passage of the Medicare and Medicaid acts (Nies & McEwen, 2022). Medicaid, Title XIX of the Social Security Act, was enacted and replaced all programs previously instituted for medical assistance. The purpose of the Medicaid program, which was jointly sponsored and financed with matching funds from federal and state governments, was to serve as medical insurance for those families, primarily women and children, with an income at or below the federal poverty level. Medicaid quickly became the largest public assistance program in the nation.

Health departments employed public health nurses to provide the bulk of the care needed by children and pregnant women in the Medicaid population. Services provided by these nurses included family planning, well-child assessments, immunizations, and prenatal care. A physician assigned as the district health officer supervised the nurses. Without the public health nurses and local health departments, many women and children in the inner city areas and rural communities would have been without access to basic health care.

Another important amendment to the Social Security Act was Title XVIII, or Medicare, passed in 1965. The Medicare program provides hospital insurance, part A, and medical insurance, part B, to all people 65 years of age and older who are eligible to receive Social Security benefits; people with total, permanent disabilities; and people with end-stage renal disease. As a result of Medicare reimbursement, many hospitals began catering to physicians who treated Medicare patients. Medicare patients were attractive to the hospitals because all hospital charges, regardless of amount or appropriateness of services, were reimbursed through the Medicare program (Nies & McEwen, 2022).

As a result of Medicare reimbursement, hospital-bed occupancy increased, which led to the need for increased numbers of nurses to staff hospitals. Nursing embraced the hospital setting as the usual practice area and moved away from the community as the preferred practice site. Nursing schools also followed the trend by reducing the number of curriculum hours devoted to community health and concentrating their efforts on hospital-based nursing (Stanhope & Lancaster, 2024).

Another outcome of the Medicare legislation was the home health movement. To receive Medicare reimbursement for home health services, patients had to have (1) home-bound status; (2) a need for part-time or intermittent, skilled nursing care; (3) a medically reasonably and necessary need for treatment; and (4) a plan of care authorized by a physician. Home health agencies were established and began to employ increasing numbers of nurses. The number of home health agencies began to grow in the mid-1960s, and the home health industry continued unprecedented growth into the 1990s as a result of Medicare reimbursement and other influences, including a growing older adult population, advances in medical technology, and public demand for increased access to health care. Home health was one of the first employment settings that provided nurses the opportunity to work weekdays only.

Nursing in the 1970s

The women's movement of the 1970s greatly influenced nursing. Nurses began to focus not only on providing quality care to patients but also on enhancing the economic benefits of the profession. Hospitals were receiving significant reimbursements for patient care; however, nurses' salaries did not reflect an adequate percentage of that reimbursement. Health care costs soared. This increase in health care costs built the framework for mandated changes in reimbursement. Nursing practice and the educational focus remained in the hospital setting.

During this time, nurses played a major role in providing health care to communities and were instrumental in developing hospice programs, birthing centers, and daycare centers for older adults (Nies & McEwen, 2022). Basic educational programs for nurse practitioners expanded during the 1970s and master's-level preparation was developed as the requirement for graduation and practice; additionally, certification was required for practice as a nurse practitioner. Before this time, only certification was required. State nursing practice acts were amended to provide for monitoring and licensing of advanced practice nurses. The numbers of men participating in this female-dominated profession also began to increase (Ellis & Hartley, 2012).

In 1974, the ANA conducted research in the area of ethnic minorities and submitted a proposal to the National Institute of Mental Health to fund a project to permit minority nurses—African Americans, Hispanics, Asians, and American Indians—to earn PhDs. Of the graduates of the project, the vast majority serves on faculties of universities and is conducting research on factors in mental health and illness related to ethnicity and cross-cultural conflict, thereby fulfilling their commitment to advance the cause of quality health care for people of all ethnicities.

Despite past laxity, the ANA House of Delegates at its 1972 convention passed an affirmative action resolution calling for a task force to develop and implement a program to correct inequities. The house also provided for the position of an ombudsman to evaluate involvement of minorities in leadership roles within the organization and to treat complaints by applicants for membership or by members of the association who had been discriminated against because of nationality, race, creed, lifestyle, color, age, or sex. It was also in the 1970s that the ANA elected its first Black president, Barbara Nichols, who served two terms.

Within the structure of many professional organizations is a unit referred to as an *academy*, which is composed of a cadre of scholars who deal with issues that concern the profession and take positions in the name of the academy. The American Academy of Nursing (AAN) was created by the ANA board in 1973. An elected group of highly accomplished leaders across all sectors of nursing (education, research, and practice), it uses the credential FAAN (Fellow, American Academy of Nursing). Through the application of visionary leadership, the intent of the AAN is to transform health care policy through nursing knowledge to optimize the well-being of the American people.

At its convention in Atlantic City in 1976, the ANA launched its Hall of Fame to pay tribute to those nurses who have paved the way for others to follow or who have made outstanding contributions to the profession.

Nursing in the 1980s

The types of patients needing health care changed in the 1980s. Homelessness became a common problem in large cities. Unstable economic developments contributed to an increase in indigent populations (Nies & McEwen, 2022). Acquired immunodeficiency syndrome (AIDS) emerged as a frightening, fatal epidemic.

Runaway health care costs became a national issue in the 1980s. Medicare was still reimbursing for any and all hospital services provided to recipients. In 1983, in an attempt to restrain hospital costs, Congress passed the Diagnosis-Related Group system for reimbursement, better known as the DRG system.

Before 1983, Medicare payments were made to the hospital after the patient received services. Although there were restrictions, the entire bill generally was paid without question. DRGs were implemented to provide prospective payment for hospital services on the basis of the patient's admitting diagnosis and thereby to reduce the overall cost to Medicare. Hospitals now were to be reimbursed one amount based on the patient's diagnosis, not on hospital charges. The system was developed by physicians at the Yale–New Haven Hospital and addressed approximately 468 diagnoses classified according to length of stay and cost of procedures associated with the diagnosis (Nies & McEwen, 2022).

As a result of the DRG reimbursement system, hospitals were forced to increase efficiency and more closely manage hospital services, including the patient's length of stay, laboratory and radiographic testing, and diagnostic procedures. Case management and critical pathways were developed to more efficiently manage patient care, and case management became a new area of specialization for the professional nurse.

Despite the high cost of health care, medicine prospered. Medical care advanced in areas such as organ transplantation, resuscitation and support of premature infants, and critical-care techniques. Physician specialization and advances in medical technology flourished. Medical specialties, such as nephrology, cardiology, endocrinology, orthopedics, neurosurgery, cardiovascular surgery, and advanced practices for obstetrics, led to improved health care services. Costs in the hospital setting increased with increased specialization and technology. The advanced technology also led to the development of outpatient surgery units.

Outpatient surgery services blossomed and provided a quick and efficient site for surgery that did not require extended hospital stays. Costs were greatly reduced because of the need for fewer staff members required for coverage, fewer supplies, and reduced facility costs. Nurses were interested in employment opportunities in outpatient facilities because they afforded a chance to work only during the day, with no weekend assignments.

As the concern over increasing health care costs heightened, use of ambulatory services increased and enrollment in health maintenance organizations grew. Advanced nurse practitioners rose in popularity as cost-effective providers of primary and preventive health care. A growing number of nurses moved from the hospital setting into the community to practice in programs such as hospice and home health. Consumers began to demand bans on unhealthy activities, such as smoking in public. Health education became more important as consumers were encouraged to take responsibility for their own care (Stanhope & Lancaster, 2024). Even the terminology changed; the individual once known as the *patient* became known as the *client* or *consumer* and was afforded respect as a person who purchases a service.

Public health programs struggled to survive as counties and states cut health department budgets. A landmark study conducted by the Institute of Medicine (IOM) in 1988, titled *Who Will Keep the Public Healthy?* (IOM, 2003), painted a dismal picture for public health. The study determined that public health had moved away from its traditional role and core functions and that no strategy was in place to bring public health back to its original purpose (Stanhope & Lancaster, 2024). Inadequate funding for public health continues to be a problem; however, it is hoped that soon public health will be restored to its original function and purpose.

Nursing enrollments dropped drastically in the late 1980s. This drop in enrollment occurred as the complexity of health care was rapidly increasing and more nurses were assuming expanded roles. As a result of these trends, a serious national shortage of nurses occurred across all settings (Ellis & Hartley, 2012).

In the late 1980s, several nursing scholars suggested that nursing research be firmly focused on the substantive information required to guide practice, rather than on philosophical and methodologic dilemmas of scientific inquiry. In 1985 the creation of the National Center for Nursing Research at the National Institutes of Health brought with it an increase in federal resources for nursing research and research training (LoBiondo-Wood & Haber, 2021).

Nursing in the 1990s

The 1990s began with alarm over the state of the US economy. Government statisticians reported an alarming increase in the national debt complicated by slow economic growth. In the early 1990s, average household incomes were stagnating. More women with families entered the workforce to afford the increasing cost of living. More nurses selected jobs in which they could work more hours in fewer days for more money, sometimes sacrificing the fringe benefits, allowing them to work a second job or earn higher pay through shift differential for working evening and night shifts. Creative shifts, such as the 10-hour day, 4-day workweek or the 12-hour day, 3-day workweek became commonplace in health care facilities. Just as in the 1980s, the cost of health care continued to rise with the technologic advancements in medical care. Men were considered a minority in nursing, and salaries were thought to be on the increase as a result of male presence in the profession (O'Lynn & Tranbarger, 2006). In 1999, Beverly Malone, the second Black President of the ANA, was named Deputy Assistant Secretary for Health.

There also were growing concerns in the 1990s about the health of the nation, which prompted the *Healthy People 2000* initiative. Many diseases associated with preventable causes characterized mortality in the United States. In 1990, more than 2 million US residents died from causes such as heart disease, cancer, cerebrovascular disease, accidents, chronic obstructive pulmonary disease, liver cirrhosis, tuberculosis, and human immunodeficiency virus infection. Disparities in rates of these diseases in the inner city due to issues related to access and quality of care became a concern (Nies & McEwen, 2022). Factors contributing to these common disease states related to lifestyle patterns, behaviors, and habits (modifiable risk factors). More youth were at risk because of behavior such as smoking cigarettes, using abusive drug substances, eating poorly balanced diets, failing to exercise, having sex with multiple partners, and being subjected to acts of violence. *Healthy People 2000: National Health Promotion and Disease Prevention Objectives* was published in 1991 by the US Department of Health and Human Services as a nationwide effort to help states, cities, and communities identify health promotion and disease prevention strategies to address these health risk problems.

The AIDS epidemic radically changed the process for infection control among health care workers in health care institutions across the nation. Recapping needles, wearing latex gloves, and using isolation precautions were issues that triggered much dialogue and debate among health care workers. Health care workers were mandated to use preventive measures in the form of Universal Precautions; all contact with blood and body fluids from all patients was considered potentially infectious.

Exposure to hazardous materials became a major issue of concern for not only health care workers but also the general public. Chemical and radioactive substances that created dangerous exposure and health risks were increasingly used in the workplace. Employers were held legally accountable for informing their employees of the actual or potential hazards and for reducing their exposure risk through training and the use of protective equipment. The hazardous materials issue was especially important in nursing and medicine, particularly with regard to exposure to carcinogenic chemicals used in drug therapy and in environmental infection control.

In 1990, the rising costs of Medicaid and Medicare triggered political action for health care reform. Findings of a federal commission appointed to evaluate the American health care system included the following (Chitty & Black, 2014):

- Fifteen percent of the gross national product was related to health care expenditures (this amounts to approximately $1 trillion annually).
- The United States spent more than twice as much as any industrialized nation for health care services.
- Americans were living longer, accounting for a growing demand for home health and nursing home care in addition to increased Medicare expenditures.

It became apparent that if health care spending continued to increase, the US economy would be in danger of collapse. Thus, the health care system moved toward managed care in an attempt to control health care expenditures. The managed care movement has had a tremendous effect on nursing.

The focus of managed care was on providing more preventive and primary care, using outpatient and home settings when possible, and limiting expensive hospitalizations. Massive downsizing of hospital nursing staff occurred, with a greater use of unlicensed assistive personnel to provide care in hospitals. There was an increasing demand for community health nurses and advanced practice nurses to provide primary care services. The nurse of the 1990s had to be focused on delivering health care services that (1) encompassed health risk assessment based on family and environmental factors, (2) supported health promotion and disease prevention, and (3) advanced counseling and health education (Nies & McEwen, 2022).

In June 1993, the National Center for Nursing Research was renamed the National Institute of Nursing Research. Moving nursing research into the National Institutes of Health enhanced the interprofessional possibilities for collaborative investigation. As a result, nursing research grew rapidly during the 1990s. Multiple research programs focused on important health issues such as health promotion across the lifespan. Nursing research began to inform health care policy through federal commissions and agency programs (LoBiondo-Wood & Haber, 2021).

In the 1990s, mandatory state licensure authorities (which set practice standards at the level of entering associate-degree graduates) and national nongovernmental bodies (which certify graduate-prepared specialists) forged a partnership. These national certifying agencies were intensely engaged in improving methods for determining the continual competence of certified nurse practitioners within the swift current of health care change. The consumer's voice in the partnership was heard via collaboration with advocacy organizations and the appointment of more public members to licensing, certifying, and accreditation boards. Voluntary credentialing bodies recognized that if they were to serve effectively, they had to engage in active public information campaigns to inform consumers about their health care choices (Buhler-Wilkerson, 2001).

Nursing in the 21st Century

It is frequently claimed that nursing is vital to the safe provision of health care and health service to our populations. It is also recognized that nursing is a costly health care resource that must be used effectively and efficiently. Therefore, there is growing recognition, from within the nursing profession, as well as by health care policymakers and society, of the need to analyze the contribution of nursing to health care and its costs. This issue becomes increasingly important in an era of staff cuts and staffing deficits, combined with higher patient expectation, escalating health care costs, and a health care system restructuring and reform agenda. Such factors make the identification and effective use of the nursing contribution to health care an issue of critical importance (Jackson et al., 2022). What are nurses' roles in modern healthcare? Jackson, Maben & Anerson (2023) conducted a qualitative interview study with twenty registered nurses and nursing students to explore how nurses understand their work. Findings revealed that nurses understand their work by its role in the healthcare system, rather than by the tasks they complete. This is significant because nurses adapt their work constantly and rigid definitions of their work would not support safe adaptation. Nurses in this study reported working across three broad roles: clinical work with patients, managing work to sustain the environment, and enabling work such as research and education that make nursing a profession.

Professional nurses in the 21st century are faced with many challenges within the dynamic state of health care. In addition to the issues of access, cost, quality, safety, and accountability in health care, nurses today are challenged by an aging population, a serious nursing shortage, generational differences in an aging workforce with poor prospects for replacements, high acuity and short staffing, conflict in the workplace, expanding technology, complex consumer health values, and an increasingly intercultural society. Nurses have identified numerous areas of concern, including insufficient staffing, inadequate salaries, effects of stress and overwork, violence in the workplace, lack of participation in decision-making, and dissatisfaction with the quality of their own nursing care.

Changing duties, responsibilities, and conflicts amid nursing shortages and public concern over patient safety and quality of care characterize present-day practice. These changes require professional nurses to have core competency in critical thinking, communication, interprofessional collaboration, assessment, leadership, and technical skills, in addition to knowledge of health promotion and disease prevention, information technology, health systems, and public policy.

Since 2001, military nurses have successfully supported military operations in deployed field hospitals in both Iraq and Afghanistan. These deployments have presented unique challenges for military nurses (Kenward & Kenward, 2015). Nursing in war is a unique experience regardless of education, preparation, and training. There are myriad variables that enter into the experience and affect outcomes, both personal and professional. Wartime deployment is a difficult challenge, as homecoming is more difficult than most nurses anticipate, and reintegration after coming home takes time and effort.

In 2008, the Robert Wood Johnson Foundation (RWJF) proposed a partnership with the IOM to assess and respond to the need to transform the nursing profession. The RWJF and the IOM established a 2-year Initiative on the Future of Nursing. The IOM report released in 2011 had the following four key messages: (1) Nurses should practice to the full extent of their education and training; (2) nurses should achieve higher levels of education and training through an improved education system that promotes seamless academic progression; (3) nurses should be full partners with physicians and other health professionals in redesigning health care in the United States; and (4) effective workforce planning and policymaking require better data collection and an improved information infrastructure (IOM, 2011). These

recommendations focus on the intersection between the health needs of diverse populations across the lifespan and the actions of the nursing workforce.

In 2010, Congress passed and President Barack Obama signed into law comprehensive health legislation. These laws, the Patient Protection and Affordable Care Act (Public Law 111–148) and the Health Care and Education Affordability Reconciliation Act (Public Law 111–152), are collectively referred to as the Affordable Care Act (ACA). The ACA represents the broadest changes to the health care system since the creation of Medicare and Medicaid programs in 1965. The ACA is expected to provide insurance coverage for 32 million previously uninsured Americans. This new demand on the health care system has significant implications for nursing, the nation's largest health care profession, with more than 3 million registered nurses (RNs) nationwide. Nurses have the potential to effect significant changes in the health care system that will meet the demand for safe, quality, patient-centered, accessible, and affordable care (IOM, 2011).

March 2016 marked the release of the report *Advancing Healthcare Transformation: A New Era for Academic Nursing*, commissioned by the AACN. This report calls for enhanced partnerships to advance integrated systems of health care, achieve improved health outcomes, and foster new models for innovation.

On January 25, 2021, leading nursing organizations launched the National Commission to Address Racism in Nursing (the Commission). The Commission examines the issue of racism within nursing nationwide, focusing on the impact on nurses, patients, communities, and health care systems to motivate all nurses to confront individual and systemic racism: https://www.nursingworld.org/practice-policy/workforce/racism-in-nursing/national-commission-to-address-racism-in-nursing/

On June 11, 2022, the ANA Membership Assembly, the governing and official voting body of ANA, took historic action to begin a journey of racial reckoning by unanimously voting 'yes' to adopt the ANA Racial Reckoning Statement.

This statement is a meaningful first step for the association to acknowledge its own past actions that have negatively impacted nurses of color and perpetuated systemic racism. For more information visit https://www.nursingworld.org/practice-policy/workforce/racism-in-nursing/RacialReckoningStatement/

A known and underreported reality for nurses in the 21st century is incivility and bullying. The American

Nurses Foundation conducted the COVID-19 Two-Year Impact Assessment Survey, in which nurses were asked if they had experienced an increase in bullying and violence in the past year, at work and outside of work. A disturbing 66% of nurses said they had experienced increased bullying at work, and 33% said they had experienced violence at work.

The issue extends beyond the doors of the organization. An alarming 23% of nurses reported bullying outside of work, and 12% reported violence outside of work (American Nurses Foundation, 2022).

The United States is projected to experience a shortage of RNs that is expected to intensify as Baby Boomers age and the need for health care grows. Compounding the problem is the fact that nursing schools across the country are struggling to expand capacity to meet the rising demand for care, given the national move toward health care reform. AACN is working with schools, policymakers, nursing organizations, and the media to bring attention to this health care concern. AACN is leveraging its resources to shape legislation, identify strategies, and form collaborations to address the shortage (AACN, 2023).

A wave of faculty retirements is expected across the United States over the next decade. Masters' and doctoral programs in nursing are not producing a large enough pool of potential nurse educators to meet the demand. Higher compensation in clinical and private-sector settings is luring current and potential nurse educators away from teaching. According to the latest Nurse Salary Research Report @ https://www.nurse.com/nursing-salary-research-report issued by Nurse.com, the median salary across advanced practice registered nurse roles is $120,000. By contrast, AACN reported in March 2022 that the average salary for master's-prepared professors in schools of nursing is $87,325.

In the winter of 2020, the COVID-19 pandemic highlighted the critical role of nurses, who were working on the frontlines to provide care for patients. While many people were avoiding situations that could expose them to the coronavirus, nurses were willing to remain at the bedside regardless of the risks. Nurses faced the fear that they not only might become infected but that they might endanger the lives of their own families. Stress and depression resulted from long work shifts, shortage of supplies, ethical dilemmas, diverse unknowns and demands of patient care, and the coexistence of countless deaths.

Although hopelessness, helplessness, and burnout occurred nurses remained on the frontlines fulfilling their ethical obligations (Al-Mandhari et al., 2020; Neto et al., 2020).

Travel nursing increased during the COVID-19 pandemic. Frequently, most travel nurses focus on how much money they can make as short-term contract workers—double or triple what their staff counterparts earn. But compensation, while important, is often not the main reason nurses leave hospitals for these contracts.

In interviews, nurses from across the country reported variations of a shared story: Working conditions, which had never been ideal in the first place—due to lack of support staff and high patient-to-staff ratios, among other factors—have dramatically deteriorated. Nurses have been asked to work to the edge of their abilities; they fear for patient safety. For many, travel contracts present a way out they never thought they'd have to take. Some nurses say that a travel contract limited to 8- or 13-week bursts protects their physical and mental health. They know that no matter how bad conditions get, for them the situation is short term. Others are using the money as a bridge to get out of nursing altogether.

Nearly one in five health care workers has quit since the pandemic began. A recent survey by the American Association of Critical Care Nurses found that 92% felt that the pandemic had "depleted nurses in their hospital, and that their career would be shorter than they had intended as a result." (DiGregorio, 2022).

ORGANIZATIONAL SOLUTIONS

The nursing profession has been under disproportionate stress due to the pandemic and typical hierarchical issues have been heightened. When comparing the Two-Year Impact Assessment Survey data to the August 2021 American Organization for Nurse Leadership (AONL) COVID Impact Longitudinal Study, a few items stand out. In the AONL study, "adding or increasing float pool" was identified as a solution considered or implemented by 56% of nurse leaders to address shortages. This can be compared to 18% of nurses in the Two-Year Impact Assessment survey who named adding or increasing float pool as a solution that has had a positive impact. Similarly, 42% of nurse leaders in the AONL study identified "flex scheduling" as a possible solution, compared to 10% of nurses in the assessment survey.

The same applies to "increased support services" such as housekeeping and transportation. In the AONL study, 17% of nurse leaders identified this as a solution, compared to 3% of nurses in this survey.

While no one-size-fits-all solution exists, this gap is significant and warrants attention. Nurse leaders are not to blame, having been tasked with responding rapidly to an unprecedented challenge. As nurse leaders strive to address shortages, these additional insights provide the needed information to help make data-driven decisions. Going forward, continued critical thinking and creative discussions on these evidence-based needs of nurses may help identify solutions that can be reasonably implemented by organizations. Ultimately, for a solution to be effective it must first be needed (American Nurses Foundation, 2022).

■ SUMMARY

To summarize the chapter let's review the questions posed at the beginning of the chapter and see what you have learned.

1. What were the challenges faced by nurses historically?

   Challenges to the nursing profession have included racism, sexism, and sometimes disgrace. Periods of war, socioeconomic change, infectious disease, and plagues have challenged the profession.

2. How has access to care and managed care affected professional nursing practice?

   The managed-care movement has had a tremendous effect on nursing. The focus of managed care was on providing more preventive and primary care, using outpatient and home settings when possible, and limiting expensive hospitalizations. Massive downsizing of hospital nursing staff occurred, with a greater use of unlicensed assistive personnel to provide care in hospitals. There was an increasing demand for community health nurses and advanced practice nurses to provide primary care services. The nurse of the 1990s had to be focused on delivering health care services that (1) encompassed health risk assessment based on family and environmental factors, (2) supported health promotion and disease prevention, and (3) advanced counseling and health education.

3. What are the challenges facing nurses in the 21st century?

   Today, nurses are challenged to practice to the fullest extent of their education and to expand their roles. The profession currently faces the daunting task of meeting the health care needs of a diverse and aging population. It is a continual effort to address the public's lack of understanding that nursing is a profession based on theory and a scientific foundation. Professional nurses in the 21st century are faced with many challenges within the dynamic state of health care. In addition to the issues of access, cost, quality, safety, and accountability in health care, nurses today are challenged by an aging population, a serious nursing shortage, generational differences in an aging workforce with poor prospects for replacements, high acuity and short staffing, conflict and incivility in the workplace, expanding technology, complex consumer health values, and an increasingly intercultural society. Nurses have identified numerous areas of concern, including insufficient staffing, inadequate salaries, effects of stress and overwork, violence in the workplace, lack of participation in decision-making, and dissatisfaction with the quality of their own nursing care. Nursing is a costly health care resource that must be used effectively and efficiently. Therefore, there is growing recognition, from within the nursing profession, as well as by health care policy-makers and society, of the need to analyze the contribution of nursing to health care and its costs.

REFERENCES

Al-Mandhari, A., et al. (2020) 2020—the year of the nurse and midwife: a call for action to scale up and strengthen the nursing and midwifery workforce in the Eastern Mediterranean Region. *Eastern Mediterranean Health Journal, 26*(4), 370–371.

American Association of Colleges of Nursing (AACN). (2006). *The essentials of doctoral education for advanced nursing practice.* https://www.aacnnursing.org/Portals/42/Publications/DNPEssentials.pdf

American Association of Colleges of Nursing (AACN). (2023). *Nursing shortage.* https://www.aacnnursing.org/News-Information/Fact-Sheets/Nursing-Shortage.

American Nurses Foundation (2022) COVID-19 Two-Year Impact Assessment.

Bahr, L., & Johnson, B. (1997). *Collier's encyclopedia,* Vol. 18: Simon and Schuster.

Buhler-Wilkerson, K. (2001). *No place like home: A history of nursing and home care in the United States.* Johns Hopkins University Press.

Buckway, A., & Sowerby, H. (2023). *Nursing in today's world: Trends, issues, and management* (12th ed.) Wolters Kluwer.

Carnegie, M.E. (1995). *The path we tread: Blacks in nursing worldwide, 1854–1994* (3rd ed.) National League for Nursing. Jones and Bartlett.

Catalano, J.T. (2015). *Nursing now: Today's issues, tomorrow's trends* (7th ed.) FA Davis.

Chitty, K.B., & Black, B.P. (2014). *Professional nursing: concepts and challenges* (7th ed.) Elsevier/Saunders.

DiGregorio, S. (2022). Hospitals desperately need staff. But capping travel nurses' pay won't help. *The Washington Post.* Perspective by Sarah DiGregorio.

Deloughery, G.L. (1998). *Issues and trends in nursing* (3rd ed.) Mosby.

Donahue, M.P. (1999). *Nursing: the finest art—an illustrated history.* Mosby.

Ellis, J.R., & Hartley, C.L. (2012). *Nursing in today's world: challenges, issues and trends* (10th ed.) Wolters Kluwer/ Lippincott Williams & Wilkins.

Fitzpatrick, M.F. (1997). The mercy brigade. *Civil War Times Illustrated,* 36(5), 34–40.

Freedman, D. (1995). *The anchor Bible dictionary.* Doubleday.

Giger, J., & Davidhizar, R. (2008). *Transcultural nursing: assessment and intervention* (5th ed.) Mosby.

Gill, G. (2004). *Nightingales: The extraordinary upbringing and curious life of Miss Florence Nightingale.* Ballantine Books.

Jackson, J., Maben, J., & Anderson, J. (2022). What are nurses' roles in modern healthcare? A qualitative interview study using interpretive description. *Journal of Nursing Research,* 27(6), 504-516. https://doi.org/10.1177/17449871211070981

Institute of Medicine (IOM). (2003). *Who will keep the public healthy? Educating public health professionals for the 21st century. Workshop summary.* In K. Gebbie, L. Rosenstock, L.M. Hernandez (Eds.), *Committee on Educating Public Health Professionals for the 21st Century, 2003, Board on Health Promotion and Disease Prevention, Institute of Medicine of the National Academies.* The National Academies Press.

Institute of Medicine (IOM). (2011). *Committee on the Robert Wood Johnson Foundation Initiative on the Future of Nursing, at the Institute of Medicine. The future of nursing: Leading change, advancing health.* National Academies Press (US). PMID: 24983041.

Joel, L. (2006). *The nursing experience: Trends, challenges, and transition* (5th ed.) McGraw-Hill.

Kalisch, P., & Kalisch, B. (1986). *The advance of American nursing* (2nd ed.) JB Lippincott.

Kalisch, P., & Kalisch, B. (1995). *The advance of American nursing* (3rd ed.) JB Lippincott.

Kalisch, B., & Kalisch, P. (2003). *American nursing: A history* (4th ed.) Lippincott Williams & Wilkins.

Karger, H.J., & Stoesz, D. (2005). *American social welfare policy: A pluralist approach* (5th ed.) Allyn and Bacon.

Katz, J.R., Carter, C., Bishop, J., & Kravits, S.L. (2009). *Keys to nursing success* (3rd ed.) Pearson/Prentice–Hall.

Kenward L.J., & Kenward, G. (2015). Experiences of military nurses in Iraq and Afghanistan. *Nursing standard.* 2015 Apr 8;29(32):34–9. doi: 10.7748/ns.29.32.34.e9248. PMID: 25850507.

Lindeman, C., & McAthie, M. (1990). *Nursing trends and issues.* Springhouse.

LoBiondo-Wood, G., & Haber, J. (2021). *Nursing research: Methods and critical appraisal for evidence-based practice* (10th ed.) Elsevier.

National Commission to Address Racism in Nursing (the Commission). The Commission examines the issue of racism within nursing nationwide, focusing on the impact on nurses, patients, communities, and health care systems to motivate all nurses to confront individual and systemic racism.

Nelson, S. (2001). "Say Little, Do Much": *Nineteenth century religious women and care of the sick.* University of Pennsylvania Press.

Neto, M., et al. (2020). When health professionals look death in the eye: The mental health of professionals who deal daily with the 2019 coronavirus outbreak. *Psychiatry Research.* 288, 112972.

Nies, M.A., & McEwen, M. (2022). *Community/public health nursing: Promoting the health of populations* (8th ed.) Elsevier Saunders.

Oermann, M.H. (1997). *Professional nursing practice.* Prentice–Hall.

O'Lynn, C.O., & Tranbarger, R. (2006). *Men in nursing: History, challenges, and opportunities.* Springer.

Robinson, T.M., & Perry, P.M. (2001). *Cadet nurse stories: The call for and response of women during World War II.* Center Nursing Press.

Small, H. (2002). *Florence Nightingale: Avenging angel.* Constable and Robinson.

Snodgrass, M.E. (2004). *Historical encyclopedia of nursing.* Diane Publishing.

Stanhope, M., & Lancaster, J. (2024). *Public health nursing: Population-centered health care in the community* (11th ed.) Elsevier.

Barondess, J., Lock, S., & Walton, J. (1994). *The Oxford medical companion.* Oxford University Press.

2

The Contemporary Image of Professional Nursing*

Leslie Moro, DNP, APRN, FNP-BC

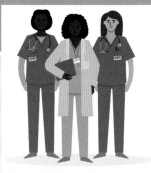

From iStock.com

ⓔ Additional resources are available online at: http://evolve.elsevier.com/Cherry/

LEARNING OBJECTIVES

After studying this chapter, the reader will be able to:
1. Describe the image of nursing in art, media, and literature over time.
2. Recognize nursing actions that convey a negative image of nursing.
3. Recommend strategies to enhance the image of nursing.
4. Explain how the IOM *Future of Nursing* report is shaping nursing's image.
5. Create a plan to promote a positive image of nursing in practice.

KEY TERMS

Antiestablishment Opposition to the conventional social, political, and economic principles of society.
Art Any branch of creative work, especially painting and drawing, that displays form, beauty, and any unusual perception.
Literature All writings in prose or verse.

Media All the means of communication, such as newspapers, radio, and television.
Stereotype A fixed or conventional conception of a person or group held by many people that allows for no individuality.

"People are always blaming their circumstances for what they are. I don't believe in circumstances. The people who get on in this world are the people who get up and look for the circumstances they want, and if they can't find them, make them."

George Bernard Shaw

*Thank you to Antoinette (Toni) Bargagliotti, PhD, RN, ANEF, FAAN for her contribution to the eighth edition.

PROFESSIONAL/ETHICAL ISSUE

John is asked to join a health care mission trip to a remote area of South Sudan that has no health care. John, the only nurse, will be joining a physician's assistant, a dentist, and multiple laypersons who will "help." They will be taking donated out-of-date medications (fourth-generation antibiotics, vials of multi-dose vaccines) as well as syringes and sterile supplies that were to be discarded because of their age and questionable sterility. When John asks who he needs to contact in this country about a temporary license to practice, the team assures him that a license isn't necessary because it would be such "a hassle" and they will only be there for 10 days. There will be minimal water and no electricity in the target village.

Response 1

Because there is no health care, the team reasons that the medications and syringes are probably fine. Following this line of reasoning, John would provide unsafe care that would place people at risk—people who have no idea of the risk that they are taking. There would be no follow-up care or referral resources. Highly sophisticated antibiotics would be introduced into an "antibiotic-naive" region to people who may not finish a course of treatment because they give the remaining pills to a needy family member or trade them for food.

Response 2

John reasons that he would be violating the ANA Code of Ethics and cannot participate in unsafe care that is disrespectful of human rights. He cannot practice without a license or the knowledge and consent of the government or bring drugs into the country in suitcases without any permission to do so. Once reconstituted, the vaccines would be unrefrigerated.

VIGNETTE

Mary, a senior nursing student, asks a faculty member, "Why can't we wear different scrubs and jewelry to clinical? Have you seen what nurses wear? Patients don't care what we're wearing. They care that we know how to take care of them. Two months after we graduate, we'll be wearing what everyone else does. Why should we look better than everyone else does?"

Questions to Consider While Reading This Chapter

1. How does the image of a nurse differ from that of a physician?
2. How does the nurse's appearance affect the patient's opinion of the quality of care the nurse provides?

CHAPTER OVERVIEW

This chapter describes how the image of nursing has been shaped and suggests strategies that nurses can use to forge a positive public and professional image of their practice. Because nurses have been the subjects of artists, sculptors, and writers for thousands of years, a historical perspective is used to illustrate the contextual background for the evolving image of the profession.

IMAGES OF NURSING

When you imagine a nurse, what mental picture comes to mind? Do you think of *LIFE* magazine's 1942 cover picture of a nurse in a starched white uniform with a cap (Life, 1942), the nurses portrayed in Johnson & Johnson's Campaign for Nursing's Future (2020a), or your colleagues with whom you practiced yesterday? All of them are architects of healing.

The contemporary image of professional nursing in the United States is an ever-changing kaleidoscope created by the 5.62 million men and women of all ages, races, and religious beliefs who have active licensure as registered nurses (RNs) (National Council of State Boards of Nursing [NCSBN], 2023a). Adding to this multifaceted collage are the numerous snapshots of nurses and nursing as portrayed in television commercials, bumper stickers, art, poetry, architecture, postage stamps, television dramas, television series, movies, newspaper comic strips, stained-glass windows, and statues. Nurses, whose profession is second in size to that of teaching, have been alternatively described as either saints or sinners, powerless or powerful, admired or ignored, and those who dare to care. Their practice has captured the attention of historians, economists, and sociologists who have studied this unusual group of people.

To whatever your image of nursing is, first add the many heroic nurses who served in Afghanistan and Iraq and in every US war. In July 1775, after the United States established the Continental Army, General George Washington requested the Second Continental Congress to provide one nurse for every 10 patients and one matron for every 100 patients to supervise the care of wounded and sick soldiers. His confidence was well placed.

In 2007, Captain Maria Ortiz, a 40-year-old clinic nurse manager, became the first nursing casualty in Iraq, dying from mortar fire to her clinic in Baghdad. Captain Jennifer Moreno was a 25-year-old University of San Francisco nursing graduate who was commissioned in the US Army upon graduation. A medical-surgical

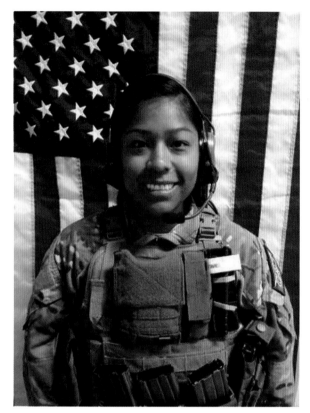

Fig. 2.1 Captain Jennifer Moreno.

nurse, she volunteered and was selected from thousands of female officers to a Special Operations Cultural Support team that included multinational, multibranch soldiers. For the first time, women were included on these male Ranger or Green Beret teams to obtain information, which was unavailable to male soldiers, from Afghan women. Every mission would be highly dangerous, especially for women. The first nurse to serve on a team, Captain Moreno served in Afghanistan with the 3rd Battalion, 75th Ranger Regiment (Fig. 2.1).

In October 2013, while Moreno was on a night mission to prevent a high-profile suicide attack in Kandahar that would have killed hundreds of civilians, an Afghan woman walked out of the compound, detonating her suicide vest and wounding six Rangers, followed by an insurgent detonating another bomb that injured others. Receiving a wounded staff sergeant's call for help and the ground commander's order for everyone to stay put to avoid detonating other bombs, Moreno heeded the call for help and ran through a heavily mined village to

rescue wounded Rangers. Her Bronze Star commendation reads, "Disregarding her own well-being, Moreno unhesitatingly moved to assist (the soldiers) upon realizing the severity of the wounds sustained by her fellow teammates. While in transit, Moreno detonated Device No. 5 and was killed in action" (Associated Press, 2014; The last moments, 2014). More than a thread in the rich tapestry of the heroic work of all nurses, Ortiz's and Moreno's courage and sacrifice illuminate the timeless commitment of all nurses to save lives and advance health.

On July 26, 2017, the arrest and assault of burn center charge nurse Alex Wubbels by Salt Lake City, Utah, Detective Payne, a 27-year veteran of the police department, enraged the American public. The body camera video released September 1, 2017, reveals Nurse Wubbels calmly explaining and providing the written protocol that the blood draw Payne was demanding from an unconscious patient required meeting one of three conditions: patient consent, a warrant, or arrest of the patient. Responding with, "I either go away with blood in vials or body in tow" (Mele & Victor, 2017) and "We're done," as Payne pushed her against a wall, held and handcuffed her, and dragged her from the hospital. Wubbels was released after being confined in a closed police car for 20 minutes. The unconscious patient—a reserve police officer with an Idaho police department—was involved in a crash and was not at fault in the accident. Following the film's release on September 1, the mayor and police chief apologized.

Since Florence Nightingale reduced mortality rates from 42% to 2% in a Crimean hospital constructed over an open sewer, nurses have been reformers who use limited resources to address unlimited "wants" for health care and to protect patients. The request for Nightingale's nursing services in the Crimea was borne out of newspaper reports about the devastating health care conditions in the Crimean War. However, the outcome that Nightingale and these nurses achieved changed conditions in the British Army, forged a system of nursing education, and continues to strongly influence the profession.

During the COVID-19 pandemic, the image of nurses became one often equated with heroism, as nurses served among the millions of health care workers in providing care to patients with COVID-19 (Bauchner & Easley, 2020). Nurses have been acknowledged for

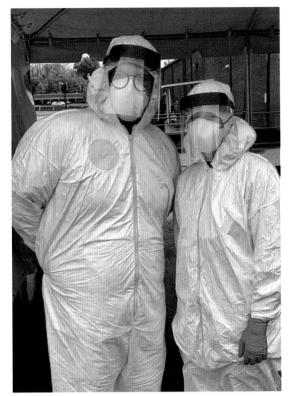

Fig. 2.2 Nurses working on the frontlines during the COVID-19 pandemic.

risking their health and lives by serving selflessly even when ill-prepared and poorly equipped, with at least 1500 nurses included in the COVID-19 death count for 2020 (International Council of Nurses, 2020). This heroic depiction of nurses, however, is not new, as nurses have been characterized as "angels of mercy" since the mid-1800s (Kalisch & Kalisch, 1983; Stokes-Parish et al., 2020) (Fig. 2.2).

Although nurses are concerned with their public image and media portrayal, Kalisch and Kalisch's (1995) extensive work outlining the image of nursing in film and media over time permanently etched the image issue into the professional radar screen.

WHY IMAGE IS IMPORTANT

Registered nurses (RNs), who account for 59% of the entire health professional workforce, are the "glue" that binds the health care of many into a more seamless experience for the patient. Safe patient care demands coordination of the armada of health professionals using many technologies and handoffs to provide care to a single person in intensive care and other technology-driven areas. How nursing is perceived inside and outside the health care system directly affects how successful nurses will be in providing and coordinating patient care.

The requirement for health care usually comes unexpectedly and without warning. When patients seek health care in a hospital, they are entrusting their life and well-being to the one person who has 24/7 direct responsibility for their care and their environment—the RN. Unlike their personal physician, with whom patients may have had a long-term relationship, or a hospitalist or intensivist the patient and family recently met, it is the RN, the coordinator of their care, who is new to them and changes every 8 to 12 hours. It is important that the public trusts and believes in this nurse and the profession the nurse represents.

REGISTERED NURSE SUPPLY

The United States averted a projected 20% shortfall (400,000 RNs) in 2020 because of the importance of nurses in health care. A combination of factors forestalled the 2020 national shortfall (Buerhaus et al., 2017b). The combined effects of the Johnson & Johnson Campaign for Nursing followed closely by other foundation initiatives and the Institute of Medicine (IOM) *Future of Nursing* report changed the image of nursing for both millennials entering college and the public. Underscoring these events were the unprecedented job losses (8.8 million) of the Great Recession (2007–2009) that happened in other fields (Goodman & Mance, 2011) as nursing saw record increases in new job growth.

RN graduates increased by more than 315% between 2002 (70,692) and 2022 (223,079) (National Council of State Boards of Nursing [NCSBN], 2003, 2022). However, the greatest growth—between 2002 and 2012—with annual increases of 7% in National Council Licensure Examination for RN (NCLEX-RN) test-takers for Associate of Science in Nursing (ASN) degrees and of 8% in test-takers for Bachelor of Science in Nursing (BSN) degrees, has levelled off to a 5% BSN annual increase and 1% ASN increase (Buerhaus et al., 2017a). Modifying the increases in new nurses is the projected retirement of one-third of the nursing workforce between 2017 and 2027 (Buerhaus et al., 2017a). In part, this change will occur because almost 24% of registered nurses remained in the workforce full-time until age 69, a trend that was mirrored among men in other professions (Auerbach et al., 2014). Later retirement ages have converted a gradual workforce loss over several years to larger losses at one time as the baby boomer majority has reached the age of 70. As Buerhaus and colleagues (2017a) noted, the significant loss when one-third of the nursing workforce retires is not one of numbers because of growth increases but rather a loss of experience and know-how. Nursing lost 1.7 million experience years to retirement in 2015 and was projected to lose an additional 2 million experience years in 2020. With the retirement of the baby boomer generation of nurses, the average age of the RN workforce has dropped from 52 years to 46 years since 2020 (National Academies of Sciences et al., 2021; NCSBN, 2023b).

Although it is important to know why an unprecedented nursing shortage was averted, the crucial issue is how it was reversed. Multiple legislative efforts began with the 2002 Nurse Reinvestment Act (Public Law 107–205), which provided nursing scholarships, public service announcements promoting nursing as a career, faculty loan cancellation programs, geriatric training grants, and nurse retention and safety enhancement grants. In 2010, the Patient Protection and Affordable Care Act increased the nursing student loan amounts, provided $50 million per year to fund nurse-managed health centers (Title V, Section 330A-1), funded gerontology nursing fellowship programs (Title V, Section 5305), provided up to $40,000 in educational loan repayment for nurse faculty and $80,000 for PhD-prepared nurse faculty, and significantly strengthened Title VIII advanced nursing education grants. Additionally, funding was made available for graduate nursing demonstration grants (Section 5509) to hospitals providing advanced nursing education clinical training to advanced practice nurses (nurse anesthetists, clinical nurse specialists, nurse practitioners, and nurse–midwives).

The image of nursing as a job growth profession continues with an expected new job growth rate from 2018 to 2028 of 12%, which is more than twice the average of all occupations (5%). Nurse practitioners are the fastest-growing occupation in health care with an anticipated growth rate of 45.7% between 2021 and 2031 (US Bureau of Labor Statistics [USBLS], 2020a, 2023).

NURSING IN ART AND LITERATURE

Although the way that nursing has been portrayed in art and literature over time may seem to be unrelated to the contemporary image of nursing, the mental image of contemporary nursing is enmeshed with the earlier images.

Art and literature have been the way in which people describe the human condition and cultural values of their time. In these earliest descriptions of nurses and nursing are found the enduring fundamental and essential tensions that exist within the profession today. Found within art and literature is the eternal question asked by those who know they will one day require nursing care: "Can I trust and entrust my life to this nurse?"

Antiquity's Image of Nursing

The earliest literary reference to nursing chronicles the actions of two nurse–midwives in approximately 1900 BC in Exodus 1 of the Old Testament, which indicates that the practice of two midwives became the vehicle through which the Israelites, the Jewish race, and the resultant Judeo–Christian heritage survived. From the 6th century until the 1800s, nurses were imaged as untrained servants, soldiers, women of religious orders, or wealthy people performing acts of Christian charity (Kalisch & Kalisch, 1995; Kampen, 1988). These meager artistic renderings of nurses convey images that continue to be familiar to contemporary nurses.

Victorian Image of Nursing

In 1844 when Florence Nightingale was "called" to become a nurse, Charles Dickens immortalized a different kind of nurse through Sairy Gamp, who nursed the sick because of the lack of other opportunities. For Sairy Gamp, a drunken, physically unkempt, uncaring nurse in *The Life and Adventures of Martin Chuzzlewit*, nursing provided a way to profit from the sick and dying. Reflecting the concern of Victorian England for untrained caregivers, Dickens writes that Sairy should be advised of the advantages of "a little less liquor, and a little more humanity, and a little less regard for herself, and a little more regard for her patients, and perhaps a trifle of additional honesty" (Dickens, 1844).

Fortunately, Sairy's literary arrival was followed by Longfellow's portrayal of the heroic Nightingale in *Santa Filomena* (1857). As important as Nightingale was to the improved health care of British soldiers and the development of modern nursing, the ever-increasing positive images of Nightingale occurred solely because she succinctly demonstrated aggregated outcomes of nursing practice. Nightingale was one of the earliest users of the emerging body of knowledge called *statistics* and developed the pie chart that remains in common use. Notably, nursing emerged at a time of turbulent social change and reform in Great Britain.

Early 20th-Century Nursing

Toward the end of the Nightingale period at the turn of the century, nurses in war settings vividly captured the attention of artists. The most compelling image is George Bellows' 1918 canvas, *Edith Cavell Directing the Escape of Soldiers from Prison Camp* (Donahue, 2010). World War I Germany shocked the world with its 1915 firing squad execution of Edith Cavell, founder of the first nursing school in Belgium, who aided soldiers escaping prison camps. The art of heroic nursing expressed in several famous paintings reflected the reality of World War I nurses, who were also the recipients of 3 Distinguished Service Crosses, 23 Distinguished Service Medals, 28 French Croix de Guerres, 69 British Military Medals, and 4 US Navy Crosses (Donahue, 2010). Notably, American nurses who served in World War I were not commissioned in the military services.

The 1930s Nurse as Angel of Mercy

On a grander scale, Warner Brothers' film *The White Angel* (1936) chronicled the professional life of Florence Nightingale (Jones, 1988). Endorsed by the American Nurses Association (ANA), *The White Angel* clearly portrayed Nightingale's persistence and head-to-head confrontation with medicine. Anticipating that the medical staff would deny rations for the nurses, she brought provisions for them. When the medical staff locked her out of the hospital, Nightingale sat outside in the snow until patients and soldiers required physicians to admit the nurses. *The White Angel* conveyed to the public that nursing is a holy vocation, nurses have professional credentials, and their career choice is opposed because popular opinion held that women belong at home (Jones, 1988).

In 1938, Francis Rich's tall and imposing white limestone statue, *The Nurses Memorial*, sometimes referred to as the *Spirit of Nursing*, was placed in Arlington National Cemetery to honor military nurses. Similarly,

Germany's postage stamp issued in 1936 commemorated nursing with a larger-than-life nurse compassionately overlooking people (Donahue, 2010).

The 1940s Nurse as Heroine

Considered to be the most positive movie about nursing, *So Proudly We Hail* is the 1942 story of nurses in Bataan and Corregidor. The film, starring Claudette Colbert, portrayed a small group of nurses rerouted to the Philippines after the attack on Pearl Harbor. Soon cut off from supplies and replacements as the Japanese captured the Philippines, these nurses provided care with few supplies and no staff to the thousands of soldiers in the Philippines. When the last nurses were to be evacuated from the occupied islands, 78 nurses (Army, Navy, and 1 Certified Registered Nurse Anesthetist [CRNA]) voluntarily stayed behind, made the march to Bataan, and were prisoners of war until 1945. Norman (1999) *We Band of Angels: The Untold Story of American Nurses Trapped on Bataan by the Japanese* (1999) tells their gritty, difficult, and heroic story from their diaries and interviews.

Nursing was depicted positively on a 1940 Australian postage stamp as a larger-than-life figure looking over a soldier, a sailor, and an aviator; on Costa Rica's 1945 postage stamp of Florence Nightingale and Edith Cavell; and in the 1945 commissioning of the USS *Higbee*, a navy destroyer named to honor a navy nurse (Donahue, 2010).

After nursing's glorious contributions to World War II, in which one in three nurses served, nurses returned home to low salaries, long hours, too few staff, and too many patients. However, the Cherry Ames book series, the Sue Barton series, and other romance novels glamorized nursing.

Nursing in the Antiestablishment Era of the 1960s

Ken Kesey developed the modern version of Sairy Gamp through the character of Nurse Ratched in *One Flew Over the Cuckoo's Nest* (1962). This best-selling novel later became a play and motion picture (1975) that won six Oscars, including Best Picture. Entrusted with the care of the mentally ill, Nurse Ratched, a militaristic nurse in a starched white uniform, was the ultimate power figure who punished patients to cure their psychosis through conformity to a "system" (Jones, 1988). However, the reality of the turbulent, antiestablishment period of the 1960s is that nursing was one of President Lyndon Johnson's first salvos in the war on poverty. The Nurse Training Act of 1964 was funded at $250 million ($1.99 billion in 2017 dollars). Although nurses also dramatically shaped the future of health care through the development of coronary care units, intensive care units, hemodialysis, and Silver and Ford's first nurse practitioner program in Colorado, a US Bureau of Labor Statistics study indicated that nursing salaries at the time were woefully inadequate in comparison with those of other, far less trained American workers (Kalisch & Kalisch, 1995).

Nursing in the Sexual Revolution of the 1970s

Media images of the nurse in the 1970s were formed amid a sexual revolution and a growing antimilitary American culture. War provided the media backdrop. The 1976 postage stamp Clara Maas, She Gave Her Life commemorated the 100th birthday of a 25-year-old nurse who died after deliberately obtaining two carrier mosquito bites so that she could continue providing care to soldiers with yellow fever in the Spanish-American War (Donahue, 2010). Her modern-day counterparts would be nurses in *M*A*S*H,* the hit television series from 1972 to 1983.

The nursing profession viewed *M*A*S*H* as professionally destructive because of the negative portrayal of Major Margaret "Hot Lips" Houlihan and the nurses of the 4077th Army MASH (Mobile Army Surgical Hospital) unit in Korea. The sexual exploits of nurses and physicians and Margaret's uncaring attitude provided few positive images. However, for the American public who were receiving a daily dose of Vietnam footage on the nightly news, *M*A*S*H* presented a glimmer of reality.

The continuous frontline exposure to the massive trauma of young men did not immunize the more than 5000 army nurses who served in Vietnam from the horrors of what they were seeing or prevent them from caring. These nurses were young (average age 23), newly graduated (only 35% having 2 years of experience, 60% having less than 6 months), and 21% were men. From 15 Army nurses in Vietnam in 1965, their numbers quickly expanded to a maximum of 900 nurses in 1969; they provided care for 5283 beds (58 patients to 1 nurse), working 12-hour shifts, 6 days a week (West, 2014). Lieutenant Sharon Lane, who was killed by mortar fire to her nursing ward, was the only

nurse killed by direct enemy fire. At the end of the war, Captain Mary Klinker, a flight nurse, was killed when her plane carrying 128 people, mostly Vietnamese orphans, was downed by enemy fire near Saigon (History Channel, n.d.).

Nurses serving in Vietnam would later be imaged in the television series *China Beach* (1988-1991).

Nursing in the 1980s to 1990s

The complexities of nursing are realistically described in the play and television movie *Miss Evers' Boys*. The character Miss Evers tells the story of actual nurse Eunice Rivers, who was hired to recruit and retain young African American men in the infamous Tuskegee experiment, designed to describe the long-term effects of untreated syphilis. Although the study began in 1932, penicillin became the treatment of choice for syphilis in 1947 in the civilian population. When subjects asked Nurse Evers to obtain the new treatment of penicillin for them and she sought to do so, the physician investigators required her to discourage them from treatment. Subjects were told they would be dropped from the study and forgo the benefits of free treatment: a free ride to the clinic, one hot meal per day, and, in case of dying, $50 for the funeral. Subjects were never told they had syphilis, only that they had "bad blood." The study, which was funded for 40 years by the US Public Health Service, ended in 1972 only because it became publicly known through the press. Ironically, Nurse Rivers was the only consistent staff person throughout the 40 years of the study. As the narrator of the story, Nurse Evers introduces nonnurses to the dilemmas of nursing practice during that era and the consequences of failing to protect patients and their descendants because of misplaced faith and trust in other health care disciplines. An outcome of the Tuskegee study was the requirement for institutional review boards to prevent this from occurring again.

In 1997, three films used war and nursing as a backdrop: *The English Patient, Love and War*, and *Paradise Road*. In these films, the nurse is knowledgeable and nonjudgmental.

Artistic views of nursing during this period focused on caring. In the Vietnam War Women's Memorial, in Washington, DC, the central figure is the nurse in battle fatigues cradling the head of a soldier. Evident in the bronze statue is the fatigue of the nurse and her care for this dying soldier.

Millennial Media

Stanley's (2008) study of nurses in film from 1900 to 2007 found that later films portrayed nurses as thoughtful, independent, intelligent professionals. The nurses in *Pearl Harbor* (2001) heroically provide care and order to the chaos following the bombing attack on Pearl Harbor. The character Greg Focker, RN, in the movies *Meet the Parents* (2000), *Meet the Fockers* (2004), and *The Little Fockers* (2010), endured his father-in-law's stereotyped views about men who are nurses. Several successful television series took place in hospitals, such as NBC's *ER* (1994–2009), ABC's *Grey's Anatomy* (2005–), Fox's *House* (2004–2012), and ABC's *Scrubs* (2001–2010), with physicians as central characters who often provide nursing care. Because their primary storylines portray physicians negatively, the scriptwriters' neglect of nursing may be professionally helpful.

Weaver and colleagues' (2013) study of the image of men in nursing in *Grey's Anatomy, Hawthorne, Mercy, Nurse Jackie,* and *Private Practice* (2007–2010) found that the men in nursing were in minor, often comedic roles in all of these shows. Questions about their sexuality and why they chose nursing reinforced every negative stereotype about men in nursing.

NBC's *Night Shift* (2014–2017) featured Kenny, an African American nurse in a San Antonio emergency department who managed physician logistics rather than sophisticated nursing practice in emergency situations (Truth About Nursing, 2017). NBC's *Chicago Med* (2015–) portrays three African American nurses positively, highlighting their nursing judgment and the safety net that nurses provide to patients.

On April 6, 2014, CBS television's *60 Minutes* traveled with two Virginia nurse practitioners, Teresa Gardner and Paula Meade, in their Health Wagon as they provided primary care to rural Appalachian people who cannot afford health care in six Virginia counties. Originally begun by Sr. Bernie Kenny from a Volkswagen Beetle, the Health Wagon has grown to include four mobile units, two freestanding medical clinics, and one dental clinic, which are funded by federal grants, donations, and the support of pharmaceutical suppliers, who provide needed medications (Fagan, 2014; The Health Wagon, 2022).

The NBC series entitled *Nurses*, which premiered in December 2020, is centered around several young nurses working in St. Mary's Hospital (NBC, 2020). However, the season premiere did not portray these nurses favorably. In this episode, the nurses are depicted in an unprofessional manner, often seen playing on their phones. In contrast to this media portrayal of nurses, the ABC series, *The Good Doctor,* is a medical drama that tends to portray physicians as professionals (ABC, 2023).

Social Media

Nurses portray nursing through their use of the social media platforms Facebook, Snapchat, Instagram, and Twitter. Although it provides an asynchronous communication medium among friends, the connection offered by "friending" or following on such platforms is often extended to unknown persons. Nurses and student nurses who have self-identified as nurses or students have posted comments about their practices, managers, or patients (whether named or not), creating serious professional issues for nursing. Some 33 state boards of nursing (SBNs) reported receiving complaints about nurses' use of social media, and 26 of these SBNs reported having disciplined the licenses of nurses (NCSBN, 2011). Nursing students have been expelled from nursing programs because of both positive and negative online postings about patients. The courts have upheld those decisions because of the significant breach of professional boundaries such postings make. Regrettably, nurses have "friended" patients and their families, leading to significant professional concerns about maintaining professional boundaries (NCSBN, 2018a).

The widespread use of candid cell phone camera pictures and video clips produces images amusing to friends but not as amusing to human resource personnel hiring nurses, to nurse managers, or to a courtroom when an error with serious consequences brings the nurse's professional judgment into question. Nurses have been terminated from positions and had their licenses disciplined or removed because they have posted pictures of patients on a social media site. They have been similarly disciplined for receiving patient pictures and not immediately reporting the problem. Removing a posting or a picture from a website does not make it unavailable because it remains retrievable (Steers & Gallups, 2020).

Nurses can positively use electronic social media to share workplace concerns or events that are emotionally charged for support and guidance, but they must always be mindful of not providing names, explicit details, or patient identifiers, including photographs, to protect patient and nurse privacy. For more information, review *A Nurse's Guide to the Use of Social Media* at https://www.ncsbn.org/public-files/NCSBN_SocialMedia.pdf.

Nursing's Response

Nursing students are the future of nursing. Taking this responsibility seriously, students began two similar programs directed toward the image of nursing: the National Student Nurses' Association's (NSNA) Image of Nursing (1993–) program and the Johns Hopkins Center for Nursing Advocacy, which has been rebranded as Truth About Nursing.org. With the theme "Healthy nurse, healthy patient," NSNA annually awards outstanding Image of Nursing projects and provides information to students. An important part of the program is the media surveillance information furnished to students. How to contact the television networks, how to most effectively transmit information to them, and sample letters are offered to enable student voices to be heard when there is negative nursing media or advertisements (NSNA, 2023a). NSNA has adopted a policy on social media that includes important examples of boundary violations.

In April 2001, seven graduate students at the Johns Hopkins University School of Nursing founded the Center for Nursing Advocacy (http://www.nursingadvocacy.org), which in 2008 became Truth About Nursing. Designed to challenge stereotypes and to monitor and positively influence the portrayal of nurses in all media venues, the organization successfully changed many negative nurse images. Skechers, Schick, Dentyne Ice, and the Lung Cancer Alliance all were persuaded by this organization to remove "naughty nurse" televised advertisements (Truth About Nursing, 2022).

Media Campaigns for Nursing

In 1990, the Tri-Council of Nursing with funding from the Pew Foundation implemented the Nurses of America (NOA) media campaign to convey to the public that nurses are expert clinicians who interpret technical data in usable ways as well as coordinate and negotiate health care. A strategically important part of the NOA campaign raised consciousness among nurses about the lack of visibility of nursing in the news media. A study of sources quoted by health coverage journalists in *The New York Times, The Los Angeles Times,* and *The Boston Globe* indicated that nurses accounted for only 10 of more than 900 citations, ranking nurses last after

patients (Buresh, 1991). Sigma Theta Tau International (STTI) published the Woodhull study (1998) of 20,000 articles from newspapers, magazines, and other health care publications, which indicated that nurses were cited only 4% of the time in the more than 2000 articles about health care. In 2018, STTI revisited the Woodhull study and found that nurses were only cited as the source of quotes in 2% of 365 reviewed articles and were never cited in articles on health policy (Mason et al., 2018). Additionally, the 2018 study revealed that nurses and the nursing profession were discussed in only 13% of the articles, and nurses appeared in just 4% of the images and photographs in the articles. Overall, this study reveals that nurses remain somewhat invisible in health news in spite of their high level of education and expertise (Mason et al., 2018).

Seeking to stem the nursing shortage and enhance the image of nursing, the pharmaceutical company Johnson & Johnson (2017) launched a $50 million multiyear media campaign (Campaign for Nursing's Future) in 2002. This project has included the issuing of more than 32 million pieces of recruitment posters, brochures, and videos in English and Spanish to junior high schools and career and community centers, as well as many television advertisements that are also available on YouTube (http://www.youtube.com). These have influenced 24% of 18- to 24-year-olds to consider nursing as a career. Additionally, there is the Nursing Notes by Johnson & Johnson Facebook fan page that launches two nursing videos per month, a comprehensive website (*Discover Nursing*) with information about nursing, an interactive program (*Your Future in Nursing*) for new graduates, and a Twitter handle (@JNJNursingNotes) (Johnson & Johnson, 2017). To commemorate the 10th year of this campaign, Johnson & Johnson invited nurses and nursing students to send pictures that became the *Art of Nursing: A Portrait of Thanks Mosaic Project*. For every picture they received, Johnson & Johnson donated $1 to the NSNA Foundation Scholarship Fund. Accompanying their marketing campaign for nursing, the ongoing Promise of Nursing galas have raised more than $20 million for nursing faculty scholarships for students planning to be nursing faculty in the states where the galas are held (Johnson & Johnson, 2020).

In response to the COVID-19 pandemic, Johnson & Johnson had a specific focus on nurses' mental health and resilience. Johnson & Johnson deployed more than $500,000 to mental health providers and organizations for services that help support the most vulnerable on the frontlines. Their #FirstResponders initiative provides support for nurses' mental health and resilience. It provided frontline health workers across the world with digital resources, online workshops, virtual training, and coaching amidst the pandemic.

The Johnson & Johnson Nurses Innovate QuickFire Challenge conducted on mental health, in partnership with the American Psychiatric Nurses Association, invited nurses and nursing students to submit potential solutions for improving mental health for patients and health care workers during the pandemic and beyond (Johnson & Johnson, 2020).

THE ENDURING PUBLIC CONCERN WITH NURSING

Against this backdrop of nursing images that extend from antiquity to the latest news broadcast is the question of the image that nurses will create today.

The Institute of Medicine's Future of Nursing

In 2010, the IOM issued a landmark report, *The Future of Nursing*, that has significantly affected the image and future of nursing. This report included four main recommendations: (1) higher levels of nursing education (80% bachelors of science degrees [BSNs] by 2020 and doubling the number of doctorates) through seamless academic progression; (2) removal of barriers to enable nurses to perform to their full scope of practice based on their educational preparation; (3) inclusion of nurses as full partners with physicians and other professionals in redesigning the health care system in the United States; and (4) improved data collection and information infrastructure to facilitate more effective workforce planning and information infrastructure (IOM, 2010). The IOM also recommended nurse residency programs that would be funded through redirection, by the Secretary of Health and Human Services, of all graduate medical education funds from diploma schools to residency programs in rural and critical access areas; a change in accreditation standards to require an assessment of clinical competency; and seamless access to higher levels of nursing education that extends beyond an articulation agreement, insuring that nurses engage in lifelong learning and prepare and enable nurses to lead change to advance health (IOM, 2010).

Much progress has been made toward the IOM's *Future of Nursing* vision for 2020. The number of nurses with bachelor's degrees has increased from 49% to 65.2%, although the goal of 80% has not been met. Additionally, the number of nurses with doctoral degrees has tripled, which exceeds the goal of doubling the number of nurses with doctoral degrees (AACN, 2023a; American Nurses Association [ANA], 2020). The National Academy of Medicine (formerly the IOM) launched a new study on the future of nursing in 2020. The Committee on the Future of Nursing 2020–2030 was established to extend the IOM vision to improve the health and well-being of the US population (ANA, 2020).

Future of Nursing 2020–2030. The National Academy of Medicine (2021) published *The Future of Nursing 2020–2030* report, which was built upon the foundation of the IOM's 2010 report. They recommended an overall goal of achieving health equity in the United States through increased nursing capacity and expertise. The strengthened nursing capacity they propose involves removing barriers that restrict nurses from practicing to the full extent of their education and training. After these barriers to practice are removed, nurses are better able to address social needs and social determinants of health and improve access to health care (National Academy of Medicine, 2021).

What the Public Believes About Nursing

Since 1999, when the Gallup Company began including nursing in its annual December public opinion poll on ethics, the public has rated nursing higher than all other professions for every year except 2001, when firefighting outranked nursing—likely representing a response to firefighters' work during and after the 9/11 attacks. For the 21st year in a row, Americans rate the honesty and ethics of nurses highest among a list of professions in the annual Gallop poll (Brenan, 2023).

THE REALITY OF THE CONTEMPORARY STAFF NURSE

"The reason for the existence of the modern health care institution—the hospital, the nursing home, the mental hospital, the home-care agency—is to deliver nursing. If surgery could be done safely and economically on the kitchen table, and if people could survive it, it would be. If diagnosis and management of serious medical illness could be done in office practices in 8.5-minute visits, it would be. If the chronically mentally ill could be taken care of at home, and protected from the world and from themselves, they would be. If the demented, the frail, the paralyzed, the very old could be cared for at home, they would be and it would be a whole lot cheaper because public policy would not contemplate channelling the money to family caregivers: they're supposed to want to do it anyway" (Diers, 1988).

Logically, it could be inferred that nurses' satisfaction with the work setting should be high because their practice settings exist to deliver their services, and new practice settings are emerging daily. The public highly values their profession. The 2018 National Sample Survey of Registered Nurses (NSSR) found that 88.7% of practicing RNs were satisfied with their job and 87.2% were with the same employer in the preceding year (HRSA, 2022). Among all RNs, nursing faculty are the most satisfied (86.6%). While nurses' satisfaction with their career choice has consistently been between 80% and 85% for the past decade, a 2021 survey of RNs—conducted in the middle of the COVID-19 pandemic—found that only 71% of RNs were satisfied with their career choice (AMN Healthcare, 2023).

FACTS ABOUT TODAY'S REGISTERED NURSE

Fifty-nine percent of all health care professionals (health diagnosing and treating occupations) in the United States are registered nurses, making nursing the largest health care professional group (World Health Organization, 2020). *US News and World Report*'s 2023 list of the 100 best jobs ranked software developer as 1st, nurse practitioner as 2nd, and registered nurse as 17th (US News and World Report, 2023). Nurse anesthetists, who are 58% of anesthesia providers in the United States; 46,540 CRNAs (USBLS, 2022a); and 37,430 anesthesiologists (USBLS, 2022b) are the major providers of anesthesia care to rural, medically underserved, and military personnel (American Association of Nurse Anesthetists [AANA], 2023). In many rural hospitals, CRNAs are the sole anesthesia providers (AANA, 2023). These are among the top

20 highest-paying occupations in the United States (USBLS, 2022c). According to AACN's report on *2022–2023 Enrollment and Graduations in Baccalaureate and Graduate Programs in Nursing*, nursing students from minority backgrounds represented 43% of students in entry-level baccalaureate programs, 40.5% of master's students, 35.8% of students in research-focused doctoral programs, and 40.7% of Doctor of Nursing Practice (DNP) students. In terms of gender breakdown, men comprised 13% of students in baccalaureate programs, 11.7% of master's students, 11.4% of research-focused doctoral students, and 14.3% of DNP students. Though nursing schools have made strides in recruiting and graduating nurses that reflect the patient population, more must be done before equal representation is realized (AACN, 2023b).

According to the 2022 National Nursing Workforce Survey (Smiley et al., 2023), the majority (71%) of practicing APRNs are NPs, 17% are clinical nurse specialists (CNSs), 9% are CRNAs, and 3% are clinical nurse–midwives (CNMs). The percent of registered nurses who are credentialed to practice as APRNs rose from 7.3% to 9.9% between the 2013 and 2017 (NCSBN, 2018b). It is anticipated that there will be a 38% increase in the number of employed APRNS between 2022 and 2032 which is much higher than the average (3%) growth rate for all occupations (USBLS, 2023b).

Men are still the minority in nursing. As Coleman's 2013 book title demands, it is past time for nursing to *Man Up!* Nurses are the problem and the solution to the low percentages of men in nursing. As Kouta and Kaite (2011) noted, women do not have female "privilege" as sole owners of empathy or caring, and we can change the subtle and not-so-subtle gender bias in nursing education and practice. A good place to begin is to recognize that men in nursing are nurses, not "male" nurses. What men think about being called a "male" nurse and how often it occurs is captured by the nurse who reported that he jokingly responds with "No, actually I started nursing school as an iguana and they put me out as a male nurse" (Rajacich et al., 2013, p. 77). The American Assembly for Men in Nursing (AAMN) is an organization dedicated to shaping the "practice, education, research, and leadership for men in nursing and advancing men's health" (AAMN, 2023). The barriers encountered by men entering nursing, such as lack of male faculty, lack of awareness of nursing as a career choice, and feminine bias in nursing textbooks, have been well documented (Guy et al., 2022; Hodges et al., 2017).

The 2022 National Nursing Workforce Study found that men now account for 11.2% of the RN workforce, which represents a 3.2% increase since 2015 and a 1.8% increase since 2020 (NCSBN, 2023b). When looking at specific nursing roles, the highest representation by men was in nurse anesthetist positions (41%) (AANA, 2022).

CREATING THE IMAGE OF 21st CENTURY NURSING

The 21st century image of nursing is one that nurses create every day as they practice and describe nursing to others. Conceptually, nursing is first and foremost "knowledge work" (Bargagliotti, 2003), and a profession for all people, not "just" a woman's profession. Knowledge workers are people who require specialized education to do work that requires judgment (Drucker, 2002). When nursing practice is conceptualized as knowledge work in which nursing judgment counts, other images of nursing fade away. For example, a randomized national study of primary care physicians (*n* = 505) and primary care NPs (*n* = 467) found that primary care physicians were more likely to advise a high-ability high school student to be a nurse practitioner rather than a primary care physician (DesRoches et al., 2015).

Consider the following data about the potential benefits of nursing judgment to patients. A meta-analysis of all mortality/morbidity/nurse staffing studies since 1990 indicated that decreasing the nurse–patient ratio in the evening was accompanied by a 90% increase in mortality and that 47% of deaths from abdominal aortic surgery were due to nursing staffing (Kane et al., 2007). Hospitals with higher percentages of BSN nurses (36%) reported a 19% to 34% lower mortality rate than hospitals with lower percentages (11%). Nurses who worked shifts lasting 12.5 hours or longer were three times more likely to make medication and other procedural mistakes. The data clearly indicate that decreased nurse–patient ratios have been associated with higher rates of mortality, shock, urinary tract infections, sepsis, hospital-acquired pneumonia, and failure to rescue, especially among surgical patients (Driscoll et al., 2018).

Aiken and colleagues' (2011) study of all hospital admissions in four of the largest states in the United States in one calendar year found that simply increasing the number of RNs is not the sole answer to reducing patient mortality. Rather, it is the educational level of the nurses and a positive work environment of the nurse, along with increasing the numbers of nurses, that matters. A "positive work environment" was defined as one in which there are positive physician–nurse relationships, management listens to the patient concerns of bedside nurses, nurses are engaged in hospital affairs, and hospitals invest in improving quality and in the continuing educational development of nurses. Nursing education matters because for every 10% increase in the percentage of BSN nurses, mortality rates decreased by 4%. These are cumulative, multiplicative effects. Similarly, increasing nurse–patient ratios in hospitals with positive work environments reduced mortality by 12% and failure to rescue by 14%.

There are tangible ways that the knowledge work of nurses is being portrayed to the public. Kalisch and associates (2007) found that on 70% of the Internet sites examined in 2001 and 2004, nurses were being imaged as intelligent and educated health professionals who are committed to patient care.

THE BASICS

At the simplest level, 5.2 million RNs create their image by ensuring that only an RN is referred to as "the nurse." Although the International Council of Nurses reserved the title of "nurse" for the RN in 1985, it is the responsibility of every nurse to ensure that the housekeeper, the untrained caregiver, the nursing assistant, and everyone else are not referred to as "the nurse." Imagine how confusing this is for patients and their families. Ensuring that patient teaching and questions about patient care are referred to "the nurse," rather than the assistant to the nurse, ensures that patients and families receive the best information possible.

A second and equally important image issue is how nurses refer to themselves and what they do. Nurses are not "medical professionals," do not practice in the "medical field," and do not provide medical care. Physicians provide medical care. Nurses practice nursing and they practice in health care, not medical care. Medicine is not the entirety of all health care, as 5.2 million RNs and a host of pharmacists, occupational therapists, physical therapists, and many other health professionals indicate. Aside from being legally incorrect, referring to nurses as medical professionals is misleading to the public.

Standardization of Entry

One barrier to the professional image of nurses is the lack of standardization of the entry-level requirement for the nursing profession. This lack of standardization causes public confusion, and potentially less respect for the profession, as there are multiple levels of degrees (e.g., diploma in nursing, associate's degree in nursing, and bachelor of science in nursing), which one may pursue in becoming a registered nurse (Institute of Medicine, 2010). This lack of standardization of entry for nursing is in contrast with other health care professions that not only require a standardized level of education for entry but also require doctorate degrees for entry into practice (i.e., medicine, pharmacy, occupational therapy, and physical therapy).

While the American Nurses Association (ANA) proposed using the BSN as standardization of entry in their 1965 position paper (ANA, 1965), the National League for Nursing (2021) supports multiple points of entry to the nursing profession, largely based on the long-standing shortage of nurses. New York state recognizes the benefit of additional nursing education, in the form of a BSN degree, for improved patient outcomes and has recently passed the Senate Bill S6768. This law, otherwise known as the "BSN in 10," requires nurses to receive a BSN degree within 10 years of obtaining their initial RN license (New York State Senate, 2017). While other states (i.e., Rhode Island and New Jersey) are working on similar BSN in 10 bills, none have passed them yet.

The Institute of Medicine (2010) echoed this need for standardization and additional education by recommending that 80% of the nursing workforce receive their BSN degrees by 2020. Hospitals seeking Magnet status, which the American Nurses Credentialing Center (ANCC) uses to recognize facilities for nursing excellence, are expected to have 80% of their nurses with BSN degrees. In addition, all nurse managers and nurse leaders within Magnet hospitals must have a BSN degree (ANCC, n.d.). While standardization of entry-level education is not characteristic of the nursing profession today, there is an increased recognition of the benefits of baccalaureate and graduate level education for nurses.

Magnet Recognition and Nursing Image

The Magnet Recognition Program, which was established by the ANCC in 1990, offers several benefits to health care organizations that receive this Magnet status. Magnet organizations promote nursing excellence, development, and education and are associated with less nurse dissatisfaction and burnout, higher levels of nurse job satisfaction, and lower nurse turnover (ANCC, n.d.). Overall, magnet organizations value nursing talent and provide excellent patient care.

Legal Cases and the Image of Nursing

Legal cases involving nurses tend to bring the image of nursing to the spotlight. Consider the recent RaDonda Vaught legal case in which a 38-year-old Vanderbilt nurse was convicted of two felonies (e.g., reckless homicide and gross neglect of an impaired adult) related to a fatal medication error at Vanderbilt University Medical Center (Feeney, 2022). The Vaught trial brought public attention to the possibility of medical errors, the potential for safeguards to fail, and the criminalization of medical errors. In the aftermath of this trial, health care organizations have had to work hard to ensure nurses promote a culture of safety.

Self-Care and PTSD in Post Pandemic Nursing

The COVID-19 pandemic revealed the dire need for nurses to engage in self-care. Nurses working during the pandemic experienced trauma related to the overwhelming number of deaths, isolation of patients who often died alone, and personal fear of being infected or infecting others. These experiences can cause post-traumatic stress disorder (PTSD) and ongoing moral injury, which negatively impact their psychological well-being. Nurses who served on the frontline of the pandemic are at increased risk for PTSD; in May 2021, the American Psychological Association reported a 49% rate of PTSD among nonphysician health care workers in 2021 (Draze, 2022). To alleviate the negative effects from COVID-19, nurses should be educated on the benefits of engaging in self-care strategies, coping mechanisms, and therapy (Hossain & Clatty, 2020).

Contributions from Nurses of Color

Mary Jane Seacole, the most renowned free Black nurse in the 19th century, is known for her work as a healer in Jamaica and as an Army nurse in the Crimean War.

Since Mary Eliza Mahoney became the first licensed African American nurse in 1879, numerous Black nurses have contributed to the advancement of American nursing. Between 1928 and 1960, more than 300 unnamed Black nurses, known as "The Black Angels," cared for more than 2000 patients infected with tuberculosis in Ney York City (Baptiste et al., 2021). While the contributions from Black nurses have been marginalized, ANA (2022) is seeking racial reconciliation in efforts to correct this. See Chapter 1 for a timeline of contributions of nurses of color to the nursing profession.

Resolving Conflicts in Nurse–Physician Interactions

An enduring mystery and common experience for nurses is how to address a medical problem with the primary customer of the hospital, the physician. Physicians generate revenue for hospitals and, in exchange for hospital privileges, agree to be self-governing and to abide by a set of medical staff bylaws, as do all advanced practice nurses in hospital practice. All medical staff bylaws include a disciplinary process that begins with the section chief, who is required to address documented patient care problems.

Too often, when nurses practice with a physician whose practice is substandard or one who is highly volatile, they believe that this behavior is a nursing problem. Rather, it is a medical problem that must be addressed by medicine via their staff bylaws. The problem can be resolved only when nurses disengage, factually document the problem in patient care terms, and forward this documentation in writing to a nurse manager and the appropriate section chief.

Just as nursing's involvement with medical problems is confined to appropriate notification, medicine's involvement with nursing must be similarly confined. When a physician notifies a nurse about a nursing problem, a more positive answer is, "Thank you. Let me investigate the problem and get back to you." Lengthy detailed discussions are unhelpful. When the nurse makes an error, a simple apology and sincere statement of corrective action is sufficient. Consider the following actual clinical situations (Case Studies 2.1 and 2.2).

CASE STUDY 2.1

A nephrologist complained in a meeting with a nursing service administrator, the chief of medical staff, and the physician liaison that he was not being notified by nursing about his patients and that nurses did not know how to take care of his dialysis patients.

Response 1

Nurse 1 told the nephrologist how well prepared the nursing staff is and that this was the first complaint of this type that had been received. (The problem was denied.) However, she indicated that nursing is short-staffed and that there are a lot of agency nurses. (Two excuses were provided.) She will investigate. (This was the first positive response.) However, without a specific incident and patient, she might not be able to correct the problem. (This was the third excuse.)

Response 2

Nurse 2 carefully took notes and limited his comments to clarifying questions while the physician became increasingly more derogatory. He concluded that there was a need to investigate, indicated that a written report would be sent to all parties, and thanked the physician for bringing this matter to his attention.

The nurse's investigation indicated that multiple nurses over time and in different units telephoned the nephrologist, who loudly announced that they had awakened his baby and abruptly hung up the phone. Additionally, the nurse learned that the complainer was a difficult physician who never had time to discuss his patients when making rounds. The nurse obtained specific examples of unanswered questions nurses had asked the nephrologist.

The written findings were prepared, and nurse 2 posed only one question: "Since the physician was not able to 'take calls' after 5:30 p.m., the patient care issue that concerned nursing is the question of who would be covering his patients."

Outcome

Within 2 weeks, the nephrologist's hospital privileges were quietly rescinded.

CASE STUDY 2.2

The nurses on a pediatric unit thought additional nursing staff was needed.

Response 1

The nurses and nurse manager "made their case" by describing to the medical staff and to nursing administration how stressed the nursing staff was. They insisted that they could not provide safe nursing care with their current level of staffing. Nothing happened.

Response 2

The nurse manager requested data from the pharmacy about the number of medications administered by nurses on this 24-bed unit for a specified period. The data indicated that nurses on the unit had administered 84,000 medications over 3 months. The only unit administering more medications was a 96-bed neonatal intensive care unit, which had administered only 10,000 more medications. Additionally, the laboratory data revealed that the pediatric unit usually administered 12 units of blood products daily, necessitating 48 additional sets of vital signs and assessments per day.

Outcome

Additional nursing staff positions were provided to the unit.

THE LOOK OF NURSING

White (2016) suggests that nursing attire is now directed more toward reflecting the nurse's individual preferences than projecting a professional image. The work attire of any professional says to the world how significant the task at hand is to that professional. Nurses are learning that a professional look encourages respect and admiration and are finding appropriate ways to express their individuality.

More recently, the nursing attire of hospital nurses has become an issue of safety for two important reasons. First, patients and families have expressed their concerns about being unable to identify who the nurse is in a hospital. When time may be a critical factor, patients and/or family members may relay critical information about a patient's condition to a housekeeper believing that person to be a knowledgeable nurse or may waste valuable time asking multiple people whether they are the nurse (White, 2016).

The second safety issue is found in the possible transmission of infectious organisms via nursing clothing that is worn in public places. Elizabeth (Betsy) McCaughey (2009), former lieutenant governor of New York and chair of a committee on infectious diseases, wrote a commentary in the *Wall Street Journal* that began as follows:

> You see them everywhere—nurses, doctors, and medical technicians in scrubs or lab coats. They shop in them, take buses and trains in them, go to restaurants in them, and wear them home. What you can't see on these garments are the bacteria that could kill you. Dirty scrubs spread bacteria to patients in the hospital and allow hospital superbugs to escape into public places such as restaurants.

Her warning was later supported by a study that cultured nurse and physician scrubs and lab coats and found pathogenic bacteria on 65% of nursing clothing. Notably, the highest colony counts were found for *Staphylococcus aureus*, with a higher colony count for methicillin-resistant *S. aureus* (MRSA) than for methicillin-sensitive *S. aureus* (Weiner-Well et al., 2011). When the public sees nurses in scrubs in public places, such as grocery stores, restaurants, and department stores, they are rightfully concerned.

Nurses should be aware that they may be asked to cover or conceal tattoos in the health care setting.

Collectively, the voices of nurses are heard through nursing professional associations, and nursing is imaged through participation rates in professional organizations. There are approximately 60,000 members of the National Student Nurses Association (NSNA, 2023b). Because 223,079 first-time takers took the NCLEX-RN in 2022 (NCSBN, 2022), it is reasonable to estimate there are at least 350,000 to 400,000 registered nursing students in the United States today. Where are the other 83% of nursing students?

These rates of participation in NSNA mirror the membership rate in the American Nurses Association (ANA). The influence that nursing could have in health policy and health legislation could be phenomenal if nurses participated more fully in their primary professional organization—the ANA. There are 61 or more specialty nursing organizations; however, the primary professional association is the ANA. At the International Council of Nursing, the national representative for the United States is the ANA.

CREATING A NEW IMAGE

Envision a new world in which nurses value nursing and image it daily. Nurses take themselves seriously and dress the part. Nurses are highly visible to patients, families, and physicians because they have reclaimed their practice. Nurses are clear about the role boundaries between themselves and those who extend their practice, and others are also. Nurses are "stuck like glue" together. Negative comments about a colleague are made to the colleague and to no one else. Professional nurses recognize tremendous value in belonging to professional nursing organizations. They look forward to annual meetings because such meetings provide an excellent opportunity to meet colleagues and discuss issues and practice innovations.

Because all nursing is valued, nurses recognize the value of caring, health promotion, and health teaching in addition to that of illness care. They celebrate that nurses save lives every day. In contemporary practice, nurses supervise assistive personnel and use their authority to ensure that patient care delivery is excellent. Nurses value the caring, knowledgeable role of the nurse because it is worn with style. To this legacy, they add the astute businessperson, advanced practice role, researcher, policymaker, legislator, and entrepreneur.

In this new world, nurses believe in nursing, in themselves, and in their colleagues. When nurses safeguard the image of nursing in local newspapers, television, media dramas, and daily practice, they protect the image of nursing.

SUMMARY

In summarizing the chapter, let's review the questions posed at the beginning of the chapter and see what learning has occurred.

1. How does the image of a nurse differ from that of a physician?

    Historically, nurses have not been as visible as physicians in health care publications and news articles, although they have been regarded as "angels of mercy" since the mid-1800s. In addition, media has often portrayed nurses in a negative manner in comparison to physicians, although this is beginning to change. The public, however, has consistently rated nurses as having the highest ethical standards, above those of medical doctors and members of other professions, for the past 21 years (Brenan, 2023). During the COVID-19 pandemic, the image of nurses became equated with heroism, as nurses served among the millions of health care workers in providing care to those with COVID-19.

2. How does the nurse's appearance affect the patient's opinion of the quality of care the nurse provides?

    As suggested in the opening Vignette, the way a nurse dresses may affect the patient's view of the quality of care they provide. Dirty scrubs have the potential to spread bacterial infections to patients. When nurses dress in a professional manner, this encourages respect and admiration from others and portrays how the individual views the significance of the task they're performing. Ensuring the public that nursing is a caring, scientifically based, quality, and safety-driven profession is essential. Everyone can care, but not everyone can be a nurse. When nurses recognize and convey to others the knowledge work that they do, nursing's role as the architect of healing is enhanced.

REFERENCES

ABC. (2023). *The Good Doctor.* https://abc.com/shows/the-good-doctor

Aides relieve nursing shortage. (1942). *Life, 12*(1), 32–34 36.

Aiken, L.H., Cimiotti, J.P., Sloane, D.M., Smith H.L., Flynn, L., & Neff, D.F. (2011). Effects of nurse staffing and nurse education on patient deaths in hospitals with different nurse work environments. *Medical Care, 49,* 1047–1053.

American Assembly of Men in Nursing (AAMN). (2023). *About us.* https://www.aamn.org

American Association of Colleges of Nursing (AACN). (2023a). *Nursing fact sheet.* https://www.aacnnursing.org/news-data/fact-sheets/nursing-fact-sheet

American Association of Colleges of Nursing (AACN). (2023b). *2022–2023 enrollment and graduations in baccalaureate and graduate programs in nursing.* American Association of Colleges of Nursing.

American Association of Nurse Anesthetists (AANA). (2023). *Certified registered nurse anesthetists fact sheet.* https://www.aana.com/membership/become-a-crna/crna-fact-sheet

AMN Healthcare. (2023). 2023 survey of registered nurses. *AMN Healthcare.* https://www.amnhealthcare.com/siteassets/amn-insights/surveys/amn-healthcare-rnsurvey-2023.pdf

American Nurses Association (ANA). (1965). *A position paper.* American Nurses Association.

American Nurses Association (ANA). (2020). *Future of nursing 2020–2030: Extending the vision.* https://www.myamericannurse.com/future-of-nursing-2020-2030-extending-the-vision/

American Nurses Association (ANA). (2022). *American Nurses Association seeks forgiveness as first step to racial reconciliation.* ANA Enterprise. Seeking Forgiveness First Step To Racial Reconciliation | ANA (nursingworld.org)

American Nurses Credentialing Center. (n.d.). *Why become Magnet?* Why Become an ANCC Magnet Recognized Organization? | ANA (nursingworld.org)

Associated Press. (2014). Madigan Army nurse killed in action in Afghanistan, KOMO News.com. https://search.yahoo.com/yhs/search?hspart=mnet&hsimp=yhs-001&type=type9097303-spa-4056-

Auerbach, D.I., Buerhaus, P.I., & Staiger, D.O. (2014). Registered nurses are delaying retirement, a shift that has contributed to recent growth in the nurse workforce. *Health affairs (Project Hope), 33*(8), 1474–1480. https://doi.org/10.1377/hlthaff.2014.0128

Auerbach, D.I. (2014). Registered nurses are delaying retirement, a shift that has contributed to recent growth in the nurse workforce. *Health Affairs, 33*(8), 1474–1480.

Baptiste, D., Turner, S., Josiah, N., Arscott, J., Alvarez, C., Turkson-Ocran, R., Rodney, T., Commodore-Mensah, Y., Francis, L., Wilson, P. R., Starks, S., Alexander, K., Taylor, J. L., Ogungbe, O., Byiringiro, S., Fisher, M. C., Charlemagne-Badal, S. J., Marseille, B., Delva, S... Hamilton, J. (2021). Hidden figures of nursing: The historical contributions of Black nurses and a narrative for those who are unnamed, undocumented and underrepresented. *Journal of Advanced Nursing, 77*(4), 1627–1632. https://doi.org/10.1111/jan.14791

Bargagliotti, L.A. (2003). Reframing nursing to renew the profession. *Nursing Education Perspectives, 24*(1), 12–16.

Bauchner, H., & Easley, T.J. (2020). Health care heroes of the COVID-19 pandemic. *Journal of the American Medical Association, 323*(20), 2021.

Brenan, M. (2023). Nurses retain top ethics rating in US, but below 2020 high. Gallup. Nurses Retain Top Ethics Rating in US, but Below 2020 High (gallup.com)

Buerhaus, P.I., Skinner, L.E., Auerbach, D.I., & Staiger, D.O. (2017a). Four challenges facing the nursing workforce in the United States. *Journal of Nursing Regulation, 8*(2), 40–46.

Buerhaus, P.I., Skinner, L.E., Auerbach, D.I., & Staiger, D.O. (2017b). State of the Registered Nurse workforce as a new era of health reform emerges. *Nursing Economic$, 35*(5), 229–237.

Buresh, B. (1991). Who counts in news coverage of health care? *Nursing Outlook, 39*(5), 204–208.

Coleman, C.L. (2013). *Man Up! A practical guide for men in nursing.* Sigma Theta Tau International.

DesRoches, C.M., Buerhaus, P.I., Dittus, R.S., & Donelan, S. (2015). Primary care workforce shortages and career recommendations from practicing clinicians. *Academic Medicine, 90*(5), 671–677.

Dickens, C. (1844). *Martin Chuzzlewit.* Chapman & Hall.

Diers, D. (1988). *The mystery of nursing: Secretary's commission on nursing support studies and background information, 2*: Department of Health and Human Services V.

Donahue, M.P. (2010). *Nursing: The finest art: An illustrated history.* Mosby.

Draze, L. (2022). COVID-19 and PTSD in frontline nurses. *American Nurse, 17*(10), 26–28.

Driscoll, A., Grant, M., Carroll, D., Dalton, S., Deatons, C., Jones, I., Lehwaldt, D., McKee, G., Munyombwe, T., & Astin, F. (2018). The effect of nurse-to-patient ratios on nurse-sensitive patient outcomes in acute specialist units: a systematic review and meta-analysis. *European Journal of Cardiovascular Nursing, 17*(1), 6–22.

Drucker, P. (2002). *Managing in the next society.* St Peter's Press.

Fagan, J. (2014). *Executive Producer: 60 Minutes Affordable health care for those still uninsured* April 6. CBS News [television broadcast].

Feeney, A. (2022). *Update: RaDonda Vaught sentenced to 3 years supervised probation.* Nurse Journal. Update: RaDonda Vaught Sentenced To 3 Years Supervised Probation | NurseJournal.org

Goodman, C.J., & Mance, S.W. (2011). Employment loss and the 2007–2009 recession: An overview. *Monthly Labor Review,* https://www.bls.gov/opub/mlr/2011/04/art1full.pdf

Guy, M., Hughes, K., & Day, P. (2022). Lack of awareness of nursing as a career choice for men: A qualitative, descriptive study. *Journal of Advanced Nursing, 78*(12), 4190–4198. https://doi.org/10.1111/jan.15402

Health Resources & Services Administration (HRSA). (2022). *Job satisfaction among registered nurses—Pre-COVID.* https://bhw.hrsa.gov/data-research/review-health-workforce-research/national-sample-survey-registered-nurses

Hodges, E., Rowsey, P.J., Gray, T.F., Kneipp, S.M., Giscombe, C.W., Foster, B.B., Alexander, G.R., & Kowlowitz, V. (2017). Bridging the gender divide: Facilitating the educational path for men in nursing. *Journal of Nursing Education, 56*(5), 295–299.

Hossain, F., & Clatty, A. (2020). Self-care strategies in response to nurses' moral injury during COVID-19 pandemic. *Nursing Ethics, 28*(1), 23–32. Self-care strategies in response to nurses' moral injury during COVID-19 pandemic - Fahmida Hossain, Ariel Clatty, 2021 (sagepub.com)

Institute of Medicine (IOM). (2010). The future of nursing: Leading change to advance health. The National Academies Press. Report Johnson & Johnson Campaign for Nursing's Future. https://nursing.jnj.com/the-johnson-johnson-i-campaign-for-nursings-future-i-celebrates-fourteen-years

International Council of Nurses. (2020, October 28). *ICN confirms 1,500 nurses have died from COVID-19 in 44 countries and estimates that healthcare workers COVID-19 fatalities worldwide could be more than 20,000.* https://www.icn.ch/news/icn-confirms-1500-nurses-have-died-covid-19-44-countries-and-estimates-healthcare-worker-covid#:;:text=more%20than%2020%2C000-,ICN%20confirms%201%2C500%20nurses%20have%20died%20from%20COVID%2D19%20in,could%20be%20more%20than%2020%2C000&text=The%20International%20Council%20of%20Nurses,up%20from%201%2C097%20in%20August

Johnson & Johnson. (2016). *About the Johnson & Johnson campaign for nursing's future.* https://search.yahoo.com/yhs/search?hspart=mnet&hsimp=yhs-001&type=type9097303-spa-4056-84481&param1=4056&param2=84481&p=Johnson+%26+Johnson.+%282016%29.+About+the+Johnson+%26+Johnson+campaign+for+nursing%E2%80%99s+fu-ture.+

Johnson & Johnson. (2017). *Preparing nurses for the future.* https://search.yoo.com/yhs/search?hspart=mnet&hsimp=yhs-001&type=type9097303-spa-4056-84481&param1=4056&param2=84481&p=Johnson+%26+Johnson.+%282016%29.+About+the+Johnson+%26+Johnson+campaign+for+nursing%E2%80%99s+fu-ture.+

Johnson & Johnson. (2020). *Why 2020 will forever be the year of the nurse: A look back on how the pandemic has impacted nursing.* (December 9, 2020). jnj.com/caring-and-giving/impact-of-covid-19-on-nursing-in-2020

Jones, A.H. (1988). *The white angel* (1936): Hollywood's image of Florence Nightingale. In A.H. Jones (Eds.), *Images of nurses: Perspectives from history, art, and literature.* University of Pennsylvania Press.

Kalisch, B.J., Begeny, S., & Neumann, S. (2007). The image of the nurse on the internet. *Nursing Outlook, 55*(4), 182–188.

Kalisch, B.J., & Kalisch, P.A. (1983). Anatomy of the image of the nurse: Dissonant and ideal models. *American Nurses Association Publications, 161*, 3–23.

Kalisch, P.A., & Kalisch, B.J. (1995). *The advance of American nursing* (3rd ed.) Lippincott.

Kampen, M.B. (1988). *Before Florence Nightingale: A prehistory of nursing in painting and sculpture.* In A.H. Jones (Eds.), *Images of nurses: Perspectives from history, art, and literature.* University of Pennsylvania Press, Philadelphia.

Kane, R.L., Shamliyan, T.A., Mueller, C., Duval, S., & Wilt, T.J. (2007). The association of registered nurse staffing levels and patient outcomes: Systematic review and meta-analysis. *Medical Care, 45*(12), 1195–1204.

Kesey, K. (1962). *One flew over the cuckoo's nest.* New American Library/Signet, New York.

Kouta, C., & Kaite, C.P. (2011). Gender discrimination and nursing: A literature review. *Journal of Professional Nursing, 27*(1), 59–63.

Longfellow, H.W. (1857). Santa Filomena. *Atlantic Monthly, 1*(11), 22–23.

Mason, D. J., Nixon, L., Glickstein, B., Han, S. Westphaln, K., & Carter, L. (2018). The Woodhull study revisited: Nurses' representation in health news media 20 years later. *Journal of Nursing Scholarship, 50*(6), 695–704. https://doi.org/10.1111/jnu.12429

McCaughey, B. (2009). Hospital scrubs are a germy, deadly mess. *Wall Street Journal.* http://online.wsj.com/news/articles/SB123137245971962641

Mele, C., & Victor, D. (2017). Utah nurse handcuffed and arrested after refusing to draw patient's blood. *New York Times.* https://www.nytimes.com/2017/09/01/us/utah-nurse-arrested-blood.html?emc=edit_tnt_20170901&nlid=10672999&tntemail0=y

National Academies of Sciences, Engineering, and Medicine, National Academies of Medicine, & Committee on the Future of Nursing 2020–2030. (2021). *The future of nursing 2020–2030: Charting a path to achieve health equity* (J.L. Flaubert, S. Le Menestrel, D. R. Williams, & M.K. Wakefield, Eds.). National Academies Press. https://www.ncbi.nlm.nih.gov/books/NBK573922/

National Council of State Boards of Nursing (NCSBN). (2003). *2002 Nurse licensee volume and NCLEX examination statistics* (Vol. 13). https://www.ncsbn.org/1236.htm

National Council of State Boards of Nursing (NCSBN). (2011). *White paper: A nurse's guide to the use of social media.* https://www.ncsbn.org/Social_Media.pdf

National Council of State Boards of Nursing. (NCSBN). (2018a). *A nurse's guide to the use of social media.* https://www.ncsbn.org/public-files/NCSBN_SocialMedia.pdf

National Council of State Boards of Nursing (NCSBN). (2018b). *Results from the 2017 national nursing workforce survey.* https://www.ncsbn.org/2018SciSymp_Smiley-Bienemy.pdf

National Council of State Boards of Nursing (NCSBN). (2020). *National nursing workforce study.* https://www.ncsbn.org/workforce.htm

National Council of State Boards of Nursing (NCSBN). (2022). *2022 NCLEX fact sheet.* NCLEX_Stats_2022-Q4-FactSheet.pdf (ncsbn.org)

National Council of State Boards of Nursing (NCSBN). (2023a). *Number of active RN licenses by state.* https://www.ncsbn.org/nursing-regulation/national-nursing-database/licensure-statistics/active-rn-licenses.page

National Council of State boards of Nursing (NCSBN). (2023b). *National nursing workforce study.* https://www.ncsbn.org/research/recent-research/workforce.page

National League for Nursing. (2021). *NLN value statement on workforce demands of the future: The educational imperative.* https://www.nln.org/detail-pages/news/2021/11/09/nln-value-statement-on-workforce-demands-of-the-future-the-educational-imperative

National Student Nurses Association (NSNA). (2023a). *Guidelines for planning: Image of nursing.* http://www.nsna.org/image-of-nursing-committee.html.

National Student Nurses Association (NSNA). (2023b). *About us.* https://www.nsna.org/about-nsna.html

NBC. (2020). *Nurses.* https://www.nbc.com/nurses

New York State Senate. (2017). *Senate bill S6768.* https://www.nysenate.gov/legislation/bills/2017/s6768

Norman, E.M. (1999). *We band of angels: The untold story of American nurses trapped on Bataan by the Japanese.* Random House.

Rajacich, D., Kane, D., Williston, C., & Cameron, S. (2013). If they do call you a nurse, it is always "male nurse:" Experiences of men in the nursing profession. *Nursing Forum, 48*(1), 71–80.

Sigma Theta Tau International. (1998). *The Woodhull study on nursing and the media: Health care's invisible partner.* STT Center Nursing Press.

Smiley, R.A., Allgeyer, R.L., Shobo, Y., Lyons, K.C., Letourneau, R., Zhong, E., Kaminski-Ozturk, N., & Alexander, M. (2023). The 2022 National Nursing Workforce Study. *Journal of Nursing, 14*(1), S1–S90. https://doi.org/10.1016/S2155-82567(23)00047-9

Stanley, D.J. (2008). Celluloid angels: a research study of nurses in feature films 1900–2007. *Journal of Advanced Nursing, 64*(1), 84–95.

Steers, M., & Gallups, S. (2020). Ethical tipping point. *Nursing, 50*(12), 52–54. https://doi: 10.1097/01.NURSE.0000694768.02007.f1

Stokes-Parish, J., Elliott, R., Rolls, K., & Massey, D. (2020). Angels and heroes: The unintended consequence of the hero narrative. *Journal of Nursing Scholarship, 52*(5), 462–466.

The Health Wagon. (2022). *Who we are.* https://thehealthwagon.org/who-we-are/

The History Channel. (n.d.). *Women in the Vietnam War.* http://www.history.com/topics/vietnam-war/women-in-the-vietnam-war

The last moments of Jennifer Moreno, an Army nurse killed in Afghanistan. (2014, April 29). *Army Times.* http://www.armytimes.com/article/20140429/NEWS/304290068/The-last-moments-Jennifer-Moreno-an-Army-nurse-killed-Afghanistan

Truth About Nursing. (2017). https://blog.truthaboutnursing.org/category/nurse-created-media.

Truth About Nursing. (2022). *Advertisements featuring nurses.* https://www.truthaboutnursing.org/media/advertisements/index.html#gsc.tab=0

US Bureau of Labor Statistics (USBLS). (2020a). *Registered nurses.* https://www.bls.gov/ooh/healthcare/registered-nurses.htm

US Bureau of Labor Statistics (USBLS).(2022a). Occupational employment and wages, 2022. *Nurse anesthetists.* https://www.bls.gov/oes/current/oes291151.htm

US Bureau of Labor Statistics (USBLS)(2022b). Occupational employment and wages, May 2022. *Anesthesiologists.* https://www.bls.gov/oes/current/oes291061.htm

US Bureau of Labor Statistics (USBLS). (2022c). *Highest paying occupations. Occupational Outlook Handbook.* https://www.bls.gov/ooh/highest-paying.htm

US Bureau of Labor Statistics (USBLS). (2023a). *Occupational projections overview, 2021–2031.* https://www.bls.gov/opub/mlr/2023/article/occupational-projections-overview-2021-31.htm#h9slgc7dcxqkkndky1k50goy1kg56hz

US Bureau of Labor Statistics (USBLS). (2023b). *Nurse anesthetists, nurse midwives, and nurse practitioners: Job outlook.* https://www.bls.gov/ooh/healthcare/nurse-anesthetists-nurse-midwives-and-nurse-practitioners.htm#tab-6

US News and World Report. (2023). *100 best jobs.* https://money.usnews.com/careers/best-jobs/rankings/the-100-best-jobs

Weaver, R., Ferguson, C., Wilbourn, M., & Salamonson, Y. (2013). Men in nursing on television: Exposing and reinforcing stereotypes. *Journal of Advanced Nursing, 70*(4), 833–842.

Weiner-Well, Y., Galuty, M., Rudensky, B., Schlesinger, Y., Attias, D., & Yinnon, A. M. (2011). Nursing and physician attire as possible source of nosocomial infections. *American Journal of Infection Control, 39*, 555–559.

West, I.J. (2014). The women of the Army Nurse Corps during the Vietnam War. *Vietnam War Memorial.* http://www.vietnamwomensmemorial.org/pdf/iwest.pdf

White, J. (2016). *Dress codes for nurses: Tool to boost professionalism.* http://www.healthcarebusinesstech.com/nursing-dress-code/

World Health Organization. (2020). *State of the world's nursing report—2020.* https://www.who.int/publications/i/item/nursing-report-2020

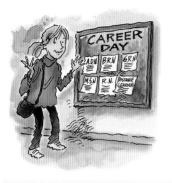

...ucational diversity promotes access and career ...velopment.

3

The Influence of Contemporary Trends and Issues on Nursing Education*

Leslie Moro, DNP, APRN, FNP-BC

ⓔ Additional resources are available online at: http://evolve.elsevier.com/Cherry/

LEARNING OUTCOMES

After studying this chapter, the reader will be able to:

1. Integrate knowledge of 10 current trends and issues in society and health care into a more holistic perception of their influence on nursing education, students, faculty, and nursing practice.
2. Create a personal philosophy and plan for ongoing professional development and practice that integrates knowledge of current trends and issues.
3. Access current information resources from the Internet related to evolving trends and issues as a component of ongoing learning and preparation for practice.
4. Differentiate among various types of conventional, mobility, and new nursing education programs and the issues associated with them.

KEY TERMS

Competency outcomes The results, or end products, of planned study and experience that are focused on specific abilities required for practice.

Contemporary issues The problems, changes, and concerns that are current for the present time.

Core competencies The essential cluster of abilities and skills required for competent nursing practice.

Diversity Wide range of individual, population, and social characteristics, such as age, gender, race, sexual orientation, religious beliefs, and socioeconomic status.

Educational mobility The progressive movement from one type or level of education to another, often based on flexible, self-directed, or advanced placement options. Examples are progression from diploma preparation to an academic degree, such as RN to BSN or MSN; BSN to doctoral degree; and nonnursing degree to BSN, MSN, or doctoral degree.

Education trends Shifts in conditions and concerns that emerge from and influence various aspects of society; broad changes in the United States and the

*We thank Dawn Vanderhoef, PhD, DNP, RN, PMHNP-BC, FAANP for her contributions to this chapter in the 8th edition, Carrie B. Lenburg, EdD, RN, FAAN for her contribution to this chapter in the 1st through 5th editions, and Susan R. Jacob, PhD, RN for her contribution to the 6th edition.

world that influence the education and practice of nurses and other providers.

Equity The quality of fairness and justice; providing resources and knowledge to individuals to allow them access to opportunities such as higher education, employment, and health care.

Inclusion Representation of organizational cultures with people who have diverse characteristics; this involves creating environments that welcome and respect the contribution from people with different perspectives and experiences.

Performance examinations Standardized evaluation based on objective demonstration of specific required competencies; used in conjunction with written tests of knowledge about those abilities. They may require performance in actual or simulated situations, related to physical psychomotor skills or the observable evidence of other skills such as critical thinking, communication, teaching, planning, writing, and analysis and integration of data.

PROFESSIONAL/ETHICAL ISSUE

Amy, a prelicensure nursing student, was in her first year of clinical and excited to begin her 5-week inpatient psychiatric rotation. Amy was considering becoming a psychiatric nurse, like her father and grandmother, and was looking forward to this clinical rotation, which she was sure would help her in making a decision about psychiatric nursing. During her fourth week on the psychiatric unit, Amy was assigned to work with Sandy, an RN on the psychiatric intensive care unit (PIC-U). During morning report, Amy learned that a female patient was placed in four-point restraints about 1 hour before the day shift nurses started. The patient, "Lindsay," was assigned to Sandy, and Amy was interested in working with a very ill psychiatric patient, but also very anxious.

After completion of her 15-minute checks, Sandy asked Amy to stay in the room with the patient while she went to the medication room to prepare Lindsay's medications, and Amy agreed. As soon as Sandy left the room, Lindsay asked Amy if she had her cell phone in her pocket, and Amy felt her face get beet red, her heart race, and her palms become sweaty; she did not know how to answer the question because she did have her cell phone in her pocket. Lindsay noticed Amy's anxiety and asked her to take her cell phone out of her pocket to take a picture of her in restraints so she could show it to her attorney. Lindsay explained how the night shift had mistreated her and said she was abused and needed documentation. She told Amy that it was okay to take the picture, that it would only be used if necessary, and if she didn't need it she could delete the photo. Lindsay

made a very logical, compelling case for needing a photo, so Amy took out her cell phone and took two photos of Lindsay. Quickly, Lindsay said, "Oh, just text the photos to me at 999-999-9999. Don't worry, you are really being a great help and I know you will make an excellent psychiatric nurse. Once you send me the pictures, you can delete them." Amy hesitated, felt uncomfortable, but sent the pictures to Lindsay.

Amy continued the shift with Sandy, and Lindsay was taken out of restraints and doing much better when Amy left for the day. Lindsay thanked Amy for her care and told her that she was doing much better and would delete the pictures from her cell when she was allowed to get her personal belongings back. Amy said good-bye to Sandy and her assigned patients and went to post conference. Amy did not tell her nursing instructor or Sandy about the pictures and deleted them from her camera as soon as she got into post conference. Amy was embarrassed that a psychiatric patient persuaded her to take her cell phone out and take pictures and feared she would be dismissed from the nursing program if she told anyone.

What ethical considerations need to be considered in the clinical experience just described? What ethical principles can be applied to this case? Provide examples.

VIGNETTE

Three students were having an animated discussion after class.

Mark: I'm tired of all this lecturing! I just want to DO nursing! Why do we always have to discuss things like EBP and critical thinking? What is it anyway? And we're always having to analyze a situation when it's perfectly clear what needs to be done! I don't get it. Just do what the doc orders or what's in the procedure book. I don't need to keep looking up stuff when I've done it before. Besides, we already have way too much to read for every class!

Katelyn: But listen to this. I heard about a student several days ago who really got into trouble because of a big mistake she made. She did just what you said, followed the provider's orders, and gave digoxin to an 80-year-old patient. She had already written a note that he was complaining of anorexia, nausea, and visual disturbances, but she didn't take time to look up "dig" toxicity or to really think things through. And guess what? The patient got into a really bad situation. It was lucky that the nurse practitioner read the note, checked the patient, put the pieces together, and got a stat serum "dig" level. She had to administer Digibind! It was so life threatening and really scary! He's not out of the woods yet. The student said the nurse practitioner was nice and helped her understand what she should have done, but the instructor pulled her off the unit and gave her a serious dressing-down because she had not taken a couple of minutes to analyze the situation, to think about what things are danger signs, or to just look up the meds and the patient's condition at the time—she just followed the provider's orders. I'd be scared to be the one being grilled at the risk management meeting! She may even fail the course.

Audrey: That sounds like a good example of what our instructors keep telling us. Nursing is about thinking as well as doing. We can seriously harm a patient if we don't know what actually needs to be done. We have to learn enough so we're competent and know how to use best practices for all kinds of situations, and where to get the information fast. We have to really study resources, use our e-books, and medical software to check things out first, and then figure out what we need to do, and fast, even if we're busy or just don't want to stop and look up something.

Katelyn: Why don't we start our own little study group to learn how to get a better understanding of each class? Nursing is a lot more than just "doing" skills. We've got to be competent in the thinking that goes with the doing. And, there's got to be a way to organize all this information and learn how to put it together for different situations. Whaddaya say? I don't want to get into trouble like that other student! Come on; let's get started on those study questions.

Questions to Consider While Reading This Chapter:

1. What are the major current trends in society and health care, and how do they influence nursing education and practice?
2. What are the most compelling reasons that nurses require ongoing development and validation of competencies for licensure and continuing practice?
3. What local, state, and national resources and Internet websites are available to learn about the trends and issues that influence nursing education?
4. What are the pros and cons of the many different types of nursing education programs that prepare students for current nursing practice?
5. What educational opportunities exist for graduates of various programs to advance beyond their current preparation, including traditional, mobility, and distance-learning programs?

CHAPTER OVERVIEW

Society as a whole is going through many significant changes, and all of them influence nursing education and health care. Nursing care is more complex, and the role of the registered nurse (RN) is more demanding, requiring nurses to be active participants in health-care decisions. Nurses need to be effective and efficient in understanding how societal, political, educational, and health care systems influence health outcomes. Our knowledge, skills, and abilities are critical to the kind of nursing care we provide, and they influence how we respond to changes in patients, families, and communities. Nurse educators must be vigilant in learning about these changes and integrating trends and changes into nursing curricula. Students also need to be aware of evolving trends and issues and must learn how they influence learning and practice. Competent nurses integrate these changes into their way of being, to become "thinking" nurses as well as "doing" nurses. Thinking nurses learn to integrate essential knowledge, skills, and abilities to provide care using best practices, evidence-based practices (EBPs) that promote patient safety and quality. As American society becomes increasingly diverse and complex, new trends precipitate different issues.

This chapter describes 10 contemporary trends that influence the way students (and nurses) learn, become competent practitioners, and meet the needs of patients.

Competent nurses integrate these changes into their way of being, to become "thinking" nurses as well as "doing" nurses. Thinking nurses learn to integrate essential knowledge, skills, and abilities to provide care using best practices, EBPs that promote patient safety and quality. Some of these trends and related issues include the following: the extreme and rapid changes of technology in patient care and education, significant changes in the demographics of our society, the economic crisis and its consequences, the globalization of knowledge and diseases, the demand for competent health care providers, the increase in domestic abuse and violence of all sorts, the complexity of physical and mental health conditions including suicide and substance use disorders, ethical issues, and the shortage of nursing faculty and nurses. This chapter also describes the types of nursing education programs, their contribution to the profession, the expansion of innovative nursing programs, the degrees and specialties available, and the multiple technologic advances that inform learning and patient care. Tables and boxes contain online resources, important organizations and associations, and some statistics related to types of programs.

Lenburg (2008) identified trends and the standards and innovation issues related to nursing education, which are used as the framework to organize this chapter (Table 3.1).

TABLE 3.1   Summary of Trends and Issues That Influence Nursing Education

Major Contemporary Trends	Related Issues for Students
Rapid knowledge expansion; increasing use of technology and informatics in education and practice	Choosing the most effective electronic and technology options. Information overload; virtually unlimited global resources, global research opportunities, issues. Identifying current and accurate information; material rapidly outdated. Expanded expectations, limited time, rapid response expected; little time for reflection. Expansion of nursing informatics, content, and skills development.
Practice-based competency; outcomes- and evidence-based content	Learning focused on core practice competency outcomes, professional skills beyond technical psychomotor skills; core practice competencies; multiple conflicting versions; which to use? Integration of evidence-based standards, research findings into practice; emphasis on critical thinking, problem solving. Changes in standards; ensuring patient safety.
Performance-based competency; learning and objective assessment methods	Multiple teaching-learning methods: interactive collaborative, in-class and out-of-class projects; problem-based learning; increasing self-responsibility; accountability for learning and competence; interprofessional learning; using electronic devices, media to access resources. Competency assessment based on performance examinations, specified portfolio documentation; standards-based assessment methods; emphasis on patient safety.
Sociodemographics, cultural, diversity, economic, and political changes	Larger aging population; increasing multicultural, ethnic diversity requires greater learning, respect for differences, preferences, customs; generational issues. Immigration conflicts, protests; consequences for access and health care. Community, faith-based projects, service-learning projects. Social, economic, and political changes influence health care delivery and access to clinical experiences; influence disrespect, conflict, abuse, violence; greater poverty and need. Multidimensional content, client care, clinical learning sites.
Community-focused interdisciplinary approaches	Interprofessional collaborative learning. Diverse alternative health practices, influence of cultures. Broad scope of nursing; clinical approach; increasing use of diverse experiences throughout community; continuum from acute care to health promotion, from hospitals to home to rural to global settings. Requires more planning, travel time, expenses, arrangements; different skills, communications; critical thinking, problem-solving strategies. Multiple teachers, preceptors, staff instructors, part-time, with varying abilities; time constraints.

TABLE 3.1   Summary of Trends and Issues That Influence Nursing Education—cont'd

Major Contemporary Trends	Related Issues for Students
Global health	Extensive global travel and commerce. Illness can arrive on any airplane, ship, or bus and spread throughout the country. Threat of epidemics. Nurses are connected globally through shared networks and technology.
Patient-centered care: engagement, safety, and privacy	All expect value, quality, individual respect, consideration, attention; privacy issues. Patient initiatives for involvement and protection; balance standards and preferences. Increased litigation, medical-nursing errors; focus on safe, competent patient care. Increased individual responsibility, accountability for learning and practice.
Ethics and bioethical concerns	Alternative solutions to ethical dilemmas; issues regarding diverse beliefs; disputes regarding biotechnology and bioengineering in health care. Many gray zones instead of black-and-white absolutes; separation of professional practice responsibilities from personal opinions, consequences for competence, and patient safety. Integrate into professional practice an acceptance of the individual's right of choice regarding life and death issues, health-care methods; respect, tolerance for patient's decisions, ethical competencies for students. Standards of quality care, patient's rights issues.
Increasing shortage of nurses and faculty	Shortage of staff results in limitations in clinical learning; heavy workload; using preceptors, part-time instructors; less one-to-one help for students; consequences for learning and patient safety. Shortage of qualified faculty; aging, retiring; increased part-time instructors, clinical staff, national and global problems, influence quality education and future nursing staff; need for more educational funding. Students need more clinical learning; more responsibility for self-directed learning, seek assistance from others. Increased use of simulation; required to validate initial and continuing competence.
Disasters, violence, and terrorism	New learning skills required for major natural disaster events; new program options, new courses, and new skills needed for emergency responders. Violence in society, homes, workplace, schools; abuse against women and children. Preparedness for terrorism; skills, programs for first responders; increased anxiety, uncertainty.
Increasing professional and personal responsibility	Lifelong learning to meet professional expectations; certification requirements. Increasing competency assessment in workplace. Changes in standards for quality-care practice. High stress from competing demands of school, home, meeting competency requirements.

TRENDS AND ISSUES IN CONTEMPORARY NURSING EDUCATION

Knowledge Expansion and Use of Technology and the Internet

With ever-expanding developments in electronic information and communication technology, the volume of information is growing exponentially on a global level. Nurses have been interacting with technology for decades. In 1994, the American Nurses Association (ANA) published nursing informatics standards, understanding that nurses interact with technology at high rates (Darvish et al., 2014). Informatics has become a major part of education and practice and is part of the American Association of Colleges of Nursing (AACN) Essentials for all levels of nursing education (AACN, 2021a). The ability to create, access, and disseminate unlimited information rapidly has enormous benefits. Individuals from across the globe use various forms of social media, including blogs, Twitter, Facebook, TikTok, YouTube, and LinkedIn. Millennials grew up using technology and are the main generation in many undergraduate nursing programs. Nursing educators must be sensitive to the learning needs of their students and incorporate innovative technologies into learning (Hay et al., 2017; Ross & Myers, 2017). Use of social media has become so common in nursing that guidelines and code of ethics statements for it have been developed by employers and by national nursing organizations (ANA, 2023a; NCSBN, 2018). The use of social media has become a concern for nurses, nursing students, and educators. Using digital forums to communicate requires an understanding of policies and potential legal implications because few understand the implications and health systems lack policies for its use (Balestra, 2018).

Websites allow for rapid access to online and printed material. Digital health-related materials can be updated quickly, allowing educators to create and revise online course content, assignments, and examinations. Nursing educators are using TED (Technology, Entertainment, Design) Talks to cover a variety of topics from science to global issues. Nursing is also engaged in various technologies that impact care. For example, nurses are now challenged with having an understanding of genetics and genomics, digital diagnostics and treatments, robotics, biometrics, and electronic health records (see Chapter 15).

Using computerized testing prepares students for computerized licensure examinations. Glasgow et al. (2019) and Montegrico (2021) found that using the RN-Comprehensive Predictor examination or Exit Evaluation at the end of a basic RN program predicts a student's success on the National Council Licensure Examination for Registered Nurse (NCLEX-RN). Students at all levels of education must be prepared to understand and manage health information technology, promote the meaningful use of electronic health records, and teach patients how to use health information wisely (Chapter 15).

Increasingly, point-of-care technology tools such as handheld computers, tablets, and smartphones are essential for the delivery of safe, efficient, high-quality patient care. Furthermore, use of technology tools in acute care settings quickly connects the nurse with the provider, allowing access to past and current patient data, references, policies, procedures, and evidence-based literature to guide clinical decisions (Chapter 15). Exposure to digital resources on mobile devices introduced early into the nursing curriculum and embedded in the classroom and clinical setting throughout the program is important (Gallegos et al., 2019; Nikpeyma et al., 2021).

With almost unlimited information available, students may actually take more time to navigate online resources than traditional print-based resources and may become overly engaged in following links, networking, and using chat rooms. Faculty and students need to work together to promote efficient and effective use of electronic learning tools and networking; reducing overload and frustration requires disciplined focus and clear guidelines and outcomes. Learning from online resources can help students develop skills in analytic thinking, decision-making, and reflective judgment that are essential for selecting valid and reliable resources; these are difficult but essential competencies for EBP (evidence-based practice) (Hughes et al., 2020). The use of blogs has been cited as a method to increase communication among nursing students and a forum to share medical information (Wolf & Morouse, 2015).

The Quality and Safety Education for Nurses (QSEN) project, funded by the Robert Wood Johnson Foundation, identified graduate and undergraduate informatics competency (QSEN, 2022a). The National Organization of Nurse Practitioner Faculties' (NONPF) core competencies also include information technology and information literacy (NONPF, 2022). Nurses, nursing students, and nursing educators must stay abreast of the rapid changes related to nursing informatics and information technology.

Artificial Intelligence in Education.   There is a growing use of artificial intelligence (AI) technology in health care today, allowing for streamlining of patient care and automated tasks (Western Governors University, 2023). Integrating AI in nursing education has the potential to transform nursing education, but there are ethical concerns associated with students' use of AI for school assignments (Abdulai & Hung, 2023). ChatGPT is a commonly used AI-based chatbot that uses learning techniques to generate natural language text. There is a growing concern surrounding students' use of ChatGPT because this practice enables them to generate written assignments, research papers, and discussion boards without engaging in original research or thought (Abdulai & Hung, 2023). Nursing faculty are now having to learn to detect the use of this type of academic dishonesty.

Practice-Based Competency Outcomes

One trend that has a powerful influence on nursing education and practice at all levels is the emphasis on competency outcomes and criteria that establish realistic expectations for clinical practice (Nalini & Aruna, 2019). The National League for Nursing (NLN) has developed outcomes and competencies for graduates of nursing programs at all levels—licensed vocational nurse (LVN), associate degree in nursing (ADN) and diploma, bachelor of science in nursing (BSN), master of science in nursing (MSN), and practice and research doctorate programs (NLN, 2022a). In 2008, the AACN (2008a) released *The Essentials of Baccalaureate Education for Professional Nursing Practice*, which serves as a guiding framework to build and transform nursing curriculum. In 2021, these *Essentials*, for both entry-level and advanced-level nursing education, were updated by the AACN. Since 2005, nurse educator competencies have been developed, mirroring student competency evaluation. The NLN identified eight competencies: facilitate learning, facilitate learner development and socialization, use assessment and evaluation strategies, participate in curriculum design and evaluation of program outcomes, function as a change agent and leader, pursue continuous quality improvements in the nurse educator role, engage in scholarship, and function within the educational environment (NLN, 2022a). Similarly, the World Health Organization (WHO, 2016) published eight nurse educator competencies: theories and principles of adult learning; curriculum and implementation; nursing practice; research and evidence; communication, collaboration, and partnership; ethical/legal principles and professionalism; monitoring and evaluation; and management, leadership, and advocacy. Nurse educators must stay current and must have a set of competencies to guide peer evaluation and professional development.

The NONPF has developed one set of core competencies for all graduating nurse practitioners (NONPF, 2022). Competency outcomes, with related criteria (critical elements), specify expected results, which are the measurable results of time and effort spent in learning. The ability to implement realistic practice-based abilities competently, therefore, is the essential outcome; competence is the target and the purpose of education.

The outcomes approach requires a mental shift from trying to memorize voluminous readings and class notes (resulting in frustration and the attitude of "Just tell me what I need to know") to actually learning to think like a nurse, to integrate information in problem-solving and decision-making, and to provide competent patient care (Billings & Halstead, 2019). Typical

objectives begin with words like *describe, discuss, list,* and *recognize*; they are directions for learning, not what nurses do. Outcomes convert the meaning of the content objectives to actions that nurses actually perform, such as implement, integrate, plan, and conduct. Accrediting and certifying organizations must mandate demonstrated mastery of skills, managerial competencies, and professional development at all levels (IOM, 2012; NONPF, 2022).

In response to the Institute of Medicine report (IOM) *To Err is Human: Building a Safer Health System* (IOM, 2000), the Robert Wood Johnson Foundation funded the national initiative, QSEN, as already mentioned, to help nursing programs reorganize curricula to focus on patient safety and quality care (QSEN, 2022a). The QSEN (2022b, 2022c) competencies at both the prelicensure and graduate levels assess the knowledge, skills, and attitudes of nurses within six areas: patient-centered care, teamwork and collaboration, EBP, quality improvement, safety, and informatics.

Performance-Based Learning and Assessment

Trends related to learning and evaluation methods are changing fundamentally, owing in part to changing technology and the greater focus on patient safety. The emphasis on competency outcomes and criteria for acceptable practice has prompted leaders in nursing education to promote innovative programs and learning methods (IOM, 2012) as well as more interactivity and engagement interspersed with lectures. Passively listening, reading, and passing written tests do not necessarily promote competence in the core performance skills expected in practice. Increased emphasis on critical thinking and learning to integrate principles is more effective than trying to remember "all the content," which often leads students to merely want to pass the test. Competency-based learning creates an atmosphere that is focused on learning concepts and encourages collaboration between teacher and learner to achieve actual practice competencies (Hodges et al., 2019).

Practice-based competence uses terms like *interactive learning, collaborative learning, experiential learning*, and *competency-based learning*. This trend requires changes in the roles of teachers and students. The teacher is less a "lecturer" and more a facilitator and coach, providing direction for learning stated outcomes; the student is more actively accountable and responsible for achieving competence in designated knowledge and practice skills.

In this new paradigm, instructors focus on the most essential content; create practice-based case studies and simulations; and set the stage for students to engage in problem-solving, critical thinking, and integration of concepts, knowledge, and evidence-based practice (Hodges et al., 2019). Nursing faculty provide feedback and validation that cannot be gained through books or the Internet. Memorization of basic facts is still important but is insufficient when nursing practice emphasizes such skills as assessment, critical thinking, communication, patient teaching, and caring and advocating for patients. The focus on practice competence helps students learn how to access and integrate everchanging information as required in actual practice, rather than trying to remember all the content.

The movement toward total adoption of competency-based nursing education is slow in part because of students' criticism that this model is expensive and requires active independent learning and faculty reports of increased workload and lack of metacognitive learning and critical thinking. Many colleges and universities have adopted a hybrid model of traditional teaching and learning pedagogies with some competency-based evaluations (Gravina, 2017).

A trend in many nursing programs is the development and incorporation of EBP courses, in addition to traditional nursing research courses. Learning about EBP includes evaluation and translation of evidence into practice. The Academic Center for Evidence-Based Practice (STAR Model | School of Nursing [uthscsa.edu]) at the University of Texas San Antonio, which was developed as a center for excellence, provides up-to-date information about evidence-based practice. In 1997, the Agency for Healthcare Research and Quality (AHRQ, 2023) developed an evidence-based practice center program.

Simulation, in various forms, is another major performance-based learning strategy. Shadow Health and vSim are technologies that use digital patient simulation to teach critical thinking. Shadow Health offers Digital Clinical Experiences such as concept labs, immersive tutorials that illustrate complex nursing subjects. Concept labs include examples of real body sounds and realistic, three-dimensional anatomic body models to compare and contrast normal and abnormal findings. The interactive interfaces of these concept labs can be used to explore body systems at an in-depth level. These experiences make classroom concepts come to life.

Designed to simulate real nursing scenarios, simulations allow students to interact with patients in a safe, realistic environment anytime, anywhere. This technology enables students to develop clinical reasoning skills, competence, and confidence in nursing. Mannequins have become more essential and incorporate sophisticated computerization to promote more realistic learning and critical thinking (Unver et al., 2018). Another form of simulation is the use of standardized patients and telemedicine technology to achieve outcomes. The use of standardized patients has the ability to bring emotions to the simulation (Farra et al., 2017). A systematic review found the objective structured clinical examinations (OSCEs) to be the most valid assessment measurement in use (Kozato et al., 2020). The use of standardized patients as a competency-based summative assessment allows faculty to assess mastery of entry-level clinical skills, some of which the student may not have access to in the clinical setting. Interprofessional simulation-based education has also been incorporated into nursing programs with favorable results in terms of student perceptions (Lee et al., 2020).

Other interactive learning strategies include portfolio learning (Mohajer et al., 2023), problem-based learning, and peer learning activities (Putri & Sumartini, 2021). Interactive strategies are even more important when the location of clinical learning is considered. More and more diverse settings are used because these are places where nurses' expertise is needed. In addition to hospitals and extended-care facilities, clinical learning often takes place in alternative settings, such as nurse-run clinics in schools, daycare and senior centers, and prisons. Over the past decade, service-learning projects have also helped students learn actual practice skills throughout the community. Another form is faith-based learning projects that put nurses in churches and congregations. Many interactive clinical-related learning strategies and more traditional clinical assignments increasingly engage practicing nurses as preceptors.

The change to competency outcomes and practice-based learning requires changes in evaluation methods that focus on valid, actual performance of required competencies in realistic scenarios; paper-and-pencil tests and inconsistent subjective clinical observations by instructors or preceptors are not adequate. Structured, objective validation of competence requires performance examinations that specify the core skills and related critical elements (the application of mandatory principles) that must be met according to established practice standards. In addition to performance of nursing skills, structured portfolios are used to document other competencies (Cope & Murray, 2018).

Needless to say, a more interactive approach in clinical and classroom courses is difficult for some students and creates issues; faculty and students have to change traditional habits and expectations of each other. Sometimes students think it is easier just to "figure out what the teacher wants" and "study for the test" rather than engage in learning to think and integrate best practices through teacher-assisted interactive exercises. Such exercises, however, help students learn to make effective decisions, to collaborate in the group process, and to manage time and resources. It may cause some anxiety, but performance examinations that require 100% accuracy of the mandatory critical elements (principles) provide more reliable evidence of practice competencies.

Sociodemographics, Cultural Diversity, and Economic and Political Changes

From rural to metropolitan areas throughout the United States, the population is undergoing significant changes in sociodemographic, cultural, and economic composition. These trends generate serious issues and consequences for education, health care, and many aspects of the socioeconomic–political systems. The following brief overview is a framework for learning how these trends and issues affect nursing education and practice.

- People are living longer, and the number of the very elderly is increasing more rapidly than other age groups. This means more people live with chronic disease and disability; many live in institutions, substandard conditions, or alone. All are subject to growing needs for health care and assistance. As a result, nursing and other provider programs have increased geriatric content and clinical experiences; geriatric patients require very different care from younger populations. The National Hartford Center of Gerontological Nursing Excellence is a collaboration of national and international nursing schools and institutions that have demonstrated the highest level of commitment to the field of gerontological nursing. Their mission is to enhance and sustain the capacity and competency of nurses to provide quality care to older adults (https://www.nhcgne.org/). The Center provides a repository of resources, funding opportunities, news, and updates about the care of older adults.
- The current political debate about health care reform is concerned about all age groups, and regardless of the outcome, nursing will continue to focus on quality care and competent practice (Bauer & Bodenheimer, 2017).
- The minority segment of the US population is growing rapidly and expected to be majority–minority by 2044 (Gest, 2022). The number of diverse ethnic minorities and illegal immigrants is expanding throughout the United States, with multiple socioeconomic consequences. The diversity often is unwanted and leads to disrespect, intolerance, conflicts, abuse, and violence. Increasingly, health care providers need to learn about different cultural values and health practices and to integrate them into care to the extent possible. Educators need to incorporate and teach tolerance and understanding of cultural diversity, as well as positive health practices. Preparing future generations of nurses to practice cultural humility is essential for improving outcomes for students, patients, and clinicians (Hughes et al., 2020). The AACN (2008b) developed end-of-program competencies for graduates of baccalaureate nursing programs for integrating cultural competencies into undergraduate education. The AACN's *The Essentials: Core Competencies for Professional Nursing Education* (2021a) mandates the inclusion of culturally diverse nursing care concepts in the curriculum.

Professional ethics requires that health care providers separate their personal values and beliefs from their professional responsibilities, even to those whose beliefs are different (Chapters 9). The number of families that become uninsured, jobless, or homeless and that survive in poverty is increasing. The economic crisis during the first decade of the 21st century has resulted in fewer financial resources for health care and ordinary expenses, and thus more people eat unhealthy diets, go without medicines or treatments, and obtain care in emergency departments. More than half of family bankruptcies are due to overwhelming health-care debt (Himmelstein et al., 2018). Jackson and Vaughn (2017) describe the incredibly difficult circle of hunger, illness, theft, and incarcerations that poor people experience in the United States.

- Domestic abuse of women and children and various forms of violence are increasing in homes, schools, and public places (The Advocates for Human Rights, 2018). The incidence of violence has increased even in nursing schools and in hospitals, including vertical abuse among nurses (ANA, 2021).

- Substance abuse, long a pervasive problem in society, has become a serious problem for college students and young adults (Patrick et al., 2022). *The CBHSQ Report*, published by the Center for Behavioral Health Statistics and Quality of the Substance Abuse and Mental Health Services Administration (Lipari & Jean-Francois, 2016), provides sobering statistics about the high rates of substance use in persons of 18 to 22 years of age. Substance use disorders have consequences for the safety and health of nurses, patients, and others; the increase in stress and anxiety often triggers violence and mental health and economic problems. The opioid epidemic in the United States affects more than 10 million Americans and leads to more than 136 deaths a day (National Center for Drug Abuse Statistics, 2023).

- In 2021, suicide was the ninth-leading cause of death in all age groups and the second-leading cause of death in persons of 10 to 34 years of age (Centers for Disease Control and Prevention [CDC], 2023a). Persons who are discharged from behavioral health facilities are at 200 times greater risk of suicide (Krause et al., 2020). Nurses are frontline providers who can screen and provide care to high-risk populations, contributing to the Zero Suicide Initiative (Education Development Center, 2023).

- The United States is experiencing an epidemic of obesity, with major consequences for health and the health care system. Obesity leads to the most prevalent health problems that strain health care facilities and financial resources. It is paramount for health care providers to teach prevention of obesity and its consequences in schools. Learning to help people change their dietary habits is a major role for nurses and other health care workers (Western Governors University, 2018).

- The traditional definition of family has changed, as evident in the number of single individuals living with other singles, single-parent households, and same-sex couples (with and without children). These nontraditional families often have limited finances and lack access to nursing and health care. They also may be resented by those with more traditional values and attitudes. Nurses must learn to respect and provide essential care regardless of differences.

- Disrespect for others, abuse of noisy mobile devices in public, and disregard for common courtesy have changed the nature of social interactions. Nursing students who use class time to send digital messages, use cell phones, or search the Internet are disrespectful of those who want to learn and the teacher who is trying to help them learn. This behavior is part of the larger trend of declining civility and integrity, with increased cheating and falsification in school and work (Ackerman-Barger et al., 2020). Such incidents trigger anger and retaliation when excessive. In health care facilities, abuse of patients is also increasing. Nurses often need to mediate health care–related situations, and effective communication skills are essential (Chapter 19). Crisis Prevention Institute offers training programs, which teach crisis prevention and verbal de-escalation skills for health care workers (2023).

- As suggested, an important part of nursing education involves trends in society and the issues that result. Nurses work with people in all aspects of society, and thus, course content and interactive practice–based learning that incorporate these issues are essential. One of the most significant issues for students is learning to distinguish the meaningful differences in beliefs, values, and expectations among patients and their responses to illness, treatments, and caregivers. This is why nursing programs include, and students need to learn from, the areas of study that support effective nursing care, such as sociology, cultural diversity, psychology, ethics, religion, economics, history, and literature. Learning the experiences of diverse peoples, including patients and coworkers, their customs, beliefs, health practices, and expectations, not only is interesting but also expands human understanding, tolerance, compassion, and the creativity essential for effective professional practice (Southern Poverty Law Center, 2020).

Community-Focused Interprofessional Approaches

The societal trends described here, along with the large-scale economic and political influences to reduce health care costs, may indirectly promote prevention and interprofessional initiatives. Many lay and professional health-conscious groups are working to change the national orientation from "illness care" to more efficient and effective "health care." Another contributing factor is the growing emphasis on health of the family as a whole and on entire communities and populations. *Healthy People 2030* has expanded on *Healthy People 2020*, with the current mission cited to identify health care initiatives, increase awareness of health, identify measurable objectives and outcomes, improve practice through evidence, and identify research, evaluation, and data collection methods (CDC, 2020b).

The changes in the health care landscape with a focus on preventive care and community care require a different philosophy of care and competencies that emphasize interprofessional and interagency collaboration (World Health Professions Alliance, 2023). The rapidly changing and expanding health-care culture incorporates concepts of shared responsibility for health prevention and promotion among individuals, family, community, and multiple care providers. Nursing education is influenced by these trends to promote family and community health and healthy lifestyles as well as increased interprofessional learning and collaboration (Romero-Collado et al., 2020).

In response to the paradigm shift to interprofessional care and the provision of care following the IOM's six aims for improvement—safe, effective, patient centered, timely, efficient, and equitable (IOM, 2001)—AACN developed core competencies for interprofessional collaborative practice. Interprofessional Education Collaborative (IPEC) updated these competencies in 2016 and in 2023. According to the AACN (2011) report, change is needed in the way health care professionals are trained, increasing didactic and clinical interprofessional collaboration. The four competency domains identified are values/ethics for professional practice, roles/responsibilities, interprofessional communication, and teams and teamwork (IPEC, 2023). Although interprofessional educational experiences are encouraged for all health care disciplines, Lucas et al. (2020) cite the importance of preparation of students for interprofessional educational experiences and the need for regular meetings when students are engaged in learning as members of a health care team.

Global Health

With extensive global travel and commerce, the health community now encompasses the world. Illness can arrive on any airplane, ship, or bus and spread throughout the country. Examples include the H1N1 "swine flu" and the coronavirus disease (COVID-19) pandemics, which have spread to every continent and continue to cause illness and deaths. COVID-19 has impacted more than 769 million people, causing nearly 7 million deaths, worldwide (WHO, 2023). Nurses are on the frontline of care and defense and have raised concerns about sufficient protection. Similarly, other infections, such as reemerging strains of tuberculosis and methicillin-resistant *Staphylococcus aureus* (MRSA), spread rapidly and are resistant to treatment; nurses and other providers need to become even more diligent in preventing the spread of organisms (CDC, 2019). With the identification of Ebola hemorrhagic fever in the United States among missionary health care providers, the Centers for Disease Control and Prevention (CDC) has reevaluated and updated the recommendations for health care providers working with patients who have symptoms of Ebola (CDC, 2023b), with nurses often at the frontline of care. Concerning the ongoing, growing COVID-19 pandemic, the CDC is continually updating information for health care providers treating patients with the virus (2023c). As new knowledge about the prevention, detection, and treatment of this novel disease is discovered, frequent updates are communicated regarding home isolation and testing recommendations (CDC, 2023c).

Consistent with the trend toward global health, nurses are engaged in the global health community through collaborative networks, research projects, and shared publications. Programs incorporate global content, and students learn to participate in international health research projects and communication through the Internet and have direct learning experiences in countries abroad (Kierkx et al., 2017).

The International Council of Nurses (ICN) provides many opportunities for students to network and learn from each other; its periodic international conferences are a major resource for students and nurses to promote world health (ICN, 2019, 2023).

These trends challenge students to prepare for a wide spectrum of nursing practice that depends on competencies such as clinical decision-making, communication, collaboration, and leadership (Marshall & Finlayson, 2018). Students need to learn how to manage illness and preventive health care for diverse clients dispersed throughout the community as well as to provide critical care to hospital patients who are sicker and go home sooner. Although very helpful, learning in diverse settings throughout the community presents some issues. For example, dispersed clinical learning requires more planning, travel, expense, and time; learning time is much shorter at each location; community-based group projects take more time; and students have less time with instructors because faculty can be at only one location at a time. In many settings, however, students work only with preceptors or staff who help them gain the competence and confidence they need but who also have other responsibilities. In addition, as students and health care leaders, nurses need to effectively communicate with other health care disciplines and to have a good understanding of their role and scope of practice to practice at the highest level of their degree and licensure.

Patient-Centered Care: Engagement, Safety, and Privacy

As patients have become more knowledgeable about illness care, health promotion, and the consequences of errors in care, they have become more assertive about their right to competent care and privacy of information. HIPAA mandates protection of an individual's privacy by health care providers and throughout society and has changed many previously careless and harmful practices. The economics and politics of health care and access to comprehensive information via the Internet have promoted more consumer activism through advocacy groups and Internet connections to influence health care policy and standards. Patients use Internet resources, sponsored by the government and private entities, to become more informed about illness and health care. As informed and engaged patients, they are better able to make effective decisions in collaboration with health care providers. This development makes critical thinking, communication, and teaching essential nursing competencies. It also means that student nurses need to change their approach from "giving patient care" to "working with the patient and family" as members of the health care team.

Another major issue affecting nursing education is the increasing number and consequences of serious medical errors, as reported in the IOM study *To Err is Human: Building a Safer Health System* (2000). These errors have led to an astonishing number of deaths and an increased number of expensive lawsuits, which further raise the cost of health care and tarnish the belief in the quality of available health care. Nursing faculty, administrators, and regulators therefore are increasingly concerned with ensuring the competence of students and nurses (Ignatavius, 2021). Medical-error issues have precipitated increased requirements for competency-based education and performance assessment in schools of nursing and other health disciplines, in annual employment evaluations, and in agency accreditation criteria, all for patient safety.

Many injuries and deaths in medical institutions are preventable, and Medicare will no longer pay for such preventable incidents, many of which are attributed to nurses. Thus, preventive care is being emphasized even more in nursing education. QSEN, Interprofessional Collaboration, and similar initiatives in every specialty organization are designed to change nursing education and practice to promote competence and patient safety (IOM, 2003, 2015).

Disasters, Violence, and Terrorism

Nurses have always worked in situations emanating from disasters, abuse, and violence in families and communities, as well as in military conflicts. Domestic violence, especially against women and children, has increased as has violence in the workplace and schools. Greater violence has precipitated an increased emphasis in nursing education (Doran & van de Mortel, 2022; Hung et al., 2021) and in state regulations for reporting and responding to violent incidents. Criminal acts and substance abuse have become more common in hospitals, other health care agencies, and schools of nursing, threatening the safety of patients and staff. As a consequence, criminal background checks are required for all students (and employees) by education programs as well as by agencies providing clinical experiences to students. Population expansion, especially in urban areas, and mass disasters, such as hurricanes, floods, and earthquakes, have precipitated the need for more nurses to become prepared to function effectively along with other first responders. Adelman and Legg (2009) describe details of preparedness and opportunities for nurses who want to learn more. See Chapter 16 for more information on emergency preparedness.

Since the terrorist attacks on September 11, 2001, in New York City, Washington, DC, and Pennsylvania, more nurses (and all other health care personnel and first responders) are more prepared to respond to acts of terrorism and disaster. Many nursing programs have added courses or even entire programs of study for specialized preparation as first responders, emergency nursing, and flight nursing (Adelman & Legg, 2009). The ANA and the American Red Cross (2023) provide educational opportunities for nurses interested in disaster preparedness. The ANA Enterprise is committed to supporting nurses through disasters, such as the coronavirus pandemic, as evidenced by their COVID-19 Resource Center, which includes online education on this infectious disease (2023b). Not all nurses will become first responders, but all nurses and students should gain enough knowledge to know their limitations, who and how to notify, and how they could work with more qualified responders. Chapter 15 provides more information about disaster preparedness for nurses.

Ethics and Bioethical Concerns

Another trend affecting nursing education is related to the multicultural, multiethnic population and patients who have different ways of responding to illness, treatment, and care providers. This development raises ethical issues as to who "is right" and who "has the right to decide." As described, one difficult issue, particularly for students and novices, is the ethical necessity to differentiate personal beliefs, values, and preferences from professional practice responsibilities. Many ethical dilemmas require students, nurses, and other providers to accept the values of others and the concept of "a gray continuum of values" instead of the black-and-white interpretations based on one's own beliefs. Some of the most controversial issues relate to the right of individual choice regarding abortion, organ transplant, stem cell research, preference in sexual partners, and the patient's right to a dignified death. Other issues emerge from the growing use of alternative health remedies outside the mainstream of traditional Western medicine, such as herbs, acupuncture, and therapeutic use of cannabis (Chapter 11).

Dishonesty among nursing students, nurses, and other professionals is increasing alarmingly and threatens patient safety. The ANA's *Code of Ethics for Nurses with Interpretive Statements* (2015) provides a succinct statement of the ethical obligations and duties of every individual who enters the nursing profession. The code of ethics for nursing has nine provisions that outline the "ethical values, obligations, duties, and professional ideals of nurses individually and collectively."

They are a nonnegotiable ethic standard as well as an "expression of nursing's own understanding of its commitment to society" (ANA, 2015). Nurses are the largest health care workforce and, for the last 21 years in a row, have been identified as having the most trusted profession, with the highest level of honesty and ethics (Brenan, 2023).

Chapter 9 presents a comprehensive discussion about ethics in health care and important issues students should be knowledgeable about for competent nursing practice.

Shortage of Nurses and Faculty

The nursing workforce shortage has challenges: aging of Baby Boomers, shortage and uneven distribution of physicians, accelerated rate of nurse retirements, and uncertainty of health care reform (Buerhaus et al., 2017). Buerhaus and Auerbach (2011) observed that during the 2008 recession, nurses older than 50 years reentered the hospital workforce. These writers assert that when this older hospital workforce retires, a hospital nursing shortage will reemerge. The nursing workforce is more than 90% female, 80% White, more than 70% prepared at the baccalaureate level or higher, 57% are employed in a hospital, and 50% are at least 50 years of age (AACN, 2023a: Smiley et al., 2023). The nursing workforce does not mirror the US population seeking care, in gender, ethnicity, or age. According to Buerhaus and Auerbach (2011), one area the RN workforce has advanced is in the percentage who have baccalaureate degrees, which now exceeds that of those with associate degrees. The percentage of those who enter BSN programs is up, but not enough to meet the workforce demands (AACN, 2023b).

Students are assigned to multiple and diverse community clinical settings, some of which may be short-staffed, making it difficult for them to find qualified preceptors. Staff nurses who act as clinical instructors or preceptors may or may not be prepared for these roles or have received adequate orientation. Students, therefore, need to learn to take more individual responsibility and initiative to gain essential core competencies. Online learning environments can be simulated to mimic real-world situations that allow for faculty to evaluate student learning from a distance. New methods are created in partnership with agencies to promote more effective clinical learning opportunities for students without overburdening staff.

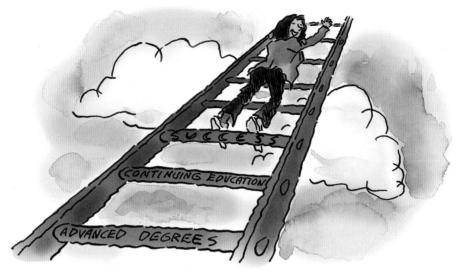

Education is the ladder to success.

Often, the causative trends related to a shortage of faculty include a limited number of nurses prepared at advanced levels, space limitations, and other administrative constraints. For example, AACN's 2022–2023 data report reveals that 66,261 qualified nursing applicants were denied admission to BSN programs in 2022 because of faculty shortages, lack of clinical sites, and limited classroom space (AACN, 2023b). According to a Special Survey on Vacant Faculty Positions released by AACN in October 2022, 2166 faculty vacancies were identified in a survey of 909 nursing schools with baccalaureate and/or graduate programs across the country (84.4% response rate) (AACN et al., 2023). In addition to the vacancies, schools acknowledged the need to create 128 new faculty positions to accommodate student demand. The data show a national nurse faculty vacancy rate of 8.8%. Most of the vacancies (84.9%) were faculty positions requiring or preferring a doctoral degree (AACN, 2022). According to AACN's 2021–2022 report on Salaries of Instructional and Administrative Nursing Faculty, the average ages of doctorally prepared nurse faculty holding the ranks of professor, associate professor, and assistant professor were 62.5, 56.7, and 50.96 years, respectively; the average ages of master's degree-prepared nurse faculty holding the ranks of professor, associate professor, and assistant professor were 55, 54.7, and 48.6 years, respectively (AACN, 2022). Some schools are expanding enrollments by using more part-time, adjunct, and clinical

faculty and by expanding the use of online courses and simulation. Moreover, the number of students in MSN or doctoral programs is not adequate to meet current needs. Nurse leaders and organizations are working vigorously with state and national governments and private entities to reverse these trends by seeking more funding and promoting recruitment and development efforts nationally (AACN, 2022).

The nursing shortage and lack of nursing faculty present many hardships for students, faculty, and nurses; however, difficult situations promote creative and innovative initiatives and solutions. For example, many organizations and associations have initiated collaborative partnerships to improve education in all types and levels of nursing education. The NLN has implemented initiatives to improve nursing education and faculty development (see AACN and NLN websites for position statements regarding innovations and transitions in nursing education).

Increasing Professional and Personal Responsibilities

Given the complexity of health-care delivery and the need for health care team members to work as an interprofessional team, another trend with multiple issues has become evident. In the current health care environment, students, teachers, and nurses confront increasing life responsibilities and associated stressful demands on time and resources. Many cope simultaneously with the expansion of information and technology; changing health care systems; more interactive and out-of-class methods of learning; multiple care settings; higher expectations for competence; shortage of nurse preceptors and teachers; and multiple cultural, ethical, and legal aspects of an ever-changing society. Many also are responsible for the care of dependent children and aging parents.

At the same time, contemporary conditions require nurses to keep current through planned, ongoing professional development. Complexities in practice, emphasis on reducing errors, and growing consumer activism increase the need for nurses to document continuing competence for initial licensure, relicensure, and recertification. Changes in state and multistate regulations increasingly focus on the need for initial and continuing competence (IOM, 2009). Current uniform licensure requirements facilitate nurses practicing in bordering states through the RN compact. As of 2023, 41 states are part of the licensure compact, which allows nurses to practice in other nurse licensure compact (NLC) states without the need to obtain an additional license (NCSBN, 2023a). The APRN Compact, which was adopted on August 12, 2020, allows advanced practice registered nurses to hold a multistate license giving them privileges to practice in compact states (NCSBN, 2023b). See Chapter 4 for more information on nursing licensure. The high stress levels associated with these professional and personal demands have consequences for nurses' own health and that of those around them. It is important for everyone involved in the educational process to be more caring, understanding, respectful, and helpful to one another. Teachers, students, administrators, staff nurses, employers, family, and friends need to learn anew the meaning of "a caring community" in the context of rapid and complex change.

These trends in society, nursing, and academic programs present the problem of how to incorporate this additional knowledge into the already overloaded program of study. The issues for students include knowing how to access and use unlimited information, prioritize learning, implement evidence-based practice, deal with ethical dilemmas professionally, and develop competencies required for effective responses to contemporary issues. Above all, students must focus on learning to think critically, reflectively, ethically, and compassionately, which are essential professional skills (IOM, 2011).

HOLISTIC ADMISSIONS REVIEW

Many nursing programs have utilized a holistic admission process to enroll a diverse group of students with the background, qualities, and skills required for success in the profession. Holistic review is an admissions strategy that considers an applicant's unique experiences in addition to traditional academic measures, such as test scores and grade point averages. It is designed to help universities view the whole person and consider a broad range of factors reflecting the applicant's academic readiness, contribution to the incoming class, and potential for success both in school and later as a professional. Holistic review, when used in conjunction with other mission-based practices, is considered a "holistic admission" process (AACN, 2023c).

DIVERSITY IN NURSING EDUCATION PROGRAMS

A brief review of the major types of education programs that prepare nurses for licensure and advanced practice sets the stage for summarizing some contemporary trends related to flexible, online, and other distance delivery methods in nursing education. A brief description of the types of programs is provided in Table 3.2.

Licensed Practical or Vocational Nurse Programs

Practical nurse (PN) or vocational nurse (VN) programs provide the shortest and most restricted option for individuals seeking a nursing license. The total number of PN licenses in the United States is 967,373, with more licenses in the Midwest, South, and Northeast regions of the country (NCSBN, 2023c). Licensed practical nurse (LPN) programs, named licensed vocational nurses (LVN) in California and Texas, usually are 9 to 12 months in length and may be offered by high school adult education programs, community colleges, vocational and proprietary schools, and hospitals. The median earnings for LPN/VNs increased from $44,000 to 50,000 between 2020 and 2022 (NCSBN, 2024).

Regardless of the increasing complexity of patient care, many individuals choose to begin a career in nursing as LPNs/LVNs. The NLN's position statement supports the role and LPN/LVN workforce, citing that this level of provider is critical to health care redesign

TABLE 3.2 Types of Nursing Education Programs

Types of Program and Credential	Type of Institution	Length of Program	Purpose and Scope
Practical (LPN) or vocational (LVN) nurse program: prepares for LVN or LPN license	High school, hospitals, vocational–technical schools; some colleges	9 to 12 months	Basic technical bedside care; hospitals, nursing homes, home care, offices in LPN positions
Diploma program: prepares for registered nurse (RN) license	Hospitals, some in conjunction with colleges	2 to 3 years	Basic RN positions; hospitals and agency care
Associate degree in nursing (ADN): prepares for RN license	Community and junior colleges	2 years; some are 1-year bridge programs for LPN/LVN graduates	Basic technical care in RN positions, primarily in institutions
Bachelor's degree in nursing (BSN): prepares for RN license	Colleges and universities	2 to 4 years (depends on type of option); some are 1- to 2-year mobility options for graduates of PN or ADN programs or accelerated options for second-degree students	Basic professional practice as RN; management, community, and public health settings; prepares for graduate school and certification; basic programs are 4 years; mobility options may be only 2 years
Master's degree in nursing (MSN)	Universities	1 to 2 years beyond BSN degree; some offer fast-track options	Advanced clinical practice, management, education, leadership positions
Doctoral degree in nursing	Universities	Varies: Doctor of Philosophy (in Nursing) (PhD), DSN, Doctor of Nursing Practice (DNP), Doctor of Nursing Science (DNSc)	Advanced nursing for research, clinical practice, education, and leadership positions

(NLN, 2014a). LPN/LVN nurses provide safe, quality, and cost-effective care (NLN, 2014a). Once licensed, many graduates continue their education in mobility programs to become RNs. Many use "1 plus 1" type of programs to earn an associate degree; others use the multiple entry–exit programs (MEEPs). For example, a MEEP is a program that allows students to enter with an ADN to obtain an MSN, or a student with a bachelor's degree to enter and obtain a master of science in nursing or an MSN. Some BSN programs accept LPN graduates on the basis of outcomes of written and performance examinations for advanced placement.

Hospital Diploma Programs

The oldest, most traditional type of program that prepares for RN licensure is the hospital-based diploma program. These programs initially were developed in the United States in the late 1800s in general hospitals in cities such as Boston, New York, Hartford, and Philadelphia and subsequently spread across the country. They followed the Nightingale model and began as training programs taught by physicians, usually only several weeks in length. In time, nurse graduates began developing and teaching courses from the nursing perspective and subsequently obtained additional education as educators and administrators. Ultimately, the length of programs was extended, and by the mid-1900s, most programs were 3 years long and had fairly uniform courses of study and clinical hours.

As the number of hospitals grew, the need for nurses likewise increased, and essentially, every hospital developed its own training program as its main source for nursing staff. At their peak from 1950 to 1960, more than 1300 diploma programs were operational. By 2014, only 67 diploma schools remained (NLN, 2014b). Diploma programs now are more similar to associate degree programs, typically 2 years in length; many have arrangements with colleges so that students can simultaneously earn an associate or baccalaureate degree. The AACN report prelicensure nursing programs at the diploma level to account for fewer than 10% of all basic RN programs, citing the transition from hospital instruction to college or university instruction (AACN, 2020; NLN, 2014b).

Associate Degree Programs

In the late 1950s, a very different trend in nursing education emerged in response to social, political, and educational changes in society and to a growing shortage of RNs. During World War II, the need for RNs who were prepared more quickly than in diploma programs became critical; the 2-year Cadet Nurse Corps was developed and proved to be very successful. From this experience, some educators realized that nurses and others could be prepared in less time and still meet RN licensure and practice requirements. After the war, Congress made funds available to publicly fund community colleges that offered 2-year associate degree programs in many technical fields. In addition, military benefits for college tuition allowed thousands of men and women to earn a 2-year college degree and fill jobs needed by burgeoning business and industry.

At the same time, the increasing complexity and expansion of medical care required more and better-prepared RNs. A few nurse educators created a new 2-year associate degree nursing program in community colleges, which required college courses in arts and sciences and a more integrated approach to nursing content and clinical learning. These pioneers reasoned that nursing belonged in a college setting, like other disciplines, to provide a better education for nurses and to establish more respect and recognition for nursing's contribution to the community's health. As the number of community colleges grew and the need for nurses increased, ADN programs became a logical program for development and expansion.

ADN education is a vivid example of how changes in society influence the evolution of nursing education; it was another significant "first" in nursing and an important part of the evolving professionalization of nursing as a discipline. For the first time, it was possible for all RNs to be educated in college settings and obtain college degrees.

In 2014, approximately 710 ADN programs were operational, a decrease of 338 programs since 2002

(NLN, 2014b). The majority of the ADN programs are found in the Midwestern and Southern regions of the United States (ADN Programs, 2023; NLN, 2014b). Of the qualified applicants to ADN programs, 35% are rejected due to difficulty with clinical placements (NLN, 2020). The trend of acceptance and growth of ADN programs, along with the slow increase in 4-year BSN programs and progressive mobility options, established the educational framework for current nursing education.

Baccalaureate Degree Nursing Programs

In 1924, Yale University offered the first separate department of nursing, whose graduates earned the baccalaureate degree. The 28-month program required scientific studies and clinical work and had the prestige and authority of other departments, with its own dean and budget (Kalisch & Kalisch, 1995).

Generic BSN programs typically require 2 years of arts and sciences followed by 2 years of nursing courses. Currently, 747 RN to BSN programs are available nationwide, including more than 650 programs that are offered at least partially online. Program length varies from 1 to 2 years, depending upon the school's requirements, the program type, and the student's previous academic achievement (AACN, 2023d). The demographic of the degree-seeking student in this program, according to AACN, is "motivated, older, and has higher academic expectations than traditional entry-level students" (2019). As in other programs, BSN courses focus on the care of patients with medical, surgical, pediatric, obstetric, and psychiatric conditions, although course sequencing and names differ considerably from school to school. BSN programs focus more emphasis on the family and community and health promotion and illness prevention; a large part of clinical experience is in diverse community settings. These programs also require courses such as research, management, leadership, and statistics.

For the BSN programs in the United States, the most common reason cited for denying an applicant is due to lack of clinical placement sites (45%), followed by a shortage of faculty (23%). Enrollment in BSN programs totaled 77,958 in 2001, contrasted with the 2022 BSN program enrollment of 353,364 (AACN, 2023e). Graduates of BSN programs take the same NCLEX-RN licensure examination as diploma and ADN graduates. Most specialty areas require the BSN degree for practice and as preparation for specialty certification. Admission into master's programs usually requires a BSN or other degree. Current NCLEX-RN data, as of December 2022, indicate the following first-time pass rates by education type: diploma 78.31% (2195), BSN 82.32% (98,942), and associate degree 77.91% (85,750) (NCSBN, 2022). The median salary for registered nurses was $77,600 (or $37.31 hourly) in 2021 (USBLS, 2022).

Master's Degree Nursing Programs

In the 1960s and 1970s, the number of BSN graduates increased; however, in response to the complexity of health care, so did the need for more qualified clinicians, educators, and administrators. The federal government responded with support for the development of MSN and BSN degree programs. Nurse leaders lobbied for and obtained federal funding for building construction and increased student tuition. Traineeship and fellowship grants were made available to thousands of RNs that enabled them to earn BSN and advanced degrees to meet these needs. Different MSN program options are available; the most typical are for BSN graduates, although an increasing number are designed for graduates of nonnursing degree programs, called accelerated or second-degree programs. Second-degree graduate nursing programs, in which graduates do not receive a BSN but are eligible to sit for the NCLEX-RN licensure examination, are growing in number. Students in these programs have been described as self-directed adult learners who pass the RN licensure examinations at high rates (Kaddoura et al., 2017).

Until the late 1960s, MSN programs primarily focused on preparing educators and administrators, but then the curriculum shifted to an overwhelming emphasis on clinical practice. By the 1990s, the negative and positive consequences of this decision became apparent, with more competent clinicians but fewer well-prepared educators and administrators. Most MSN programs are designed to prepare advanced nurse practitioners and clinical specialists in various specialty areas. The extraordinary and rapid changes in health care since the early 1990s highlighted the cost-effective and quality care benefits of using advanced practice nurses in primary health care and other specialty areas. With intensive and persistent legal activities, nurses won battles to change state laws to permit nurse practitioners to write prescriptions, receive reimbursement for care, and operate independent nurse practices and health centers.

As a result of this expanded scope of practice, an increasing number of nurses has obtained MSN degrees and advanced practice certification. Most specialty practice nurses, managers, administrators, and educators now are required to have master's or doctoral degrees. The AACN and NLN offer descriptions and numbers of different types of programs on their websites. Additionally, the consensus model for advanced practice registered nurse regulation, which included licensure, accreditation, certification, and education, was published in 2008 (AACN, 2008c). *Consensus Model for APRN regulation: Licensure, accreditation, certification and education* outlines four APRN roles—nurse anesthetist, nurse–midwife, clinical nurse specialist, and nurse practitioner—followed by six population foci. This document provides data to guide nursing licensure, accreditation of programs, certification, and educational programs.

Clinical Nurse Leader

In 2000, the national movement to enhance quality and safety in health care inspired discussions among the AACN, nurse executives, and other health care leaders that led to the development of a new nursing role—the clinical nurse leader (CNL). In July 2002, the AACN board created the Task Force on Education and Regulation (TFER 2). Its focus was the nurse competencies needed in current and future health care systems to improve patient care and what the "new nurse" role might look like. This work resulted in the publication of the *White Paper on the Role of the Clinical Nurse Leader (CNL)* in 2007 (NCSBN, 2016). The CNL is a master's-prepared generalist clinician, not an advanced practice nurse, who oversees the care coordination of a distinct group of patients, evaluates patient outcomes, and has the decision-making authority to change care plans when necessary. The CNL actively provides direct patient care in complex situations, serves as a lateral integrator who provides centralized care coordination for a distinct group of patients, and puts evidence-based care into practice to ensure that patients benefit from the latest innovations. A CNL is a leader in the health care delivery system, with expertise in quality improvement and cost-effective resource utilization (AACN, 2023f). The CNL is not an advanced practice nurse, nor is the CNL prepared in an area of clinical specialty; however, the CNL can consult with a clinical nurse specialist as needed; further, the CNL can provide evidence-based care to complex patients (AACN, 2023f). The Commission on Nurse Certification, an autonomous arm of the AACN, began certifying CNLs in 2007.

Doctoral Programs

Changes in society and health care have necessitated an increase in the educational preparation of nurse leaders. Both clinical and research leaders are charged with the development, implementation, and leadership of nursing doctoral programs. In 1934, New York University offered a PhD program for nurses. More than 30 years elapsed before doctoral programs *in nursing* (instead of *for nurses*) were offered (e.g., the doctor of nursing science degree [DNS or DNSc]).

For the past few decades, three types of doctoral degrees in nursing have been available: (1) the doctor of philosophy (PhD) for those interested in research; (2) the DNS or DNSc for those interested in advanced clinical nursing practice; and (3) the doctor of nursing (ND) for those with BS or higher degrees in nonnursing fields who want to pursue a career in nursing leadership. The ND degree, which prepared nurses for basic licensure (NCLEX-RN), was first offered at Case Western Reserve University in 1979. Shortly thereafter, Rush University, the University of Colorado Health Sciences Center, and others offered this degree. Nursing schools have transitioned to doctor of nursing practice or PhD programs.

Beginning in 2000, AACN leaders developed and implemented a new clinical-focused doctoral degree: the doctor of nursing practice (DNP) (AACN, 2023g). The DNP is conceived as preparation for contemporary advanced nurse practitioners; it is viewed as the clinical equivalent to the research-oriented PhD nursing degree. Although the DNP prepares clinicians and does not formally prepare nurse educators, many individuals who complete a DNP degree frequently shift from practice to a dual role and serve in faculty roles in addition to clinical roles. The AACN and NONPF have recommended that all advanced practice education programs move from the masters to the doctoral level by 2025. In 2023, the AACN reported that in the 974 schools that offer nursing degrees, the number of DNP programs increased from 156 in 2010 to 426 in 2023. The growth in programs is impressive, and this important trend is consistent with the NONPF statement that the entry into advanced practice nursing should be at the doctoral level.

Diversity, Equity, and Inclusion in Nursing Education

The AACN (2023h) strongly advocates for promoting diversity, equity, and inclusion (DEI) in nursing education. Their position statement on DEI sets three goals for academic nursing, which serve to: improve the quality of education; address inequities in health care; and enhance the civic readiness and potential of nursing students (AACN, 2021b).

DEI initiatives are key to providing equitable, patient-centered care to diverse populations. Nurses from minority backgrounds only represent 19.4% of the RN workforce, which does not reflect the more diverse patient population (AACN, 2023a). Increasing the diversity of the nursing workforce is believed to reduce health disparities, as minority nurses are more likely to work in underserved areas and provide health care to those experiencing health disparities (AACN, 2023a). Overall, diversity in the workforce will increase access to care for minority patients and be more equipped to care for a diverse patient population. One way nursing programs have increased diversity in their student enrollment is through the use of holistic admissions (AACN, 2023e). In spite of progress in this area, the nursing profession has been unable to recruit and retain a workforce that reflects the diversity of the patient population (Morrison et al., 2021).

In addition to the need to attract diverse nursing students, there is a similar need to recruit minority faculty. In 2021, only 19.2% of full-time nursing faculty members indicated they were from minority backgrounds, and only 7.4% were male (AACN, 2023a). Diversifying nursing faculty is associated with better educational experiences for students (AACN, 2020).

Scholarship and Funding for Nursing Education

Several organizations provide scholarships and grants for nursing education, and many of these opportunities are for minority students, with the goal of increasing the diversity of the nursing workforce. Health Resources and Services Administration (HRSA) provides scholarships to those willing to work in a Critical Shortage Facility or a health professional shortage area (HRSA, 2023a). HRSA (2023b) not only provides scholarships to nursing students, but also awards grants to schools; these funds help support nursing education. The NLN was the first national organization to fund nursing education research and offer scholarships for nursing education (NLN, 2022b).

Many hospitals also provide tuition reimbursement for nurses willing to sign a work agreement. This benefit serves to both attract and retain talented nurses. Additional state-funded opportunities for loan forgiveness are available for those seeking to become nurse educators and administrators within colleges and universities. Many of these graduate nursing loan forgiveness programs require the recipient to work for a specified period after completing their education (Tennessee Higher Education Commission & Student Assistance Corporation, 2023).

The military also awards undergraduate and graduate nursing scholarships for health care professionals willing to serve in the military upon graduation. The Air Force offers scholarships for nurse training and education, providing opportunities for graduate education (US Air Force, n.d.). The Army Nurse Corps Association (2023) and Navy Nurse Corps (2018) also award scholarships that pay for both undergraduate and graduate nursing education and training.

FLEXIBLE EDUCATION, MOBILITY, AND DISTANCE-LEARNING PROGRAMS

Various and nontraditional educational mobility programs now are commonplace. The AACN and NLN websites attest to the growing number of programs that offer some form of flexible, alternative program in addition to position statements on technology in nursing education, distance-learning, and online programs. Distance or mobility programs include those for LPN or LVN to ADN and BSN; diploma and ADN graduates to BSN and MSN; and BSN to MSN and doctoral programs. Almost all use some form of Internet-based courses, and some are entirely online. Some require periods of intensive on-campus classes or assigned clinical experiences with preceptors. Distance nursing education at all levels is another important trend to track.

The most controversial but pace-setting distance-learning program in nursing was developed under the New York Board of Regents as "the external degree program." Initially named the NY Regents External Degree Program (NYREDP), it later was renamed Excelsior College. Its ADN program, initiated in 1972, and the BSN program, in 1976, were fully accredited by the NLN shortly thereafter. This innovative college provides quality degree programs in many disciplines for adult learners underserved by traditional programs by using assessment methods to document prior learning and theory and performance examinations to validate current knowledge and competence. The nursing programs enroll thousands of students and are accessible regardless of geographic location; the students are primarily LPNs or RNs, some of whom also have other degrees or health-related certificates. Over the years, many nursing programs have accepted and modified the distance-learning and assessment approach originally developed by the NYREDP and continued as Excelsior College. The integration of electronic learning technology with assessment methods makes nursing degrees accessible to an increasing number of nurses seeking additional preparation.

Career ladder programs designed as "1 plus 1" or "2 plus 2" options, which allow students to acquire two degrees at the same time, have been offered for many years by some schools and through several statewide programs. Multiple mobility programs are available for LPNs to obtain an ADN degree. Fortunately, an increasing number of registered nurses are recognizing the need to advance their education, and many employers are providing funding and support to facilitate academic progression. To accommodate the growing demand, the number of RN to BSN programs has also increased dramatically over the last decade. There are approximately 800 RN to BSN programs available nationwide, including more than 650 programs that are offered at least partially online. Program length ranges from 1 to 2 years, depending on the school's requirements, the program type, and the student's previous academic achievement (AACN, 2023d).

Changes in social, political, financial, and philosophic trends; the extensive use of communication and learning technology; verified success from past experiences; and the continuing shortage of nurses have combined to make education mobility and distance-learning opportunities a necessity and a reality both nationally and internationally. Whereas the NLN continues to support all levels of education programs, the AACN and other organizations vigorously support the BSN for "entry into practice" and the professionalization of nursing (IOM, 2010).

In October 2010, the IOM released the report *The Future of Nursing: Leading Change, Advancing Health,* which provides a blueprint for transforming the nursing profession. A key message of this IOM report was that nurses should achieve higher levels of education and training through an improved education system that promotes seamless academic progression (IOM, 2011). A variety of innovative strategies that include online education and simulation have been developed to create a seamless pathway from ADN to BSN, ADN to MSN, and BSN to DNP and PhD. The National Academy of Medicine (formerly the IOM) recently published a new study to extend the vision of the Future of Nursing. The Committee on the Future of Nursing 2020–2030 was created to achieve the task of extending this vision with the goal of improving the overall health and well-being of the US population (National Academy of Medicine et al., 2021).

On December 18, 2017, New York passed legislation (S6768/A1842B) that requires future RN graduates of associate degree and diploma nursing programs to finish a baccalaureate completion program in nursing within 10 years after initial licensure in New York State. This legislation took effect immediately, and the requirement that nurses obtain a baccalaureate degree in nursing within 10 years of licensure became effective in June 2020, only 30 months after the legislation became law (ANA New York & New York Organization of Executives and Leaders, 2017).

The US Bureau of Labor Statistics estimated an average of 194,500 registered nurse job openings annually between 2020 and 2030, anticipating an employment growth rate of 9% for nurses. The need for new nurses is largely related to the aging workforce, with more than one-quarter of RNs stating their intent to retire over the next 5 years (ANA, 2023c; Smiley et al., 2023). The escalating nursing shortage and the aging of the current nursing workforce and nurse educators have prompted more schools to offer flexible mobility options and types of programs. Some target potentially underrepresented groups, such as men, minority groups, and those with existing academic degrees.

The most rapidly growing programs are the accelerated, fast-track, or second-degree programs, designed for nonnurses with other degrees. These are intended to try to meet the increased workforce need. In 2023, the AACN reported the availability of 321 accelerated BSN programs and 51 accelerated master's programs available at nursing schools nationwide. For a list of accelerated nursing programs, visit http://www.aacnnursing.org/Nursing-Education-Programs/Accelerated-Programs.

Trends and issues that influence nursing education make it even more important to comply with quality standards that emphasize competency outcomes. Educational trends include changes in number, diversity, and qualifications of students, and shortage of faculty and finances make it necessary to develop more efficient and effective learning strategies for on-campus and distant students. Although mobility and electronic options are more convenient, they present issues. In addition to learning to access multiple digital resources, students also need discipline and determination to pursue courses and clinical learning when a teacher is not physically present or accessible. Regardless of methods, they must achieve required competencies despite other responsibilities and learn to integrate critical thinking, reflective judgment, and evidence-based practices in patient care. In contrast to previous decades, organizations and schools now require more creative, responsive programs and expect more documented competence from students and faculty. Nursing organizations (Box 3.1) set the standards and innovation that assist in the evolution of nursing education at all levels. Although these trends pose challenges for nursing students, faculties, and employers, they move nursing toward more competent professional practice and improved patient safety.

◼ SUMMARY

To summarize the chapter let's review the questions posed at the beginning of the chapter and see what you have learned.
1. What are the major current trends in society and health care, and how do they influence nursing education and practice?
    This chapter describes 10 major trends and related issues in nursing education programs and offers an overview of multiple types of nursing programs. Current trends in society include changes in sociodemographic, cultural, and economic composition. Nursing education responds to sociodemographic changes (e.g., increase in the older adult population) by increasing geriatric content and clinical experiences in curricula. Due to a multicultural patient population with increased

BOX 3.1   Selected Organizations Relevant to Nursing Education: General Description and Purpose

American Academy of Nursing (AAN)—The organization of leaders in all facets of nursing: practice, education, administration, research, organizations, and government; the think tank of the profession; promotes advancement of all aspects of nursing; and publishes position papers, conference proceedings, and documents to advance nursing.

American Association of Colleges of Nursing (AACN)—The organization of deans and directors of baccalaureate and higher-degree nursing programs: establishes standards for programs concerned with legislative issues that pertain to professional nursing education and publishes the *Journal of Professional Nursing, The Essentials of Entry-Level and Advanced-Level Professional Nursing Education* (2021a), and other related documents pertaining to the BSN and higher-degree education.

American Nurses Association (ANA)—The major national nursing organization concerned with a broad scope of practice issues: standard of practice, scope of practice, ethics, legal, and employment issues; a federation of state nurses associations; and publications relate to an array of practice issues and standards.

Commission on Collegiate Nursing Education (CCNE)—A subsidiary of the AACN with responsibility for establishing and implementing standards and criteria and for accreditation of baccalaureate and graduate degree programs in nursing.

National Council of State Boards of Nursing (NCSBN)—The organization of all state boards: coordinates licensure activities on a national level; creates and administers licensure examinations (NCLEX); develops computerized licensure examinations; and works with other organizations to promote nursing standards and regulations and establish interstate licensure protocols.

National League for Nursing (NLN)—The national organization of nurse educators, with long-standing commitment to four types of basic programs (LPN, diploma, ADN, and BSN): includes lay citizens concerned with nursing and health care on its board; has councils for nursing informatics, research in nursing education, wellness centers, and multiple types of print publications; initiated a certification program and examination to certify excellence of nursing educators; and established the Centers for Excellence for nursing programs that meet designated standards.

NLN Accreditation Commission (NLNAC)—Formed in 1997, with responsibility for establishing and implementing standards and criteria and for accrediting all types of schools of nursing, is now the Accreditation Commission for Education in Nursing (ACEN).

National Organization of Nurse Practitioner Faculties (NONPF)—An organization of nurse practitioners in multiple specialties: sets national standards and criteria for programs and certification.

National Student Nurses Association (NSNA)—A national organization of statewide student nurse associations: concerned with education and career issues and provides student perspectives to other national nursing organizations.

ethnic diversity, contemporary education prepares students for culturally competent care, allowing them to care for diverse populations and respect cultural, ethnic differences, preferences, and customs. The increasing complexity of health care also has an impact on education and practice. As health care has become more complex, there is a resulting demand for a higher number of BSN graduates in practice, as well as a need for more qualified clinicians, educators, and administrators.

Changes in social, political, financial, and philosophic trends; the extensive use of communication and learning technology; verified success from past experiences; and the continuing shortage of nurses have also made education mobility and distance-learning opportunities a necessity. The trends have a significant influence on the content, learning process, and evaluation methods used in all types of programs and have influenced the development of new degrees and majors. Additionally, they have had a remarkable effect on the persistence of various types of programs for entry into practice and on the increasing acceptance of diverse mobility and distance-learning programs. Regardless of the type of program, most students now use the Internet to access courses, electronic databases, and other e-learning resources and integrate evidence-based practice and critical thinking. As students integrate current trends and attempt to resolve issues, they create the trends for the next generation and are participating in nursing history in the making. The most profound trend in nursing education is learning to learn, to reason, and to access relevant resources to solve problems.

Contemporary trends include a greater use of social media, informatics/technology, and use of AI. Nursing education and practice has had to incorporate these and apply ethics to the use of social media, informatics, and AI. Education has adapted to current trends by adopting competency-based education, interactive education, experiential learning, simulation, and interprofessional education in nursing curricula. These more contemporary forms of education better equip students to provide quality patient care in practice and prepare them to appropriately use technology and social media in practice.

2. What are the most compelling reasons that nurses require ongoing development and validation of competencies for licensure and continuing practice?

Nurses need ongoing development and validation of competencies for licensure due to changes in technology and standards for quality care practice. Contemporary conditions require nurses to keep current through continuing education and professional development. Complexities in practice, the need for reducing errors, and growing consumer activism increase the need for nurses to demonstrate competence for initial licensure, relicensure, and recertification. Due to changes in state regulations, there is an increased need to validate nurses' continuing competencies.

3. Which local, state, and national resources and Internet websites are available to learn about the trends and issues that influence nursing education?

Organizations relevant to nursing education include: American Academy of Nursing (AAN), American Association of Colleges of Nursing (AACN), American Nurses Association (ANA), Commision on Collegiate Nursing Education (CCNE), National Council of State Boards of Nursing (NCSBN), National League for Nurses (NLN), National Organization of Nurse Practitioner Faculties (NONPF), and National Student Nurses Association (NSNA). State boards of nursing serve as resources for each state regarding licensure requirements and education requirements for certification and recertification. These organizations all have websites for individuals to easily access information.

4. What are the pros and cons of the many different types of nursing education programs that prepare students for current nursing practice?

There are various nursing education programs that differ in terms of type of program and credential, type of institution, length of program, and purpose and scope (Table 3.2). Aspects to consider when evaluating programs include length of program, flexibility (e.g., distance-learning) of learning platform/clinical opportunities, and funding opportunities (i.e., grants/scholarships). Different programs vary in terms of flexibility based on their teaching platform (e.g., online/hybrid/face-to-face learning) and prerequisites/degree required (i.e., traditional degree, second-degree/accelerated, and bridge programs). While some prefer the flexibility of an online degree, this advantage requires greater discipline on the part of the enrolled students. In considering the type of program and credential, one needs to remember that while higher levels are typically longer programs, they confer a bigger scope of practice. For example, an LPN program is shorter than a BSN degree program, but BSN graduates have broader scopes of practice. Additionally, accelerated programs allow second-degree students to complete their degrees in a faster period of time; however, students in these programs need to be self-directed and disciplined due to the quick pace of the program.

5. What educational opportunities exist for graduates of various programs to advance beyond their current preparation, including traditional, mobility, and distance-learning programs?

Different types of programs exist for those seeking to advance their education, which include traditional, as well as accelerated and second-degree programs. Several of these options include distance-learning or mobility programs for LPN or LVN to ADN and BSN; diploma and ADN graduates to BSN and MSN; and BSN to MSN and doctoral programs. Many employers, as well as government organizations (i.e., HRSA grant), are also providing funding and support to facilitate this academic progression.

REFERENCES

Abdulai, A., & Hung, L. (2023). Will ChatGPT undermine ethical values in nursing education, research, and practice? *Nursing Inquiry, 30*(3), e12556. Will ChatGPT undermine ethical values in nursing education, research, and practice? - PubMed (nih.gov)

Academic Center for Evidence-Based Practice. (2016). *STAR model.* STAR Model | School of Nursing (uthscsa.edu).

Ackerman-Barger, K., Dickinson, J.K, & Martin, L. (2020). Promoting a culture of civility in nursing learning environments. *Nurse Educator, 46*(4), 234–238. https://doi.org/10.1097/NNE.0000000000000929

Adelman, D.S., & Legg, T.J. (2009). *Disaster nursing: A handbook for practice.* Jones and Bartlett.

ADN Programs (2023). *ADN programs by state.* ADN Programs by State

Agency for Healthcare Research and Quality (AHRQ). (2023). Evidence-based practice centers. https://effectivehealthcare.ahrq.gov/about/epcAmerican

Association of Colleges of Nursing (AACN). (2007). *Competencies.* http://qsen.org/competencies/

American Association of Colleges of Nursing (AACN). (2008a). *The essentials of baccalaureate education for professional nursing practice.* http://www.aacn.nche.edu/education-resources/BaccEssentials08.pdf

American Association of Colleges of Nursing (AACN). (2008b). *Cultural competency in baccalaureate education.* http://www.aacn.nche.edu/education-resources/cultural-competency

American Association of Colleges of Nursing (AACN). (2008c). *Consensus model for APRN regulation: Licensure, accreditation, certification and education (LACE).* http://www.aacn.nche.edu/education-resources/APRNReport.pdf

American Association of Colleges of Nursing (AACN). (2011). *Core competencies for interprofessional collaborative practice.* http://www.aacn.nche.edu/education-resources/ipecreport.pdf

American Association of Colleges of Nursing (AACN). (2020). Promising practices in holistic admissions review: Implementation in academic nursing [White paper]. https://www.aacnnursing.org/Portals/42/News/White-Papers/AACN-White-Paper-Promising-Practices-in-Holistic-Admissions-Review-December-2020.pdf

American Association of Colleges of Nursing (AACN). (2021a). *The essentials: Core competencies for professional nursing education.* AACN. https://www.aacnnursing.org/Portals/0/PDFs/Publications/Essentials-2021.pdf

American Association of Colleges of Nursing (AACN). (2021b). *Diversity, equity, and inclusion in academic nursing: AACN position statement.* https://www.aacnnursing.org/Portals/0/PDFs/Position-Statements/Diversity-Inclusion.pdf

American Association of Colleges of Nursing (AACN). (2022). *Fact sheet: Nursing faculty shortage.* https://www.aacnnursing.org/Portals/42/News/Factsheets/Faculty-Shortage-Factsheet.pdf

American Association of Colleges of Nursing (AACN). (2023a). Fact sheet: Enhancing diversity in the nursing workforce. https://www.aacnnursing.org/Portals/0/PDFs/Fact-Sheets/Enhancing-Diversity-Factsheet.pdf

American Association of Colleges of Nursing (AACN). (2023b). *New data show enrollment declines in schools of nursing, raising concerns about the nation's nursing workforce.* https://www.aacnnursing.org/news-data/all-news/new-data-show-enrollment-declines-in-schools-of-nursing-raising-concerns-about-the-nations-nursing-workforce

American Association of Colleges of Nursing (AACN). (2023c). Holistic admissions. https://www.aacnnursing.org/our-initiatives/diversity-equity-inclusion/holistic-admissions#:,:text=AACN%20now%20offers%20Holistic%20Admissions,and%20later%20as%20a%20professional

American Association of Colleges of Nursing (AACN). (2023d). *RN to baccalaureate programs.* Degree Completion Programs for Registered Nurses: RN to Master's Degree and RN to Baccalaureate Programs (aacnnursing.org)

American Association of Colleges of Nursing (AACN). (2023e). *2022-2023 Enrollment and graduations in baccalaureate and graduate programs in nursing.* AACN. https://www.aacnnursing.org/news-data/research-data-center/standard-data-reports

American Association of Colleges of Nursing (AACN). (2023f). *Clinical nurse leader.* https://www.aacnnursing.org/CNL

American Association of Colleges of Nursing (AACN). (2023g). *Fact sheet: The doctor of nursing practice (DNP).* http://www.aacn.nche.edu/News-Information/Fact-Sheets/DNP-Fact-Sheet

American Association of Colleges of Nursing. (2023h). *Diversity, equity, and inclusion.* Diversity, Equity, & Inclusion (aacnnursing.org)

American Association of Colleges of Nursing, Byrne, C. Keyt, J., & Fang, D. (2023). *Special survey on vacant faculty positions for academic year 2022–2023.* https://www.aacnnursing.org/Portals/42/News/Surveys-Data/2022-Faculty-Vacancy-Report.pdf

American Nurses Association (ANA). (2015). *Code of ethics for nurses with interpretive statements.* http://www.nursingworld.org/about/01action.htm#code

American Nurses Association (ANA). (2021). *Workplace violence.* http://www.nursingworld.org/workplaceviolence

American Nurses Association (ANA). (2023a). *Social media.* https://www.nursingworld.org/social/

American Nurses Association (ANA). (2023ba). *Disaster preparedness.* https://www.nursingworld.org/practice-policy/work-environment/health-safety/disaster-preparedness/coronavirus/

American Nurses Association (ANA). (2023c). *Nurses in the workforce.* https://www.nursingworld.org/practice-policy/workforce/

American Nurses Association (ANA) New York, & New York Organization of Executives and Leaders. (2017). *Coalition for advancement of nursing education.* Press Release: New York State Governor Cuomo signs legislation to strengthen educational requirements for future registered nurses. https://www.foundationnysnurses.org/wp-content/uploads/2018/01/Nursing-Press-Release-final.pdf

American Red Cross. (2023). *Disaster training.* https://www.redcross.org/take-a-class/disaster-training

Balestra, M.L. (2018). Social media missteps could put your nursing license at risk. *American Nurse, 13*(3), 21–23. https://www.myamericannurse.com/social-media-nursing-license-risk/

Bauer, L., & Bodenheimer, T. (2017). Expanded roles of registered nurses in primary care delivery of the future. *Nursing Outlook, 65,* 624–632.

Billings, D.M., & Halstead, J.A. (2019). *Teaching in nursing: A guide for faculty* (6th ed.). Elsevier.

Brenan, M. (2023, January 10). *Nurses retain top ethics rating in U.S. but below 2020 high.* Gallup. https://news.gallup.com/poll/467804/nurses-retain-top-ethics-rating-below-2020-high.aspx

Buerhaus, P.I., & Auerbach, D.I. (2011). The recession's effect on hospital registered nurse employment growth. *Nursing Economics, 29*(4), 163–167.

Buerhaus, P.I., Skinner, L.E., Auerbach, D.I., & Staiger, D.O. (2017). Four challenges facing the nursing workforce in the United States. *Journal of Nursing Regulation, 8*(2), 40–46. https://doi.org/10.1016/S2155-8256(17)30097-2

Centers for Disease Control and Prevention (CDC). (2019). *Methicillin-resistant Staphylococcus aureus (MRSA).* https://www.cdc.gov/mrsa/community/index.html

Centers for Disease Control and Prevention (CDC). (2020a). *Preventing suicide.* https://www.cdc.gov/violenceprevention/suicide/fastfact.html

Centers for Disease Control and Prevention (CDC). (2020b). *Healthy people 2030.* https://www.cdc.gov/nchs/healthy_people/hp2030/hp2030.htm

Centers for Disease Control and Prevention (CDC). (2023a). *Facts about suicide.* Facts About Suicide | Suicide | CDC

Centers for Disease Control and Prevention (CDC). (2023b) *Ebola disease.* https://www.cdc.gov/vhf/ebola/index.html

Centers for Disease Control and Prevention (CDC). (2023c). *Coronavirus disease 2019 (COVID-19) treatment guidelines.* https://www.covid19treatmentguidelines.nih.gov/

Cope, V., & Murray, M. (2018). Use of professional portfolios in nursing. *Nursing Standard, 32*(30), 55. https://doi.org/10.7748/ns.2018.e10985

Crisis Prevention Institute. (2023). *Our programs.* https://www.crisisprevention.com/Our-Programs

Darvish, A., Bahramnezhad, F., Keyhanian, S., & Navidhamidi, M. (2014). The role of nursing informatics on promoting quality of health care and the need for appropriate education. *Global Journal of Health Science, 6*(6), 11–18.

Doran, F., & van de Mortel, T. (2022). The influence of an educational intervention on nursing students' domestic violence knowledge and attitudes: A pre and post intervention study. *BMC Nursing, 21*(1), 109. https://doi.org/10.1186/s12912-022-00884-4

Education Development Center. (2023). *Zero suicide.* https://solutions.edc.org/solutions/zero-suicide-institute/zero-suicide

Farra, S.L., Smith, S.J., & Ulrich, D.L. (2017). The student experience with varying immersion levels of virtual reality simulation. *Nursing Education Perspectives, 39*(2), 99–101. https://doi.org/10.1097/01.NEP.0000000000000258

Gallegos, C., Gehrke, P., & Nakashima, N. (2019). Can mobile devices be used as an active learning strategy? Student perceptions of mobile device use in a nursing course. *Nurse Educator, 44*(5), 270–274. https://doi.org/10.1097/NNE.0000000000000613

Gest, J. (2022). *What happens when White people become a minority in America? Foreign Policy.* https://foreignpolicy.com/2022/03/22/us-white-majority-minority-nation-demographic-change/#:,:text=So%2C%20despite%20four%20years%20of,becomes%20one%20of%20multiple%20minorities

Glasgow, M.E.S., Dreher, H.M., & Schreiber, J. (2019). Standardized testing in nursing education: Preparing students for NCLEX-RN and practice. *Journal of Professional Nursing, 35*(6), 440–446. https://doi.org/10.1016/j.profnurs.2019.04.012

Gravina, E. (2017). Competency-based education and its effect on nursing education: A literature review. *Teaching & Learning in Nursing, 12*(2), 117–121. https://doi.org/10.1016/j.teln.2016.11.004

Hay, B., Carr, P. J., Dawe, L., & Clark-Burg, K. (2017). I'm ready to learn: Undergraduate nursing students' knowledge, preferences, and practice of mobile technology and social media. *Computers, Informatics, Nursing, 35*(1), 8–17.

Health Resources & Services Administration (HRSA). (2023a). *Apply for a scholarship.* https://bhw.hrsa.gov/funding/apply-scholarship#nurse-corps-sp

Health Resources & Services Administration (HRSA). (2023b). *Apply for a grant.* https://bhw.hrsa.gov/funding/apply-grant#nursing

Himmelstein, D.U., Woolhandler, S., Lawless, R.M., Thorne, D., & Foohey, P. (2018). Medical bankruptcy: Still common despite the Affordable Care Act. *American Journal of Public Health, 109,* 431–433. https://doi.org/10.2105/AJPH.2018.30491

Hodges, A.L., Konicki, A.J., Talley, M.H., Bordelon, C.J., Holland, A C., & Galin, F.S. (2019). Competency-based education in transitioning nurse practitioner students from education into practice. *Journal of the American Association of Nurse Practitioners, 31*(11), 675–682. https://doi.org/10.1097/JXX.0000000000000327 PMID: 31584507

Hughes, V., Delva, S., Nkimbeng, M., Spaulding, E., Turksun-Ocran, R., Cudjoe, J., Ford, A., Rushton, C., D'Aoust, R., & Han, H. (2020). Not missing the opportunity: Strategies to promote cultural humility among future nursing faculty. *Journal of Professional Nursing, 36*(1), 28–33.

Hung, M.S., Lam, S.K.K., Chow, M.C.M., Ng, W.W.M., & Pau, O.K. (2021). The effectiveness of disaster education for undergraduate nursing students' knowledge, willingness, and perceived ability: An evaluation study. *International Journal of Environmental Research and Public Health, 18*(19), 10545. https://doi.org/10.3390/ijerph181910545

Ignatavius, D. (2021). *Developing clinical judgment for professional nursing and the next-generation NCLEX-RN Examination.* Elsevier.

Institute of Medicine (IOM). (2000). *To err is human: Building a safer health system.* National Academies Press. http://www.iom.edu.

Institute of Medicine (IOM). (2001). *Crossing the quality chasm a new health system for the 21st century.* National Academies Press. http://www.iom.edu

Institute of Medicine (IOM) (2003). *Health professions education: A bridge to quality.* National Academies Press.

Institute of Medicine (IOM). (2009). *Redesigning continuing education in the health professions.* National Academies Press.

Institute of Medicine (IOM). (2010). *The future of Nursing: Leading change, advancing health.* National Academies Press.

Institute of Medicine (IOM). (2011). *The future of nursing: Leading change, advancing health.* National Academies Press.

Institute of Medicine (IOM). (2012). The future of nursing: Accomplishments a year after the landmark report (Editorial). *Journal of Nursing Scholarship, 44*(1), 1.

Institute of Medicine (IOM). (2015). *Measuring the impact of interprofessional education on collaborative practice and patient outcomes.* https://harvardmedsim.org/blog/institute-of-medicine-releases-report-on-interprofessional-education/

International Council of Nurses (ICN). (2019). *Student nurses gather in Singapore at International Council of Nurses' Congress.* https://www.icn.ch/news/student-nurses-gather-singapore-international-council-nurses-congress

International Council of Nurses (ICN). (2023). *ICN mission, vision, and strategic plan.* https://www.icn.ch/who-we-are/icn-mission-vision-and-strategic-plan

International Professional Education Collaborative. (2023). *IPEC core competencies revision, 2021–2023.* https://www.ipecollaborative.org/2021-2023-core-competencies-revision

Kaddoura, M.A., Flint, E.P., Van Dyke, O., Yang, Q., & Chiang, L. (2017). Academic and demographic predictor of NCLEX-RN pass rates in first- and second-degree accelerated BSN programs. *Journal of Professional Nursing, 33*(3), 229–240. https://doi.org/10.1016/j.profnurs.2016.09.005

Kalisch, P.A., & Kalisch, B.J. (1995). *The advance of American nursing* (3rd ed.) Lippincott.

Kierkx, L., Seuneke, P., de Wolf, P., & Rossing, W.A.H. (2017). Replication and translation of co-innovation: The influence of institutional context in large international participatory research projects. *Land Use Policy, 61,* 276–292.

Kozato, S., Patel, N., & Shikino, K. (2020). A randomised controlled pilot trial of the influence of non-native English accents on examiners' scores in OSCEs. *BMC Medical Education, 20,* 268. https://doi.org/10.1186/s12909-020-02198-y

Krause, T.J., Lederer, A., Sauer, M., Schneider, J., Sauer, C., Jabs, B., Etzersdorfer, E., Genz, A., Bauer, M., Richter, S., Rujescu, D., & Lewitzka, U. (2020). Suicide risk after psychiatric discharge: Study protocol of a naturalistic, long-term, prospective observational study. *Pilot and Feasibility Studies.* 6, 145. https://doi.org/10.1186/s408140-020-00685-z

Lee, W., Kim, M., Kang, Y., Lee, Y., Kim, S. M., Lee, J., Hyun, S., Yu, J., & Park, Y. (2020). Nursing and medical students' perceptions of an interprofessional simulation-based education: A qualitative descriptive study. *Korean Journal of Medical Education, 32*(4), 317–327. https://doi.org/10.3946/kjme.2020.179.

Lenburg, C.B. (2008). *The influence of contemporary trends and issues on nursing education.* In B. Cherry, S. Jacob (Eds.), *Contemporary nursing: Issues, trends, and management* (4th ed.). Mosby.

Lipari, R.N., & Jean-Francois, B. (2016). A day in the life of college students aged 18 to 22: Substance use facts. The CBHSQ Report. Center for Behavioral Health Statistics and Quality, Substance Abuse and Mental Health Services Administration.

Lucas, C., Power, T., Kennedy, D. S., Forrest, G., Hemsley, B., Freeman-Sanderson, A., Courtney-Harris, M., Ferguson, C., & Hayes, C. (2020). Conceptualization and development of the RIPE-N model (reflective interprofessional education-network model) to enhance interprofessional collaboration across multiple health professions. *Reflective Practice, 21*(2), 712–730. https://doi.org/10.1080/14623943.2020.1784866

Marshall, D.C., & Finlayson, M.P. (2018). Identifying the nontechnical skills required of nurses in general surgical wards. *Journal of Clinical Nursing, 27*(7), 1475–1487. https://onlinelibrary-wiley-com.proxy.lib.utc.edu/doi/full/10.1111/jocn.14290

Mohajer, S., Li Yoong, T., Chan, C. M., Danaee, M., Mazlum, S.R., & Bagheri, N. (2023). The effect of professional portfolio learning on nursing students' self-concepts in geriatric adult internship: A quasi-experimental study. *BMC Medical Education, 23*(1), 114. https://doi.org/10.1186/s12909-023-04097-4

Montegrico, J. (2021). Standardized tests as predictors of NCLEX-RN success. *Philippine Journal of Nursing, 91*(1), 22–31. https://www.researchgate.net/publication/352907399_Standardized_Tests_as_Predictors_of_NCLEX-RN_Success/link/60df3e3e92851ca944a2a71f/download

Morrison, V., Hauch, R.R., Perez, E., Bates, M., Sepe, P., & Dans, M. (2021). Diversity, equity, and inclusion in nursing: The pathway to excellence framework alignment. *Nursing Administration Quarterly, 45*(4), 311–323. doi: 10.1097/NAQ.0000000000000494

Nalini, S.J., & Aruna, S. (2019). Competency-based clinical programme for baccalaureate nursing graduates: A need-based analysis. *Nursing Journal of India, 110*(3), 142–144. https://proxy.lib.utc.edu/login?url=https://www-proquest-com.proxy.lib.utc.edu/docview/2267676241?accountid=14767

National Academy of Medicine, National Academies of Science, Engineering, and Medicine, & Committee on the Future of Nursing, 2020–2030. (2021). *The future of nursing 2020–2030: Charting a path to achieve health equity.* https://nam.edu/publications/the-future-of-nursing-2020-2030/.

National Center for Drug Abuse Statistics. (2023). Opioid epidemic: Addiction statistics. https://drugabusestatistics.org/opioid-epidemic/

National Council of State Boards of Nursing (NCSBN). (2016). The 2015 national nursing workforce survey. *Journal of Nursing Regulation, 7*(1), S4-S6. Executive Summary (ncsbn.org)

National Council of State Boards of Nursing (NCSBN). (2018). *A nurse's guide to the use of social media.* https://www.ncsbn.org/public-files/NCSBN_SocialMedia.pdf

National Council of State Boards of Nursing (NCSBN). (2022). *2022 NCLEX pass rates.* https://www.ncsbn.org/publications/2022-nclex-pass-rates

National Council of State Boards of Nursing (NCSBN). (2023a). *Nurse licensure compact.* https://www.nursecompact.com

National Council of State Boards of Nursing (NCSBN). (2023b). *APRN compact.* https://www.ncsbn.org/aprn-compact.htm

National Council of State Boards of Nursing (NCSBN). (2023c). *Active PN licenses.* https://ncsbn.org/active-pn-licenses

National Council of State Boards of Nursing (NCSBN). (2024). *National nursing workforce study.* https://www.ncsbn.org/research/recent-research/workforce.page

National League for Nursing (NLN). (2014a). *A vision recognition of the role of licensed practical/vocational nurses in advancing the nation's health.* http://www.nln.org/docs/default-source/about/nln-vision-series-%28position-statements%29/nlnvision_7.pdf?sfvrsn=4l

National League for Nursing (NLN). (2014b). *Number of basic RN programs by program type: 2005–2014.* http://www.nln.org/docs/default-source/newsroom/nursing-education-statistics/number-of-basic-rn-programs-total-and-by-program-type-2005-to-2014.pdf?

National League for Nursing. (2020). Biennial survey of schools of nursing, 2020. Microsoft PowerPoint - NLN Biennial Survey of Schools of Nursing 2020 Slides Power point.pptm

National League for Nursing (NLN). (2022a). *NLN core competencies for academic nurse educators.* Core Competencies for Academic Nurse Educators (nln.org)

National League for Nursing (NLN). (2022b). *NLN Nursing education scholarships.* https://www.nln.org/nln-foundation/foundationoverview/nursing-education-scholarship-awards

National Organization of Nurse Practitioner Faculties (NONPF). (2022). *Nurse practitioner role core competencies.* https://www.nonpf.org/page/NP_Role_Core_Competencies

Nikpeyma, N., Zolfaghari, M., & Mohammadi, A. (2021). Barriers and facilitators of using mobile devices as an educational tool by nursing students: A qualitative research. *BMC Nursing, 20*(1), 1–11. https://www.ncbi.nlm.nih.gov/pmc/articles/PMC8579623/pdf/12912_2021_Article_750.pdf

Patrick, M.E., Schulenberg, J.E., Miech, R.A., Johnston, L.D., O'Malley, P.M., & Bachman, J.G. (2022). *Monitoring the future panel study annual report: National data on substance use among adults ages 19 to 60, 1976–2021.* University of Michigan Institute for Social Research. doi:10.7826/ISRUM.06.585140.002.07.0001.2022

Putri, S.T., & Sumartini, S. (2021). Integrating peer learning activities and problem-based learning in clinical nursing education. *SAGE Open Nursing, 7*, 23779608211000262. https://doi.org/10.1177/23779608211000262

Quality and Safety Education for Nurses (QSEN). (2022a). *Project overview.* Project Overview (qsen.org)

Quality and Safety Education for Nurses (QSEN). (2022b). QSEN competencies. QSEN Competencies | QSEN.

Quality and Safety Education for Nurses (QSEN). (2022c). *Graduate QSEN competencies.* Graduate QSEN Competencies | QSEN.

Romero-Collado, A., Baltasar-Bagué, A., Puigvert-Viu, N., Rascón-Hernán, C., & Homs-Romero, E. (2020). Using simulation and electronic health records to train nursing students in prevention and health promotion interventions. *Nurse Education Today, 89*, 104384.

Ross, G.J., & Myers, S.M. (2017). The current use of social media in undergraduate nursing: A review of the literature. *Computers, Informatics, Nursing, 35*(7), 338–344. https://doi.org/10.1097/CIN.0000000000000342

Smiley, R.A., Allgeyer, R.L., Shobo, Y., Lyons, K.C., Letourneau, R., Zhong, E., Kaminski-Ozturk, N., & Alexander, M. (2023). The 2022 national nursing workforce survey. *The Journal of Nursing Regulation, 14*(1), S1-S90. https://doi.org/10.1016/S2155-8256(23)00047-9

Southern Poverty Law Center. (2020). *What anti-racism really means for educators.* https://www.tolerance.org/magazine/what-antiracism-really-means-for-educators

Tennessee Higher Education Commission & Student Assistance Corporation. (2023). Graduate nursing loan forgiveness program. https://www.tn.gov/collegepays/money-for-college/loan-forgiveness-programs/graduate-nursing-loan-forgiveness-program.html

The Advocates for Human Rights. (2018). *Stop violence against women: A project by the advocates for human rights.* http://www.stopvaw.org

The Army Nurse Corps Association. (2023). Scholarships. https://e-anca.org/Scholarships

Unver, V., Basak, T., Ayhan, H., Cinar, F. I., Iyigun, E., Tosun, N., Tastan, S., & Kose, G. (2018). Integrating simulation-based learning into nursing education programs: Hybrid simulation. *Technology and Health Care, 26*(2), 263–270. https://doi.org/10.3233/THC-170853

US Air Force. (n.d.). *Healthcare professionals caring for those protecting the nation.* https://www.airforce.com/careers/specialty-careers/healthcare/training-and-education?&&gclid=EAIaIQobChMI4NnPlbeJgAMVjDjUAR3f-QuWEAAYAyAAEgL0PPD_BwE&gclsrc=aw.ds

US Bureau of Labor Statistics (USBLS). (2022). *Registered nurses.* Registered Nurses: Occupational Outlook Handbook: US Bureau of Labor Statistics (bls.gov)

US Navy (2018). *Nurse corps.* https://www.navy.com/sites/default/files/2018-03/nurse-brochure.pdf

Western Governors University. (2018). *How nurses help fight the obesity epidemic.* https://www.wgu.edu/blog/how-nurses-help-fight-obesity-epidemic1811.html#close

Western Governors University. (2023). How AI is influencing nursing education. How AI Is Influencing Nursing Education (wgu.edu)

Wolf, D.M., & Morouse, K.M. (2015). Using blogs to support informatics nurses' curriculum needs. *Online Journal of Nursing Informatics, 19*(2). http://cjni.net/Journal_original/V11N4/My%20Editorial/Using%20Blogs%20to%20Support%20Informatics%20Nurses%27%20Curriculum%20Needs%3A%20EBSCOhost.pdf

World Health Organization (WHO). (2016). *Nurse educator core competencies.* http://who.int/hrh/nursing_midwifery/nurse_educator050416.pdf

World Health Organization (WHO). (2023). *WHO coronavirus disease (COVID-19) dashboard.* https://covid19.who.int/"://covid19.who.int/

World Health Professions Alliance. (2023). *Interprofessional collaborative practice.* https://www.whpa.org/activities/interprofessional-collaborative-practice

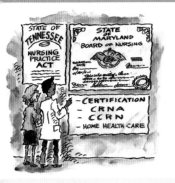

Nursing Licensure and Certification

Susan R. Jacob, PhD, MS, RN*

al regulations and professional certification
ire safe, competent nursing care.

Additional resources are available online at: http://evolve.elsevier.com/Cherry/

LEARNING OUTCOMES

After studying this chapter, the reader will be able to:

1. Explain the development of licensure requirements in the United States.
2. Summarize current licensure requirements in the context of historical developments.
3. Analyze the various components of a **nurse practice act**.
4. Discuss the **mutual recognition model** and identify Nurse Licensure Compact states.
5. Describe the development of certification requirements for advanced practice.
6. Identify requirements for certification for advanced practice in different specialties.
7. Use appropriate resources to obtain current information on licensure and certification.

KEY TERMS

Accreditation Voluntary process by which schools of nursing are approved to conduct nursing education programs.

Advanced practice nurse (APN) Legal title for nurses prepared by education and competence to perform independent practice.

American Nurses Association (ANA) Professional organization that represents all registered nurses.

American Nurses Credentialing Center (ANCC) An independent agency of the American Nurses Association that conducts certification examinations and certifies advanced practice nurses.

Certification Process by which nurses are recognized for advanced education and competence.

Compact state A term of law. In the context of the Nurse Licensure Compact, a state that has established an agreement with other states allowing nurses to practice within the state without an additional license. The interstate compacts are enacted by the state legislatures.

Continued competency program A variety of initiatives to ensure nurses' knowledge, skills, and expertise beyond initial licensure.

Grandfathered In nursing, the statutory process by which previously licensed persons are included without further action in revisions or additions in nurse practice acts.

International Council of Nurses (ICN) Professional organization that represents nurses in countries around the world.

Licensure by endorsement The original program whereby nurses licensed in one state seek licensure in another state without repeat examinations. The requirements are included in state nurse practice acts or accompanying rules and regulations.

*We thank Janet C. Scherubel, PhD, RN, for her contribution to this chapter in the fourth edition.

Mandatory continuing education Educational requirements imposed by individual states for renewal of a license.

Mutual recognition model Program developed by the National Council of State Boards of Nursing in 2012. The Nurse Licensure Compact program establishes interstate compacts so that nurses licensed in one jurisdiction may practice in other compact states without obtaining duplicate licensure.

National Council of State Boards of Nursing (NCSBN) Organization whose membership consists of the board of nursing of each state or territory.

Nurse practice act Statute in each state and territory that regulates the practice of nursing.

State board of nursing Appointed board within each state charged with the responsibility to administer the nurse practice act of that state.

Sunset legislation Statutes that provide for revocation of laws if not reviewed and renewed within a specified time.

PROFESSIONAL/ETHICAL ISSUE

Russell and Rudy were working as needed in a very busy comprehensive home-health agency. The agency had recently experienced high registered nurse (RN) turnover and numerous changes in administrative personnel. Mary, the efficient staff person with whom they had worked from the beginning of their employment, resigned 6 months ago, and temporary staff had been sporadically doing her job. Russell and Rudy discussed how they both missed Mary because she always reminded them of important things such as insurance enrollment periods, cardiopulmonary resuscitation (CPR) certification expiration dates, and the date their nursing licenses were about to expire. Rudy stated, "I'm afraid critical things have been slipping through the cracks lately and going unnoticed since Mary resigned." Russell, who had told Rudy he was way over the limit on all of his credit cards and overdue on many of his bills, responded, "I know my RN license is about to expire, but I have no money to spend on that in the near future, so I am really hoping no one checks up on this detail. Then I might get away with not having a current license for a few months until I can get my financial issues worked out."

- How should Rudy respond to Russell?
- What are the implications for practicing as an RN without a current nursing license?

VIGNETTE

Three nurses are discussing their nursing practice licenses. Joe Branch, a senior nursing student, is preparing for initial licensure. Mary Stone's license is due for renewal. Carmella Larkin just moved into the state. As the three are talking about these changes in their practice, Giorgio Gonzales, a nurse practitioner, joins the group. Giorgio recently completed a certification examination and is interested in becoming certified for advanced practice. All the nurses have a general knowledge of the requirements for licensure and certification, but lack the specific information needed to legally practice within the state.

Mary suggests contacting the state board of nursing. The nurses agree that this is a sensible idea, and Mary leaves to phone the board of nursing. Upon returning, Mary informs the group that the answers to all of their questions can be found in the state's nurse practice act and accompanying rules and regulations, which can be accessed online. She tells them that the state board of nursing office will also send free copies of both documents to individuals who request them.

The situation described here is not uncommon. Nurses need specific, current information on licensure and renewal of licensure. The most comprehensive sources for this information are the state nurse practice act and the state board of nursing. These resources provide accurate descriptions of the law governing nursing practice within each state and the US territories.

Every nurse and nursing student will benefit from obtaining a copy of his or her state's nurse practice act and becoming familiar with its contents.

Questions to Consider While Reading This Chapter:

1. Who establishes the "rules" for nursing practice—the state or the employer?
2. Do graduates from different types of nursing education programs require different types of licenses?

3. If a nurse graduate passes the NCLEX-RN examination, does this person still need a license?

4. What happens if a nurse's license expires? Can the nurse still practice?

5. Must a nurse complete graduate school and take an examination to be an advanced practice nurse?

6. Are the regulations governing advanced practice the same in all states?

CHAPTER OVERVIEW

To practice nursing as an RN is the goal of every student nurse. It is a goal achieved through study, clinical practice, and successful completion of the National Council Licensure Examination–Registered Nurse (NCLEX-RN) exam. This chapter discusses how and why nursing licensure was developed, steps necessary to become licensed, licensure regulations, and the responsibilities of an RN.

After licensure as RNs, nurses must still maintain and increase their knowledge and skills. Many nurses may wish to specialize in a particular area of nursing and expand their practice. Nurses with these goals may seek certification in a specialty field. This chapter describes certification, the means to achieve certification, and the organizations that administer certifying examinations. Whether it is licensure or certification, the nursing profession is constantly progressing. Legal requirements to practice are continually being revised to ensure the public's protection. Throughout history and in the current health care environment, nurses face complex issues and new challenges as they seek to increase their competence and ensure the delivery of excellent nursing services to patients. This chapter explores issues related to licensure and certification, as well as some of the challenges nurses and students will face.

THE HISTORY OF NURSING LICENSURE
Recognition: Pins and Registries

The aim of caregivers throughout history has been to be recognized and acknowledged for their skills and achievements. Early caregivers, particularly in the monasteries and convents of the medieval period, were identified by the habits they wore. Frequently, special insignias designated health personnel. During the Crusades, a large Maltese cross adorned the habits of the Knights Hospitalers of St. John of Jerusalem on the battlefield (Kalisch & Kalisch, 2003). These forms of identification allowed others to recognize their particular skills in caregiving and healing. More recently, nurses around the world wore a readily identifiable symbol of their school of nursing—the nursing cap.

Today, as in the past, the school of nursing pin identifies graduates from a particular school of nursing. Early in each school's history, the students and faculty crafted the pin. The pin's emblems and text symbolize the philosophy, beliefs, and aspirations of the nursing program. Students receive their own pins at graduation in a special pinning ceremony. Nurses wear their pins proudly, as evidence of their achievement, learning, and skill. It is one way that nurses distinguish themselves as distinct health care providers with a specialized body of knowledge and clinical skills.

Although White Coat Ceremonies have been an important rite of passage at medical schools for more than 20 years, it is now common to offer similar events at schools of nursing. In 2014, nursing schools in 43 states, plus the District of Columbia, were given financial support and guidance by The Arnold P. Gold Foundation and the American Association of Colleges of Nursing to offer a White Coat Ceremony. This ceremony usually consists of the recitation of an oath, cloaking of students in a white coat, an address by an eminent role model, and a reception for students and invited guests. Students typically also receive their nursing pins at the White Coat Ceremony.

Nursing programs also maintain a record of all graduates. Florence Nightingale started this practice in 1860, when she created a list of graduates of the St. Thomas's School of Nursing in England. This list became known as the "registry" of graduate nurses. The registry of nurses initiated by Nightingale provided institutions, as well as patients, with a system of identifying graduates of particular nursing programs. These lists proclaimed to all the skills and knowledge of graduates. These nurses could then be distinguished from lay practitioners and local citizens who provided care to the ill and infirm. Today, nursing programs around the world continue the tradition started by Nightingale and maintain registries or listings of all of their graduates. In addition, state and international agencies maintain lists of nurses practicing in their jurisdictions.

Purpose of Licensure

As nursing programs proliferated, variations developed among the programs. Entry criteria differed, and many educational programs were structured to meet specific employer needs. A simple registry of nurse graduates was no longer sufficient to ensure minimal levels of competency in all nurses, regardless of the school where the nurses were educated. Another system was necessary to distinguish those sufficiently trained to provide nursing care from untrained or lesser-trained individuals. Graduate nurses, physicians, and hospitals met to resolve this confusion. The outcome was criteria for the licensure of nurses in the United States. Then, as now, the primary purpose of licensure was protection of the public.

Early Licensure Activities

US nursing programs developed in much the same manner as was the pattern in England. As early as 1867, Dr. Henry Wentworth Acland encouraged licensure of English nurses. However, it was not until 1896 that attempts were made to license nurses in the United States. Prior to the late 1800s, many hospitals established training programs to prepare nursing staff for their own institutions. The programs varied with the needs of the hospital, the availability of physicians and nurses for training students, and the resources devoted to the training. It became apparent to many nurses that consistent minimum standards to practice across settings were necessary. These standards would provide for safety of the public and improve the mobility of nurses among institutions. A key advocate for these standards was the Nurses Associated Alumnae of the United States and Canada. This organization later became the American Nurses Association (ANA). However, the group met with resistance from hospitals, physicians, and even nurses. The early attempts at nursing licensure failed for lack of broad-based support (Joel, 2006).

Nurses worldwide mounted an extensive educational campaign explaining the purposes and safeguards inherent in licensure. Success was achieved, and in 1901 the International Council of Nurses (ICN) passed a resolution that each nation and state examine and license its nurses. Several US states responded shortly thereafter. In 1903 North Carolina, New Jersey, New York, and Virginia were the first to institute permissive licensure. The licensure rules were voluntary. These permissive licenses permitted but did not require nurses to become registered.

Under permissive licensure, educational standards were set at a minimum of 2 years of training for nurses.

State boards of nursing were established with rules for examinations, as well as revocation of the license. Nurses who did not pass the examination could not use the title of RN. These early regulations served two purposes: first, to protect the public from unskilled practitioners; and, second, to provide legal sanctions to protect the title of RN. The New York State Board of Regents began a registry of nurses who had successfully completed all requirements. In 20 years, by 1923, all states had instituted examinations for permissive licensure. Each state's licensure examinations varied in content, length, and format and had written, oral, and practice components. The early work in examinations for licensure was the forerunner of today's licensure and certification requirements (Kalisch & Kalisch, 2003).

The early state efforts in licensing nurses were commendable. Nonetheless, there was considerable variability among states in the requirements for nursing education, the licensure examinations, and the nurse practice acts themselves. The widespread variability in nurse practice acts prompted the ANA (and later the National Council of State Boards of Nursing [NCSBN]) to design model nurse practice acts. The model acts provided a template for states to follow. The first was published in 1915. These model practice acts are revised and updated as nursing practice advances. The NCSBN Model Act and Rules are exemplary legislation that can be adopted by a state board of nursing (BON).

The model nurse practice act is composed of many sections, including a definition of nursing and the scope of practice for the RN, descriptions of advanced practice nursing, requirements for prescriptive authority of nurses, nursing education, compact guidelines, and processes for disciplinary actions against nurses who violate sections of the act. Separate sections of the model act provide guidelines for state boards of nursing and the necessary requirements for entry into practice. The latest model practice act (NCSBN, 2021) is available online at the NCSBN website (https://www.ncsbn.org/3867.htm).

From these model acts, each state or jurisdiction developed a unique practice act. Although individual states and territories' practice acts address the needs of the developing jurisdiction, every practice act includes the sections described in the model act. Students and practicing nurses may obtain the nurse practice act for any jurisdiction by contacting that state or territorial board of nursing.

Mandatory Licensure

Once each state had established permissive licensure, the next movement was toward a requirement that all nurses must be licensed. This practice is termed *mandatory licensure*. New York was the first state to require mandatory licensure, although this requirement was not in place until 1947. At the same time, nursing groups moved to standardize nursing licensure testing procedures.

After World War II, the ANA formed the NCSBN. The council was composed of a representative of each state and jurisdiction in the United States. As part of its original activities, the council advocated a standardized examination for licensure. These varied activities culminated in the National League for Nursing, which administered the first State Board Test Pool Examination in 1950. The written examination had separate sections on medical–surgical nursing, maternity nursing, nursing of children, and psychiatric nursing. This format for the examination continued for more than 30 years, and many of today's nurses took them.

The next major event in licensure efforts occurred in 1982 with the development of the first NCLEX-RN examination. The test was revised to include all nursing content within one section of the examination. In addition, the format was changed to present questions in a nursing process format. Just as with previous versions of licensing examinations, the NCLEX-RN examination has evolved over time. Paper-and-pencil testing was replaced with computerized adaptive testing in 1994. Extensive information on the NCLEX-RN examination may be found in Chapter 28 of this text.

COMPONENTS OF NURSE PRACTICE ACTS

Each state develops rules and regulations to govern the practice of nursing within that state. These rules are in the nurse practice acts or in their accompanying rules and regulations to administer the act. Many nurse practice acts are patterned after the ANA or NCSBN model practice act, and all contain comparable information.

Purpose of Act

Each act begins with a purpose. All nurse practice acts include two essential purposes. First, each act has statements that refer to protecting the health and safety of the citizens in the jurisdiction. The act describes the qualifications and responsibilities of those individuals covered by the regulations. Likewise, the act delineates

those excluded from the practice of nursing. These provisions also serve to ensure protection of the public. The second purpose is to protect the title of RN. The legal title RN is reserved for those meeting the requirements to practice nursing. Only those licensed may use the designation RN. Thus unlicensed personnel are prevented from using the title RN.

Definition of Nursing and Scope of Practice

In each state or jurisdictional nurse practice act, the practice of professional nursing is defined. The definition of nursing is of utmost importance because it delineates the scope of practice for nurses within the jurisdiction. That is, each act outlines the activities nurses may legally perform within the jurisdiction. Many states follow the guidelines incorporated in the model practice act, although each is specific and delineates practice within that state or jurisdiction. For example, some states describe nursing as a process that includes nursing diagnosis, whereas other states list broad areas of nursing activities. To avoid becoming outdated, the acts contain no lists of skills or procedures. As nursing knowledge and practices advance, new techniques are frequently allowable because of the comprehensive nature of the definition of nursing.

Many jurisdictions incorporate definitions of advanced practice nursing within one definition of nursing. In other states the definitions of advanced practice nursing, and the scope of practice for the advanced practice nurse, are separate.

Each state or jurisdiction establishes laws regulating practice within its borders. Therefore it is imperative for the nurse to know and understand the definition of nursing in the states in which they practice. Further, each jurisdiction retains the right to govern practice within that jurisdiction. This right supersedes the presence of a mutual recognition agreement with other compact states. The retention of states' rights is an essential component in the mutual recognition model.

There are other important reasons for becoming familiar with the definition of nursing practice. Frequently, nurses are asked to perform in ways that are beyond the legal definition of nursing. This is illegal, and if the nurse complies, they could lose the privilege of practicing nursing. In other situations, labor laws or other statutes affect nurses. Definitions may include or exclude nurses on the basis of their legal definitions of nursing practice. As nursing practice becomes more complex and sophisticated, states may revise their nurse practice acts. Nurses are accountable for knowing the definition and scope of practice within their jurisdictions and practicing accordingly. To know and understand the laws regulating their practice, nurses should obtain copies of and become familiar with nurse practice acts for the states or jurisdictions in which they plan to practice.

Licensure Requirements
Entry Into Practice Licensure

A section of each nurse practice act describes the requirements and procedures necessary for initial entry into nursing practice or nursing licensure. An initial requirement in all jurisdictions is graduation from both high school and an accredited nursing program. Candidates for licensure must submit evidence of graduation as defined by each state.

To verify an applicant's graduation from a nursing program, a transcript of coursework, a diploma, or a letter from the dean of the program is frequently necessary. Additional requirements for licensure may include a statement regarding the mental and physical health status of the applicant. Some jurisdictions conduct a review of prior legal convictions; this is especially important in reference to felony convictions. Some states also require declaration of misdemeanors, even those that have been expunged. Other states have appended provisions related to recreational drug abuse, and some states require declaration of termination and disciplinary action from a nursing or health care employer. Finally, most states require statements from the school of nursing attesting to the eligibility of the candidate for licensure. The requirements for licensure are detailed in each nurse practice act and the accompanying rules and regulations for practice.

In the past it was customary for nurses to practice in only one state or territory. More than ever, nurses are practicing in more than one jurisdiction, either by their physical presence in that jurisdiction or through technological advances such as telephone and computer access to patients across state and territory lines. As laws are continually being revised to reflect the current practice of nursing, it is incumbent on the individual to be cognizant of the current licensure requirements in all states and territories in which they intend to practice.

Regardless of individual state requirements, all nurse practice acts require candidates to successfully complete the NCLEX-RN licensure examination before they can practice. In some states it is possible to obtain a temporary permit to practice, pending receipt of success on the licensure examination. This arrangement was especially prevalent in past years because it took several months for results of the licensure examinations to be reported. Now, however, with computer testing and the prompt response from the testing services, the use of temporary permits to practice is becoming less frequent.

Temporary permits are still available for nurses moving from one jurisdiction to another. To obtain a license to practice in another state, the nurse applies for licensure by endorsement. Nurses licensed in one jurisdiction may apply for licensure in a second jurisdiction by submitting a letter to the second state board of nursing. Typically, evidence for the new license is similar to that for initial licensure. In addition, proof of the nurse's current license to practice, as well as any restrictions imposed on the license by the first state, is required. These procedures will continue for all states not participating in the Nurse Licensure Compact (NLC). For any state designated as a compact state, the nurse should contact the state board of nursing to determine the appropriate procedures for initiating nursing practice in that jurisdiction.

In 2020 the unprecedented number of patients affected by COVID-19, and the overwhelming effect it had on health care providers, resulted in all states, territories, and the District of Columbia issuing emergency declarations and lifting state licensure regulations. In some states several health care industry regulations, including suspending the collaborating physician requirement for nurse practitioners and waiving some licensure requirements for nursing school graduates, were enacted. In some cases emergency license waivers were issued to allow nurses licensed in other states to hasten their ability to practice and assist with disaster relief. The loosening of licensing restrictions to enable cross-border practice resulted in confusing state emergency orders available on the NCSBN website (NCSBN, 2022).

Advanced Practice Nursing Licensure

Advanced practice nurses must obtain separate nursing licensure in addition to licensure for entry into practice. State requirements vary; therefore, advanced practice nurses should contact the state board of nursing to determine the criteria and procedures.

Renewal of Licensure

In addition to outlining requirements for initial licensure, each nurse practice act includes the requirements and information necessary to renew one's nursing license. These regulations define the length of time a license is valid, generally from 2 to 3 years, as well as any specific requirements for renewal of licensure.

Mandatory Continuing Education

The nurse will find information on mandatory continuing education requirements for renewal of licensure in the section on license renewal. All nurses are expected to maintain continued competency to practice through various means of continuing education. In 1976 California was the first state to institute mandatory continuing education for renewal of licensure. Since that time, a number of states have instituted requirements of continuing education for renewal of licensure. The number of hours necessary varies depending on the jurisdiction, ranging from 20 to 40 hours over a 2- to 3-year period.

A few jurisdictions require specific continuing education coursework in the areas of health care ethics, the state nurse practice act, or other content specific to that jurisdiction. Clinical course content may be designated for specific health problems, such as sexually transmitted diseases, human immunodeficiency virus/acquired immunodeficiency syndrome, and family violence. In other states the board of nursing allows the nurse a wide latitude in meeting the requirements for renewal of licensure. Details of specific continuing education requirements are found in the nurse practice act and the accompanying rules and regulations.

ROLE OF REGULATORY BOARDS TO ENSURE SAFE PRACTICE

Membership of the Board of Nursing

An important section of every nurse practice act is the designation of a regulatory board of nurses and consumers to administer the act. Frequently, this responsibility is assigned to a state board of nursing. The practice act outlines guidelines for membership on the board. In addition, procedures by which members are appointed to the board of nursing are designated. In most cases the members are appointed by the governor's office. Interested individuals or organizations, such as the state nurses' association, may submit names to the governor for consideration.

Duties of the Board of Nursing

The responsibilities and duties of the board of nursing are delineated in detail. Specific duties of the board may be outlined in the act itself or in the enabling laws. These enabling administrative statutes are frequently designated as rules and regulations for the practice of nursing. It is through the work of the board of nursing that nursing licenses are granted and renewed, and disciplinary action is taken when provisions of the act are violated. Just as all nurses need to be cognizant of their nurse practice acts, nurses should also become familiar with the role of the state board of nursing.

A major responsibility of the board of nursing is addressing concerns about a nurse's practice. The review of a nurse's potential malfeasance, or violation of the act or other state or federal laws, is within the responsibilities of the board of nursing. The nurse practice act describes the due process and procedures for this review. The board of nursing then assigns appropriate disciplinary action. These activities are a key responsibility of the board of nursing. Actions may include restrictions on a nurse's license or its suspension or revocation. Just as all nurses need to be cognizant of their nurse practice acts, nurses should become familiar with the role of the state board of nursing.

SPECIAL CASES OF LICENSURE

Military and Government Nurses

There are many nurses whose practice takes them throughout the country on a regular basis. For example, many nurses are members of the military, or join the military nursing services after graduation. The Veterans Administration and US Public Health Service employ thousands of nurses who serve in many jurisdictions, as well as outside US boundaries. It is not necessary for these nursing personnel to obtain a nursing license in each jurisdiction in which they practice. The graduate takes the NCLEX-RN examination in one state. Upon successful completion, as an employee of the US government, they may practice in other jurisdictions without additional licensure requirements. Nurses should obtain the current requirements for licensure because rules are updated to reflect current practices.

Internationally Educated Nurses

Internationally educated nurses (IENs) have become an integral part of the US registered nurse workforce. Top countries represented by IENs passing the NCLEX-RN examination in 2019 include Philippines, India, Puerto Rico, Kenya, and Korea (NCSBN, 2023a). IENs are another pipeline for the US nursing workforce, especially in times of shortage in the domestic supply. Health workforce migration, a critical issue for many years, has received increased attention as a result of the 2010 World Health Organization's (WHO) Global Code of Practice on the International Recruitment of Health Personnel (Global Code). The Global Code represents an effort to promote ethical principles in the recruitment of international health personnel, with a particular focus on minimizing recruitment from countries experiencing critical shortages (WHO, 2010).

IENs have met the requirements for practice in their own countries. When nurses move to the United States, they must show evidence of completing their original educational program and restrictions of their licenses. In addition, nurses need to demonstrate competency in English, and the ability to take and pass the NCLEX-RN examination. Foreign nurses take a special examination administered by the Commission on Graduates of Foreign Nursing Schools. The examination is given in English, and tests the knowledge required to practice in the United States. Upon successful completion, the foreign nurse graduate may apply for a license to practice in the United States. The intent of these regulations is not to be punitive or obstructive to the nurse. The regulations are yet another example of two key principles: first, the protection of the public and, second, the protection of the title of RN.

International Practice

In a similar manner, nurses licensed in the United States may want to practice in other countries. Nurses interested in these opportunities may contact either the ICN or the nursing regulatory board of the country in which they wish to practice. The ICN is composed of representatives of organized nursing worldwide. One of its functions is to assist nurses in obtaining licensure in other countries.

Each country has specific laws and regulations governing nursing practice that must guide the practice of the US nurse. Just as a foreign nurse must demonstrate competency to practice in the United States, the US nurse should be prepared to submit documentation on education, NCLEX-RN examination results, and proof of licensure and practice to officials in the foreign country. Advanced planning and contact with the appropriate regulatory agency will ease the transition for the nurse.

In an increasingly connected world, nursing care, more and more often, transcends the boundaries of countries and continents. NCSBN's Global Regulatory Atlas is the first comprehensive resource on the regulation of nurses in countries around the world. This tool allows regulators and educators to easily compare regulations in their own jurisdictions with those of their neighbors; researchers can access data from around the world; and nurses considering immigration can view the policies of the countries to which they might migrate. Free to use and built with the assistance of health care regulators worldwide, the Global Regulatory Atlas puts the world's nurses at your fingertips. NCSBN (2023b) data from 320 jurisdictions, and information relating to more than 22 million nurses around the world, is available on this site.

REVISION OF NURSE PRACTICE ACTS

Nurse practice acts, just as other sections of states' codes, are written and passed by legislators. As in any legislative endeavor, many governmental agencies, administrators, consumers, and special-interest groups seek to influence the legislation. These groups become actively involved in developing the accompanying rules and regulations. For example, physicians, dentists, pharmacists, licensed practical nurses, certified nursing assistants, emergency personnel, and physician assistants are just a few of the health care providers directly affected by the scope and definition of nursing practice. Likewise, organizations such as schools, hospitals, home health agencies, and extended-care facilities are vitally concerned with the role of nurses today. Equally important, citizen groups are interested in determining nurses' roles and responsibilities. For this reason, the nurse practice act, as finally passed or amended by the state legislature, represents the aims and concerns not only of nurses but of many individuals and multiple-interest groups.

Review of a state's practice act reveals the influential parties involved in creating the act. Each group participates in defining the scope and practice of nursing, as well as regulations affecting nursing practice within the jurisdiction. Because of these varied interests, it is essential for nurses to understand the practice act and the additional legislation that influences and controls their practice. Further, as proposals to amend the nurse practice act are promulgated at the state level, it is imperative for all nurses to be involved in the process. The resulting laws affect their profession, their practice, and their livelihood.

Sunset Legislation

One example of legislative activity affecting nurse practice acts is sunset legislation. Sunset laws, found in many states, are intended to ensure that legislation is current and reflects the needs of the public. When sunset provisions are included in a nurse practice act, the act must be reviewed by a specific date. If the act is not renewed, it is automatically rescinded. This review process allows for revisions to update practice acts to be consistent with current nursing practice. Many nurse practice acts contain sunset provisions. It is through these activities that the scope of nursing practice is updated, and components, such as the diagnosis of nursing problems, have been incorporated into definitions of nursing. Other changes include changes in requirements for mandatory continuing education for licensure renewal. Equally important, sunset laws have provided the means to define advanced practice nursing and incorporate prescriptive authority for advanced practice nurses. Nurses should determine whether sunset regulations affect the nurse practice act in the state in which they practice. Likewise, nurses should be aware of, and involved in, activities to amend the nurse practice act.

DELEGATION OF AUTHORITY TO OTHERS

The rapid expansion of an array of health care providers, changes in health care delivery systems, and efforts to control health care costs have led to participation of many types of unlicensed personnel in the provision of health care. These personnel present a challenge to RNs working with them. Questions arise as to who can delegate what activities to which unlicensed provider groups. Guidelines for delegation have been developed by many nursing organizations, including the NCSBN and ANA (NCSBN, 2019). Although the professional organizations' guidelines are helpful, it is the nurse practice acts of individual states that establish the legal definitions of appropriate delegation practices. Because regulations differ among states, each nurse must identify and understand the regulations for the state in which they practice. Chapter 20 presents a detailed discussion of delegation and supervision.

CURRENT LICENSURE ACTIVITIES
Mutual Recognition Model

Efforts to provide common definitions of nursing practice, equivalent educational standards for practice, and uniform testing for entry into practice through the NCLEX-RN examination have been very successful. Nonetheless, most nurses are still required to apply for licensure in each state in which they practice. With the increased mobility of nurses, the telehealth movement, and the necessity of caring for patients across long distances, state boards of nursing have recognized the need to provide practicing nurses with more than procedures of endorsement of their initial licenses. This need has led to further changes in nursing licensure.

In 1997 the Delegate Assembly of the NCSBN moved to a new level of nursing regulation. The assembly endorsed a mutual recognition model of nursing regulation. Through this model, state boards of nursing formed the NLC.

The original NLC allowed nurses with a multistate license to practice physically, telephonically, or electronically in their home state and other original NLC states without obtaining additional licenses. In 2015 the NLC underwent revisions that led to new legislation known as the enhanced NLC (eNLC) (NCSBN, 2023c). At this time, most NLC states and many noncompact states are moving forward with the process of joining the enhanced NLC. "Under the eNLC, nurses are able to provide care to patients in other eNLC states, without having to obtain additional licenses. 'The newly enhanced compact or eNLC was approved by the BONs on May 4, 2015, as a licensure model of the future. It replaces the original NLC and adds extra protections. The original NLC states are currently enacting state legislation enabling them to transition into the eNLC. New states, not previously members of the original NLC, are also enacting state legislation to become members of the eNLC.'" For a current map of **eNLC** states, visit https://www.nursecompact.com/

"Nurses with an original NLC multistate license will be grandfathered into the eNLC" (NCSBN, 2023d): https://www.ncsbn.org/public-files/Grandfathering_Guidelines_(3).pdf

The APRN Compact, adopted August 12, 2020, allows an advanced practice registered nurse (APRN) to hold one multistate license with a privilege to practice in other compact states. The APRN Compact (NCSBN, 2023e) will be implemented when seven states have enacted the legislation. Visit the NCSBN website or https://www.aprncompact.com for key provisions of the APRN Compact.

A number of issues associated with mutual recognition concerns nurses. On the one hand, mutual recognition greatly facilitates interstate practice, telehealth programs, and movement of nurses to areas of shortage. In addition, a national nursing database provides information on individual nurses' practice and disciplinary actions taken against nurses.

Nursys is "the first-ever comprehensive source of nursing licensure statistics for the US and its territories" (NCSBN, Nursys, 2023f). Compiled by NCSBN's database, Nursys "is an electronic information system where boards of nursing enter licensure data on a frequent basis. Nursys e-Notify is a free, innovative nurse licensure notification system. The system helps nurses track their license and discipline status and provides license renewal reminders. The information is provided as it is entered into the Nursys database by participating boards of nursing. This database supports a key licensure goal—to protect the public health and safety. These advantages have resulted in support for the NLC by many nursing organizations" (Tri-Council for Nursing, 2020).

On the other hand, concerns relate to monitoring nurses' practice in multiple jurisdictions, nurse privacy, and due process rights. Issues related to disciplinary action in home and distant states are still being resolved. In addition, differences in practice requirements in different states may cause nurses confusion as to their rights and responsibilities. The NLC is increasingly affecting all nurses. Nursing students and graduates must remain apprised of changing conditions. Because changes occur frequently in this area, the most comprehensive and current sources of information are the websites for the ANA, the NCSBN, and the state boards of nursing for individual jurisdictions.

Continued Competency

As discussed earlier in the chapter, the primary purpose of nurse licensure is protection of the public. Thus mandatory continuing education was instituted as a strategy to ensure that nurses were competent to remain in practice. These programs have continued for many years. However, a growing number of nurses believe that more is required than just attending seminars to demonstrate continued competency. Consortiums of nurses in several states are examining alternatives for renewal of licensure. These requirements may include designated numbers of clinical practice hours, portfolios of achievements in clinical practice, and other exemplars of practice. Nurses and students are encouraged to become aware of continued competency initiatives so that they may be prepared for changes in future licensure requirements.

There is increasing concern for patient safety and treatment in today's health care system. Models of continued competency are but one attempt by professional nurses to ensure that patients receive safe, effective nursing care. Another strategy in this quest is establishing programs for certification of advanced practice nurses.

CERTIFICATION

History of Certification

There are distinct differences between licensure and certification. At the most basic level, licensure establishes minimal levels of practice, whereas certification recognizes excellence in practice. Because of this difference, the background, requirements, and practice opportunities for licensure and certification differ markedly.

Just as with the development of nursing licensure, at its inception, certification was not legally required; rather, it was voluntary. In an effort to recognize nurses who had completed additional education and demonstrated competency in clinical practice, numerous nursing graduate schools and nursing specialty organizations offered certification programs. In the 1970s and later, advanced clinical courses were designed for nurses as certificate programs. The programs varied in length and content and did not offer a full master's course of study in nursing.

A second distinct difference in licensure and certification pertains to the organizations that grant certification. Whereas licensure is granted and governed by legislation, and administered through the state boards of nursing, certification is awarded by nongovernmental agencies. The first field of nursing practice to certify advanced practitioners was nurse anaesthesiology in

1946. Similarly, in 1961 the American College of Nurse-Midwives began certifying nurse-midwives. As certificate programs developed, it became apparent that program standardization was a necessity. In 1975 the ANA convened a national study group at the University of Wisconsin, Milwaukee, to explore the issue. This meeting was attended by 75 nursing specialty organizations. The report of the group recommended the formation of a central organization for certification of nurses. This report, in conjunction with efforts of many nurses, resulted in the formation of the American Nurses Credentialing Center (ANCC, 2023). More than a quarter million nurses in more than 40 areas of specialty practice have been certified by the ANCC since 1990. More than 80,000 advanced practice nurses are currently certified by the ANCC. Today, many of the ANCC's examinations are open to nurses with a variety of educational backgrounds.

In addition to the ANCC, other professional specialty nursing organizations (Box 4.1) offer certification examinations. These organizations have created certification boards that are separate from the parent organizations, to maintain an independent role and to conform to department of education requirements. Nurses may contact these specialty nursing organizations directly for current guidelines and information.

All APRNs should be certified through a nationally recognized nursing certifying body, and they should understand that the examinations offered by these certification agencies will be used by state boards to grant APRNs the authority to practice. The lengths to which organized nursing has invested in certification of advanced practice in nursing are further indications of nurses' commitment to protection of the public and the patients they serve.

Certification began as a voluntary effort controlled by professional nursing organizations. State agencies were not involved in the credentialing process. This is still the case, although state nurse practice acts do include requirements for nurses to practice in advanced roles. Thus state practice acts first contained provisions requiring certification for nurse anaesthesiologists and nurse-midwives. With the development of additional advanced practice roles, all states have included requirements for certification in their regulations for advanced practice nurses in all specialty roles.

Purpose of Certification

The purpose of advanced practice laws is, first and foremost, protection of the public. Within the acts are definitions of advanced practice nursing. Several states further differentiate the advanced practice of nursing by including separate titles for nurse practitioners and clinical nurse specialists. The scope of practice of the advanced practice nurse is well defined. States describe supervisory or collaborative practice with physicians, with differences existing among states as to the regulations governing these relationships. Requirements for practice vary among states. Although many states require a master's degree in the specialty area for practice, this is not the case in all jurisdictions. All states require evidence of certification in the specialty area, and many require periods of practice in the specialty prior to awarding of certification status. All states incorporate specific provisions for prescribing medications.

Steps to Certification

The best strategy for a nurse wishing to practice in an expanded role is to become informed of specific

---

BOX 4.1 Other Nursing Certification Organizations

Advanced Diabetes Management—Association of Diabetes Care & Education Specialists https://www.diabeteseducator.org/education/certification/bc_adm

Advanced Practice Palliative Nurse—National Board for Certification of Hospice and Palliative Nurses https://www.nhpco.org/palliativecare/palliative-care-accreditation/

Certified Nurse Educator—National League for Nursing https://www.nln.org/awards-recognition/certification-for-nurse-educators-overview

Clinical Nurse Leader—Commission on Nurse Certification https://www.aacnnursing.org/our-initiatives/education-practice/clinical-nurse-leader/cnl-certification/about

Flight Nurse—Board of Certification for Emergency Nurses Board of Certification for Emergency Nurses https://bcen.org/

Nurse Anesthetist – National Board of Certification & Recertification of Nurse Anesthetists https://www.nbcrna.com/

Public Health—National Board of Public Health Examiners https://www.nbphe.org/

School Nurse—National Board for Certification of School Nurses https://www.nbcsn.org/

Nurse Midwife-The American Midwifery Certification Board (AMCB) https://www.midwife.org/The-Certification-Exam

requirements in the chosen field. The nurse should examine carefully the roles and responsibilities inherent in advanced practice nursing. First, the nurse should contact both the ANCC and the specialty organization in his or her area of practice to determine the education, experience, and examination requirements for certification. Concurrently, every nurse should contact the state boards of nursing in the state(s) in which they wish to practice and should obtain information on legal requirements to practice in those jurisdictions. After gathering the requirements to practice, the nurse will be able to develop a plan of action to complete the necessary advanced coursework, clinical practice requirements, and examinations. Upon completion of the requirements of these agencies, the advanced practice nurse may practice in an expanded role. In addition to the certifying agencies, the nurse may wish to contact other advanced practice nurses who will serve as valuable colleagues for the new advanced practice nurse.

Current Issues in Certification

Despite tremendous strides in fewer than 40 years, certification processes for the advanced practice nurse continue to evolve. As with any new endeavor, advances are made in small steps and great leaps.

Nurses in advanced practice face changing educational requirements for licensure and relicensure. Professional and legal issues regarding the scope of nursing practice, and the independence of advanced practice nursing, must change along with changes in the health care environment. Advanced practice nurses develop professional relationships with their physician colleagues, as do all nurses; however, the advanced practice nurses must define their legal relationships with physician practitioners and other caregivers. These issues are not uncommon to nurses in any practice setting; yet, the advanced practice nurse is charting new territory.

A unique challenge to advanced practice nurses is reimbursement for nursing services. As advanced practice continues to expand, nurses have moved from secondary to independent billing for services. Federal regulations allow direct reimbursement for some nursing services, while state and local practices vary. There are ongoing efforts at the state and national levels to resolve these issues. Advanced practice nurses are in constant communication with their peers and professional organizations. They look to all nurses to become involved in issues facing the advanced practice nurse.

The Consensus Model for APRN Regulation, Licensure, Accreditation, Certification, and Education

"With approximately 300,000 advanced practice registered nurses (APRNs) in the United States, APRNs represent a powerful force in the health care system. The Consensus Model provides guidance for states to adopt uniformity in the regulation of APRN roles. Today, many states have adopted portions of the Model elements but there still may be variation within states. APRNs moving from state to state need to ask themselves the following:

- "Have I met the requirements to practice in this state?"
- "Do I have the appropriate certification required to practice in this state?"
- "Does my training/experience match within the scope of practice required to practice?"

During the COVID-19 pandemic, the need for nurses and other health professionals across the United States greatly exceeded the supply. Many health care facilities took advantage of regulatory flexibilities that expand the workforce to include recently retired health care providers and nursing students. Yet, the strain that COVID-19 put on US hospitals is not showing any signs of abating in the near future (Rashid et al., 2023). The COVID-19 pandemic prompted some state governors to temporarily remove unnecessary restrictions on APRNs. Lifting these barriers, which do not follow the Consensus Model, allowed APRNs to practice across state lines to meet the need for health care providers in surge areas (NCSBN, 2022).

"As long as regulatory requirements differ from state to state, each state border represents an obstacle to portability—potentially preventing access to professionals and access to care. The *Consensus Model for APRN Regulation* (NCSBN, 2023g) has the potential to harness this power by outlining regulatory requirements in licensure, accreditation, certification, and education that should be adopted by every state." Visit the Consensus Model toolkit, a compendium of resources for understanding the Consensus Model at https://ncsbn.org/739.htm"(NCSBN, 2023h)

SUMMARY

To summarize the chapter, let's review the questions posed at the beginning of the chapter and see what you have learned.

1. Who establishes the "rules" for nursing practice—the state or the employer?

   Each state develops rules and regulations to govern the practice of nursing within that state. These rules are in the nurse practice acts or in their accompanying rules and regulations to administer the act. Many nurse practice acts are patterned after the ANA or NCSBN model practice act, and all contain comparable information.

2. Do graduates from different types of nursing education programs require different types of licenses?

   All candidates for entry into practice as a registered nurse are required to successfully complete the NCLEX-RN licensure examination. Advanced practice nurses have a separate advanced practice license.

3. If a nurse graduate passes the NCLEX-RN examination, does this person still need a license?

   Registered nurses are required to have licenses to practice. The requirements for licensure are detailed in each state's nurse practice act and the accompanying rules and regulations for practice.

4. What happens if a nurse's license expires? Can the nurse still practice?

   If a nurse's license expires, the nurse cannot practice until the license is renewed. In addition to outlining requirements for initial licensure, each nurse practice act includes the requirements and information necessary to renew one's nursing license. These regulations define the length of time a license is valid, generally from 2 to 3 years, as well as any specific requirements for renewal of licensure.

5. Must a nurse complete graduate school and take an examination to be an advanced practice nurse?

   Advanced practice nurses must complete graduate school and obtain separate nursing licensure in addition to licensure for entry into practice.

6. Are the regulations governing advanced practice the same in all states?

   State requirements vary; therefore, advanced practice nurses should contact the state board of nursing to determine the criteria and procedures.

Nurse practice acts provide protection for both the public and the title of RN. This is accomplished through the development of specific regulations regarding education and examination of competence to practice. Each act contains guidelines for disciplinary action to protect both the public and professional nursing. The nurse practice act of each jurisdiction addresses the needs of the state and the responsibilities of nurses practicing within that state. It is important for all nurses and students of nursing to become familiar with the regulations guiding their own practice.

As health care delivery evolves and nursing practice advances, new issues and initiatives arise. It is imperative to update nurse practice acts so that they remain responsive to the needs of all and allow nurses to practice to the full extent of their education and training. Nurses must be part of this process. Collaboration among professional nursing organizations, state boards of nursing, and individual nurses will enable nursing to continually meet the needs of patients.

REFERENCES

American Nurses Credentialing Center (ANCC). (2023). *Certifications available.* https://www.nursingworld.org/our-certifications/

Joel, L.A. (2006). *The nursing experience: Trends, challenges, and transitions* (5th ed.) McGraw-Hill.

Kalisch, B.J., & Kalisch, P.A. (2003). *The advance of American nursing* (4th ed.) Lippincott.

National Council of State Boards of Nursing (NCSBN) and American Nurses Association (ANA). (2019). *National Guidelines for Nursing Delegation.* https://www.ncsbn.org/public-files/NGND-PosPaper_06.pdf

National Council of State Boards of Nursing (NCSBN). (2021). *Model act.* https://www.ncsbn.org/3867.htm

National Council of State Boards of Nursing (NCSBN). (2023a). *2023 NCLEX Fact Sheet.* https://www.ncsbn.org/exams/exam-statistics-and-publications.page

National Council of State Boards of Nursing (NCSBN). (2023b). *Global regulatory atlas.* https://www.regulatoryatlas.com/

National Council of State Boards of Nursing (NCSBN). (2023c). *Enhanced Nurse Licensure Compact (eNLC) implementation. For a current map of eNLC states, visit* Home | NURSECOMPACT

National Council of State Boards of Nursing (NCSBN). (2023d). *Guidelines for Grandfathering APRNs by Endorsement.* https://www.ncsbn.org/public-files/Grandfathering_Guidelines_(3).pdf

National Council of State Boards of Nursing (NCSBN). (2023e). *APRN compact.* https://www.aprncompact.com/

National Council of State Boards of Nursing (NCSBN). (2023f). *Nursys database.* https://www.nursys.com/

National Council of State Boards of Nursing (NCSBN). (2023g). *APRN consensus model: The consensus model for APRN Regulation, licensure, accreditation, certification, and education.* https://www.ncsbn.org/aprn-consensus.htm

National Council of State Boards of Nursing (NCSBN). (2023h). *APRN consensus model toolkit.* https://ncsbn.org/739.htm

National Council of State Boards of Nursing (NCSBN). (2022). *State response to COVID-19 as of May 2, 2022.* https://www.ncsbn.org/public-files/APRNState_COVID-19_Response.pdf

Rashid, K., Ansar, F., Khan, Y., Rashid, N., Rehman, H., Shah, S.Z., Ullah, S., & Waheed, M. Impact of staffing levels and resources of intensive care units on compliance to standard mechanical ventilator guidelines: A city-wide study in times of COVID-19 pandemic. *Nurs Crit Care* (2023). March 28 (2): 218–224.

Tri-Council for Nursing. (2020). *Statement from the Tri-Council for Nursing on the status of the U.S. health care workforce during the COVID-19 pandemic.* https://www.nln.org/detail-pages/news/2020/12/04/Statement-from-the-Tri-Council-for-Nursing-on-the-Status-of-the-U-S-Health-Care-Workforce-during-the-COVID-19-Pandemic

World Health Organization (WHO). (2010). *World Health Organization's global code of practice on the international recruitment of health personnel (global code).* https://www.who.int/publications/i/item/wha68.32

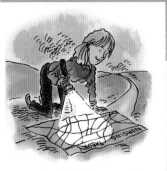

5

Theories of Nursing Practice

*Susan R. Jacob, PhD, MS, RN**

*rsing theory provides the direction for nursing
ctice and research.*

Ⓔ Additional resources are available online at: http://evolve.elsevier.com/Cherry/

LEARNING OUTCOMES

After studying this chapter, the reader will be able to:
1. Differentiate between a science and a theory.
2. Identify the criteria necessary for science.
3. Identify the criteria necessary for theory.
4. Explain a nursing theory and a nursing model.

5. Discuss two early and two contemporary nursing theorists and their theories.
6. Explain the effect of nursing theory on the profession of nursing.

KEY TERMS

Concept An idea or a general impression. Concepts are the basic ingredients of theory. Examples of nursing concepts include pain, quality of life, health, stress, and adaptation.

Conceptual model A group of concepts that are associated because of their relevance to a common theme.

Nursing science The collection and organization of data related to nursing and its associated components. The purpose of this data collection is to provide a body of scientific knowledge, which provides the basis for nursing practice.

Theory The compilation of data that define, describe, and logically relate information that will explain past nursing phenomena and predict future trends. Theories provide a foundation for developing models or frameworks for nursing practice development.

Proposition A statement that proposes the relationship between and among concepts.

Schematic model A diagram or visual representation of concepts, conceptual models, or theory.

"Science is built up with facts, as a house is with stones. But a collection of facts is no more a science than a heap of stones a house."
Jules Henri Poincaré, 1909, French scientist and mathematician

---

*We thank Margaret Soderstrom, PhD, RN, CS-P, APRN, and Linda C. Pugh, PhD, RNC, FAAN, for their contributions to this chapter in the 4th edition.

PROFESSIONAL/ETHICAL ISSUE

Bachelor of science in nursing (BSN) students Matt, Toni, and Britainy were studying together for their theory class when Matt spoke up and said, "I think all this theory is just a bunch of junk. Nurses in practice don't have time to learn about theories, and they sure don't use them to guide their practice."

Britainy spoke up and said, "My aunt is an RN on the cancer unit at Memorial Hospital and she has told me that on her unit they use Jean Watson's caring theory to guide their interactions with patients."

Toni said, "Really? Then maybe there is something to this theory stuff. I think we should take this class more seriously."

Britainy agreed and suggested that they divide the material among themselves and meet again the next day to prepare for the upcoming test.

Matt said, "You guys can do that if you want, but count me out. My plan is to skim the information and take my chances on the test. I am amazed you two really think we will ever need to know any of this stuff after we graduate. Nursing theory is never going to help me start an IV."

Is there a way for Britainy and Toni to show Matt he is wrong? If so, how?

How can Britainy and Toni persuade Matt to divide the theory material with them to prepare for the upcoming test?

VIGNETTE

When I was a nursing student, it was hard for me to understand why I needed to know anything about nursing theory, but now that I am in practice, I see that theories provide a way for me to organize, deliver, and evaluate the care I provide. On our labor and delivery unit, we use Roy's adaptation model to guide our practice as we provide care to laboring moms. The use of this theory allows us to assess how well they are coping and provides guidance as we plan nursing interventions that promote their successful coping.

Questions to Consider While Reading This Chapter:

1. What is nursing theory?
2. How is nursing theory different from the theory of other disciplines?
3. How does theory relate to nursing practice?
4. Why is it important to understand nursing theory?
5. Why is it important for nurses to develop theory?

CHAPTER OVERVIEW

Explicit, detailed knowledge is the keystone, the foundation, and the carefully laid support that are critical to the classification of a discipline. In a seminal paper titled "The Discipline of Nursing," Donaldson and Crowley (1978) note that a discipline "is characterized by a unique perspective, a distinct way of viewing all phenomena, which ultimately defines the limits and nature of its inquiry" (pp. 113–120). Nursing, long ranked an art and a science, is actually quite young in its continuing struggle for professional and public recognition as a matchless, expert, and commanding profession. This notion is readily supported as one marks nursing's ongoing effort to define itself as a distinct discipline that is exclusive from other disciplines, particularly the medical practice model. Only when a substantial body of nursing knowledge is collected, organized, and developed will the profession be defined and its scope of practice differentiated. Key to this accomplishment is the development and practice of nursing theory.

It is important for nurses to study the development of nursing theory because without an idea of where you have been, how can you know how, why, when, or where to go? Nursing theory provides nurses with a focus for research and practice. You may consider using a theory as similar to using a map that provides direction while making available a variety of ways to get where you are going. As logical as this seems, the worth of studying nursing theorists, their theories, and the role of responsibility these theories contribute to the evolution of nursing science has been curiously underappreciated. Even more surprising, many of the naysayers are nursing students. Nursing theory is not usually the favorite subject of undergraduates, who would rather learn technical, hands-on skills. Whether this is a maturation issue or an issue of knowledge and experience remains undetermined by nursing faculty and the profession itself.

This chapter in no way reflects the breadth and depth of nursing theorists and their theories. There are many scholarly works devoted to this topic. Instead it is a survey, a general overview, a smattering of nursing theories, with chosen segments intended to assist in providing the idea, the notion, and indeed, the semblance of what a theory is and how it is critical to the profession of nursing. Readers interested in examining the theoretic basis for nursing practice will find resources for further exploration at the end of the chapter.

SCIENCE AND THEORY

Science is a method of bringing together facts and giving them coherence and integrity. Science assists us in understanding how the unique, yet related, parts of a structure fit and become more than the sum of individual parts. In the opening metaphor, the stones represent the facts, the process of laying the stones represents the science, and the future ideas and new directions represent the theory.

Science is dynamic and static—dynamic in figuring out how a phenomenon happens, static in describing what happens. Scientific inquiry involves five steps: (1) hypothesis, (2) method, (3) data collection, (4) results, and (5) evaluation. These five steps are described in Box 5.1.

"Nursing theory is defined as an abstract generalization that presents a systematic explanation about the relationships among phenomena" (Polit & Beck, 2017, p. 746). Theory development functions in a parallel manner to scientific process, although theory generally applies to a more specific area of the larger scientific process. Even though Sigmund Freud and Carl Jung each had their individual theories about the psychology of humans, their theories were focused on specific ideas taken from the entire knowledge base surrounding psychology and psychotherapy and its scientific premise. Similarly, Albert Einstein's theory of relativity was but a fraction of the existing scientific knowledge base of mathematics at the time. Nevertheless, it is an undisputed fact that these theorists changed the thinking of their time and were responsible for the evolution of

> ### BOX 5.2   Criteria for Theory Acceptance
>
> **Inclusiveness:** Does the theory include all concepts related to the area of interest?
> **Consistency:** Can the theory address new entities without having its founding assumptions changed?
> **Accuracy:** Does the theory explain retrospective occurrences? Does the theory maintain its capacity to predict future outcomes?
> **Relevance:** Does the theory relate to the scientific foundation from which it is derived? Is it reflective of the scientific base?
> **Fruitfulness:** Does the theory generate new directions for future research?
> **Simplicity:** Does the theory provide a road map for replication? Is it simple to follow? Does it make sense?

their philosophic and scientific interests (Anastasi, 1958). For a proposed theory to be accepted as a theory, it must meet the following six criteria: (1) inclusiveness, (2) consistency, (3) accuracy, (4) relevance, (5) fruitfulness, and (6) simplicity. These criteria are further explained in Box 5.2.

The importance of theories in the evolution of science is unquestioned. Nursing has evolved as a profession and a science in a similar manner. Nursing theories have explained, explored, defined, and delineated specific areas. They are foundational to nursing, helping to accumulate further knowledge and give indications of what direction nursing should take to develop the discipline. In practice, nursing theories help nurses by describing, explaining, and predicting everyday experiences. Theories can guide nurses in their assessments, interventions, and evaluations of nursing care.

Beginning with the work of Florence Nightingale in 1860, nursing theorists have taken the vast pool of scientific information available and focused on precise target areas of interest. In so doing, theoretic models have been conceptualized to guide nursing actions, interventions, and implementation. Specific nursing theories are discussed later in the chapter.

Nursing Science

As might be expected, there are several definitions of nursing science (Abdellah, 1969; Jacox, 1974). Although these definitions differ, they generally support the premise that nursing science is a collection of data related to

> ### BOX 5.1   The Five Steps of the Scientific Process
>
> **Hypothesis:** Ask the question that is to be the main focus. It usually includes independent and dependent variables.
> **Method:** Decide what data will be collected to answer the question. Decide on and identify the step-by-step procedure that will be used to collect these data. Make sure this process can be easily replicated.
> **Data collection:** Implement the step-by-step procedure that has been determined to answer the question.
> **Results:** On the conclusion of the data collection, statistically identify the outcomes. Establish parameters (e.g., level of significance) that will determine whether the data are relevant.
> **Evaluation:** Examine the results to determine the relevance of outcome data in answering the hypothesis. Determine the significance and identify the potential for future research.

nursing that may be applied to the practice of nursing. These data encompass a vast array of knowledge that spans all of nursing and its diversity. This knowledge guides the practice of nursing to better serve patients through healing, prevention, education, and health maintenance.

Theories, Models, and Frameworks

Researchers use theories and conceptual models as their primary method to organize findings into a broader conceptual context (Polit & Beck, 2022). Different terms are used in relation to conceptual contexts for research. These terms include *theories, models, frameworks, schemes,* and *maps.* Different writers often use terms differently, resulting in a blurring of distinct terms (Polit & Beck, 2017).

Theory. Theory is generally considered an abstract generalization that presents a systematic explanation about how phenomena are interrelated. Therefore, traditionally, a theory must have at least two related concepts that support it (Polit & Beck, 2022).

Conceptual Model. A conceptual model deals with concepts that are assembled because of their relevance to a common theme. The term *conceptual framework* is used interchangeably with the term *conceptual model.* Conceptual models, or frameworks, also provide a conceptual perspective regarding interrelated phenomena, but they are more loosely structured than theories. There are many conceptual models of nursing that offer broad explanations of the nursing process. Four concepts basic to nursing that are included in these models are: (1) nursing, (2) person, (3) health, and (4) environment. The various nursing models define these concepts differently, link the concepts in various ways, and emphasize the relationships among the concepts differently. For example, Roy's adaptation model emphasizes the patient's adaptation as a central phenomenon, whereas Martha Rogers emphasizes centrality of the individual as a unified whole. These models are used by nurse researchers to formulate research questions and hypotheses.

The terms *conceptual model* (or *framework*) and *nursing theory* are often used interchangeably. In this chapter, the nursing theories described may also be referred to as conceptual models. The term *model* is also used in reference to a diagram depicting the theory.

In this chapter, *model* refers to a schematic model, which is a diagram or visual representation of the conceptual model or theory.

Nursing Theory

Theory and theoretic thinking guide research and practice. The basic ingredients of theory are concepts. Examples of nursing concepts include health, stress, and adaptation. Propositions are statements that propose the relationship between and among concepts (Polit & Beck, 2022). Theories provide us with a frame of reference, the ability to choose concepts to study, or ideas that are within one's practice. A theory helps guide research, and research helps validate theory.

In the research model, the researcher decides what to study and how and why the area of interest is important to the practice of nursing. In the practice model, the clinician decides what areas to directly assess, when to assess, and which intervention to implement. These decisions may or may not be knowingly based on a model or theory. Regardless, often the outcome supports the notion that behavior replicates a theoretic model, even though the nurse may be unaware that they are using a theoretic model in the practice process. Evidence-based theories (i.e., theories that are empirically supported through well-designed studies) are used by nurses for clinical decision-making (Melnyk & Fineout-Overholt, 2019). Nurses use critical thinking to adapt theories as needed to their patient situations.

Just as in any other discipline, nursing theory has its own unique language. The words of this language identify linkages between the database of scientific nursing knowledge and the extracted information taken from this source for nursing theory. The interpretation of these words translates uniquely to the theory investigated. This application, or language of nursing theory, is the structure, or framework, from which one understands the theory. Table 5.1 presents the language of nursing theory along with definitions and examples.

Schematic Models

A schematic model is something that demonstrates concepts, usually with a picture. It is a visual representation of ideas. The model depicts concepts and shows how the concepts are related with the use of images, such as arrows and dotted lines (Polit & Beck, 2022). For example, a blueprint is a pictorial demonstration of a particular type of house someone might build. A model

TABLE 5.1	**The Language of Nursing Theory**	
Term	**Definition**	**Examples**
Concept	Labels given to ideas, objects, events; a summary of thoughts or a way to categorize thoughts or ideas	Comfort, fatigue, pain, depression, environment
Conceptual model	A structure to organize concepts (ideas)	Roy's adaptation model
Philosophy	Values and beliefs of the discipline	Watson's philosophy and science of caring
Theory	The organization of concepts or constructs that shows the relationship of the ideas with the intention of describing, explaining, or predicting. The purpose is to make scientific findings meaningful and generalizable. Our goal in science has been to explain, predict, and control.	Self-care, adaptation, caring, behavioral system, unitary man, hierarchy of needs, interpersonal relationships, humanistic, nurse–client transactions

airplane is a detailed miniature replication of the original full-sized version. Diagramming a sentence outlines the specific parts (adverb, adjective, verb, subject, object, phrases) that make that particular sentence complete. Similarly, a nursing model gives a visual diagram or picture of concepts. Whether that is a critical pathway, decision tree, medication protocol, or other nursing-related practice, the model allows one to view the interrelated parts of the whole in picture form. A model of a nursing theory does the same thing. From the earliest model offered by Florence Nightingale, nursing theory has been described and explained using this medium. Schematic models are used for clarifying complex concepts. The language of theory is translated into picture form, offering a comprehensive view, or model, of the theory. The schematic model shows how the concepts are related. A model, like a blueprint of a building, allows one to see the layout, including outlines of all features specific to the theory. Although it is not the same as understanding every little detail about the structure, its intent is to provide an overview, which at a glance is informative and descriptive.

Levels of Theory

Many people refer to the level of a nursing theory, which can range from broad in scope to a smaller, more specific scope. For example, grand theory is often broad in scope and may describe and explain large segments of human experience. Rogers theory of unitary man describes the entire nursing process. Other levels include middle-range theory and practice theory, which are smaller in scope and may refer to a specific population,

such as Jacob's theory of the grief process in older women whose husbands received hospice care (Jacob, 1996), or to a specific situation, such as Beck's theory of postpartum depression (Beck, 2012), or Pender's Health Promotion Model (Pender et al., 2015). Another example of a middle-range theory is the theory of unpleasant symptoms (Lenz & Pugh, 2003), which examines symptoms that are influenced by physiologic, psychologic, and situational factors as they relate to performance. The model of this theory is presented in Fig. 5.1. Nurses often use these middle-range theories, which are smaller in scope and simpler to understand, to guide their daily practice.

To better illustrate the application of theory to nursing practice, Case Study 5.1 presents a case example of middle-range theory application using Mishel's uncertainty in illness theory (Mishel, 1997). In examining nursing theories, students may be surprised to discover that they are already using some of the concepts in their individual practices. Nursing theories assist with further defining and organizing these concepts into an underpinning that explains and details nursing practice and claims it as a unique discipline.

FLORENCE NIGHTINGALE: THE FIRST NURSING THEORIST

If *theory* means to put concepts in a form in which relationships are described and predictions are made, then Florence Nightingale was the first nursing theorist. Nightingale did not deliberately set out to develop theory; rather, her goal was to ease the suffering

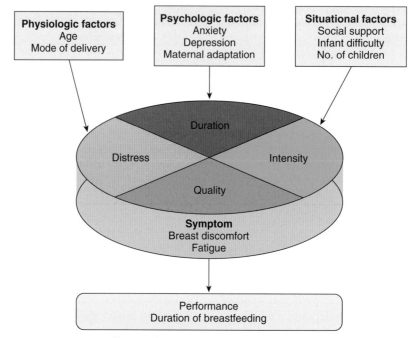

Fig. 5.1 Theory of unpleasant symptoms.

CASE STUDY 5.1   Application of Theory to Practice

Mishel's Uncerta`inty in Illness Theory

A 9-year-old female client, Christine, is admitted to the pediatric unit for evaluation of a new onset of abdominal pain. The admission diagnosis is "intermittent abdominal pain, rule out appendicitis." It is her first time as a patient in a hospital. Her father, who is a surgeon, and her mother, who is a nurse, accompany Christine to the unit. Her mother will stay with her. After talking with the parents, you as the nurse, are confident that Christine is well informed, well cared for, and well prepared for her admission. While her parents are speaking with Christine's attending physician in a nearby office, you talk with Christine, who goes from smiling and chatting to bursting into tears. You observe that she is quite upset as she expresses to you that she is afraid because her father told her that if she did need surgery she would not feel anything because she would be asleep. Christine tells you that when she sleeps she wakes up sometimes and that she is sure that if her appendix is "cut out" she will wake up during the operation and it "will hurt a lot." She tells you she has not told her parents she is afraid because they have told her how proud they are that she is so brave. You realize Christine is terrified. Using Mishel's

uncertainty in illness theory, you apply the four-stage framework:

1. *Stimuli frame:* Inadvertently, Christine, who concretely has understood the word "sleep" using her own filter for life experience, has misinterpreted the positive intention of the language used by her father. This misinterpretation has resulted in Christine's negative cognitive schema. Christine notably does not understand "sleep" and its use (or adult misuse, in this case) as a synonym for, or definition of, surgical anesthesia. This is the root cause of Christine's current uncertainty in illness.

   Nursing intervention: Listen carefully and caringly; explain in simple, understandable language what *sleep* means in the context her father presented; initiate, seek, and clarify Christine's concerns and questions; use the term *anesthesia* to differentiate it from *sleep*. Inform and involve her parents in the overall process.

2. *Appraisal stage:* As a result of Christine's concrete experiential interpretation of "sleep," she has applied a negative value to the environmental conditions surrounding her abdominal pain. This is particularly so as it relates to surgical anesthesia.

Nursing intervention: Follow up with Christine to make sure she comprehends the newly provided information. Elicit the support of Christine's parents and hospital staff. If there are appropriate postsurgical patients on the unit, have them talk with Christine about their positive anesthesia experience.

3. *Initiation of coping mechanisms:* Christine is 9 years old. Her coping skills are limited to those used in her 9 years of life experience.

   Nursing intervention: Check with Christine and observe verbal and nonverbal cues. Have her verbalize any uncertainties she may be experiencing. Some of this process will be influenced by the progress of the illness.

4. *Adaptation:* Dependent on steps 1, 2, and 3.

   Nursing intervention: As Christine accepts the new information, new schema will follow. Although the

outcome of her abdominal pain may initially be uncertain, her acceptance of the new schema will hopefully result in an increased comfort zone and decreased fear.

SUMMARY

A central tenet of Mishel's theory is the core position that uncertainty in illness must be addressed. If it is left unheeded, negative perceptions will escalate and clients will suffer. Their quality of life may be affected and positive outcomes may be compromised. Nursing's responsibility in applying Mishel's theory is to reframe the client's perceived loss of control, or uncertainty, and assist the client in developing new skills of assimilation and accommodation. The client will then be able to identify, develop, and master those targets capable of control.

---

of soldiers and citizens of England. However, many important influences in her life directed her toward theory development:

- A classical education (philosophy [science], French, Italian, Greek, Latin, the arts, and history)
- Upper-class background, great wealth, and a prominent social life (operas, parties, balls)
- Religion and spirituality (spent much time daydreaming about how she could serve God and experienced four visions from God)
- Era of reform throughout England (Industrial Revolution and great divisions among the classes)

Despite her wealth and upper-class status, Nightingale was very dissatisfied with life. In 1852, she wrote a monograph titled "Cassandra," in which she pointed out the hopelessness inherent in being a woman in her day. "The family? It is too narrow a field for the development of an immortal spirit . . . The system dooms some minds to incurable infancy, others to silent misery. Marriage is the only chance [and it is but a chance] offered to women for escape from this death; and how eagerly and how ignorantly it is embraced" (Nightingale, 1992, pp. 37–38). Her diary writings have been interpreted at times to be suicidal. Often depressed, Nightingale resorted to dreams as an escape from her unhappiness and discontent. Her personality and her lifestyle (dogmatic, practical, a critical observer who was fascinated by numbers and recorded everything she saw and

experienced) set her apart. She was self-willed, unhappy, and dissatisfied at times in spite of having beauty, a brilliant social career, and an education of which few men of her day could boast.

She had enjoyed the best of music and art and the companionship of charming and important people. However, in refusing marriage and the round of social gaiety, she was revolting against the restrictions placed on women of her day, and she struggled to be allowed to work in a serious way.

Florence Nightingale eventually persuaded her family to allow her to attend nurses' training, and so began her distinguished career in the development of professional nursing. Nightingale is well remembered for her significant contributions to professional nursing in the areas of theory of practice, nursing education, scholarship, and statistics. Box 5.3 provides Nightingale's definitions of professional nursing.

BOX 5.3   Nightingale's Definition of Nursing

Nursing is an art—an art requiring organized, practical, and scientific training.

Nursing is putting us in the best possible conditions for nature to preserve health—to prevent, restore, or cure disease or injury.

Nursing is, therefore, to help the patient live.

Nightingale's Theory of Practice

Nightingale's theory of practice, an environmental adaptation theory, was documented for nurses and laypersons alike and served as the foundation for the promotion of health. She referred to this theory as the canons of nursing that guided the practice of professional nursing. A description of these canons, or standards, follows.

Ventilation and Warming. In the concept of ventilation and warming, Nightingale is very precise to "keep the air he breathes as pure as the external air without chilling him" (Nightingale, 1859, p. 8). She believed that good ventilation is necessary to carry off noxious elements from a sick person's lungs and skin.

Noise. "Unnecessary noise, or noise that creates an expectation in the mind is that which hurts a patient" (Nightingale, 1859, p. 25). The idea is that the nurse should guard against sudden noise, thoughtless chatter, and whispering in a patient's room. Nightingale believed that the effect of music may be beneficial.

Variety. Variety is another concept that helps alleviate suffering. Beautiful objects, brilliant colors, cut flowers, perhaps different things to do (e.g., handwork), and even pets may alleviate the boredom felt by those suffering.

Diet. The fourth concept is diet. "Sick cookery should half do the work of your poor patient's weak digestion" (Nightingale, 1859, p. 38). Nightingale reviews some of the common substances (gruel, arrowroot puddings, and egg flip) given to the sick.

Light. "It is the unqualified result of all my experience with the sick that second only to their need of fresh air is their need of light" (Nightingale, 1859, p. 47). Nightingale suggested taking the patient outside for direct sunlight, and keeping rooms well lighted with no bed curtains or dark windows.

Chattering Hopes and Advices. According to Nightingale, "chattering hopes and advices" are attempts by attendants and friends to cheer the patient. Nightingale warns against these attempts because she determines them to offer false hope and hollow advice. She clearly appeals, "Leave off this practice of attempting to cheer the sick by making light of their danger and by exaggerating their probabilities of recovery" (Nightingale, 1859, p. 54).

Cleanliness (Health of Houses). Nightingale's attention to cleanliness takes up a large portion of her book. She writes that health depends on this principle. Describing the care of bed, bedding, rooms, and walls, she states the exact steps needed to clean each. In addition, she details how to clean the sick person so as to prevent poisoning by the skin. She describes the patient's feeling of well-being after washing and drying. The nurse needs to wash her own hands with friction as well. Some believe that Nightingale's success was based primarily on cleaning up the hospitals.

Because of these significant contributions to nursing and to improving the health of soldiers and citizens alike, Nightingale was highly recognized. Her honors, decorations, medals, and citations may be seen in the United Services Museum in Whitehall, London. She was the first woman to receive the British Order of Merit, which was bestowed by King Edward VII. One of her biographers (Cook, 1942) said, "She was not only 'The Lady with a Lamp' throwing light into dark places but also a kind of galvanic battery stirring and sometimes shocking the dull and sluggish public to life and action."

SURVEY OF SELECTED NURSING THEORIES

A brief discussion of selected nursing theories follows. The date identified for each indicates the year in which the theory was first presented. However, most theories have continued to be refined and modified. A summary of the major nursing theorists, with a brief description of their theory or conceptual model, is presented in Table 5.2, which provides the reader with information to guide further exploration of nursing theory.

A useful nursing theory will make assumptions concerning health problems, environment, behaviors, and target populations that are logical, consistent, research supported, and similar to ones that have proved to be successful in previous programs.

Betty Neuman (1970)—The System Model

The system model focuses on the response of the client system to actual or potential environmental stressors and on the use of several levels of nursing prevention intervention for attaining, retaining, and maintaining

TABLE 5.2 Summary of Major Nursing Theorists and Theory Description

Theorist and Date	Theory Description
Florence Nightingale, 1860	Investigates the effect of the environment on healing.
Hildegard E. Peplau, 1952	Interpersonal relations model explores the interpersonal relationship of the nurse and the client and identifies the client's feelings as a predictor of positive outcomes related to health and wellness.
Faye Abdellah, 1960	Twenty-one nursing problems. Client-centered interventions.
Ida Jean Orlando, 1961	Theory of the nursing process. Deliberate nursing approach that stresses the action of the individual client in determining the action of the nurse; focus is on the present or short-term outcome.
Virginia Henderson, 1966	Definition of nursing. Nursing assists patients with 14 essential functions toward independence.
Myra Estrin Levine, 1967	Conservation model. Four conservation principles of inpatient client resources (energy, structural integrity, personal integrity, and social integrity).
Martha E. Rogers, 1970	Science of unitary human beings: energy fields, openness, pattern, and organization; nurse promotes synchronicity between human beings and their universe or environment.
Betty Neuman, 1970	Systems model: wellness–illness continuum; promotes the nurse as the agent in assisting the client in adapting to and, therefore, reducing stressors; supports the notion of prevention through appropriate intervention.
Dorothea Orem, 1971	Self-care model. Nursing facilitates client self-care by measuring the client's deficit relative to self-care needs; the nurse implements appropriate measures to assist the client in meeting these needs by matching them with an appropriate supportive intervention.
Imogene King, 1971	Goal attainment theory. Goal attainment using nurse–client transactions; addresses client systems and includes society, groups, and the individual.
Sister Callista Roy, 1974	Adaptation model. Client's adaptation to condition using environmental stimuli to adjust perception.
Madeline Leininger, 1977	Theory of cultural care diversity and universality. Transcultural and caring nursing; concepts are aimed toward caring and the components of a culture care theory; diversity, universality, worldview, and ethnohistory are essential to the four concepts of care, caring, health, and nursing.
Jean Watson, 1978	Philosophy and science of caring and humanistic nursing; there are 10 "carative" factors that are core to nursing; this holistic outlook addresses the impact and importance of altruism, sensitivity, trust, and interpersonal skills.
Margaret Newman, 1979	Central components of this model are health and consciousness followed by concepts of movement, time, and space; all components are summative units, described in relationship to health and to each other.
Dorothy E. Johnson, 1980	Behavioral system model for nursing; separates the psychologic and physiologic aspects of illness; role of the nurse is to provide support and comfort to attain regulation of the client's behavior.
Rosemarie Rizzo Parse, 1981	Theory of human becoming proposes that quality of life from each person's individual perspective should be the goal of nursing practice. Parse first published the theory in 1981 as the "man-living-health" theory; however, the name was officially changed to "the human becoming theory" in 1992 to remove the term *man* after the change in the dictionary definition of the word from its former meaning of "humankind"; individual, by existing, actively participates in creating health according to environmental influences; individual is regarded as an open system wherein health is a process.

optimal client system wellness. Neuman defines the concern of nursing as preventing stress invasion. If stress is not prevented, then the nurse should protect the client's basic structure and obtain or maintain a maximum level of wellness. Nurses provide care through primary, secondary, and tertiary prevention modes.

Hildegard E. Peplau (1952)—Interpersonal Relations as a Nursing Process: Man as an Organism That Exists in an Unstable Equilibrium

When the client incurs an insult that renders her or him incapable of moving forward because of stressful environmental conditions, anxiety increases. This condition creates a situation wherein the option is to either move in a backward direction or remain on a plateau. Nursing intervention in Peplau's model focuses on reducing the related incapacitating stressors through therapeutic interpersonal interaction. Intervention involves the nurse's assisting the client with mutual goal setting. These goals may address exploration of the identified problem, identification of viable options, and implementation of available resources for resolution. The interpersonal nursing process is present and interactive, using associated and appropriate nursing intervention skills, which incorporate the roles of the nurse as resource person, educator, mentor, transfer agent, and counselor. Peplau's model requires that the nurse have self-awareness and insight regarding her or his own behaviors. This awareness may be applied in identifying and working through those behaviors unique to the client's schema. Fig. 5.2 presents Peplau's psychodynamic nursing model.

Martha E. Rogers (1970)—Science of Unitary Human Beings: Humans as Energy Fields That Interact Constantly With the Environment

According to Rogers theory, when the client-human unit incurs an insult that renders them out of balance with the universe, nursing interventions must be geared toward helping the client-human unit attain an increasingly complex balance and synchronicity with the universe. Essential to Rogers theory is the belief that each being is unique and consists of more than the collective sum of parts, and that each being is constantly evolving in a forward momentum as they interact continually with the surrounding environmental field. Rogers's theory states that a brain integration is necessary to support the notion of human-environmental synergy, using the right side of the brain to recognize every human unit's capacity for imagery, sensation, and emotion and the left side of the brain for language, abstraction, and thought.

Dorothea Orem (1971)—Self-Care Deficit Model: Self-Care, Self-Care Deficits, and Nursing Systems

When a client incurs an insult that renders them incapable of fully functioning, deficient self-care occurs, which makes nursing intervention necessary. The object of Orem's theory is to restore the client's self-care

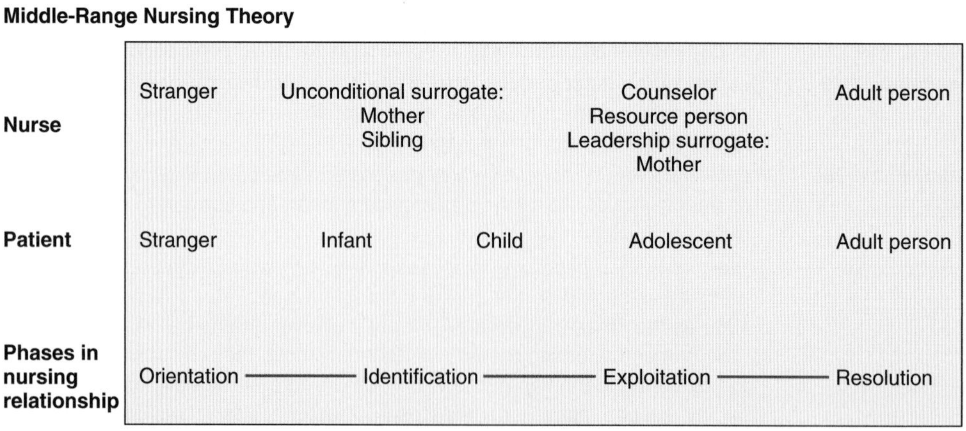

Middle-Range Nursing Theory

Nurse	Stranger	Unconditional surrogate: Mother Sibling	Counselor Resource person Leadership surrogate: Mother	Adult person
Patient	Stranger	Infant Child	Adolescent	Adult person
Phases in nursing relationship	Orientation ———— Identification ———— Exploitation ———— Resolution			

Fig. 5.2 Peplau's psychodynamic nursing model: Phases and changing roles in nurse–patient relationships. (From Peplau, H.E. [1952]. *Interpersonal relations in nursing* [p. 54]. GP Putnam.)

capability to enable them to sustain structural reliability, performance, and growth through purposeful nursing intervention. The aim of such intervention is to help the client cope with unmet care needs by acquiring the maximal level of function. This would be to either regain previous function or maximize available function present after the insult, hence restoring a sense of well-being.

Sister Callista Roy (1974)—Adaptation Model: Assistance With the Adaptation to Stressors to Facilitate the Integration Process of the Client

When the client incurs an insult that renders them in need of environmental modification, the nurse is the agent of change to assist the individual with this adaptation. Helping the "biopsychosocial" client to modify external stimuli allows adaptation to occur. In the case of illness, the outcome is a diminution or absence of integration of the constantly changing setting known as the *illness environment* with the constantly changing human, who is interacting with the existing outside surroundings. To attain wellness, adaptation must occur through this integration. The nurse's role is to promote this adaptation by modifying and regulating peripheral stimuli to enable the client's adaptation and integration with a supportive, healing environment. In so doing, the nurse is instrumental in assisting the client with the areas of health and well-being, life worth and value, and self-respect and dignity. See Sister Callista Roy's adaptation model at https://nursingtheoryandtheoristsroyorem. weebly.com/roy-theory-analysis.

Madeline Leininger (1977)—Theory of Cultural Care Diversity and Universality

Transcultural nursing and caring nursing concepts are aimed toward caring and the components of a culture care theory. In Leininger's theory, diversity, universality, worldview, and ethnohistory are essential to the four concepts of care, caring, health, and nursing.

Jean Watson (1978)—Theory of Human Caring: Transpersonal Caring as the Fulcrum; Philosophy and Science as the Core of Nursing

When the client incurs an insult that renders them in need, the transpersonal process between the client and the nurse is considered a healing nursing intervention.

An assumption of Watson's theory is that everyone requires human caring to quell need. Hence, the transpersonal process of "caring," or the caring among nurse, environment, and client, is essential to healing. Caring promotes the notion that every human being strives for interconnectedness with other humans and with nature. The nurse who implements these "carative" factors is the facilitator in the goal of restoring congruence between the client's perceived self and the existent self through the promotion of health and equilibrium. The expectation is that the client will experience balance and harmony in mind, body, and soul. Harmony, or wellness, will prevail, whereas disharmony, or illness, will be altered, eliminated, or circumvented.

Margaret Newman (1979, Revised 1986)—Health as Expanding Consciousness

Margaret Newman's theory defines health as "expanding consciousness," or increasing complexity. The theory of health as expanding consciousness was stimulated by concern for those for whom health, defined as the absence of disease or disability, is not possible. Nurses often relate well to people facing the uncertainty, debilitation, loss, and eventual death associated with chronic illness. The theory has progressed to include the health of all persons regardless of the presence or absence of disease. The theory asserts that every person in every situation, no matter how disordered and hopeless it may seem, is part of the universal process of expanding consciousness—a process of becoming more of oneself, of finding greater meaning in life, and of reaching new dimensions of connectedness with other people and the world. For more information, visit https://nursology. net/nurse-theories/newmans-theory-of-health-as-expanding-consciousness/.

Merle Mishel (1981, Revised 1990)—Uncertainty of Illness

Uncertainty in illness is frequently a stress-producing incident that is capable of contributing to negative physical and/or psychologic outcomes. Uncertainty exists when the client is unsure about a diagnosed illness. This uncertainty renders the client incapable of assigning a concrete value either to the illness itself or to a predictable outcome. Uncertainty can occur when a client misperceives a diagnosed illness because the information received is inadequate, the health care provider incorrectly presumes client knowledge, or the health care informant fails to recognize the client's individual unique filtering of provided illness information. Mishel's theory is used in chronic illness and other practice settings. Mishel's model outlines a four-step approach in defining her theory: (1) stimuli frame: antecedents generating client uncertainty; (2) appraisal stage: client assignment of a value (positive or negative) to the uncertainty; (3) initiation of coping mechanisms: client ability to develop, improvise, and implement skills to cope with uncertainty; and (4) adaptation: positive client assimilation and accommodation to uncertainty, resulting from effective coping. Mishel's theory establishes a framework that guides nursing practice by assisting nurses to work with clients in establishing interventions that promote positive outcomes.

Gisele Saraiva Bispo Hirano, Alba Lucia Bottura, Leite de Barros, Viviane Martins Silva (2023)—Situation-Specific Theory for Health Management in Heart Failure

This situation-specific theory was developed by linking concepts from Orem's Self-Care Deficit Nursing Theory and standardized nursing languages with the purpose of explaining and describing the health management of outpatients with heart failure. This theory suggests that the health management of these patients is influenced by basic conditioning factors, which may affect individuals' health management capability and may interfere with the ability to present health management behaviors. Knowing the ability of these patients to manage their health will allow nurses to plan their interventions, which will reflect directly on a patient's quality of life, and reduce the chances of hospitalization and health costs (Hirano et al., 2023).

History of Nursology.net

This website project was conceived and developed by members of the Theory-Guided Practice Expert Panel of the American Academy of Nursing in the fall of 2017. The members of the Expert Panel recognized a growing crisis of confidence in the discipline. This website was unveiled in September 2018. Nursology.net is a web site for nurse scholars, developed and maintained by nurse scholars. Founders of the website chose the word nursology to denote knowledge development and testing. Specifically, the web site is a repository for resources about nursing conceptual models, grand theories, middle-range theories, and situation-specific theories, philosophies, and associated methodologies.

The mission of nursology.net is to provide access to sentinel, contemporary, comprehensive, and authentic nursing knowledge development to facilitate advancement of nursing science and humanistic initiatives worldwide and across time.

Specifically, the purposes of this site are to:
- Be the nurse-led, nurse-developed repository providing the most current and accurate information about nursing discipline-specific knowledge that advances human betterment globally.
- Promote nursing discipline-specific knowledge that will advance human betterment globally.
- Facilitate accessibility to historic and contemporary nursing knowledge across time.
- Provide access to links to nursing theory-based organizations, conferences, notable and foundational publications, and ongoing work in practice, research, education, and health policy.
- Foster collaboration among nurse scholars at local, regional, national, and international levels.

Nursing Theory Institutes. According to Nursology.net, there are 18 theory-focused organizations globally, chiefly comprised on societies, associations, institutes, and groups with a mission to support nursing knowledge development through theory, research, practice and education. Watson's Caring Science Institute https://www.watsoncaringscience.org/, the Anne Boykin Institute for the Advancement of Caring in Nursing housed in Florida Atlantic University—Christine E. Lynn College of Nursing, https://nursing.fau.edu/outreach/anne-boykin-institute/index.php, and The Dr. Margaret A. Newman Center for Nursing Theory, which opened in May 2023, are the three nursing theory institutes worldwide. As a physical and virtual space, the Newman Center is unique as it is supported by an endowment from the theorist with an archive of more than 15 cubic feet of a special collection of Dr. Newman's scholarly work and personal items designed and organized by her.

Nursology https://nursology.net/resources/organizations/theory-focused-groups/

FUTURE OF NURSING THEORIES AND THEORISTS

At no time in history have so many health care concerns been the primary focus of federal and state legislative agendas. New questions are being asked in the 21st century about how health care is being conducted and managed. It is imperative that nurses be on the front-lines to provide testimony in response to these queries.

The current nursing shortage, scarce resources, patient safety and medical errors, managed care, Medicare, welfare-to-work plans, confidentiality issues, parity of reimbursement, advanced practice nurses and their scope of practice, mandatory overtime, whistle-blower protection, prescriptive authority, licensure, multistate compacts, telemedicine, and many other policy issues that directly affect nursing practice are coming before the US Congress and individual state legislative bodies for practice-related decisions. The direct effect on nursing cannot be overemphasized.

As nursing continues to operate in an environment of ongoing change, outcome data will be analyzed in an effort to provide quality care and access to that care for all clients in need of health care services. Therefore, one may predict that established nursing theories will be reevaluated and modified accordingly. New theories will be created and developed that may help answer the health care questions of the 21st century. Simply put, nursing theories in the 21st century will embrace complex environmental changes that incorporate new technologies such as genetics, computers, noninvasive surgery, robotics, decreasing energy sources, increasing pollutants under a thinning ozone layer, environmental hazards, new diseases, and antibiotic-resistant illness. These changes have already resulted in client needs that differ from those that occurred in the past.

SUMMARY

To summarize the chapter, let's review the questions posed at the beginning of the chapter and see what you have learned.

1. What is nursing theory?

   The compilation of data that define, describe, and logically relate information that will explain past nursing phenomena and predict future trends. Theories provide a foundation for developing models or frameworks for nursing practice development.

2. How is nursing theory different from the theory of other disciplines?

   Just as in any other discipline, nursing theory has its own unique language. The words of this language identify linkages between the database of scientific nursing knowledge and the extracted information taken from this source for nursing theory. The interpretation of these words translates uniquely to the theory investigated. This application, or language of nursing theory, is the structure, or framework, from which one understands the theory.

3. How does theory relate to nursing practice?

   In the practice model, the clinician decides what areas to directly assess, when to assess, and which intervention to implement. These decisions may or may not be knowingly based on a model or theory. Regardless, often the outcome supports the notion that behavior replicates a theoretic model, even though the nurse may be unaware that they are using a theoretic model in the practice process. Evidence-based theories (i.e., theories that are empirically supported through well-designed studies) are used by nurses for clinical decision-making (Melnyk & Fineout-Overholt, 2019). Nurses use critical thinking to adapt theories as needed to their patient situations.

4. Why is it important to understand nursing theory?

   Nursing theory can guide research and practice by serving as a roadmap.

5. Why is it important for nurses to develop theory?

   As nursing continues to operate in an environment of ongoing change, outcome data will be analyzed in an effort to provide quality care and access to that care for all clients in need of health care services. Therefore, one may predict that established nursing theories will be reevaluated and modified accordingly. New theories will need to be developed and tested that may help answer the health care questions of the 21st century. Client needs differ from those that occurred in the past and new theories are needed to help guide client care.

   Practice and theory are interdependent entities. In other words, practice and theory cannot efficiently or effectively exist one without the other. As in the metaphor at the beginning of this chapter, without the existence of the scientific data (stones) the organization of specific, concentrated yet related areas (house, theory) could not have happened.

REFERENCES

Abdellah, F.G. (1969). The nature of nursing science. *Nursing Research, 18*(5), 393.

Anastasi, A. (1958). Heredity, environment, and the question "how"?. *Psychological Review, 65*(4), 197–208.

Beck, C.T. (2012). *Exemplar: Teetering on the edge: A second grounded theory modification.* In P.L. Munhall (Ed.), *Nursing research. A qualitative perspective* (5th ed.) Jones & Bartlett, pp. 257–284.

Cook, E. (1942). *The life of Florence Nightingale.* Macmillan.

Donaldson, S.K., & Crowley, D.M. (1978). The discipline of nursing. *Nursing Outlook, 26*(2), 113–120.

Hirano, G.S.B., Barros, A.L.B.L., Silva, V.M.D. (2023). Situation-specific theory for health management in heart failure. *Nursing Science Quarterly, 36*(3):264–272. doi: 10.1177/08943184231169757. PMID: 37309148.

Jacob, S. (1996). The grief process of older women whose husbands received hospice care. *Journal of Advanced Nursing, 24*(2), 280–286.

Jacox, A.K. (1974). Theory construction in nursing: An overview. *Nursing Research, 23*(1), 4.

Lenz, E.R., & Pugh, L.C. (2003). *Theory of unpleasant symptoms.* In M.J. Smith, P. Liehr (Eds.), *Middle range theory for nursing.* Springer.

Melnyk, B.M., & Fineout-Overholt, E. (2019). *Evidence-based practice in nursing and healthcare: A guide to best practice* (4th ed.) Lippincott Williams & Wilkins/Wolters Kluwer.

Mishel, M.H. (1981). The measurement of uncertainty in illness. *Nursing Research, 30*(5), 258–263.

Mishel, M.H. (1997). Uncertainty in acute illness. *Annual Review of Nursing Research, 15*, 57–80.

Nightingale, F. (1859). *Notes on nursing: What it is, and what it is not.* Harrison and Sons.

Nightingale, F. (1992). *Notes on nursing: What it is, and what it is not* (commemorative edition). Lippincott.

Murdaugh, C., Parsons, M., & Pender, N.J. (2015). *Health promotion in nursing practice* (7th ed.) Prentice Hall.

Polit, D., & Beck, C. (2017). *Nursing research* (10th ed.) Wolters Kluwer Health/Lippincott.

Polit, D., & Beck, C. (2022). *Nursing research* (10th ed.) Wolters Kluwer Health/Lippincott.

Sacred Heart University. (2013). Nursing grand theory and theorists: Roy and Orem - Roy: Theory Analysis (weebly.com). Retrieved August 31, 2023.

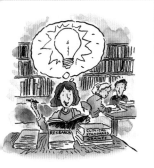

6

Nursing Research and Evidence-Based Practice

Leslie Moro, DNP, APRN, FNP-BC*

*~sing research provides the foun-
~ion for evidence-based nursing
~ctice.*

ⓔ Additional resources are available online at: http://evolve.elsevier.com/Cherry/

LEARNING OUTCOMES

After studying this chapter, the reader will be able to:
1. Summarize major points in the evolution of nursing research in relation to contemporary nursing.
2. Evaluate the influence of nursing research on current nursing and health care practices.
3. Differentiate among nursing research methods.
4. Critically appraise the quality of research studies using established criteria.
5. Participate in the research process.
6. Use research findings to improve nursing practice.

KEY TERMS

Abstract A brief overview of a research study.

Clinical nurse leader (CNL) An advanced practice nurse who provides clinical leadership and promotes safe, quality patient care.

Clinical nurse specialist (CNS) An advanced practice nurse who provides direct care to clients and participates in health education and research.

Clinical practice guideline (CPG) An evidence-based guide to clinical practice developed by experts in a particular field for direct application in clinical environments.

Control group Subjects in an experiment who do not receive the experimental treatment and whose performance provides a baseline against which the effects of the treatment can be measured. When a true experimental design is not used, this group is called a comparison group.

Data collection The process of acquiring existing information or developing new information.

Empirical Having a foundation based on data gathered through the senses (e.g., observation or experience) rather than purely through theorizing or logic.

Ethnography A qualitative research method for the purpose of investigating cultures that involve data collection, description, and analysis of data to develop a theory of cultural behavior.

Evidence-based practice (EBP) The process of systematically finding, appraising, and using research findings as the basis for clinical practice.

Experimental design A design that includes randomization, a control group, and manipulation between or among variables to examine probability and causality among selected variables for the purpose of predicting and controlling phenomena.

Generalizability The inference that findings can be generalized from the sample to the entire population.

Grant Proposal developed to seek research funding from private or public agencies.

6

*We thank Rosemary A. McLaughlin, PhD, CNE, RN-NIC, and Zoila V. Sanchez, PhD, FNP, for their contributions to this chapter in the 8th edition.

Grounded theory A qualitative research design used to collect and analyze data aiming to develop theories grounded in real-world observations.

Integrative research review (IRR) Methodology that simultaneously synthesizes several experimental and nonexperimental research findings to provide a comprehensive understanding of the phenomena of interest.

Meta-analysis Statistical method of quantitative synthesis of findings from several studies to determine what is known about a phenomenon.

Meta-synthesis Interpretive translations produced from the integration or comparison of findings from qualitative studies.

Methodologic Research design used to develop the validity and reliability of instruments that measure research concepts and variables.

Naturalistic paradigm Holistic view of nature and the direction of science that guides qualitative research.

Needs assessment Study in which the researcher estimates the resource needs of a group.

Peer review A process by which a scholarly work (such as a paper or a research proposal) is checked by a group of experts in the same field to make sure it meets the necessary standards before it is published or accepted.

Phenomenology Qualitative research design employing inductive descriptive methodology to describe the lived experiences of study participants.

Pilot study Conduct of a smaller version of a proposed study that develops or refines methodology prior to use in a larger study.

Practice guidelines Research-based recommendations stated as standards of practice, procedures, or decision algorithms.

Qualitative research Systematic, subjective approach used to describe life experiences and give them meaning.

Quantitative research Formal, objective, systematic process used to describe and test relationships and examine cause-and-effect interactions among variables.

Quasiexperimental research A type of quantitative research study design that lacks one of the components of an experimental design (i.e., randomization, control group, manipulation of one or more variables).

Randomization The assignment of subjects to treatment conditions in a random manner (determined by chance alone).

Secondary analysis A research design in which data previously collected in another study are analyzed for different aims than the original study.

Survey A nonexperimental research design that focuses on obtaining information regarding the status quo of a situation, often through direct questioning of participants.

Translational research The work of interprofessional teams in applying research findings to practice.

Triangulation The use of a variety of methods to collect data on the same concept.

PROFESSIONAL/ETHICAL ISSUES

Issue 1

Mary Smith is a 19-year-old female who comes to the health department women's center complaining about vaginal itching, foul-smelling discharge, and pain with sexual intercourse. She admits to being sexually active for the last 2 years with multiple partners and a prior history of trichomoniasis infections, twice within the last year. Ms. Smith has been on an oral contraceptive pill for the last 2 years and her last menstrual cycle was 4 days ago. Ms. Smith admits that there is family history of cervical cancer. Her mother was diagnosed

and treated in 1992 for this condition. Ms. Smith has never had a Pap test. Ms. Smith stated, "The family planning center just did blood work to make sure I was not pregnant and gave me a prescription for oral contraceptive pills."

As a registered nurse, you are aware that family history of cervical cancer needs further inquiry and follow-up. A vaginal examination is performed by a nurse practitioner, with findings of multiple fleshy, soft, pale-colored growths on the vagina and perianal area. As a nurse, you are aware that most cervical cancers are caused by certain oncogenic (cancer-causing) strains of the human papillomavirus (HPV). Owing to the family history of cervical cancer, you anticipate that the nurse practitioner will follow up with a Pap test on this patient.

However, the current practice guidelines of the American Cancer Society and the American Society for Colposcopy and Cervical Pathology recommend that women younger than 21 years should not be screened (Pap test) for cervical cancer or HPV, regardless of whether they are sexually active.

Issue 2

One of the latest epidemics in the United States involves the use and misuse of opioid analgesics. Although opioids can be safe and effective for certain pain conditions, such as postoperative acute pain and end-of-life pain, the long-term use of opioids to treat chronic pain is highly debatable. As a result, these conflicting reports have led to an increase in the misuse of opioids that has resulted in opioid hyperalgesia and an increase in opioid-related deaths.

Your friend in nursing school is getting her wisdom tooth removed and you have gone with her to drive her home. An opioid is offered for pain control. As a nurse, what would you do?

VIGNETTE

I did not understand why I had to take a research class when all I wanted to do was be a staff nurse in a critical care unit. Research? Evidence-based practice? Why are these topics in the nursing program? I have enough to do just learning all the content in my clinical courses. What do research and evidence have to do with developing my nursing abilities? I trust the faculty, the textbooks, and clinical experience to prepare me for nursing. I'm already getting what I need to know.

That was my earlier attitude. Now that I am practicing, I have a new appreciation for nursing research and the evidence it provides for application to practice. I have an entirely different way of addressing clinical questions. I'm starting to ask questions about how I can improve the care I give to patients and how I can be involved in my workplace's efforts to improve care for the patients it serves. I have discovered by purposeful reading in my practice area that research reports and research summaries contain many implications that apply to practice in the critical care unit.

Questions to Consider While Reading This Chapter:

1. How can a desire to read research and evidence-based practice literature in students be facilitated?
2. How does research affect nursing practice?
3. How can nurses motivate colleagues to base their practice on research?

CHAPTER OVERVIEW

This chapter provides basic knowledge regarding the research process and the ultimate importance of evidence-based nursing practice. The intent is to inspire an appreciation for nursing research and to show both how it can improve nursing practice and how results can be translated into health policy. *Nursing research* is defined as a systematic approach used to examine phenomena important to nursing and nurses. A summary of major points in the evolution of nursing research in relation to contemporary nursing is presented. A description of private and public organizations that fund research is given, and their research priorities are listed. Major research designs are briefly described, and examples of each are given. Nurses of all educational levels are encouraged to participate in and promote nursing research at varying degrees. Evidence-based practice (EBP) is the use of the best scientific evidence, integrated with clinical experience and incorporating patients' values and preferences in the practice of professional nursing. Competencies have been developed to ensure that nurses are competent in providing EBP care and its uniformity in the application and generation of evidence. The process of locating research and evidence, including practice guidelines, is reviewed. Students are introduced to the research process and guided in the process of critically appraising published research and research syntheses. Ethical issues related to research are examined, and historical examples of unethical research are given. The functions of the institutional review board (IRB) and the use of informed consent in protecting the rights of human subjects are emphasized.

DEFINITION OF NURSING RESEARCH

Research is a process of systematic inquiry or study to build knowledge in a discipline. The purpose of research is to develop an empirical body of knowledge for a discipline or profession. Specifically, research validates and refines existing knowledge and develops new knowledge (LoBiondo-Wood & Haber, 2021). The results of the research process provide a foundation on which practice decisions and behaviors are laid. Research results create a strong scientific base for nursing practice, especially when deliberately and carefully evaluated for application to specific clinical topics (Melnyk & Fineout-Overholt, 2023).

Nursing research is a systematic approach used to examine phenomena important to nursing and nurses. Because nursing is a practice profession, it is important that clinical practice be based on scientific knowledge. Evidence generated by nursing research provides support for the quality and cost-effectiveness of nursing interventions. Thus, recipients of health care—and particularly nursing care—reap benefits when nurses attend to research evidence and introduce change based on that evidence into nursing practice. The introduction of evidence-based change into the direct provision of nursing care may occur at the individual level, with a particular nurse, or at varied organizational or social levels. Research within the realms of nursing education, nursing administration, health services, characteristics of nurses, and nursing roles provide evidence for effectively changing these supporting areas of nursing knowledge (LoBiondo-Wood & Haber, 2021).

EVOLUTION OF NURSING RESEARCH

Nursing research began with the work of Florence Nightingale during the Crimean War. After Florence Nightingale's work, the pattern that nursing research followed was closely related to the problems confronting nurses. For example, nursing education was the focus of most research studies between 1900 and 1940. As more nurses received their education in a university setting, studies regarding student characteristics and satisfactions were conducted. As more nurses pursued a college education researchers became interested in studying nurses. Questions such as what type of person enters nursing and how are nurses perceived by other groups guided research investigations. Teaching, administration, and curriculum were topics that dominated nursing research until the 1970s. By the 1970s, more doctorally prepared nurses were conducting research, and there was a shift to studies that focused on the improvement of patient care. The 1980s brought nursing research to a

new stage of development. There were many more qualified nurse researchers, widespread availability of computers for collection and analysis of data, and a realization that research is a vital part of professional nursing (Polit & Beck, 2021). Nurse researchers began conducting studies based on the naturalistic paradigm. These studies were qualitative rather than quantitative. In addition, instead of conducting many small, unrelated research studies, teams of researchers, often interdisciplinary, began conducting programs of research to build bodies of knowledge related to specific topics, such as urinary incontinence, decubitus ulcers, pain, and quality of life. The 1990s brought increasing concern about health care reform, and now, in the 21st century, research studies focus on important health care delivery issues such as cost, quality, and access. With the developing educational emphasis on the doctorate in nursing practice degree, research emphasis on patient care foci is gaining momentum, especially in view of the quality gaps highlighted by sentinel reports from the Institute of Medicine (2001, 2011).

Increasingly, research findings are being used as the basis for clinical decisions. Evidence-based practice can be defined as the process of systematically finding, appraising, and using research findings as a basis for making decisions about patient care (Dang et al., 2022). The rise of technology and the worldwide access to and flow of information have transformed the decision-making processes of practitioners. No longer do nurses and other health care professionals simply compare outcomes of patient care between units in the same hospital; solutions, choices, and outcomes are sought on an international level. Hospitals must show improved outcomes and clinical practice based on current evidence. In recent decades, the nursing discipline is paying greater attention to the necessity of participating in research, as evidenced by the maintenance of magnet status for facilities (Dang et al., 2022).

RESEARCH PRIORITIES

Why set priorities for research in the nursing discipline? Can nurses do research in areas that match personal areas of interest? The answer to the second question is yes, certainly. But nursing exists to provide high-quality nursing care to individuals in need of health-promoting, health-sustaining, and health-restoring strategies. The main outcome of research activity for a nurse is to put the knowledge gained to work in health care delivery. Research priorities, often set by groups that fund research, encourage nurse researchers to invest effort and money into those areas of research likely to generate the most benefit to recipients of care.

Two major sources of funding for nursing research are the National Institute of Nursing Research (NINR) and the Agency for Healthcare Research and Quality (AHRQ), which are both funded by federal congressional appropriations. Private foundations and nursing organizations also provide funding for nursing research.

National Institute of Nursing Research

As part of the National Institutes of Health (NIH), NINR supports research on the biologic and behavioral aspects of critical health problems that confront the nation. The NINR's focus is designed to advance the "science of health" by encompassing four key themes: symptom science (promoting personalized health strategies); wellness (promoting health and preventing illness); self-management (improving quality of life for individuals with chronic illness); and end-of-life and palliative care (the science of compassion) (NINR, 2022).

The areas of research emphasis published by the NINR are useful guides for investigators developing proposals but are not considered prescriptive in nature. Investigators bring to bear their own unique expertise and creativity when proposing research in harmony with NINR priority research areas. Recently, the NINR Innovative Questions Initiative was launched to encourage new research questions, new thinking, and creativity in nursing to promote results-oriented innovations. This allowed for identification, discussion, and debate (Grady, 2014).

The NINR's 2022–2026 Strategic Plan identifies their guiding principles and research lenses. Guiding principles for NINR-supported research describe valued qualities of research. These principles state that: NINR research is innovative; promotes equity, diversity, and inclusion; addresses current challenges; and focuses on solutions for health improvement (NINR, 2022). The NINR research lenses focus on health equity, social determinants of health, population and community health, disease prevention and health promotion, and systems and models of care (NINR, 2022).

Agency for Healthcare Research and Quality

The AHRQ broadly defines its mission as producing evidence to make health care "safer, higher quality, more accessible, equitable, and affordable" (AHRQ, 2023). As an agency of the US Department of Health and Human Services, the AHRQ has health-related aims: to reduce the risk of harm by promoting delivery of the best possible health care, improve health care outcomes by encouraging the use of evidence to make informed health care decisions, transform research into practice to facilitate wider access to effective health care services, and reduce unnecessary costs (AHRQ, 2022). Since the inception of the agency in 1989, strategic goals have centered on supporting improvements in health outcomes, strengthening measurement of health care quality indicators, and fostering access to and cost-effectiveness of health care. The 1999 reauthorizing legislation expanded the role of the agency by directing the AHRQ to:
- Improve the quality of health care through scientific inquiry, dissemination of findings, and facilitation of public access to information.
- Promote patient safety and reduce medical errors through scientific inquiry, building partnerships with health care providers, and establishing centers for education and research on therapeutics.
- Advance the use of information technology for coordinating patient care and conducting quality and outcomes research.
- Establish an office on priority populations to ensure that the needs of low-income groups, minorities, women, children, older adults, and individuals with special health care needs are addressed by the agency's research efforts.

The research-related activities of the AHRQ are quite varied, but a recent shift emphasizes a more deliberate translation of research evidence into practice. In a process similar to that used by the NIH, investigators are invited to submit research proposals for possible funding through grant announcements. A listing of current areas of the agency's research interests can be found online at https://www.ahrq.gov/innovations/index.html.

The AHRQ actively promotes EBP, partially through the establishment of nine evidence-based practice centers (EBPCs) in the United States and Canada. EBPCs conduct research on assigned clinical care topics and generate reports on the effectiveness of health care methodologies. Health care providers may then use the evidence in developing site-specific guidelines that direct clinical practice. Another addition to AHRQ's initiatives is the Healthcare Innovations Exchange (AHRQ, 2021), which provides a public source of information about innovations taking place in health care delivery. Submitted innovations are reviewed for the quality of achieved outcomes, providing evidence as a foundation for decision-making by others who may be searching for or considering similar innovations. Although most AHRQ activities are intended to support health care professionals and institutions, the agency supports health care recipients by designing some information specifically for dissemination to the lay public (AHRQ, 2021).

Private Foundations

Obtaining money for research is becoming increasingly competitive, so voluntary foundations and private and community-based organizations should be investigated as possible funding sources. Many foundations and corporate direct-giving programs are interested in funding health care projects and research. Computer databases and guides to funding are available in local libraries. In addition, grant-seeking enterprises often purchase subscriptions that allow computer access to enhanced listings of funding foundations that include information about the types of projects those foundations typically fund. Although such subscriptions are expensive, costs are often balanced by the efficiency with which suitable funding prospects are identified. An example of such a service is Prospect Research Online that can be accessed at https://www.prospectresearchinstitute.org/.

Private foundations, such as the Robert Wood Johnson Foundation (2023a, 2023b) and the W.K. Kellogg Foundation (https://www.wkkf.org/grantseekers), offer program funding for health-related research. Investigators are encouraged to pursue funding for small projects through local sources or private foundations until they establish a track record in research design and implementation, which will then lead to securing of funding from public sources.

Nursing Organizations

Sigma Theta Tau International (STTI), the American Nurses Association (ANA), and the Oncology Nurses Society (ONS) are a few of the nursing organizations that fund research studies. STTI makes research grant awards to increase scientific knowledge related to nursing practice. This organization supports creative interdisciplinary research and places importance on identifying best practices and benchmark innovations. Awards are made at the international and local chapter levels. The ANA

awards small grants through the American Nurses Foundation. Specialty nursing organizations offer grants to support research related to their specialty. For example, the ONS awards grants that focus on issues related to oncology. A list of current nursing organizations offering funding opportunities can be found online at http://nursingworld.org/research-toolkit/Research-Funding.

Summary

Multiple potential sources of funding are available for research projects. The individual or group wishing to conduct research will need to carefully develop a proposal, search for a possible funding source, and submit the proposal. Libraries and the Internet provide ample information about the many foundations and organizations interested in funding research endeavors. Most research institutions establish offices that help in the search and procurement of funding that supports researchers in their work of knowledge building.

COMPONENTS OF THE RESEARCH PROCESS

The research process involves conceptualizing a research study, planning and implementing that study, and communicating the findings. The process involves a logical flow as each step builds on the previous steps. These steps should be included in published research reports so that the reader has a basis for understanding and critiquing the study (Box 6.1).

BOX 6.1   Components of the Research Process

Research is a process that takes place in a series of steps:
1. Formulating the research question or problem.
2. Defining the purpose of the study.
3. Reviewing related literature.
4. Formulating hypotheses and defining variables.
5. Selecting the research design.
6. Selecting the population, sample, and setting.
7. Conducting a **pilot study**.
8. Collecting the data.
9. Analyzing the data.
10. Communicating conclusions.

STUDY DESIGNS

Study designs are plans that tell a researcher how data are to be collected, from whom data are to be collected, and how data will be analyzed to answer specific research questions. Research studies are classified into two basic methods, quantitative and qualitative, two distinctly different approaches to conducting research. The researcher chooses the method on the basis of the research question and the current level of knowledge about the phenomena and the problem to be studied. Quantitative research is a formal, objective, systematic process in which numeric data are used. Qualitative research is a systematic approach used to describe and promote understanding of human experiences related to health in a nonnumeric fashion. The qualitative approach to research focuses on understanding the human experience as it is lived, thus complementing quantitative methodologies (LoBiondo-Wood & Haber, 2021).

Artificial Intelligence and Nursing Research

Artificial intelligence (AI) has the potential to impact nursing research with the recent increase in usage of AI-based chatbots, such as ChatGPT. Nurses need to reflect on the potential for ChatGPT to undermine values and principles that serve as the foundation for nursing research. There are ethical concerns with using such AI tools because they enable users to generate research papers without engaging in original thought or research. ChatGPT has been cited as a coauthor in recently published peer-reviewed nursing papers. This practice prompts many to question the suitability of an AI author who lacks accountability possessed by a human author (Abdulai & Hung, 2023).

Quantitative Designs

Arising from early scientific models for doing research, the nursing discipline directly adopted the quantitative method of conducting research. Thus, quantitative design has traditionally been prevalent in nursing research studies. Deriving meaning from the statistical analysis of numeric data obtained from samples and populations has yielded significant contributions to nursing knowledge. The usual intent of quantitative study is to apply or generalize knowledge from a smaller sample of subjects to a larger population. The most common quantitative designs used in health care research are survey, needs assessment, experimental,

quasiexperimental, methodologic, meta-analysis, and secondary analysis. A brief overview of these mostly quantitative study designs is given in Table 6.1. For in-depth understanding of particular methods and their suitability for studying particular phenomena, the reader should consult research methods texts.

Qualitative Designs

Qualitative research is designed for discovery rather than verification. It is used to explore little-understood or ambiguous phenomena rather than to verify a cause-and-effect issue. Qualitative methods can be important to the complex study of humans. Concepts that are important to health care professionals often are difficult to reduce in a quantitative way. Interviewing is the main technique used in qualitative methods to explore the meaning of certain experiences to individuals. This method is time-consuming and costly and uses small samples; therefore, generalizations cannot be made from findings. However, in an exploration of issues such as caregiver burden, it might be more appropriate to interview participants with open-ended questions to get their perspective rather than to send out a standard questionnaire, thereby broadening the data gathered. The main types of qualitative research designs include phenomenology, ethnography, and grounded theory. Table 6.2 provides brief descriptions of these methods. For a more complete understanding, the reader should refer to qualitative research texts.

Although there is a need for qualitative research studies in health care, qualitative one-on-one interviews take time; they must be recorded, typed, transcribed, and analyzed. Data analysis is conducted by the researcher, who then reviews each transcribed interview line by line to group common conceptual meanings. Concepts are combined to describe the experience for the particular group being studied. The researcher cannot assert that findings from a small unique sample would be the same in a large, diverse population. However, findings should be transferable. The researcher should give a thorough description of the sample and setting so that findings could be expected to occur in similar individuals in a similar setting. In addition, triangulation studies may provide the strength needed to increase generalizability of the findings.

Triangulation

Triangulation is the use of various research methods or different data collection techniques in the same study.

TABLE 6.1 A Sample of Quantitative Research Methodologies

Method	Description
Survey	Survey research designs are popular in nursing research studies that are designed to obtain information regarding the prevalence, distribution, and interrelationships of variables within a population. This is a useful design for the collection of demographic information, social characteristics, behavioral patterns, and information bases.
Needs assessment	Needs assessments are used to determine what is most beneficial to a specific aggregate group. This design can be used by organizations, communities, or groups to establish priorities for their respective client groups (Polit & Beck, 2021).
Methodologic	Methodologic research focuses on the development of data collection instruments, such as surveys and questionnaires. The goal is to improve the reliability and validity of instruments. This work is time-consuming and tedious, but necessary for the implementation of research studies. However, when quality instruments are developed, they can be used in multiple studies.
Meta-analysis	Meta-analysis is an advanced process whereby multiple research studies on a specific topic are reviewed and the findings of these studies are statistically analyzed. Meta-analysis synthesizes quantitative data from multiple similar studies, thus enlarging the power of the results and allowing more confident generalizations than a single study.
Experimental study	Experimental studies, having several subtypes, include the manipulation of one or more independent variables, random assignment to either a control group or treatment group, and observation of the outcome or effect that presumably is a result of the independent variable. Rigor and control of extraneous variables allow researchers to establish cause-and-effect relationships, testing causal relationships (Polit & Beck, 2021).
Quasiexperimental design	A quasiexperimental design is lacking one of the required components of the experimental design. This is a useful design when randomization, a control group, or the manipulation of one or more variables is not possible. Several subtypes exist.
Secondary analysis	Secondary analysis involves asking new questions of data collected previously. The data may have been generated from previous formal research or may have resulted from any prior systematic collection of data. Examples of prior nonresearch data include the many inevitable records generated as a by-product of health care delivery systems.

TABLE 6.2 A Sample of Qualitative Research Methodologies

Method	Description
Phenomenology	Phenomenology is designed to provide understanding of the participants' "lived experience." This method is a valuable approach for studying intangible experiences such as grief, hope, and risk taking.
Ethnography	Ethnography is a method used to study phenomena from a cultural perspective. Ethnographers spend time in the cultural setting with the research participants to observe and better understand their experience.
Grounded theory	Grounded theory is designed to explore and describe a social process. This method is used to explore a process that people use to deal with problematic areas of their lives, such as coping with a terminal illness or adjusting to bereavement.

Triangulation commonly refers to the use of qualitative and quantitative methods in the same study. This method can be useful when data from multiple sources and methods are necessary to provide a holistic understanding of the subject matter.

Pilot Studies

Pilot studies are small-scale studies used to identify the strengths and limitations of a planned larger-scale study. Pilot work is preliminary research that can be used to assess the design, methodology, and feasibility of a study, and typically includes participants who are similar to those who will be used in the larger research study. By performing each step, the researcher can evaluate the effectiveness of the proposed data collection methods to improve and assess the feasibility of the study (LoBiondo-Wood & Haber, 2021). Pilot studies can serve to discover preliminary trends in outcomes for a particular agency, personnel, and clients.

EVIDENCE-BASED PRACTICE AND RESEARCH UTILIZATION

From the beginnings of the nursing research endeavor, nurses have been interested in using nursing research to effectively affect the care of individuals and aggregate groups. Despite other incentives for the conduct of research, none is more powerful for a nurse than the difference that might be made in the lives of individuals and aggregates for the betterment of health. Thus, early emphasis in the 1980s on research utilization has been expanded, with the increasing emphasis on EBP. Although the terms *research utilization* and *evidence-based practice* are related, research utilization has been described as a subset of EBP (LoBiondo-Wood & Haber, 2021). EBP encompasses multiple types of evidence, such as research findings, research reviews, and evidence-based theory, and the integration of that evidence with clinician's expertise and patient preferences and values (Melnyk & Fineout-Overholt, 2023) (Box 6.2).

In this third decade of the 21st century, EBP has become a major driving force in the disciplinary life of clinicians, students, educators, administrators, and policymakers. Discussion on barriers to research utilization and EBP has shifted to how to actively promote implementation of EBP. Extensive work is being done on the best ways to translate research into practice, spawning a new area of health care science called *translation science*. The promise of translation science is eventually to provide guidance on the best ways to incorporate best evidence into health care, including nursing. As an example of translation strategy, White (2011) describes "nurse champions" as key agents in the "timely integration of discovery" into daily practice. Nurse champions will take ownership of a practice project and personally oversee a practice innovation process from discovery to adoption and dissemination. Table 6.2 provides brief

> ## BOX 6.2 Seven Steps of Evidence-Based Practice
>
> Here is a brief overview of the multistep process involved in evidence-based practice (EBP):
> 1. Cultivating a spirit of inquiring.
> 2. Asking a clinical question in the PICOT format (P, population; I, intervention or interest area; C, comparison intervention or group; O, outcome; and T, time).
> 3. Searching for and collecting the most relevant best evidence to answer the question. Reliable sources include systematic reviews, preappraised literature and studies from peer-reviewed journals, and practice guidelines.
> 4. Critically evaluating the evidence. Making rapid critical appraisal of the findings (evidence) for validity, reliability, and applicability, then synthesizing that evidence.
> 5. Integrating the best evidence with one's clinical expertise and patient preferences and values in making a practice decision regarding whether a practice change should be made.
> 6. Evaluating outcomes of the practice decision or change on the basis of the evidence. Outcomes should be measured to determine the positive or negative outcomes of the change.
> 7. Disseminating the outcomes of the EBP decision or change through presentations or publications so that others can benefit from the process.

descriptions of the steps involved in the EBP process. Whole texts are available that explain the multiple aspects of EBP, and various models have been proposed that more carefully detail the process of incorporating evidence into practice (Christenbery, 2018; Melnyk & Fineout-Overholt, 2023).

Advancing Evidence-Based Practice

How does one get started with EBP? A list of strategies for encouraging a climate of EBP is likely to look somewhat different depending on the context of care—a clinic, a hospital, or a conglomerate. A short list of broad strategies suggested by Melnyk and Fineout-Overholt (2023) applies regardless of the setting:

- Assessing barriers to EBP
- Correcting misperceptions about EBP goals and processes
- Questioning current clinical practices

Assessment should be as comprehensive as possible to identify the knowledge, beliefs, and behaviors that are common in the existing system and to raise the awareness of a need for shifting decision-making about clinical care toward a consideration of current best evidence. Raising questions about current clinical practices provides a strategy for getting the critical thinking juices flowing about particular clinical practices and problems. Individuals with common interests may form collaborative groups that further strengthen the EBP culture through bonding around specific patient problems and the discovery of evidence-based solutions. The specific tactics, processes, and events that undergird an EBP initiative require allocation of resources, creativeness, and dedication. Of particular significance to EBP initiatives is the availability of individuals in clinical environments who have the specific responsibility and expertise to understand and translate evidence into practice (Melnyk & Fineout-Overholt, 2023).

To facilitate and advance the use of EBP by nurses, specific EBP competencies have been developed for the practicing registered nurses (RNs) and advance practice nurses (APNs) (Tables 6.3 and 6.4). The online Merriam-Webster Dictionary generally defines competency as the quality of being competent to perform or capable of performing a function. ANA (2010) defines competency as "an expected and measurable level of nursing performance that integrates knowledge, skills, abilities, and judgement, based on scientific knowledge and expectations for nursing practice." Melnyk et al. (2016) outline 13 EBP competencies for RNs and APNs, and 11 EBP competencies specifically for APNs (Tables 6.3 and 6.4). The EBP competencies' goal is to ensure competency of nurses in providing EBP care and uniformity in the application and generation of EBP.

Nurse Researcher and Evidence-Based Practice Roles

Three nursing roles are specifically focused on research and EBP: the clinical nurse specialist, the clinical nurse leader, and the clinical research nurse.

Clinical Nurse Specialist. The clinical nurse specialist (CNS) is a registered nurse with graduate preparation in a specialized area of nursing practice and an expert clinician with additional responsibility for education and research. A CNS is in an ideal position to link research to practice by assessing an agency's

TABLE 6.3 Evidence-Based Practice (EBP) Competencies for Registered Nurses

Competency	Description
1	Questions clinical practices for the purpose of improving the quality of care
2	Describes clinical problems based on patient assessment date, outcomes management, and quality improvement data
3	Participates in the formulate clinical question using PICOT (P, population; I, intervention/area of interest; C, comparison/intervention group; O, outcome; T, time)
4	Systemically searches current evidence (evidence generated from research) to address clinical question
5	Participates in critical appraisal of preappraised evidence (i.e., clinical practice guidelines, EBP policies and procedures, evidence syntheses)
6	Participates in critical appraisal of published clinical research studies
7	Participates in the evaluation and synthesis of evidence retrieved
8	Systematically collects practice data (e.g., internal patient data, quality improvement, outcome data) for clinical decision-making used in providing patient care
9	Integrates evidence gathered from internal and external sources to plan EBP changes
10	Implements practice changes based on evidence and clinical expertise and patient's preferences to improve care processes and patient outcomes
11	Evaluates outcomes of evidence-based decisions and practice changes to determine best practices
12	Disseminates best practices supported by evidence to improve quality care and patient outcomes
13	Participates in strategies to sustain an evidence-based practice culture

From Melnyk, B.M., et al. (2016). *Implementing the evidence-based practice (EBP) competencies in healthcare*: A practical guide for improving quality, safety, and outcomes. Sigma Theta Tau International.

TABLE 6.4 **Evidence-Based Practice Competencies for Advance Practice Nurses**	
Competency	**Description**
14	Systematically conducts an exhaustive search for external evidence* (clinical research studies) to address clinical questions
15	Critically appraises relevant preappraised evidence (i.e., clinical guidelines, summaries, synthesis of external evidence)
16	Integrates external evidence from nursing and related fields with internal evidence (i.e., patient data, outcomes management, and quality improvement data)
17	Leads transdisciplinary teams in applying synthesized evidence to initiate clinical decisions and practices changes to improve the health of individuals, groups, and populations
18	Generates internal evidence through outcome management and EBP implementation projects
19	Measures process and outcomes of evidence-based clinical decisions
20	Formulates evidence-based policies and procedures
21	Participates in generation of external evidence with other health care professionals
22	Mentors others in evidence-based decision-making and EBP process
23	Implements strategies to sustain an EBP culture
24	Communicates best evidence to individuals, groups, colleagues, and policymakers

*External evidence refers to evidence generated from research. From Melnyk, B.M., et al. (2016). *Implementing the evidence-based practice (EBP) competencies in healthcare*: A practical guide for improving quality, safety, and outcomes. Sigma Theta Tau International.

readiness for research utilization, consulting with staff to identify clinical problems, and helping staff to discover, implement, and evaluate findings that improve health care delivery (National Association of Clinical Nurse Specialists, 2018).

The CNS also may need to communicate results to legislators or other policymakers if the results potentially affect health policy. Research evidence is important to policymaking because it provides a logical foundation for policy change. The process of writing brief summaries of evidence or personally testifying about particular topics should be approached carefully. One should know the target audience, the exact policy issue, the background of the issue, and the full range of pertinent evidence (Melnyk & Fineout-Overholt, 2023).

If agencies do not have a CNS, they should be encouraged to develop relationships with researchers in university settings or other agencies. Professors in academic settings are expected to conduct research and often are interested in collaborating with health care agencies that might serve as a site. These agencies often have the patient population that can serve as a study sample. For example, a university professor interested in home health care issues might collaborate with an agency to examine the efficacy of various health care delivery models for patients with congestive heart failure. In today's care environment, it would be essential for the agency to offer care that is the most effective and efficient. Therefore, this collaborative relationship would reward the researcher and the health care agency.

Case Study 6.1 is an illustration of how a CNS led efforts to use research findings to improve practice.

Clinical Nurse Leader. The clinical nurse leader (CNL) is a registered nurse with a master's level education who provides patient care and is prepared to practice in all clinical settings. The CNL serves as a leader in health care and implements EBP to improve patient-care processes and health care outcomes (AACN, 2024).

Clinical Research Nurse. The clinical research nursing role focuses on the care of research participants. "In addition to providing and coordinating clinical care, clinical research nurses have a central role in assuring participant safety, ongoing maintenance of informed consent, integrity of protocol implementation, accuracy of data collection, data recording and follow up" (Hastings, 2009, para. 2).

Emerging Roles. In addition to the CNS and CNL, there are emerging role definitions for the doctor of nursing practice (DNP). Given the specified role definitions published by the American Association of Colleges of Nursing (AACN), the CNL and DNP are considered to be major contributors to the advancement of nursing research and EBP (AACN, 2021a). CNLs use quality improvement methods in evaluating individual and aggregate client care and for self-improvement.

Nurses prepared at the DNP level provide leadership for EBP in nursing and translate evidence-based nursing research into their own practice. They are expected to disseminate and integrate new knowledge. Regardless of the official role definition, nurses at the point of care and nursing division leaders increasingly may be called upon to lead and contribute to collaborative research and EBP initiatives at the health care agency level (Melnyk & Fineout-Overholt, 2023).

The DNP-Prepared Nurse and Evidence-Based Practice. The AACN identified *Essentials for Advanced-Level Nursing Education*, or the curricular requirements and essential competencies for advanced practice registered nurses. The fourth essential refers to clinical scholarship and analytic methods for EBP (AACN, 2021a). The AACN acknowledges the role of the DNP-prepared nurse as a leader in translating research into practice or applying EBP to clinical practice. By teaching graduate students to critically analyze literature, DNP programs prepare graduates to discover and implement the best evidence for practice. The DNP-prepared nurse is taught to evaluate the need for quality improvement and practice guidelines and then apply research findings to develop practice guidelines and ultimately improve practice. In addition, these nurse leaders should disseminate findings from EBP and research to improve patient outcomes (AACN, 2021b).

About the Evidence

Practice decisions made from a foundation of evidence are more likely to be clear, rational, and motivational than those made from the foundation of mere authority. Although research evidence forms the backbone of EBP, other evidence types, such as patient values and preferences, expert opinion, theory-based information, evidence-based theories, and compiled database information, are also useful (Melnyk & Fineout-Overholt, 2023). When care is being delivered to an individual, evidence regarding patient assessment and resource availability must also be considered (Melnyk & Fineout-Overholt, 2023).

CASE STUDY 6.1

Mary, a CNS in a medical center, asks the staff nurses on a pediatric oncology unit to identify patient care problems that need to be investigated. The nurses identify pain control as a major problem for the children admitted to the unit. In talking with the nurses on the unit, Mary discovers that the nurses routinely use physiologic measures, such as heart rate and blood pressure, as indicators of pain. Occasionally, the nurses rely on parents' reports, but rarely do they consult the child.

Mary conducts a systematic review of the literature/evidence to determine proven ways to assess pain in children. In the *Western Journal of Nursing Research*, Mary discovers a meta-analysis of pediatric pain assessment techniques. Findings from this study indicate that self-report tools are appropriate for most children 4 years and older and provide the most accurate measure of children's pain. Mary discovers a pediatric pain interview tool in the literature that she thinks would be practical and feasible for use on the unit.

She then writes a utilization memo to the nurse manager citing the problem (inadequate pain control), the research findings documented in the literature, and a suggestion for change in practice (use of the self-report pain assessment) on the pediatric oncology unit. Next, Mary organizes a meeting with the nurses to discuss conducting a pilot study on the unit for the purpose of comparing the effectiveness of the pediatric pain assessment interview tool and their usual procedures for assessing pain in the pediatric oncology patients. Findings from this study are incorporated into practice through documentation of the preferred method of pain assessment in the unit's protocol.

The change instituted by the pediatric oncology unit is cited in the medical center's accreditation report as an example of how the medical center is meeting standards of care in pain management.

Locating Published Research and Evidence Summaries for Evidence-Based Practice

The health care literature is continually and rapidly expanding; the task of keeping up with relevant health care information is daunting. Strategies to facilitate access to research evidence include formulating a clear and concise clinical question, identifying the research design that would best answer the question, and identifying the most appropriate place to look for studies that answer the question.

Many health care practitioners routinely read clinical practice journals but are unfamiliar with research or EBP journals. Computerized databases aid the process of locating research relevant to current practice. These databases list article information, provide a short summary, identify key words, and provide links to similar articles. *Cumulative Index to Nursing and Allied Health Literature* (CINAHL, 2024) is an index of selected journal articles about nursing, allied health, biomedicine, and health care. MEDLINE (Medical Literature Analysis and Retrieval System Online) is the most comprehensive online resource for national and international medical literature (US National Library of Medicine, 2021). Multiple other useful databases may be available from academic and health care libraries. These databases consist largely of primary or original research studies, as well as guidelines and best practices (National Guideline Clearinghouse; https://www.thecommunityguide.org/index.html).

University and public libraries are the major access points to these databases and journals, which are available online directly from publishers. Because of online availability, novice users may be tempted to limit searches only to those articles that are available online as full text. *This is a serious mistake that any investigator of published literature should avoid.*

The search for literature should be conducted with the intent of procuring all or most of the current articles appropriate to answer the clinical question. A truly comprehensive reading of the literature may include all articles of current and historical relevance to the topic.

Even though nurses may have access to computerized databases to assist with a literature search, they often are unaware of the journals that are entirely devoted to the publication of research studies. Box 6.3 contains a list of research journals and other health-related journals that publish research and evidence summaries.

Other important sources for locating evidence are:
- *Clinical practice guidelines* are systematically developed statements to assist practitioner and patient decisions about appropriate health care for specific clinical circumstances. In the United Kingdom, the Cochrane Collaboration (Cochrane Library, 2023) (https://www.cochrane.org) is an electronic resource for locating high-quality information quickly. This resource has published hundreds of intervention guidelines based on meta-analyses and research reviews of health care practice areas. *Evidence-Based Nursing* (http://www.

BOX 6.3   Nursing and Health-Related Journals

Nursing
- *Advances in Nursing Science*
- *Applied Nursing Research*
- *Biological Research for Nursing*
- *Clinical Nursing Research*
- *Evidence-Based Nursing*
- *International Journal of Nursing Studies*
- *Journal of Nursing Scholarship*
- *Journal of Advanced Nursing*
- *Journal of Transcultural Nursing*
- *Nursing Clinics of North America*
- *Nursing Economics*
- *Nursing Research*
- *Nursing Science Quarterly*
- *Qualitative Health Research*
- *Research in Nursing and Health*
- *Western Journal of Nursing Research*
- *Worldviews on Evidence-Based Nursing*

Health
- *American Journal of Public Health*
- *Hastings Center Report*
- *Health Affairs*
- *Health Care Management Review*
- *Health Services Research*
- *Heart & Lung*
- *Journal of Pain & Palliative Care Pharmacotherapy*
- *International Journal of Evidence-Based Healthcare*
- *Journal of Health Economics*
- *Journal of the American Medical Association*
- *New England Journal of Medicine*
- *Oncology Nursing Forum*
- *Social Science and Medicine*

---

evidencebasednursing.com) selects original studies from more than 100 health care journals and presents critical appraisal and summary in brief abstracts.
- *The Internet* is a useful source of health care information for both health care professionals and consumers. However, the potential for harm from inaccurate information is substantial. As a result, it is important to evaluate the quality of web-based materials on the Internet.

Types and Levels of Evidence

Evidence exists in many forms. Perhaps the most obvious form is the journal article describing a single research study. Prior to the current disciplinary emphasis on EBP, it would have been the responsibility of the reader of these reports to critique each article and decide which, if any, of the research findings could be used in practice (research utilization). Though this technique continues to be somewhat useful, more systematic methods have been developed for synthesizing multiple research reports on a single topic. These systematic review methods include meta-analysis, integrative research reviews (IRR), and meta-synthesis.

In a meta-analysis the findings of multiple quantitative randomized controlled trials (RCTs), studies on a single topic, are statistically analyzed to produce a summary statistic. A meta-synthesis takes the findings of multiple qualitative studies on a single topic and synthesizes and amplifies the narrative information contained in the reports. An IRR takes the findings from experimental and nonexperimental studies on a single topic and synthesizes them to provide a comprehensive understanding of the phenomena. The importance of such reviews is that they represent a meticulous integration of the best evidence available at the time the review was conducted and are considered to provide the highest possible evidence (Polit & Beck, 2021; Melnyk & Fineout-Overholt, 2023). Therefore, individuals or agencies with clinical questions are able to consult well-prepared knowledge syntheses for possible application in the practice arena. Fig. 6.1 illustrates an evidence hierarchy based on levels of evidence regarding the effectiveness of interventions and/or findings.

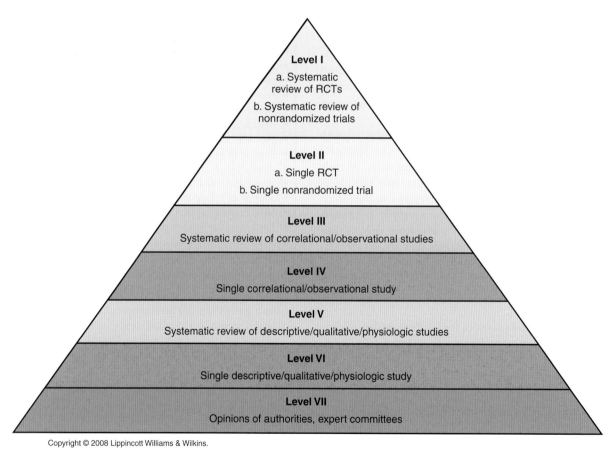

Level I
a. Systematic review of RCTs
b. Systematic review of nonrandomized trials

Level II
a. Single RCT
b. Single nonrandomized trial

Level III
Systematic review of correlational/observational studies

Level IV
Single correlational/observational study

Level V
Systematic review of descriptive/qualitative/physiologic studies

Level VI
Single descriptive/qualitative/physiologic study

Level VII
Opinions of authorities, expert committees

Fig. 6.1 Quick guide to an evidence hierarchy of designs for cause-probing questions. *RCT,* Randomized controlled trial. (From Polit, D.E., & Beck, T.C. [2021]. *Nursing research: Generating and assessing evidence for nursing practice* (11th ed.). Lippincott Williams & Wilkins.)

With such an array of evidence types, it is not surprising that evidence is viewed as requiring an assessment of just how strong it is. The terms *evidence hierarchy, levels of evidence,* and *strength of evidence* are used to refer to the categorical classifications that have been proposed to rate evidence along a continuum from best evidence to worst evidence. Most rating schemes rate meta-analyses of well-conducted RCTs as best evidence, with other evidence types sitting lower in the hierarchy (Melnyk & Fineout-Overholt, 2023; Polit & Beck, 2021).

Clinical Practice Guidelines

A clinical practice guideline (CPG) is an evidence-based guide to clinical practice developed by experts in a particular field for direct application in clinical environments (Melnyk & Fineout-Overholt, 2023). Like systematic reviews, guidelines gather, appraise, and combine evidence. Guidelines, however, go beyond systematic reviews in attempting to address all the issues relevant to a clinical decision and all the values that could sway a clinical recommendation. Guidelines make explicit recommendations and, in some circumstances, may be used to define "standard of care." In this scenario, a CPG *may* have legal ramifications. Several court cases have addressed the use of CPGs, but there are no set judicial standards for how these documents may be used and interpreted in individual cases (Melnyk & Fineout-Overholt, 2023). This is an evolving discussion because practice guidelines are playing important roles in guiding health care practices. In theory, any professional association, government agency, or health system can produce CPGs; however, practice guidelines are to be researched and driven by evidence. Practice guidelines are based on the consensus of a group of decision-makers—ideally experts and front-line clinicians.

Critical Appraisal

Nurses at all levels of educational preparation should critically read research journal articles and research summary articles. These articles are accepted on a competitive basis and undergo a *blind review* because the reviewers are unaware of who wrote the article. Therefore, readers can assume that experts have scrutinized it for merit and relevance to nursing; however, the reader should critically appraise the findings for validity. This is accomplished through detailed analysis of study design and measurement strategies. The abstract gives an overview of the study, and the discussion or conclusion provides suggestions for nursing practice based on the findings of the research study.

Preappraised evidence such as systematic reviews also require appraisal, but the emphasis is on whether the review provides ample and trustworthy evidence for answering a particular clinical question. The appraisal of various types of research and research summary articles for application to practice is best approached by using defined appraisal guidelines that may be located on the Internet, such as those from the EQUATOR network (http://www.equator-network.org). Careful appraisal may or may not lead one to make a change in practice. If change is implemented, the health care provider has an ethical and moral responsibility to evaluate the quality of patient outcomes derived from the change.

Rather than being a simple process of implementing the practice suggestions found at the end of a research report, use of research requires careful and complex analysis, wise implementation, and patient outcome assessment. CPGs can be methodologically weak or strong and thus may yield either valid or invalid recommendations. When considering using a practice guideline as a basis for an agency protocol, or as a guide for providing patient care, health care providers need to critically assess the credibility, clinical significance, and applicability of the guideline's recommendations. To facilitate the review process, there are instruments for appraising the quality of a CPG. The Appraisal of Guidelines for Research and Evaluation (AGREE) Instrument is a reliable and valid instrument that evaluates the process of practice guideline development and quality of reporting (Melnyk & Fineout-Overholt, 2023). AGREE can be accessed at http://www.agreetrust.org.

Nurses and Utilization of Evidence-Based Practice.
It is quite evident that there is a need for all nurses to understand and implement EBP in their clinical settings to improve health care outcomes. When staff nurses learn to critically evaluate the literature and clinical findings and begin to apply them to their patient care, there is great potential for improved patient outcomes.

An example of how nurses have implemented EBP in the hospital setting is through change from shift report at the nurses' station to bedside shift report (BSR). This practice change was part of a quality improvement project, which began with a research question and subsequent literature review on the topic of the potential benefits of BSR in terms of patient safety and patient and nurse satisfaction. Overall, BSRs have been found to be associated with improved patient safety, patient satisfaction, and nurse satisfaction (Dorvil, 2018; McAllen et al., 2018).

How to Utilize Evidence-Based Practice. There are many ways in which nurses can use EBP. For example, nurses can generate clinical questions and then search (and critically appraise) the literature in answering these questions. Nurses should also seek areas in need of quality improvement within their areas of clinical practice. We can also encourage the use of EBP by helping to implement practice changes that are based on evidence or clinical expertise (see Tables 6.3 and 6.4 for a list of EBP competencies for RNs and APNs).

Barriers to Evidence-Based Practice. While it is well-known and recognized that there are many benefits to the use of EBP, there are many significant barriers to EBP. These include both individual and institutional barriers. Individual barriers include lack of time, overwhelming patient loads, lack of value for research in practice, lack of time and resources to search for and critically appraise evidence, lack of competencies for implementing EBP, lack of electronic search skills, lack of knowledge about research, and lack of skills for critiquing and synthesizing the literature (Melnyk & Fineout-Overholt, 2023) (see Box 6.4 for Barriers to Evidence-Based Practice). Institutional facilitators for EBP include expectations and incentives, evidence-based policies and procedures, clinical promotion systems, and performance evaluations that include EBP, journal clubs and EBP rounds, EBP mentors, and a certification credential (see Box 6.5 for Facilitators for Evidence-Based Practice).

Overcoming Barriers to Evidence-Based Practice. Overcoming the barriers to EBP involves training in the areas of: computer skills; the use of electronic databases; the importance of research; and skills for critiquing and synthesizing literature. This training needs to be done on an institutional and organizational level. Health care facilities and management are responsible for creating an organizational culture that values research in practice and declares the use of EBP as an institutional priority, which should be reflected in their training budgets and in their provision of access to

---

BOX 6.4   Barriers to Evidence-Based Practice

- Lack of evidence-based practice (EBP) knowledge and skills
- Misperceptions or negative attitudes about EBP and research
- Lack of time and resources to critically search for and appraise evidence
- Resistance to change
- Lack of administrative support and incentives
- Demands from patients for certain kinds of treatments
- Lack of autonomy and power to change practice
- Inadequate EBP content and skills included in educational programs
- Lack of mentors
- Overwhelming patient loads
- Lack of knowledge about research

Adapted from Melnyk, B.M., & Fineout-Overholt, E. (2023). *Evidence-based practice in nursing and healthcare: A guide to best practice* (5th ed.). Wolters Kluwer. p. 28.

BOX 6.5   Facilitators of Evidence-Based Practice

- A culture that makes evidence-based practice (EBP) the standard or norm
- Support and encouragement from leadership/administration
- Time to critically appraise studies and implement their findings
- Proper tools to assist with EBP at the point of care (e.g., computers dedicated to EBP)
- Integrating EBP into health professions curricula
- Evidence-based clinical practice policies and procedures
- Clinical performance and promotion systems that incorporate EBP competencies
- Journal clubs and EBP rounds
- A certification credential and high level of education

Adapted from Melnyk, B.M., & Fineout-Overholt, E. (2023). *Evidence-based practice in nursing and healthcare: A guide to best practice* (5th ed.). Wolters Kluwer. p. 29.

---

electronic databases. From an academic standpoint, all nursing schools should implement research courses, beginning in baccalaureate programs and continuing through graduate programs. This equips nurses with the research skills needed to understand, value, and implement EBP.

Creating a Culture of Clinical Inquiry. Clinical settings capable of implementing EBP are those with cultures that support clinical inquiry. Such cultures are those that encourage clinicians to ask clinical questions; open communication and mutual respect must be present across all disciplines. Collaboration among interdisciplinary team members is key for optimal outcomes. Units with high turnover or those resistant to change often serve as a barrier for EBP implementation. In addition, the unit (or facility) leadership and environment need to support continual learning and provide adequate resources and time for accessing research and implementing EBP. Continuing education is one way that institutions can promote and support EBP (Hall & Roussel, 2020).

Translational Research. Translational research highlights the value of multiple disciplines working together as a team with the goal of translating research into clinical practice more quickly (Christenbery, 2018). The National Institute of Health (NIH) launched the NIH Roadmap for Medical Research in 2004 to transform the process of biomedical research (NIEHS, 2019). The Roadmap initiatives support high-risk, high-reward research, encourage the development of transformative methodologies, and help fill knowledge gaps. The goal of the Roadmap was to increase attention to "translating basic science research more quickly into human studies, leading to treatment or tests for clinical practice that would benefit patients" (Hall & Roussel, 2020, p. 263). This initiative led to the development of translational research centers within NIH institutes. The goal of these centers is to aid institutions in creating a home for Clinical and Translational Science with resources for interdisciplinary research teams to support the application of new knowledge and techniques to clinical practice.

Evolution of Evidence-Based Practice: Some Examples

Though much work remains, the potential effect of research on health care knowledge and practice can be demonstrated by two examples:
1. The use of heparinized saline for flushing capped peripheral intravenous catheters was compared with saline only. Saline only was found to be clinically effective in maintaining patency of peripheral catheters (Goode et al., 1991, 1993) and in neonates (Cook et al., 2011; Shah et al., 2005). As a result of this research, many acute care facilities revised their institutional policies to recommend saline only as a flush for peripheral intravenous catheters.
2. Pressure ulcers are a significant problem for multiple populations. It should not be surprising that many groups are interested in their prevention and treatment. An online search of the National Guideline Clearinghouse (NGC) yielded multiple clinical guideline statements contributed by groups, public and private, nursing and medical. In the case of pressure ulcers, much research evidence is available for implementing prevention and management strategies.

From these two examples, it can be seen that research evidence can play a significant role in health care practice. However, the process of spreading the "good news" about new or refined practice-related knowledge is a complex one. Researchers must make the knowledge they generate available and understandable. Practitioners must access, interpret, and carefully apply research evidence. The scientific process may take years to yield enough data to make clinical recommendations and more years to evaluate the effect of evidence-based changes through outcomes research. For instance, peptic ulcer disease was researched for many years before the discovery and acceptance of the presence of *Helicobacter pylori* in the stomach and duodenum (Marshall, 2002).

ETHICAL ISSUES RELATED TO RESEARCH
Institutional Review

In institutional review, a committee called an *institutional review board (IRB),* or human subjects committee, examines research proposals to ensure the ethical rights of those individuals participating in the research study are protected. Participants must sign an informed consent that explains the study and assures them of their rights, including their right to refuse to participate or to withdraw from the study. Institutions that receive federal funding or conduct drug or medical device research regulated by the US Food and Drug Administration (FDA) are required by federal regulations to establish an IRB. Federally funded studies have to meet strict guidelines to ensure the protection of the human rights of subjects, such as self-determination, privacy, anonymity and confidentiality, fair treatment, and protection from discomfort and harm. The informed consent must include essential study information and statements about potential risks and benefits, protection of anonymity and confidentiality, voluntary participation, compensation, alternative treatment, and specific information on how to contact the investigator (Polit & Beck, 2021).

Historical Examples of Unethical Research

In addition to the institutional review process, numerous codes and regulations have been implemented to ensure ethical conduct in research. The two historical documents are the Nuremberg Code and the Declaration of Helsinki, which were developed in response to unethical acts such as the Nazi experiments. These experiments, which occurred in the 1930s and 1940s, used untested drugs, sterilization, and euthanasia on prisoners of war. The experiments were unethical because they caused grievous harm to the subjects and denied them the opportunity to refuse participation (Polit & Beck, 2021).

Another famous incident of unethical research that prompted the need to oversee the conduct of research is the famous Tuskegee syphilis study. This study, which was initiated by the US Public Health Service, continued for 40 years. The study was conducted to determine the natural course of syphilis in African American men. Many participants were not adequately informed about the purpose and procedures of the study. The subjects periodically were examined but did not receive treatment for syphilis, even after penicillin was determined to be effective. The study was not stopped until 1972, when published reports of it sparked public outrage (Centers for Disease Control and Prevention, 2017). *Bad Blood*, a comprehensive documentary account of the Tuskegee syphilis study, clearly relates the study's adverse effects on research participation by African Americans and on race relations in the United States (Jones, 1993).

As late as the 1960s, another famous study that violated human rights took place. The Jewish Chronic Disease Hospital in New York was the setting for a study to determine patients' rejection of liver cancer cells. Twenty-two patients were injected with liver cancer cells without being informed that they were taking part in the research. In addition, the physician directing the study did not have institutional approval for a study that had the potential to cause the subjects harm or even death (Murphy, 2004).

In institutions in which IRB approval is not required for nonfederally funded programs, the researcher should seek external advice regarding ethical considerations. When IRB approval is an option, researchers should seek it because IRB approval demonstrates scientific rigor.

▋ SUMMARY

Educators must prepare health care professionals to have an appreciation of research and to participate in research at the level of their preparation. Practicing nurses must seek, develop, and adopt EBP protocols while encouraging affiliated institutions to support this effort. Health care administrators must facilitate an environment that supports research efforts. Collaborative arrangements between health care agencies and universities must be developed for such activities as student projects, continuing education, development of clinical practice guidelines, and research endeavors. Consumers must be educated about the value of health care research, and policymakers must be informed of pertinent findings so results can be translated into health policy.

To summarize the chapter, let's review the questions presented at the beginning of the chapter to see what you've learned.

1. How can a desire to read research and evidence-based practice literature in students be facilitated?

As visualized in the opening Vignette, integrating EBP into nursing curricula promotes an understanding and appreciation for nursing research and evidence-based practice literature. There are many facilitators to EBP, which are important to consider when seeking to inspire others to read research and EBP literature. These include:

A culture that makes EBP the standard or norm

Support and encouragement from leadership/administration

Time to critically appraise studies and implement their findings

Proper tools to assist with EBP at the point of care (e.g., computers dedicated to EBP)

Integrating EBP into health professions curricula

Evidence-based clinical practice policies and procedures

Clinical performance and promotion systems that incorporate EBP competencies

Journal clubs and EBP rounds

A certification credential and high level of education (Melnyk & Fineout-Overholt, 2023).

2. How does research affect nursing practice?

As previously discussed, evidence-based practice (EBP) is the retrieval, appraisal, and use of research findings as the basis for clinical practice. Evidence generated by nursing research supports quality, cost-effective nursing interventions in clinical practice. Recipients of nursing care benefit from nurses who attend to research evidence and introduce evidence-based changes in practice. The introduction of evidence-based change into nursing care may occur at the individual, organizational, or social levels.

3. How can nurses motivate colleagues to base their practice on research?

As discussed in facilitators to EBP, nurses can encourage colleagues to base their practice on research through supportive leadership and administration. In addition, they can contribute to a culture that promotes EBP and makes basing practice on research the norm. Journal clubs and EBP rounds can also help inspire others to apply evidence to their clinical practice.

REFERENCES

Abdulai A.F., & Hung, L. (2023). Will ChatGPT undermine ethical values in nursing education, research, and practice? *Nursing Inquiry, 30*(3):e12556. doi: 10.1111/nin.12556. Epub 2023 Apr 26. PMID: 37101311.

Agency for Healthcare Research and Quality (AHRQ). (2022). *Agency for Healthcare Research and Quality: A profile.* Agency for Healthcare Research and Quality: A Profile | Agency for Healthcare Research and Quality (ahrq.gov)

Agency for Healthcare Research and Quality (AHRQ). (2023). *Our mission.* http://integrationacademy.ahrq.gov

American Association of Colleges of Nursing (AACN). (2021a). *The essentials: Competencies for professional nursing education.* https://www.aacnnursing.org/Portals/0/PDFs/Publications/Essentials-2021.pdf

American Association of Colleges of Nursing (AACN). (2021b). *About the Doctor of Nursing Practice (DNP).* https://www.aacnnursing.org/our-initiatives/education-practice/doctor-of-nursing-practice/about-the-dnp

American Association of Colleges of Nursing (AACN). (2024). Clinical nurse leader. Clinical Nurse Leader (CNL) (aacnnursing.org)

American Nurses Association. (2010). *Nursing: Scope and standards of practice* (3rd ed.)

Centers for Disease Control and Prevention. (2017). *U.S. Public Health Service syphilis study at Tuskegee.* https://www.cdc.gov/tuskegee/timeline.htm

Christenbery, T. (2018). *Evidence-based practice in nursing: foundations, skills, and roles.* Springer.

CINAHL Information Systems. (2024). *Nursing resources from EBESCO.* https://www.ebsco.com/products/research-databases/cinahl-complete

The Cochrane Collection. (2023). *Cochran library.* http://www.cochrane.org/

Cook, L., Bellini S., & Cusson R.M. (2011). Heparinized saline vs normal saline for maintenance of intravenous access in neonates: An evidence-based practice change. *Advances in Neonatal Care, 11*(3), 208–215.

Dang, D., Dearholt, S., Bissett, K., Ascenzi, J., & Whalen, M. (2022). *Johns Hopkins nursing evidence-based practice for nurses and healthcare professionals: Model and guidelines* (4th ed.) Sigma Theta Tau International.

Dorvil, B. (2018). The secrets to successful nurse bedside shift report implementation and sustainability. *Nursing Management, 49*(6), 20–25. https://www.ncbi.nlm.nih.gov/pmc/articles/PMC5976230/

Goode, C.J., Titler, M., Rakel, B.A., Ones, D.S., Kleiber, C., Small, S., & Triolo, P.K. (1991). A meta-analysis of effects of heparin flush and saline flush: Quality and cost implications. *Nursing Research, 40*(6), 324–330.

Goode, C.J., Kleiber, C., Titler, M., Small, S., Rakel, B., Steelman, V., Walker, J.B., & Buckwalter, K. (1993). Improving practice through research: The case of heparin vs. saline for peripheral intermittent infusion devices. *Medsurg Nursing, 2*(1), 23–27.

Grady, P.A. (2014). Charting future directions in nursing research: NINR's innovative questions initiative. *Journal of Nursing Scholarship, 46*(3), 143.

Hall, H.R., & Roussel, L.A. (2020). *Evidence-based practice: An integrative approach to research, administration, and practice* (3rd ed.) Jones & Bartlett Learning.

Hastings, C. (2009). *Nursing at the NIH Clinical Center: Clinical research nursing: Background and overview.* https://www.cc.nih.gov/nursing/crn/crn_2010.html

Institute of Medicine (US) Committee on Quality of Health Care in America. (2001). Crossing the quality chasm: A new health system for the 21st century. Washington (DC): National Academies Press (US). PMID: 25057539

Institute of Medicine (IOM). (2011). *The future of Nursing: Leading change, advancing health.* The National Academies Press. https://www.nap.edu/catalog/12956/the-future-of-nursing-leading-change-advancing-health

Jones, J. (1993). *Bad blood: The Tuskegee syphilis experiment* (rev. ed.) Free Press.

LoBiondo-Wood, G., & Haber, J. (2021). *Nursing research: Methods and critical appraisal for evidence-based practice* (10th ed.) Elsevier.

Marshall, B. (2002). *The discovery that Helicobacter pylori, a spiral bacterium, caused peptic ulcer disease.* In J. Barry, B. Marshall (Eds.), *Helicobacter pioneers: Firsthand accounts from the scientists who discovered helicobacter, 1892–1982.* Blackwell, pp. 165–202.

McAllen, E.R., Stephens, K., Swanson-Bierman, B., Kerr, K., & Whiteman, K. (2018). Moving shift report to the bedside: An evidence-based quality improvement project. *The Online Journal of Issues in Nursing, 23*(2), pp. 1–12. https://doi.org/10.3912/OJIN.Vol23No02PPT22

Melnyk, B.M., Gallagher-Ford, L., & Fineout-Overholt, E. (2016). *Implementing the evidence-based practice (EBP) competencies in healthcare: A practical guide for improving quality, safety, & outcomes.* Sigma Theta Tau International.

Melnyk, B.M., & Fineout-Overholt, E. (2023). *Evidence-based practice in nursing and healthcare: A guide to best practice* (5th ed.) Wolters Kluwer.

Murphy, T.F. (2004). *Case studies in biomedical research ethics.* MIT Press.

National Association of Clinical Nurse Specialists. (2018). *Statement on clinical nurse specialists practice and education* (3rd ed.) http://nacns.org/wp-content/uploads/2018/05/3rd-Edition-Statement-on-Clinical-Nurse-Specialist-Practice-and-Education-2018-line-numbers.pdf

National Institute of Environmental Health Services (NIEHS). (2019). NIH roadmap and roadmap-affiliated initiatives. https://www.niehs.nih.gov/funding/grants/announcements/roadmap/index.cfm.

National Institute of Nursing Research (NINR). (2022). *NINR 2022-2026 strategic plan.* https://www.ninr.nih.gov/aboutninr/-mission-and-strategic-plan

Polit, D., & Beck, C. (2021). *Essentials of nursing research: Appraising evidence for nursing practice* (11th ed.). Lippincott Williams & Wilkins.

Robert Wood Johnson Foundation. (2023a). *About RWJF.* https://www.rwjf.org/en/about-rwjf.html

Robert Wood Johnson Foundation. (2023b). *Explore our grants.* http://www.rwjf.org/en/grants.html#q/maptype/grants/II/37.91,-96.38/z/4

Shah, P.S., Ng, E., & Sinha, A.K. (2005). Heparin for prolonging peripheral intravenous catheter use in neonates. *The Cochrane Database of Systematic Reviews, 4,* CD002774. https://doi.org/10.1002/14651858.CD002774

U.S. National Library of Medicine. (2021). *MEDLINE.* MEDLINE Home (nih.gov)

White, C.L. (2011). Nurse champions: A key role in bridging the gap between research and practice. *Journal of Emergency Nursing, 37*(4), 386–387.

7

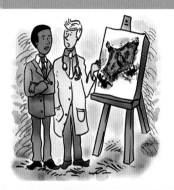

Paying for Health Care in America: Rising Costs and Challenges

Barbara Cherry, DNSc, MBA, RN, NEA-BC

...re than ever, nurses and business leaders need
...work together to manage the health care dollar.

Additional resources are available online at: http://evolve.elsevier.com/Cherry/

LEARNING OUTCOMES

After studying this chapter, the reader will be able to:

1. Analyze major factors that have influenced health care access and financing since the middle of the 20th century.
2. Articulate causes of rising health care costs and related health care reform measures that are being implemented to reduce health care costs.
3. Understand the public and private insurance programs that pay for health care in the United States and the consequences of not having health insurance coverage.
4. Describe how evolving health care reimbursement models have created new opportunities for professional nursing practice.

KEY TERMS

Centers for Medicare & Medicaid Services (CMS) The federal government agency that administers Medicare and Medicaid.

Diagnosis-related groups (DRGs) A common method of reimbursement for health care services based on a predetermined fixed price-per-diagnosis.

Effectiveness Taking the right action to achieve the desired outcome.

Efficiency Achieving the desired outcome while using resources, such as energy, time, and money, in the best way possible.

Gross domestic product (GDP) The measure of the total value of goods and services produced within a country; the most comprehensive overall measure of economic output; provides key insight into the driving forces of the economy.

Health Insurance Exchange Also known as the "Health Insurance Marketplace," an online marketplace for individuals to shop for and purchase health insurance at affordable rates and to identify whether they qualify for cost assistance subsidies to help pay the cost of the insurance; states established health insurance exchanges as a component of the Patient Protection and Affordable Care Act to provide access to affordable health insurance options for American citizens and legal residents.

Medicaid A jointly sponsored state and federal program that pays for medical services for persons who are elderly, poor, blind, or disabled and for certain families with dependent children who meet specified income guidelines.

Medicare A federally funded health insurance program for the disabled, persons with end-stage renal disease, and persons 65 years of age and older who qualify for Social Security benefits.

Patient Protection and Affordable Care Act (ACA) A federal statute enacted in 2010 that requires US citizens and legal residents to have health insurance through comprehensive health care reform.

Private health insurance A method for individuals to maintain insurance coverage for health care costs through a contract with a health insurance company that agrees to pay all or a portion of the cost of a set of defined health care services such as routine, preventive, and emergency health care; hospitalizations; medical procedures; and/or prescription drugs. Typically, the private insurance is provided through an individual's employer, with a portion of the cost paid by the employer and a portion paid by the employee. Private insurance policies can also be purchased by individuals but are generally more expensive than when provided through an employer's group plan.

Prospective payment system A method of reimbursing health care providers (e.g., physicians, hospitals) in which the total amount of payment for care is predetermined on the basis of the patient's diagnosis; encourages increased efficiency in the use of health care services because providers are reimbursed at a predetermined level regardless of how many services are rendered or procedures performed to treat a particular diagnostic category; the most common method of payment in today's health care system.

Provider A licensed health care professional (e.g., physician or nurse practitioner) who or an organization (e.g., hospital) that receives reimbursement for providing health care services.

Retrospective payment system A method of reimbursing health care providers (e.g., physicians, hospitals) in which professional services are rendered and charges are billed based on the basis of the individual services provided; also known as the "fee-for-service" payment system. This system may encourage overuse of health care services because the more services rendered or procedures performed, the more revenue received by providers.

Single-payer system A method of reimbursement in which one payer, usually the government, pays all health care expenses for citizens; funded by taxes; decisions about covered treatments, medications, and services are made by the government. Though the terms universal health care and single-payer system are sometimes used interchangeably, universal health care could be administered by many different payer groups; both offer all citizens health insurance coverage.

Third-party payer An organization other than the patient and the provider (e.g., hospital, physician, nurse practitioner), such as an insurance company, that assumes responsibility for payment of health care charges. An individual's health insurance plan provided by his or her employer is considered a third-party payer.

PROFESSIONAL/ETHICAL ISSUE

Claudia and Matt Taylor have a 2-year-old daughter, Carmen. Claudia worked full time as a nurse in a local clinic until Carmen was born. So far the Taylors have been able to budget for Claudia to work only 1 day a week so she can stay home and care for Carmen. They downsized to a smaller home and adjusted their spending to address the changes in the economy and rising costs of basic living such as food, gas, and utilities.

The Taylors have health insurance through Matt's employer, a small local business. The premiums and copays have increased over the past few years, stressing their tight budget. The Taylors believe that all people should have access to quality health care; as a nurse, Claudia has been an advocate for those who needed care, with or without insurance. However, the Taylors question why their insurance costs continue to increase and strain their already tight family budget. Matt and Claudia did not anticipate the yearly increases in health insurance costs and are struggling with many questions. Is it fair that the Taylors' lifestyle should be negatively affected by the rising cost for health insurance, especially since they are a healthy family and practice good health behaviors? How are small businesses like Matt's employer affected by the cost of health insurance for their employees? Are there less-expensive insurance alternatives available to the Taylors? What would happen if the Taylors chose not to carry health insurance?

VIGNETTE

As a home care nurse for many years, Callie Thompson primarily provides care to older adults. Knowledge of Medicare coverage guidelines (i.e., which services would be paid or not paid by Medicare) is critical to the financial success of the home-care agency where she works since the majority of patients they serve are covered by Medicare. Callie must understand how many days and which types of nursing care will be covered by Medicare for each patient's specific condition. She also needs to know if her patients may qualify for other needed services such as physical therapy or occupational therapy. In applying her understanding of financial issues related to home health care, Callie knows that providing education and preventive care (for example, addressing wound complications as early as possible) may help her patients avoid a trip to the hospital or emergency department. Such actions by a professional nurse make a major contribution toward reducing health care costs, both for patients and the overall health care system. Callie's advocacy for patient education and preventive care also provides the best possible health outcomes for her patients and allows them to remain in their own homes. In addition to her clinical skills, Callie's knowledge of the financial aspects of health care has helped her to be successful in her role as a home health nurse.

Questions to Consider While Reading This Chapter:

1. What changes are occurring in our health care system to help reduce overall health care costs?
2. Why do I need to understand health care reimbursement and its implications for individuals who do not have health insurance?
3. What do health care economics and finance have to do with me as I provide patient care?

CHAPTER OVERVIEW

In the past several decades, the costs of health care have continued to increase, with economic issues taking a central role in health care decision-making. Hospital leaders know that for most patients the hospital will receive a predetermined payment, regardless of length of stay and specific treatments; leaders also know that payment from Medicare and health insurance companies is very often tied to a quality component such as patient satisfaction (more on this later in the chapter). Physicians and nurse practitioners recognize that the prescribed course of treatment for their patients may be analyzed by a peer review committee and that the costs their patients incur may be compared with those of other providers or against cost benchmarks. Businesses require employees to pay higher costs for their health insurance premiums and/or pay larger deductibles and copayments. Health insurance companies "manage" care, sometimes placing limits on which health care services will be covered, on which providers a patient may be treated by, and/or on the site of care delivery. The Patient Protection and Affordable Care Act (ACA) of 2010 added a new dimension to health care financing with various insurance options for universal coverage of American citizens and different models of reimbursement to promote quality and cost-effective health care.

The objective of this chapter is to provide an overview of the major economic issues and trends driving changes in health care delivery, how health care is paid for, and how these issues affect nursing practice. This chapter presents information about historical trends in health care finance, the problem of the uninsured and underinsured, methods of paying for health care, and the effect of health care finance on professional nursing practice.

HISTORY OF HEALTH CARE FINANCING

The high costs of health care did not occur overnight. To understand current health care financing, it is necessary to understand its history (Table 7.1). Historically, several underlying themes have driven health care financing in the United States. Among these are:
- the physician's role as being primarily responsible for health care decision-making
- the fee-for-service payment method that encouraged overuse of health care services
- the rapidly increasing sophistication and cost of medical technology.

For many years, physician domination in decision-making and the fee-for-service payment method were intertwined and contributed to the lack of cost consciousness in health care. Physicians made all decisions about what health care services were needed; costs were rarely discussed between physician and patient, so the cost of care was not considered.

Beginning in the 1960s, the attitude that "if it might help, do it" flourished as the rapid pace of sophisticated technologies enhanced providers' abilities to deliver treatment. The more tests or procedures performed, the greater the earnings for providers (i.e., hospitals and physicians) because they were paid according to the number of procedures performed or services provided. Instead of attempting to allocate medical resources to the highest medical need, the financial incentive was to provide as much care as possible using the most technically advanced methods of care. Overuse of health services and rapid cost inflation resulted.

Another cause of rising costs was that the general public remained insulated from the cost of health care. Most patients had some form of insurance or third-party payment and did not pay the full cost for their care or

TABLE 7.1	Historical Highlights of Health Care Finance
1847	Massachusetts Health Insurance of Boston offers a group policy.
1861–1865	Insurance plans become available during the Civil War.
1890	Individual disability and/or illness policies become available.
1929	First group health coverage is offered for a monthly charge; teachers in Dallas, Texas, contract with Baylor Hospital. This is the beginning of Blue Cross/Blue Shield insurance.
1932	Blue Cross insurance forms.
1934	Hospitals receive payment through Blue Cross, a prepaid health insurance plan to protect hospitals during the Great Depression.
1950s	Employee benefit packages are initiated to attract workers.
1954	Government disability program with Social Security coverage becomes available.
1965	Medicare and Medicaid programs are created, making comprehensive health care available to millions of Americans.
1980–1990	Managed care plans emerge.
1983	Hospitals become answerable to the diagnosis-related group (DRG) system.
2010	Patient Protection and Affordable Care Act (ACA), the most significant health reform legislation since Medicare and Medicaid, is enacted with three primary goals: (1) make affordable health insurance available to more people and provide subsidies to help reduce health insurance costs for low-income households; (2) expand Medicaid to cover more adults; and (3) support innovative health care delivery models to reduce the overall cost of health care (US Department of Health and Human Services, 2022)

even for their health insurance premiums. The full cost of care remained hidden from people because costs were subsidized by employers through private insurance or by taxpayers through such programs as Medicare and Medicaid. Providers had little incentive to contain costs and patients rarely considered costs. Thus, the demand for medical care generated "perverse" economic incentives in which providers received more income for using more services, with no financial risk for their use of additional resources, and patients did not question the appropriateness of treatments ordered by the provider.

These perverse economic incentives had a drastic effect on the Medicare program. Medicare was established by the US Congress in 1965 to provide health insurance coverage for persons 65 years and older who are eligible for Social Security benefits, persons with end-stage renal disease, and the eligible disabled population. By the early 1980s, increased medical usage (increased intensity of care) and high inflation combined with a growing older adult population generated substantial increases in Medicare costs. The rapid growth of Medicare expenditures became a major factor in the federal budget deficit, causing the Centers for Medicare & Medicaid Services (CMS) to rethink the entire Medicare payment system. This process led to a revolution in how the government and private health insurance companies paid for health care.

Health Care Financing Revolution

The rising cost of health care over the last 70 years is a dangerous trend that continues today and poses a significant threat to the US economy. Consider the following facts about rising health care expenditures in the United States (CMS, 2023a):

- In 1970, annual health care expenditures were **$353** per person.
- In 2021, annual health care expenditures were **$12,914** per person.
- Total health care spending increased from $1.3 trillion in 2000 to $4.3 trillion in 2021.

National health expenditures as a percentage of the gross domestic product (GDP) were 18.3% in 2021 and are projected to be 19.6% by 2031 (CMS, 2023a). This means that for every dollar a person spends buying products or services in the United States, more than 18 cents goes to pay for health care. In contrast, health care spending in neighboring Canada was $8,563 per Canadian in 2022, with a health care GDP of 12.2% (Canadian Institute for Health Information, 2022).

To control rapidly rising health care costs, in 1983 Medicare moved from a retrospective (fee-for-service) payment system to a prospective payment system (PPS) based on diagnosis-related groups (DRGs). This shift was critical for hospitals because Medicare is the largest single payer of hospital charges. Under DRGs, each Medicare patient is assigned to a diagnostic grouping on the basis of his or her primary diagnosis at hospital admission. Medicare limits total payment to the hospital to the amount preestablished for that DRG, unlike with the previous approach, in which hospitals billed Medicare for any and all services provided to patients, and Medicare reimbursed these charges with a generous payment schedule.

If hospital costs exceed the DRG payment for a patient's treatment, the hospital incurs a loss, but if costs are less than the DRG amount, the hospital makes a profit. Thus, hospitals face a strong financial incentive to reduce the patient's length of stay and minimize procedures and tests performed. Although DRGs originally applied only to hospital payments for Medicare patients, similar reimbursement arrangements were initiated by private insurance companies. Implementation of the DRG system created a new role for nurses as utilization review experts to review medical records and determine the most appropriate DRGs for patients.

The Development of Managed Care

With the shift to prospective payment under Medicare, private insurance companies followed Medicare's lead and developed managed care. Managed care organizations (MCOs) encompass several different approaches, such as health maintenance organizations (HMOs), preferred provider organizations (PPOs), and point-of-service (POS) plans (Table 7.2). The primary commonality among all of these health plans is that they use some method to review and approve (or deny) the use of health care services. For example, a physician wants a patient with shoulder pain to have a CAT (computerized axial tomography) scan. Before the CAT scan can be done, the patient's insurance company must first review the appropriateness of the CAT scan. In this review process, the patient's medical options are reviewed by a nurse or physician employed by the health insurance company, and a judgment is made as to the necessity of the service being considered. Coverage may be denied for unnecessary, excessive, or experimental procedures, in strong contrast to the previous "if it might help, do it" approach. The goal of managed care is to

TABLE 7.2 **Common Types of Health Insurance Plans in the United States**	
Fee-for-service (FFS)/ indemnity plan	Member (covered individual) pays a premium for a fixed percentage of expenses covered Plan requires the member to pay deductible and copayment amounts Allows member to choose physician and specialists without restraint May cover only usual or reasonable and customary charges for treatment and services, with member responsible for charges above that payment Pays for preventive care as required by the Affordable Care Act
Preferred provider organization (PPO)	Member (covered individual) pays a premium for a fixed percentage of expenses covered Plan requires the member to pay deductible and copayment amounts Member may select physician, but pays less for physicians and facilities on the plan's preferred list Pays for preventive care as required by the Affordable Care Act
Point of service (POS)	Offered by HMO or FFS Allows use of providers outside the plan's preferred list or network, but requires higher premiums and copayments for services
Health maintenance organization (HMO)	Member (covered individual) pays a premium There is a fixed copayment Member must select a primary care provider approved by the HMO Member must be referred for treatments, specialists, and services by the primary care provider Services outside of "network" must be preapproved for payment Plan may refuse to pay for services not recommended by primary care provider Plan encourages use of preventive care
Medicare	Federal health insurance plan for Americans 65 years of age and older and certain disabled persons Member must be eligible for Social Security or railroad retirement Part A covers hospital stays and care in skilled nursing facilities (does not cover long-term care) Part B requires payment of a premium by the individual and covers physician services and supplies Plan offers a prescription drug benefit
Medicaid	Health care coverage for low-income persons who are aged, blind, or disabled and for certain families with dependent children Combined federal and state program delivered and managed by each state for eligibility and scope of services offered Plan covers long-term care (i.e., nursing home care) for qualifying individuals
TRICARE: Military health insurance (formerly CHAMPUS)	Civilian health and medical health insurance program for military, spouses, dependents, and beneficiaries Program offered through Military Health Services System

minimize payment of charges for inappropriate or excessive health care services.

As health care costs rise, the costs for businesses to provide health insurance for employees also rise; these increasing costs are then passed to consumers by increasing the price of the products or services produced by the business. US businesses benefit from the approach

used by MCOs to reduce the overall costs of health care. The primary goals of managed care plans are to:

- limit unnecessary health care services
- use the least expensive service (but equal in quality) when care is needed
- use the least expensive medication (but equal in quality) available.

ACCESS TO HEALTH CARE: THE PROBLEM OF THE UNINSURED AND EFFORTS TO PROMOTE ACCESS

As health care costs continue to rise dramatically in the United States, one major issue that must be addressed is access to health care for the uninsured or underinsured. The lack of access to health care primarily reflects a lack of insurance coverage, so access is an issue of financial access. The uninsured and underinsured include the working poor employed by small businesses without employer insurance coverage, part-time workers, unemployed persons, and the homeless. Individuals without health insurance are more likely to lack a usual source of care, less likely to use preventive services, and more likely to be hospitalized for avoidable conditions than those who have health insurance.

Consider these statistics: The number of uninsured, nonelderly individuals in 2021 was 27.5 million compared to 46.5 million nonelderly people in 2010 (Tolbert et al., 2022). The focus of data on the number of uninsured is for those people under the age of 65 years because those 65 years and older are covered by Medicare. Children are less likely to be uninsured due to the availability of coverage through Medicaid and the Children's Health Insurance Program (CHIP) (Tolbert et al., 2022). This reduction in uninsured adults is a result of the availability of more affordable health insurance options through the ACA.

The uninsured and underinsured populations generate uncompensated or indigent care costs and bad debt for health care providers. Unpaid costs must be covered by those who do pay so the hospital can continue operating, a process known as *cost shifting*. Providers increase their charges to public and private insurers who pay for care to make a contribution for the care of the uninsured population. This practice raises insurance premiums, making it even more difficult for many households and businesses to afford coverage. The problem of uncompensated care and cost shifting was a major factor leading to health care reform and the passage of the ACA.

Despite advances in providing health insurance through the ACA, in 2022 there were still more than 27 million people in the United States without health insurance (Tolbert et al., 2022). People most likely to be uninsured are low-income adults and people of color; the major barrier to obtaining and maintaining health insurance is the cost of coverage (Tolbert et al., 2022). Lack of health insurance is perhaps the greatest barrier to accessing health care services and has a tremendous negative effect on an individual's overall health status. Consider that people without health insurance:

- Are more likely to go without needed care due to cost;
- Have an increased risk of being diagnosed at the later stages of a disease, leading to higher mortality rates;
- May not receive preventive care;
- Are less likely to receive care for chronic diseases; and
- May often seek treatment in emergency departments at a much higher cost to the health care system.

People without health insurance weigh their costs for daily living expenses, such as food, housing, and transportation, against the cost of health insurance coverage and are simply not able to meet the financial demands for health insurance, even with the assistance provided through the ACA. The ACA does not provide health insurance for every person for several reasons: a person's income may make him or her ineligible for financial assistance through the ACA, yet he or she is still unable to afford the insurance premiums or has made a conscious decision not to purchase health insurance; the person is subject to immigrant eligibility restrictions; or the state in which the person lives did not expand Medicaid to his or her income level.

Medicaid, a combined state and federal health insurance program administered by each state, is intended to improve access to health care for the poor, covering approximately 18.8% of the population in 2022 (Keisler-Starkey, Bunch & Lindstrom, 2023). The ACA expanded federal Medicaid support to any state that accepted this assistance, allowing those states to increase the number of people who meet the qualifications for Medicaid. The following section provides a more detailed discussion of the ACA.

The Patient Protection and Affordable Care Act (ACA)

The Patient Protection and Affordable Care Act (Public Law 111–148) (ACA) was signed into law in 2010, making it the most significant health care legislation passed since Medicare and Medicaid were established in 1965. The ACA represents the first major effort to reform the US health care system by expanding health insurance coverage to uninsured populations and slowing unsustainable growth in health care costs, improving quality, and moving health care to a focus on prevention and population health rather than acute illness treatment. In

---

BOX 7.1   **Key Components of the Affordable Care Act**

- Low-income individuals and families receive financial assistance either through tax credits or subsidies to help make health insurance more affordable.
- Employers with more than 200 employees must offer health insurance.
- State-based health insurance exchanges, also known as the ACA Marketplace, are offered whereby individuals and small businesses can purchase qualified coverage at more affordable rates.
- The health plan must cover specified benefits including ambulatory patient services, emergency services, hospitalizations, maternity and newborn care, mental health and substance abuse treatment, prescription drugs, rehabilitative services, laboratory services, preventive and wellness services, chronic disease management, and pediatric services to include vision and oral care.

- Insurers cannot deny coverage for preexisting conditions, charge higher premiums based on health status or gender, revoke coverage when someone gets sick, or impose annual or lifetime limits.
- Dependent coverage for children up to age 26 years must be included for all individual and group policies.
- Insurance companies must spend 80% of premiums on medical care, a requirement that forces them to reduce their administrative expenses.
- Medicare will no longer pay hospitals to treat hospital-acquired conditions (e.g., falls, decubitus ulcers, infections).
- The value-based purchasing program pays hospitals on the basis of their performance on quality measures, including patient satisfaction.
- Medicare payments to hospitals for preventable hospital readmissions are reduced.

From U.S. Department of Health and Human Services. (2022). About the Affordable Care Act. https://www.hhs.gov/healthcare/about-the-aca/index.html

---

its broadest view, the ACA is the plan for a comprehensive national health insurance program to provide funding for US citizens and legal residents to secure health insurance beyond the current programs such as Medicare and Medicaid. Even more than 10 years since this legislation was signed into law, it remains important for nurses to understand the key components of the ACA noted in Box 7.1

Future Health Care Reform Proposals

Because costs for health care are a significant portion of the federal budget, health care reform initiatives will continue to be developed and debated in Congress. Thus, it is important for nurses to understand and evaluate any new health care reform proposals that come forward for possible legislative consideration. Key questions that need to be considered in any proposals regarding health care reform are (Buerhaus, 2020):

- Does the proposal help to improve health care delivery systems (improve quality, control costs, reduce waste, improve care coordination, and promote community and population health)?
- Does the proposal expand access to health care beyond what is currently available to individuals and populations?

- Does the proposal increase emphasis on disease prevention and social determinants of health to improve community and population health outcomes?
- Does the payment system address and reward the value of health care services over the volume of services provided?
- How would the proposal affect the well-being of patients and the environment in which care is provided?

Nurses, considered for decades to be the most trusted professionals, should be able to speak as knowledgeable voices about potential proposals to reform to the US health care system based on the above-noted criteria.

HOW HEALTH CARE IS PAID FOR

A combination of private and public sources pays for health care services and supplies for individuals in the United States. Most individual health care is paid for either by households through direct out-of-pocket payments or by third-party public or private insurers (Table 7.3). Third-party payers include private insurance companies and government health programs, such as Medicare, Medicaid, and the Veterans Administration (VA) health system.

TABLE 7.3 Health Insurance Coverage in the United States (2022)	
People with health insurance (for all or part of the year)	92.1% of the US population
People without health insurance (for the entire year)	7.9% of the US population
Children younger than 19 years without health insurance	5.0% of children
People covered by private health insurance plans (for all or part of the year)	65.6% of the US population (54.3% employer-based; 9.9% had direct-purchase health coverage; 2.4% covered by TRICARE)
People with government insurance (for all or part of the year)	36.1% of the US population (18.8% Medicaid; 18.7% Medicare; 1% military and VA) (some people may be covered by both Medicare and Medicaid)

Keisler-Starkey, K., Bunch, L.N., & Lindstrom, R.A. (2023). *Health insurance coverage in the United States: 2022.* U.S. Census Bureau. https://www.census.gov/content/dam/Census library/publications/2023/demo/p60-281.pdf

Private Insurance

Private insurance accounts for the largest percentage of coverage for health care, with the cost of providing health insurance to employees passed on by the employer to the consumer in the pricing of goods and services. This means that everyone pays a part of the country's health care costs in every purchase made. Individuals still must pay a portion of their health care costs directly from their own pockets, through payments for insurance premiums, deductibles, and copayments.

With managed care products, such as HMOs, PPOs, and POS arrangements, the premium the consumer pays for coverage has continued to rise. In response to these concerns, some companies now offer their employees high-deductible health plans (HDHPs), health reimbursement accounts (HRAs), health savings accounts (HSAs), or a combination of these. These plans offer more flexibility and consumer discretion over their health care dollars and provide a tax-free way to save for future health care needs.

Public Insurance: Medicare and Medicaid

The US government is the biggest influence in the health insurance market, generating half of hospital revenues and more than one-fourth of physician incomes. The largest government health insurance program is Medicare. Medicare is an entitlement program based on age or disability criteria, rather than on need, with these key components:

- Medicare Part A covers inpatient hospital services, skilled nursing facilities (SNFs), and home health benefits;
- Medicare does not cover long-term care;
- Medicare hospital coverage requires the individual to pay deductible and coinsurance amounts and has some coverage limitations;
- Medicare Part B covers physician and outpatient services; and
- Medicare Part D provides coverage for prescription medications.

Medicaid is a joint federal–state program to provide health insurance coverage for impoverished families, particularly those with children. Medicaid, along with the Children's Health Insurance Program (CHIP), offers health coverage to almost 20% of Americans (Keisler-Starkey, Bunch & Lindstrom, 2023). Those eligible for health care services include pregnant females, children and parents, persons with disabilities, and seniors who meet certain income criteria. Each state administers its own Medicaid program within minimal federal income guidelines, so some variances can occur from state to state. Medicaid is a primary payer of long-term care nationwide. It represents the fastest-growing component in most states' budgets.

PAYMENT METHODS TO REDUCE HEALTH CARE COSTS AND IMPROVE QUALITY

Various methods of reimbursing providers for health care services have emerged in attempts to control the rapid growth in health care costs and improve the safety and quality of health care. Hospitals and providers can now be financially rewarded for achieving improved health outcomes and are not paid for certain medical errors. Value-based payment models, "never events," value-based purchasing, and readmission reduction programs focus on aligning reimbursement with patient outcomes. Nurses are at the center of helping hospitals and other health care organizations successfully manage these payment mechanisms by ensuring that errors are prevented, health and quality outcomes are achieved, and financial rewards are realized.

Improving Quality through Value-Based Payment Models

Medicare and private insurance companies have shown success with various methods of reimbursing providers (hospitals and physicians) based on quality measures that reflect the quality of care provided, with an emphasis on providing evidence-based care, preventing complications, coordinating care to reduce costs and meeting standards of care for certain conditions such as diabetes, myocardial infarction, pneumonia, and heart failure. To be successful with value-based payment models, hospitals leaders, nurses, and providers must work toward improved health in communities and put systems in place to care for people earlier to prevent them from getting very sick (Davis et al., 2023).

To promote innovative models of care designed to improve care quality, reduce costs, support patient-centered practices, and keep people healthier, the Centers for Medicare and Medicaid Services (CMS) established its Innovation Center, which allows for creating and testing of new care delivery models (CMS, n.d.). New models include Accountable Care Organizations, Medical Home Models, and Episode-based payment initiatives. Several innovative models focus on specific disease treatments such as:

- Comprehensive Care for Joint Replacement Model to improve care and reduce costs for patients receiving hip and knee replacements
- Oncology Care Model to improve quality and coordination of care for patients receiving chemotherapy. Students are encouraged to visit the CMS Innovation Center at https://innovation.cms.gov/ to learn more about these new models of care delivery.

Preventing "Never Events" (Serious Reportable Events)

To save lives and millions of dollars, CMS adopted a policy that it will no longer pay hospitals for the extra costs of treating preventable errors. Medicare will no longer pay hospitals for the cost of treating *never events*—medical errors that are largely preventable and have serious consequences for patients. The purpose of the never events payment policy is to eliminate payments for certain medical errors and encourage hospitals to direct resources to preventing errors rather than being paid for them. Never events include hospital-acquired infections, injuries from falls, wrong-site surgery, and mismatched blood transfusions. Nurses have a highly visible and important role to play in preventing such complications and helping to control costs for hospitals. The full list of Never Events, also known as "Serious Reportable Events," can be found on the National Quality Forum website at www.qualityforum.org.

Rewarding Quality Care and Patient Satisfaction—Value-Based Purchasing

Value-based purchasing (VBP) is a CMS reimbursement model that rewards inpatient hospitals for providing quality care to include patient satisfaction (CMS, 2023b). The incentives for VBP arise from two domains: (1) the patient experience of care and (2) clinical processes of care. The patient experience of care is based on the hospital's scores on the Hospital Consumer Assessment of Healthcare Providers and Systems (HCAHPS), which is essentially a standardized patient satisfaction survey (Box 7.2). Clinical process of care measures include such items as discharge instructions delivered to heart failure patients, receiving fibrinolytic therapy given within 30 minutes of hospital arrival to patients with acute myocardial infarction, and prophylactic antibiotic received within 1 hour prior to surgical incision.

In addition to affecting hospital reimbursement, data from the VBP program is used to provide information to the public about hospital quality, nursing home quality, and even quality of care provided by individual

---

BOX 7.2 Components of the Hospital Consumer Assessment of Health Care Providers and Systems (HCAHPS) Patient Experience Survey

- Communication with nurses
- Communication with doctors
- Responsiveness of hospital staff
- Communication about medicines
- Cleanliness and quietness of hospital environment
- Discharge information
- Overall rating of hospital

From CMS. (2021). HCAHPS: Patients' Perspectives of Care Survey. https://www.cms.gov/medicare/quality-initiatives-patient-assessment-instruments/hospitalqualityinits/hospitalhcahps

BOX 7.3 **Economic Issues and Trends**		
From		**To**
Illness treatment	→	Prevention and population health driven
Acute care	→	Preventive care, home care
Hospital or institution based	→	Noninstitution based (clinic or home)
Fee-for-service (cost based)	→	Value-driven payment models
If it might help, use it	→	Outcomes measurement and cost-effectiveness
Independent decisions (practice variation)	→	Protocols and guidelines (evidence-based practice)

providers. Visit the CMS Hospital Compare website at https://www.medicare.gov/care-compare to learn more about how quality measures are reported to the public. As the reader can easily see, nurses are at the center of addressing the clinical processes of care and the patient experience to enhance the VBP financial rewards and also its publicly available quality indicators.

Reducing Readmissions

A provision of the ACA established the *Hospital Readmissions Reduction Program*, which reduces Medicare payments to hospitals with excessive readmissions. A *readmission* is defined as admission to a hospital within 30 days of a discharge from the same or another hospital (CMS, 2023c). The provision is currently focused on readmissions for acute myocardial infarction, heart failure, pneumonia, chronic obstructive pulmonary disease, elective total hip arthroplasty, elective total knee arthroplasty, and coronary artery bypass graft surgery. Again, nurses caring for patients with these conditions have a highly important role in ensuring effective discharge planning and education so the patient and family are fully prepared for recovery at home or in a transitional care setting. New roles for nurses as patient care navigators and transition care providers are rapidly emerging both in community settings and as part of the hospital's services to prevent readmissions. Just as with VBP models and never events, nurses are at the center of the efforts to prevent readmissions and avoid costly financial penalties to the hospital.

IMPLICATIONS FOR NURSES: MANAGING COST-EFFECTIVE, HIGH-QUALITY CARE

Nurses represent the largest health professional discipline in the United States and have an extremely important role in influencing the delivery of high-quality, lower-cost health care while also promoting health for individuals and communities. Never has there been a greater opportunity to advance the practice of professional nursing. Innovation and excellence in all nursing practices are needed to contain costs while attaining positive, measurable outcomes. As the reader can see from the various methods of reimbursement discussed earlier, nurses are at the center of ensuring quality patient outcomes, maximizing reimbursement, and decreasing financial penalties for errors and readmissions. Every setting in which professional nurses practice holds challenges in providing and managing care that is efficient, affordable, and high quality. Box 7.3 summarizes the trends occurring in health care that affect professional nurses. These trends mandate that nurses have a clear understanding of the economic and financing issues underlying their continually evolving roles.

Care Coordination

One key to improving quality and reducing costs is to ensure that health care is coordinated to decrease duplication of services and reduce wasted resources. Effective care coordination requires the use of case management and other emerging practice models, such as a patient care navigator and a transition care coordinator, all with the same goals: to ensure care is delivered in the community through home care, outpatient clinics, and ambulatory care centers at less costly rates; to decrease more expensive hospital-based care; and to prevent readmissions to the hospital. Nurses as care coordinators, case managers, patient care navigators, or transition care coordinators demonstrate cost-effectiveness by ensuring that patients have the resources they need to get effective treatment at the appropriate level of care across the continuum of care.

Expansion of Technology

Improved technology for diagnostic and therapeutic practice is under examination for cost-efficiency in comparison with outcome delivery. Leaders must balance the health contributions of the improved technology and the accompanying costs with issues of quality of life, access to care, risk–benefit analysis, and individual consumer choice.

US consumers have had access to high levels of technology with little concern for costs. Nurses are key players in educating patients and their family members about the cost-to-benefit ratio of certain technologies and can assist in selecting alternative treatment options. One example is the increased use of pharmaceuticals; more advanced drugs are marketed although they have varying degrees of actual documented benefit in comparison with existing, less–expensive drugs. Patients may not trust generic drugs, although they are less expensive. The nurse should be an advocate for educating patients and the public regarding the implications of using a less-expensive drug instead of a more expensive alternative.

The technology of the Internet offers promise for information and education that allows people to access health care resources more effectively. Some health care plans offer subscribers free newsletters and/or online programs that highlight ways to prevent disease and to manage chronic illness for improved quality of life and lower costs.

Information technology provides the professional nurse the ability to gather and analyze health-related information and data for improved care. Health care information systems and electronic health records offer many opportunities for managing health care costs. Combining clinical skills with information technology skills can be a significant advantage in the success of professional nurses as they demonstrate their ability to provide cost-effective outcomes measurement. See Chapter 15 for a more detailed discussion of information technology in the clinical setting.

Consumer Empowerment

Health care customers should demand quality health care services at affordable rates. Economic forces to reduce health care costs are motivating the shift toward health promotion and preventive care to achieve cost-effectiveness. This relationship with the consumer emphasizes cost sharing through individual choices in health practices. For instance, the presence of unhealthy personal practices, such as smoking, illegal drug use, and a sedentary lifestyle, may lead to a higher insurance rate for an individual. Smokers may pay higher rates and have to be smoke-free for 1 year to qualify for lower rates. Box 7.4 shows ways consumers can reduce their health care costs.

BOX 7.4   Ways Consumers Can Reduce Health Care Costs

- Practice good health behaviors—healthy eating, regular exercise, good sleep.
- Use reputable Internet sites to learn more about your health and preventing disease.
- Recognize early warning signs of disease and get prompt treatment.
- Practice preventive health with health screenings and routine self-examinations. Take advantage of free screenings offered at community sites, hospitals, or churches.
- Develop an active relationship with health care providers to improve communication. Ask providers to explain the purpose of all prescribed tests and medications. Become an informed consumer.
- Use emergency care only in emergencies. See your health care provider during office hours.
- Know health risks for lifestyle choices, such as alcohol and drug use, dietary habits, sedentary behaviors, and safety at home and while driving.
- Understand and use the health care benefits of your insurance plan to stay healthy. Take advantage of all preventive benefits offered.
- Determine whether the health care treatment is really necessary. Choose nonhospital alternatives for treatment whenever possible. Comparison shop for health care alternatives.
- Choose generic drugs when possible. Question expensive drugs or devices.
- Review your health care bills carefully, and notify the provider and/or facility of errors.

SUMMARY

To summarize the chapter, let's review the questions posed at the beginning of the chapter and see what you have learned.

1. What changes are occurring in our health care system to help reduce overall health care costs?

    Changes in the US health care system bring new challenges for professional nurses. Health care has moved from an emphasis on illness to an emphasis on wellness and prevention and is shifting from acute care services to preventive and community-based services, such as ambulatory care and home care, which are less expensive sites for care than the acute-care setting. Financing of health care services has gone from retrospective, fee-for-service payment systems to prospective payment and managed care and continues to evolve through implementation of the ACA to expand insurance coverage and new models of financial rewards and incentives (e.g., never events, value-based purchasing, readmission reduction programs) to improve quality and reduce costs. US leaders and legislators agree that health care costs are too high, but they differ in the best ways to stop the increased cost of health care. Most agree that when citizens practice healthy lifestyles they require less health care and enjoy a better quality of life.

2. Why do I need to understand health care reimbursement and its implications for individuals who do not have health insurance?

    As visualized in the opening Vignette, Callie's understanding of the reimbursement mechanism for home health allows her to advocate for her patients to ensure they are receiving care that is paid for by Medicare while also helping her to educate her patients about actions to better manage their chronic illnesses or prevent readmissions. Nurses should also understand that uninsured patients may lack preventive care, poorly manage their chronic conditions, and/or not seek care until the later stages of a disease. Finding innovative strategies to help uninsured patients achieve better health is an important role for the nurse in conjunction with the interprofessional team. Regardless of nurses' practice settings, they must understand how health care services are being paid so they can contribute to leading and implementing nursing practices that promote health and reduce costs.

3. What do health care economics and finance have to do with me as I provide patient care?

    Nursing practice in a cost- and quality-conscious environment is here to stay. Nurses must constantly challenge current practice for quality improvement and cost-effectiveness. Accurate data must be collected to show cost containment and positive patient outcomes. Roles on clinical teams, in administration, with insurance companies, and with the government hold promise for empowered change. Nurses can take the lead by being healthy role models, educating consumers, and encouraging personal responsibility for improved health practices. Managing care brings nurses back to the basics as society recognizes that healthy people are good business.

CASE STUDY

Clinical Judgment and Next-Generation NCLEX® Examination-Style Questions

Ava Elizabeth, RN, BSN, has been a nurse for 18 months, working in the emergency department (ED) of a large teaching hospital. She feels she is becoming competent in her role as an ED nurse and has become especially adept at assessing patients and discussing her observations with the providers to help develop the treatment plan. She has noticed a troubling trend over the past several months, where some patients who are chronically ill with congestive health failure (CHF) come to the ED frequently for exacerbations of their CHF. Ava realizes that these patients who visit the ED frequently for the same complaints have a poor quality of life and have higher health care costs because of being treated frequently in the ED and sometimes being hospitalized. Through discussions with the ED providers, Ava is aware that there are probably better ways to manage these patients in outpatient settings to improve their quality of life and reduce costs, but there is not an outpatient program for CHF patients. Ava recently read an article in a nursing journal about the creation of a CHF clinic to more closely monitor and manage CHF patients in

Continued

CASE STUDY—cont'd

Clinical Judgment and Next-Generation NCLEX® Examination-Style Questions

their home or clinic, prevent their CHF exacerbations, reduce ED visits and hospitalizations, and improve their quality of life. Ava is excited about this option to have such a clinic in her community that will reduce costs for the hospital and ED while also helping her patients have a better quality of life. She begins to promote the idea of a CHF clinic to her supervisor and to the ED Medical Director, who both agree that something should be done and are willing to work on a proposal to present to the hospital executive leaders to establish a CHF outpatient clinic. What key points can Ava make to add strength to the proposal for an outpatient CHF clinic?

For each action step, use an X to indicate if it was Effective (helped to meet expected outcomes), Ineffective (did not help meet expected outcomes), or Unrelated (not related to the expected outcomes).

Action	Effective	Ineffective	Unrelated
Uninsured patients with CHF are less likely to use preventive services and more likely to be hospitalized for avoidable exacerbations of their chronic condition.			
Reducing readmissions to the hospital for a CHF patient discharged within 30 days of a discharge from the same or another hospital can create cost savings for the hospital.			
Nurses should be able to recognize the clinical signs of a patient with an exacerbation of CHF.			
Patients without health insurance often seek treatment for their CHF in emergency departments at a much higher cost to the health care system.			
Some patients with CHF are not able to manage their disease and are expected to make frequent visits to the ED.			
Nurses can be an important resource in coordinating care and providing supportive, comprehensive education for CHF patients about how to manage their disease and avoid ED visits and hospitalizations.			
Early treatment in an easy-to-access outpatient clinic can help CHF patients to keep their disease in better control and prevent costly visits to the ED.			
Routine follow-up by nurses with CHF patients to reinforce health behaviors and monitor medication management can be key in helping these patients manage their disease and have a better quality of life.			
Nurses are not expected to make recommendations about innovative models that can reduce costs and improve quality of care for patients; this is the responsibility of the health care executive leadership team.			
Nurses should provide discharge teaching before allowing a patient to leave the hospital or the ED.			

REFERENCES

Buerhaus, P.I. (2020). Demystifying national healthcare reform proposals: Implications for nurses. *Nursing Economics, 38*(2), 58–64.

Canadian Institute for Health Information. (2022). *National health expenditure trends.* https://www.cihi.ca/en/national-health-expenditure-trends#:~:text=Prior%20to%20the%20pandemic%2C%20from,total%20health%20spending)%20in%202022

Centers for Medicare and Medicaid Services (CMS). (n.d.). *The CMS Innovation Center.* https://innovation.cms.gov/.

Centers for Medicare and Medicaid Services (CMS). (2023a). *National health expenditure fact sheet.* https://www.cms.gov/research-statistics-data-and-systems/statistics-trends-and-reports/nationalhealthexpenddata/nhe-fact-sheet

Centers for Medicare and Medicaid Services (CMS). (2023b). *The Hospital Value-Based Purchasing (VBP) Program.* https://www.cms.gov/medicare/quality-initiatives-patient-assessment-instruments/value-based-programs/hvbp/hospital-value-based-purchasing

Centers for Medicare and Medicaid Services (CMS). (2023c). *Hospital readmissions reduction program.* https://www.cms.gov/medicare/medicare-fee-for-service-payment/acuteinpatientpps/readmissions-reduction-program

Davis, M., et al. (2023). Taking action in value-based-care: Intermountain Health's ambulatory care approach. *Voice of Nursing Leadership*, September 2023, 18–21.

Keisler-Starkey, K., Bunch, L.N., & Lindstrom, R.A. (2023). *Health insurance coverage in the United States: 2022.* US Census Bureau. https://www.census.gov/content/dam/Census/library/publications/2023/demo/p60-281.pdf

Tolbert, J., Drake, P., & Damico, A. (2022). *Key facts about the uninsured population.* Kaiser Family Foundation. https://www.kff.org/uninsured/issue-brief/key-facts-about-the-uninsured-population.

US Department of Health and Human Services. (2022). *About the Affordable Care Act.* https://www.hhs.gov/healthcare/about-the-aca/index.html

8

Legal Issues in Nursing and Health Care

Laura Mahlmeister, PhD, RN

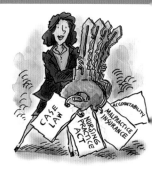

Knowledge of the law enhances the nurs[e's] ability to provide safe and effective care

@ Additional resources are available online at: http://evolve.elsevier.com/Cherry/

LEARNING OUTCOMES

After studying this chapter, the reader will be able to:

1. Differentiate among the three major categories of law on which nursing practice is established and governed.
2. Analyze the relationship between accountability and liability for one's actions in professional nursing practice.
3. Outline the essential elements that must be proven to establish a claim of negligence or malpractice.
4. Distinguish between intentional and unintentional torts in relation to nursing practice.
5. Identify causes of nursing error and patient injury that have led to claims of criminal negligence.
6. Incorporate fundamental laws and statutory regulations that establish the patient's right to autonomy.
7. Incorporate laws and statutory regulations that establish the patient's right to privacy and privacy of health records.

KEY TERMS

Accountability Being responsible for one's actions; a sense of duty in performing nursing tasks and activities.

Advance directives Written or verbal instructions created by the patient that describe specific wishes about medical care in the event they become incapacitated or incompetent. Examples include living wills and durable powers of attorney.

Breach of duty Occurs when one person or company has a duty of care toward another person or company but fails to live up to that standard.

Case law Body of written opinions created by judges in federal and state appellate cases; also known as judge-made law and common law.

Civil law A category of law (tort law) that deals with conduct considered unacceptable. It is based on societal expectations regarding interpersonal conduct. Common causes of civil litigation include professional malpractice, negligence, and assault and battery.

Common law Law that is created through the decisions of judges as opposed to laws enacted by legislative bodies (e.g., Congress).

Comparative negligence A type of liability in which damages may be apportioned among two or more defendants in a malpractice case. The extent of liability depends on the defendant's relative contribution to the patient's injury.

Criminal negligence Negligence that indicates "reckless and wanton" disregard for the safety, well-being, or life of an individual; behavior that demonstrates a complete disregard for another, such that death is likely.

Damages Monetary compensation the court orders paid to a person who has sustained a loss or injury to their person or property through the misconduct (intentional or unintentional) of another.

Defendant The individual who is named in a person's (plaintiff's) complaint as responsible for an injury;

the person who the plaintiff claims committed a negligent act or malpractice.

Disclosure A process in which the patient's primary provider (physician or advanced practice nurse) gives the patient, and when applicable, family members, complete information about unanticipated adverse outcomes of treatment and care.

Durable power of attorney for health care An instrument that authorizes another person to act as one's agent in decisions regarding health care if one becomes incompetent to make one's own decisions.

Error A failure of a planned action to be completed as intended or the use of a wrong plan to achieve a specific aim.

Ethical issues A problem that requires a person or organization to choose between alternatives that must be evaluated as right (ethical) or wrong (unethical).

Gross negligence A legal concept that means extreme carelessness showing willful or reckless disregard for the consequences to a person (patient).

Health care law Federal, state, and local laws and associated rules and regulations applicable to the health care industry and health care workers.

Immunity Legal doctrine by which a person is protected from a lawsuit for negligent acts or an institution is protected from a suit for the negligent acts of its employees.

Legal liability Failure of a person or an entity to meet legally defined responsibilities and allows a lawsuit for resulting damages.

Liability Being legally responsible for harm caused to another person or property as a result of one's actions; compensation for harm is normally monetary.

Licensing laws Laws that establish the qualifications for obtaining and maintaining a license to perform particular services. Persons and institutions may be required to obtain licenses to provide particular health care services.

Malpractice Failure of a professional to meet the standard of conduct that a reasonable and prudent member of their profession would exercise in similar circumstances that results in harm. The professional's misconduct is unintentional.

Negligence Failure to act in a manner that an ordinary, prudent person (either a layperson or professional) would act in similar circumstances that results in harm. The failure to act in a reasonable and prudent manner is unintentional.

Nursing case law The body of written legal opinions developed by judges through court decisions that eventually contribute to the expected standard of nursing conduct.

Nursing malpractice An incident in which a nurse fails to competently perform their legal duty owed to a patient and that failure harms the patient.

Nursing Practice Act The body of state law that sets out the scope of practice and responsibilities of the registered nurse to protect the health and welfare of individuals or communities under the care of the registered nurse.

Plaintiff The complaining person in a lawsuit; the person who claims they were injured by the acts of another.

Preventable adverse event An injury caused by medical management rather than the patient's underlying condition. An adverse event attributable to error is a preventable adverse event.

Punitive damages Monetary compensation awarded to an injured person (patient) that goes beyond what is necessary to compensate for losses (e.g., the ability to function, death, income) and is intended to punish the wrongdoer.

Res ipsa loquitur Legal doctrine applicable to cases in which the provider (e.g., the physician) had exclusive control of events that resulted in the patient's injury; the injury would not have occurred ordinarily without a negligent act; a Latin phrase meaning "the thing speaks for itself."

Respondeat superior Legal doctrine that holds an employer indirectly responsible for the negligent acts of employees carried out within the scope of employment; a Latin phrase meaning "let the master answer."

Risk management Process of identifying, analyzing, and controlling risks posed to patients; involves human factor and incident analysis, changes in systems operations, and loss control and prevention.

Sentinel event As defined by The Joint Commission, an unintended adverse outcome that results in death, paralysis, coma, or other major permanent loss of function. Examples of sentinel events include patient suicide while in a licensed health care facility, surgical procedure on the wrong organ or body side, and a patient fall.

Standard of care In civil cases the legal criteria against which the nurse's (and physician's) conduct is compared to determine whether a negligent act or malpractice occurred; commonly defined as the knowledge and skill that an ordinary, reasonably prudent person would possess and exercise in the same or similar circumstances.

Statute or statutory law Law enacted by a legislative body; separate from judge-made or common law.

Strict liability A legal doctrine, sometimes referred to as absolute liability, that can be imposed on a person or entity (e.g., a hospital) without proof of carelessness or negligence.

Vicarious liability Legal doctrine in which a person or institution is liable for the negligent acts of another because of a special relationship between the two parties; a substituted liability.

PROFESSIONAL/ETHICAL ISSUE

All health care systems are challenged to provide safe patient care when employees, physicians, or other providers report illness while at work. Although health care workers are advised to stay home if they are febrile and have signs of respiratory infection that may be spread to patients and coworkers, anecdotal evidence suggests that workers are in fact pressured to "tough it out" and come to work. The following is a scenario illustrating ethical issues and challenges related to working with sick colleagues.

A pregnant woman arrives in a labor and delivery unit at 6:45 a.m. for a scheduled repeat cesarean delivery. Her obstetrician, Dr. Mary Smith, is on call and planning to perform the surgical birth. The obstetrician is completing her preoperative documentation at the nurses' station. The charge nurse notes that Dr. Smith has obvious symptoms of a severe respiratory illness. She is coughing, sneezing, has copious nasal secretions, and looks quite ill. The patient's nurse observes Dr. Smith drinking about a third of a bottle of a liquid cold and flu remedy and pocketing the rest of the medication in her lab coat. The nurse knows that one of the side effects of the medication is significant drowsiness.

She approaches the physician and says, "Dr. Smith, you look quite ill. I am concerned about you and whether you are up to performing surgery this morning. Can we call your partner who is scheduled to start at 8:00 a.m. to come in and relieve you?"

Dr. Smith responds, "Look, it's just a bad cold. I've taken a large dose of a cold remedy. I will double-mask and use a splash shield. Let's get going. I'm off duty at 8:00 a.m. If we move fast I'll be out of here before then. Call me when the patient's on the table." Dr. Smith then walks into the physician's lounge and reclines on a couch.

Questions

1. What is the nurse's ethical duty to the patient and coworkers at this time?
2. What danger does complying with Dr. Smith's plan to proceed with surgery pose to the patient and coworkers?
3. Does the nurse have an ethical duty to the physician?

PROFESSIONAL/LEGAL ISSUE

There is a broad range of health care laws underpinning nursing practice. The nurse must be familiar with these legal imperatives and how they affect professional nursing care. Ignorance of the law is not a defense against charges of negligence, malpractice, or criminal misconduct. An increasing number of cases have been filed alleging a violation of health care statutes by nurses.

VIGNETTE

On July 26, 2017, an unconscious man injured in a motor vehicle accident was conveyed to the University of Utah Hospital in Salt Lake City (Smart, 2017). A registered nurse was directed by a police officer, who had entered the emergency department (ED), to draw blood from the man who was still unresponsive. The blood sample would be tested for alcohol, drugs, and illicit substances that could alter mentation. A charge nurse explained to the officer that neither she nor the police were permitted to obtain the sample because the patient had not given consent. The police officer telephoned his supervisor, who supported the officer's directive to draw the blood sample. The nurse had alerted a hospital supervisor about the unresolved disagreement, but that person had not yet arrived in the ED.

A videotape captured the encounter between the nurse and officer. It was released in September of 2017 to the media (*The Salt Lake Tribune*, 2017). The nurse was able to contact a hospital representative to speak telephonically with the police officer. When the nurse continued to respectfully refuse the order the officer arrested her, forcefully removed her from the ED, handcuffed her, and conveyed her to the police department.

Questions to Consider While Reading This Chapter:

1. What was the nurse's legal duty in this situation?
2. What legal principles underlie the nurse's obligations to the patient?
3. What laws, if any, would govern the nurse's decision-making process in this case?
4. In this situation does the police officer's order to draw the blood supersede the nurse's right to refuse the order?
5. Could the patient sue the charge nurse if she had drawn the blood sample and given it to the police officer?
6. What would the likely claims of nursing negligence be if a lawsuit had been filed on behalf of the patient?

CHAPTER OVERVIEW

The preceding vignettes highlight growing clinical dilemmas that nurses and patients face in an ever-changing health care system. In an increasingly complex health care environment the nurse's ability to make appropriate decisions about the provision of patient care services is assisted by a sound knowledge of ethical principles (Khoshmehr et al., 2020) and the laws governing practice. In the case of the ED charge nurse, consent and diagnostic testing are regulated by a federal law known as the Emergency Medical Treatment and Active Labor Act (EMTALA) (CFR, 42 U.S.C. §1395dd). Furthermore, the Fourth Amendment to the US Constitution, prohibiting unreasonable searches and seizures, underpins the patient's right to refuse drug testing under certain circumstances.

There also may be a specific state law regarding drug testing in the ED as well as other departments such as inpatient psychiatric units and obstetric departments. Additionally, sections of the state's Nursing Practice Act or professional and business code often describe professional conduct of the RN. They would assist the nurse in responding to a concern about possible physician impairment or a request by an officer of the law to obtain blood samples for drug testing. The role of the nurse as patient advocate also informs the nurse's actions when the patient's rights are jeopardized.

Each nurse must be able to describe their professional duty to the patient or client under the law and associated health care rules and regulations and to recognize legal risks in practice. Knowledge of the law enhances the nurse's ability to provide safe, effective, and humane care in all settings. This chapter examines the legal aspects of nursing practice. The concepts of law, professional accountability, legal liability, negligence, malpractice, and criminal offense are defined. Specific laws or statutes governing nursing practice are also reviewed. The reader is introduced to current, relevant information about case law, also known as common law or judge-made law, as it applies to professional nursing practice. Patients' rights are explored within the context of law and court opinions. Finally, the ongoing reports about medical errors published by organizations such as the Institute of Medicine (IOM), The Joint Commission (TJC), the Agency for Healthcare Research and Quality (AHRQ), and the Institute for Safe Medication Practices (ISMP) are discussed, and specific strategies to reduce errors and legal risk are detailed.

SOURCES OF LAW AND NURSING PRACTICE

The actions of all individuals are regulated through two systems of principles known as laws and ethics. *Laws* enforce a minimal level of conduct by imposing penalties for violations of acceptable behavior (DeMarco et al., 2019). Laws are expressed in terms of "must" and "shall" and are based on a society's interest in prohibiting or controlling certain behaviors. *Ethics* are described in terms of "should" and "may" and address beliefs about appropriate behaviors within a societal context (Butts & Rich, 2019). Chapter 9 presents an in-depth discussion about nursing ethics. Along with ethics professional nursing conduct is regulated by a variety of laws. The two major sources of law are statutory law and common law. The standards for professional nursing practice are in great part derived from statutory as well as common law. The following section deals with statutory law and describes how it governs and indirectly influences nursing practice.

STATUTORY LAW

The terms *law* and *statute* are used interchangeably in this chapter. Laws that are written by legislative bodies, such as Congress or state legislatures, are enacted as statutes. The previously mentioned law, EMTALA, is an example of a federal statute. Violation of law is a criminal offense against the general public and is prosecuted by government authorities. Crimes are punishable by fines or imprisonment. The list of federal and state statutes that govern nursing practice has multiplied over the past 25 years. Nurses at all levels of practice must develop a greater depth and breadth of knowledge about laws related to patient safety, professional practice, their specific practice setting (e.g., the ED in the case of EMTALA), and health care systems in general. Ignorance of the law is never a defense when a nurse violates a health care statute. A nurse who violates the law is subject to penalties, including monetary fines, suspension or revocation of their license, and even imprisonment in some instances (Berglund, 2019).

Federal Statutes

Conditions of Participation for Hospitals in Medicare (42 CFR Part 482).

Federal laws, rules, and regulations have a major effect on nursing practice and hospital operations. In the *U.S. Code of Federal Regulations* (CFR) Title 42 is the principal set of rules and regulations issued by federal agencies regarding public health. Title 42, Part 482, contains the Conditions of Participation for Hospitals in Medicare (CoPs) and is abbreviated in references as "42 CFR Part 482." The CoPs delineate the minimal standards of care required in all health care settings that receive federal reimbursement for treatment of Medicare beneficiaries. Medicare is administered by the Centers for Medicare & Medicaid Services (CMS), which has the authority to establish new rules and regulations to enhance patient safety and quality and reduce the cost of care. For instance, the CoPs require nurses to develop an individualized written nursing care plan for each patient and to revise the plan as necessary. Other CoPs mandate that hospitals properly train nurses for their stated roles and responsibilities, provide adequate staff to meet patient needs, and begin discharge planning as soon as possible after the patient's admission to the hospital.

Hospitals that are not in compliance with the CoPs may lose their federal funding if the CMS determines

the violations place a patient in "immediate jeopardy" of harm. The hospital or units within the hospital may be prohibited from accepting patients until corrective actions are taken to ensure the safety of all patients (Mahlmeister, 2015). Likewise, nurses engaged in unprofessional conduct that violate CoPs may be barred from employment in hospitals that participate in the Medicare program. Nurses can access information about the CoPs online and without cost at the CMS website: http://www.cms.gov/Regulations-and-Guidance/Legislation/CFCsAndCoPs/Hospitals.html. The CoPs can be downloaded from the site as a pdf file, *Appendix A of the State Operations Manual. The State Operations Manual* delineates each of the 23 CoPs pertaining to hospitals and provides Interpretive Guidelines for each of the requirements in language that can be easily understood by nurses and consumers of health care. The major revisions the CMS proposed in the CoPs took effect on July 16, 2012. Under these rules nurses are required to develop greater expertise in the provision of evidence-based patient care, case management, and discharge planning.

In 2008 the CMS issued new rules that halt payment to hospitals for treatment of preventable patient complications and injuries, often referred to as "never events." The CMS identified 10 categories of hospital-acquired conditions (HACs) that studies have demonstrated are "reasonably preventable" (CMS, 2008). The CMS added four additional HACs in 2016. Box 8.1 lists 14 categories of adverse events that are subject to nonpayment. The new rules have made a significant impact on hospital nursing care through the introduction of evidence-based practices to prevent complications such as falls, infections, and the development of stage III and stage IV pressure ulcers.

The CMS has also developed a methodology to calculate and display overall hospital quality using a "Star Rating System." One goal of the Hospital Star Rating is to improve the usability and interpretability of information about a hospital's incidence of complications (HACs). The information is posted on the CMS website, "Hospital Compare," designed to assist consumers in making decisions about where to seek inpatient care. Consumers can access information about Hospital Compare at: https://www.cms.gov/Medicare/Quality-Initiatives-Patient-Assessment-Instruments/HospitalQualityInits/HospitalCompare. Furthermore, the "Hospital-Acquired Condition (HAC) Reduction Program," mandated by the

---

BOX 8.1   Categories of Hospital-Acquired Conditions Subject to Nonpayment

1. Foreign object retained after surgery (e.g., instruments, surgical sponges)
2. Air embolism
3. Blood incompatibility (blood transfusion error)
4. Development of stage III or stage IV pressure ulcer
5. Falls and trauma:
   - Fractures
   - Joint dislocation
   - Intracranial injuries
   - Crushing injuries
   - Burns
   - Electric shock
6. Manifestations of poor glycemic control:
   - Diabetic ketoacidosis
   - Nonketotic hyperosmolar coma
   - Hypoglycemic coma
   - Secondary diabetes with ketoacidosis
   - Secondary diabetes with hyperosmolarity
7. Catheter-associated urinary tract infection (UTI)
8. Vascular catheter-associated infection
9. Surgical site infection following:
   - Coronary artery bypass graft—mediastinitis
10. Surgical site infection following bariatric surgery for obesity:
    - Laparoscopic gastric bypass
    - Gastroenterostomy
    - Orthopedic procedure
11. Surgical site infection following certain orthopedic procedures:
    - Spine
    - Neck
    - Shoulder
    - Elbow
12. Surgical site infection following cardiac implantable electronic device (CIED)
13. Deep vein thrombosis (DVT)/pulmonary embolism (PE) following certain orthopedic procedures:
    - Total knee replacement
    - Hip replacement
14. Iatrogenic pneumothorax with venous catheterization

Data from Centers for Medicare & Medicaid Services (CMS). (2020). *Medicare program: Changes to the hospital inpatient prospective payment system and fiscal year 2016 rates.* 81 FR 56761. https://www.cms.gov/Medicare/Medicare-Fee-for-Service-Payment/HospitalAcqCond/Hospital-Acquired_Conditions.html

---

Affordable Care Act, required the CMS to reduce hospital payments by 1% for hospitals that ranked among the lowest-performing 25% with regard to HACs.

Legal concerns have been raised about a possible increase in malpractice claims related to HACs. It may be more difficult for a hospital to defend a malpractice claim if "strict liability" is applied to these hospital-acquired events. In other words, if the federal government deems the HAC a cause for levying penalties or denying reimbursement, does the decision constitute negligence per se? Case law has yet to determine whether the courts will accept the "strict liability" claim. However, hospitals will still face serious financial losses when hospital-acquired events occur.

Federal laws have also established rules and regulations to ensure the confidentiality of patients' personal health information (Health Insurance Portability and Accountability Act [HIPAA]). Several federal laws protect the rights of patients who participate as subjects in research by mandating the creation of institutional review boards and an appropriate informed consent process. The Americans with Disabilities Act (ADA) requires health care entities to provide interpreter services and communication devices for patients who are unable to effectively communicate their needs or wishes. The Federal False Claims Act makes it an offense to submit a false claim to the government for payment of health care services. The US Department of Justice recovered more than $2.2 billion in settlements and judgments from civil cases involving fraud and false claims against the government in fiscal year 2022 (US Department of Justice, Public Affairs Office, 2023). Furthermore, the person who reports the false or fraudulent claim (often referred to as a "whistleblower") is entitled to 15% to 25% of any monetary amount recovered by the federal government if the government wins the case in court. Nurses have been the recipients of these "bounties" in several recent false claims cases in which the federal government recovered several million dollars.

Three federal statutes that nurses must be familiar with and clearly understand are discussed in this section. The list is not comprehensive but it includes examples of federal laws that directly affect nursing practice. Many federal laws are relevant to specific health care settings (e.g., mental health hospitals, nursing homes, EDs, maternity settings). When nurses are knowledgeable about the federal laws applicable to their area of practice they are able to more effectively advocate for patients in that setting. Unfortunately, most nurses are unfamiliar with health care law and rely on authorities in their employment setting to know what is legal and therefore permissible. Automatically deferring to administrators or nurse managers about the legality of a particular issue is no longer acceptable behavior for the professional nurse. Each RN must take accountability for knowing the law and understanding how it relates to patient care and nursing practice.

Emergency Medical Treatment and Active Labor Law (CFR, 42 U.S.C. §1395dd).

The federal statute known as EMTALA, often referred to as the "antidumping" law, was enacted in 1986 to prohibit the refusal of care for indigent and uninsured patients seeking medical assistance in an ED (Moffat, 2023). This law also prohibits the transfer of unstable patients, including women in labor, from one facility to another. The law states: "All persons presenting for care must receive the same Medical Screening Examination (MSE)." The MSE must be performed by a Qualified Medical Personnel (QMP), a physician, advanced practice nurse, or physician assistant, after the required education and training is completed and competence to conduct the MSE is confirmed and recorded (CMS, 2020a). The patient must be stabilized, regardless of their financial status or insurance coverage, before discharge or transfer. An EMTALA exception permits registered nurses who work in Obstetric Triage units to perform the MSE with the same requirements for training and competency validation.

EMTALA is applicable to people coming to nonED settings, such as urgent care clinics and obstetric triage units. It even governs the transfer of a patient from an inpatient setting to a lower level of care in some parts of the United States (*Roberts v. Galen of Virginia, Inc.*, 1997). Significant penalties can be levied against a facility that violates EMTALA, including a $25,000 to $50,000 fine (not covered by liability insurance). The federal government also can revoke the facility's Medicare contract, an action that could result in a major loss of revenue for the institution, or even insolvency. In light of the substance abuse crisis in the United States EMTALA also requires QMP to perform an appropriate medical screening exam for "Substance Use Disorder" (SUD) when the person presents to the ED with "a range of acute SUD-related symptoms, withdrawal, overdose, organ damages, and/or infections." The ED personnel must also provide care to prevent deterioration of a patient's SUD upon discharge (Yaboah-Sampong et al., 2023).

Many legitimate concerns that nurses have about the discharge or transfer of patients could be promptly addressed if the nurses had a solid understanding of EMTALA. A 2006 case illustrates the importance of understanding EMTALA. In *Love v. Rancocas Hospital* (2006) a woman was transported by ambulance to the ED after losing consciousness at home. She had a history of hypertension and continued to have high blood pressure readings in the ED. The woman also fell off the bed twice while being monitored but the ED nurse did not report these events to the physician. The nurse received a discharge order from the physician and sent the woman home in an unstable condition, thus violating the stabilization requirement of EMTALA. The woman returned 2 days later after experiencing a stroke. Understanding EMTALA is not a daunting task for nurses engaged in the triage and medical screening of patients presenting to the ED or obstetric triage department (Brent, 2017).

EMTALA and disaster response. During the COVID-19 pandemic of 2020–2021 many EDs struggled to comply with EMTALA as they were overwhelmed with critically ill patients seeking care. In response the Department of Health and Human Services/Centers for Medicare and Medicaid Services (CMS, 2020b) declared a "Public Health Emergency" (PHE). Hospitals were allowed to temporarily eliminate some of the required EMTALA ED regulations. In addition, hospitals were expected to initiate approved "Disaster Protocols" to address the COVID-19 crisis. In 2023 the White House declared the PHE ended and by the end of the year certain EMTALA waivers ended (American Hospital Association [AHA], 2023). Nurses working in EDs and obstetric triage units are expected to review EMTALA hospital policies, procedures, and protocols.

Americans with Disabilities Act of 1990 (Public Law No. 101-336; 42 U.S.C. Section 12101).

The intent of the ADA is to end discrimination against qualified persons with disabilities by removing barriers that prevent them from enjoying the same opportunities available to persons without disabilities. Court cases have established that, as a place of public accommodation, a health care facility must provide reasonable accommodation to patients (and family members) with sensory disabilities, such as vision and hearing impairment *(Abernathy v. Valley Medical Center*, 2006; *Boyer v. Tift County Hospital*, 2008). In another case *(Parco v. Pacifica Hospital*, 2007) a nurse was caring for a ventilator-dependent quadriplegic patient who was unable to speak or use his call light. She requested a special pillow that activated the patient's call light when he turned his head but was told that all the pillows were in use. The patient subsequently experienced three episodes of respiratory distress that he was unable to alert the nurse about and could only hope that someone would discover his problem before he suffered brain damage or death (Snyder, 2007). The patient sued for emotional distress and mental anguish. The court affirmed that the ADA requires hospitals to provide assistive devices to patients with communication problems related to a disability. The hospital settled the lawsuit for $295,000.

This statute has relevance for all nurses. As patient advocates nurses have a legal and ethical duty to provide appropriate patient and family education and to support the process of informed consent. In *Parco v. Pacifica Hospital* the court noted that it was a basic tenet of nursing practice that patients be given the ability to communicate with caregivers. The health care facility must have a policy that defines how it will meet the need for education and information of a client with a vision or hearing disability. The policy also describes how a nurse can obtain translators and special types of equipment needed to facilitate communication with clients who have physical disabilities or language barriers.

Patient Self-Determination Act of 1990; Omnibus Budget Reconciliation Act of 1990 (Public Law No. 101-508; Sections 4206 and 4751).

The Patient Self-Determination Act of 1990 is a Medicare and Medicaid amendment intended to support individuals in expressing their preferences about medical treatment and making decisions about end-of-life care. The law requires all federally funded hospitals to give patients written notice on admission to the health care facility of their decision-making rights and policies regarding advance health care directives in their state and in the institution to which they have been admitted. Under the Patient Self-Determination Act, patients have the right to:

- Participate in their own health care decisions
- Accept or refuse medical treatment
- Make advance health care directives

These choices include collaborating with the physician in formulating "do not resuscitate" (DNR) orders. Facilities must inquire as to whether the patient already has an advance health care directive, and they must make note of this in the patient's medical record. The institution must also provide education to their staff about advance health care directives. The law provides guidance to nurses, who often are in the best position to discuss these issues with the patient (e.g., while completing a comprehensive admission assessment). (Legal considerations related to living wills, durable power of attorney, and DNR orders are discussed in "The Law and Patient Rights," the last section of this chapter.)

Health Insurance Portability and Accountability Act of 1996 (Public Law No. 104-191).

The intent of HIPAA is to ensure confidentiality of the patient's health information. Legitimate concerns regarding the uses of and release of medical information, particularly to private entities such as insurance companies, led to the passage of this law. The introduction of electronic medical records provided additional impetus for introduction of this legislation. The statute sets guidelines for maintaining the privacy of health data. It provides explicit guidelines for nurses who are in a position to release health information. To maintain confidentiality of the patient's health information all nurses must have a basic understanding of this federal law. Nurses should also take note that the HIPAA confers whistleblower protection for individuals who report in good faith any illegal disclosure of patients' health. In 2005 a federal statute, the Patient Safety and Quality Improvement Act (Public Law No. 109–41), was enacted to allow certain disclosures of patient safety data. The law permits a provider to disclose *nonidentifiable* patient data to a qualified patient safety organization (PSO) for the purpose of analyzing medical errors. The law prohibits an accreditation body, such as TJC, from taking any action against a provider who reports patient safety data to an approved PSO (Public Law No. 109–41).

With the continued rise in the number of nurses using social media such as blogs, social networking sites, video sites, and online chat rooms and forums, a patient's right to privacy is threatened. In 2011 the American Nurses Association (ANA) published the Principles of Social Networking Toolkit for Nurses (ANA, 2011) and the National Council of State Boards of Nursing (NCSBN) published a complementary brochure, "A Nurse's Guide to the Use of Social Media" (NCSBN, 2018a). The publications review the benefits and risks of using social media in the workplace and bringing workplace issues to social media sites during free time. The release of private health data, either inadvertent or intentional, is a violation of HIPAA and is punishable by significant fines and a term of imprisonment. It may also result in suspension or revocation of the nurse's license (Basen, 2021). Civil actions may arise from a violation of patient confidentiality, alleging failure to maintain security and confidentiality of protected patient health data, unprofessional conduct, and violation of hospital policies and procedures that restrict access to patient information on a "need-to-know" basis. Posting photographs or videotapes of patients, or even ostensibly unidentifiable body parts, is expressly forbidden and also violates the ANA's *Code of Ethics for Nurses* (2015a). Discussing conflicts with managers or coworkers on social networking sites or posting unauthorized photos or videos of professional colleagues opens the nurse to claims of invasion of privacy, slander, intentional infliction of harm, and emotional distress, among other things. Further risks to livelihood and future employment as a nurse are presented when the nurse publicly airs dissatisfaction with their employer or discusses problems at work that make the employer vulnerable to ridicule or loss of reputation in the community or larger health care arena.

State Statutes

In addition to federal laws nursing practice is governed by state laws that delineate the conduct of licensed nurses and define behaviors of all health care professionals in promoting public health and welfare.

State Nurse Practice Act and Board of Nursing Rules and Regulations.

One of the most important state laws governing nursing practice is a Nursing Practice Act (NPA), which defines the scope and limitations of professional nursing practice. The aim of regulating practice in this manner is to protect the public and make the individual nurse accountable for their actions. State legislatures authorize the nurses' licensing board to promulgate administrative rules and regulations necessary to implement the NPA. Once these administrative rules and regulations are formally adopted they have the same force and effect as any other law.

Although NPAs vary from state to state, they usually contain the following information:

- Definition of the term *RN*
- Description of professional nursing functions
- Standards of competent performance
- Behaviors that represent misconduct or prohibited practices
- Grounds for disciplinary action
- Fines and penalties the licensing board may levy when an NPA is violated

For further exploration, excerpts from three separate state NPAs, illustrating how an NPA defines the scope of practice for nurses, can be found on the Evolve site at http://evolve.elsevier.com/Cherry/.

Surprisingly, many nurses are not even aware that the NPA is a law, and they unknowingly violate aspects of this statute (Russell, 2017). They are not familiar with the administrative rules and regulations enacted by the licensing board. This is an unfortunate lack because these administrative rules and regulations answer crucial questions that nurses have about the day-to-day aspects of practice and unusual occurrences. For example, the increasing complexity of health care requires effective communication, collaboration, and planning of care among many licensed health team members. Rules promulgated by the Ohio Board of Nursing Section 4723.03, which refer to the competent practice as an RN, direct the nurse in appropriate reporting and consultation, as follows:

> "A registered nurse shall in a timely manner:
>   Implement any order for a client unless the registered nurse believes or should have reason to believe the order is:
> 1. Inaccurate
> 2. Not properly authorized
> 3. Not current or valid
> 4. Harmful, or potentially harmful to a client
> 5. Contraindicated by other documented information; and
>   Clarify any order for a client when the registered nurse believes or should have reason to believe the order is: [a through e as delineated in (1)]"

Ohio Administrative Code, Section 4723-4-03, E, 2019

According to this section, an RN in Ohio who does not clarify a questionable order before administering a medication or carrying out the prescribed action is in violation of the law.

Each nurse should own a current copy of the NPA and the licensing board's administrative rules and regulations for the jurisdiction in which they practice. The nurse also must know how to access the licensing board online and by telephone to clarify issues related to nursing practice. The dramatic changes occurring in health care often lead to uncertainty among nurses about which functions constitute the exclusive practice of registered nursing and which patient care tasks may be lawfully delegated to a licensed practical nurse/licensed vocational nurse (LPN/LVN) or unlicensed assistive personnel. The NPA and licensing board rules and regulations provide essential information that clarifies these important questions. In 2008 the Texas Board of Nursing approved a new rule requiring all nurses to take and pass a Nursing Jurisprudence Exam prior to initial licensure. The examination tests knowledge regarding nursing board statutes, rules, position statements, disciplinary action, and other resource documents accessible on the Texas Board's website (http://bon.state.tx.us/index.html). The NCLEX Exam for licensure also includes questions regarding legal issues and nursing jurisprudence.

Nurses may also have questions and concerns regarding the legal aspects of floating to unfamiliar units. An NPA provides information regarding the scope of practice, the required competencies, and the responsibilities of a nurse who accepts an assignment or agrees to carry out any task or activity in the clinical setting. The NPA broadly defines the practice of registered nursing in accordance with nursing's rapidly evolving functions. In recent years, with the expansion of basic nursing functions and the development of advanced nursing practice, many states have revised their NPAs. Licensing boards also have been authorized in some states to provide guidelines for the development of "standardized procedures." Standardized procedures are a legal means by which RNs may expand their practice into areas traditionally considered to be within the realm of medicine. The standardized procedure is actually developed within the facility where the expanded nursing functions have been approved. It is developed in collaboration with nursing, medicine, and administration. An example of a standardized procedure is a written protocol authorizing a nurse to implement a peripherally inserted venous catheter for any patient in the neonatal intensive care unit. The NCSBN provides additional online resources for nurses covering diverse topics, including licensure and regulation (NCSBN, 2023a).

Violations of an NPA. State legislatures have given licensing boards the authority to hear and decide administrative cases against nurses when there is an alleged violation of an NPA or the nursing board's rules and regulations. Nurses who violate the NPA or board's administrative rules and regulations are subject to disciplinary action by the board. Table 8.1 contains a synopsis of the licensing board procedure for a complaint made about a nurse. Courts have consistently affirmed board of nursing decisions to restrict, suspend, or revoke the nurse's license when nurses have challenged the decision.

Box 8.2 presents the more common grounds for disciplinary action by state boards of nursing. Penalties that licensing boards may impose for violations of an NPA include:
- Issuing a formal reprimand
- Establishing a period of probation
- Levying fines
- Limiting, suspending, or revoking a nurse's license.

It is estimated that 10% to 15% of RNs in the United States are chemically dependent (Cares et al., 2015; NCSBN, 2018b). The majority of disciplinary actions by licensing boards are related to misconduct resulting from chemical impairment, including the misappropriation of drugs for personal use and the sale of drugs and drug paraphernalia to support the nurse's addiction. For a nurse whose license is limited or suspended because of problems related to chemical impairment, the ability to practice in the future is often predicated on successful completion of a drug rehabilitation program and evidence of abstinence. An increasing number of state licensing boards have established programs to identify nurses with substance abuse disorders, refer them for treatment, and guide them through rehabilitation to reestablish licensure (Toney-Butler & Siela, 2022; NCSBN, 2018b).

Nurse–Patient Ratios and Mandatory Overtime Statutes

Inadequate and often unsafe nurse–patient ratios continue to plague nursing and result in missed nursing

TABLE 8.1   Licensing Board Procedure When a Complaint Is Filed

Action	Consequence
Complaint is made (initial complaint may be lodged by a telephone call or a letter mailed to the licensing board) by: • Consumer (patient) • Family member • Nurse or nurse manager or employer • Professional nursing organization • State board of nursing • Federal or state authority (i.e., CMS or Department of Health & Human Services)	Sworn complaints must be filed
Licensing board reviews complaint: • Examines evidence • Reviews reports	Insufficient evidence—no action; administrative review scheduled • Nurse notified
Board makes determination	Nurse summoned • Rules of proceeding explained • Witnesses called to testify • Further evidence examined
Licensing board makes decision	Nurse exonerated Nurse guilty of violating the NPA
Board takes disciplinary action	Possible actions • Board issues formal reprimand • Fines levied against nurse • Nurse placed on probation • License suspended or revoked • License not renewed
Nurse may challenge licensing board's actions	Nurse must file appeal in court
Court reviews case (court action depends on jurisdiction) • Reviews conduct of proceedings • Reviews board's decision	Licensing board ruling is reversed
Licensing board can appeal ruling	Court reviews case
Court renders a decision	Licensing board ruling is upheld
OR	OR
Court renders a decision	Licensing board ruling is overturned Licensing board can appeal to a higher court
Case scheduled for trial	Licensing board ruling is upheld OR Licensing board ruling is reversed

CMS, Centers for Medicare & Medicaid Services; *NPA,* Nurse Practice Act.

care (PS Net, 2019a). A growing body of evidence confirms a strong association between nurse–patient ratios and patient outcomes (Lasater, et al., 2021; Griffiths et al., 2018; Silber et al., 2016). The ANA launched its "Safe Staffing Saves Lives Campaign" in 2008, publishing the results of a poll conducted to examine nurses' perceptions of staffing problems (ANA, 2009). More

than 50% of respondents were considering leaving their current nursing position, and 42% indicated that the reason for leaving was associated with inadequate staffing. Another study surveyed direct-care nurses about nursing errors of omission. More than 70% of respondents reported the inability at times to plan and implement required care and intervene in a timely

BOX 8.2 Grounds for Disciplinary Action by State Boards of Nursing

- Practicing without a valid license
- Failure to use appropriate nursing judgment
- Guilty of a felony
- Falsification of records
- Failure to complete nursing documentation
- Incorrect nursing documentation
- Failure to practice in accordance with nursing standards
- Inappropriate behavior or occurrence at work
- Medicare fraud
- Misappropriation of personal items

manner. Forty-four percent of respondents missed essential assessments (Kalisch & Lee, 2012). Eighty-five percent of the nurses indicated that lack of human resources (nurse and support staff) was the primary reason for omissions in essential components of the nursing process. In 2014 the ANA responded to these findings, publishing a white paper to assist nurse leaders in developing effective staffing strategies and in 2019 released the third edition of Principles for Safe Staffing to provide additional guidance. In 2023 the National Council of State Boards of Nursing (NCSBN) published data that revealed the current and future challenges in nurse staffing (NCSBN, 2023b):

- Approximately 100,000 registered nurses (RNs) left the workforce during the COVID-19 pandemic.
- Approximately 610,300 RNs report an intent to leave the workforce by 2027.
- An additional 188,900 RNs under age 40 report the same intention to leave.

The primary reasons for leaving were stress, burnout, emotionally drained, fatigue, and retirement.

Nurse staffing is influenced to some degree by federal law through the CoPs and, increasingly, by state laws. Hospitals risk losing federal Medicare and Medicaid funding for a confirmed pattern of understaffing that has not been properly addressed by managers and administrators and the hospital's Board of Directors. The CMS has fined hospitals for understaffing, in part owing to increased patient census. Hospital administrators and clinical leaders must prepare a corrective action plan and submit it to the CMS within a specified time when cited by the CMS for safety violations such as unsafe staffing levels. Nurses can positively affect nurse staffing levels when armed with knowledge regarding

federal and state laws. When concerns about work-related issues arise (e.g., a reduction in RN staffing, mandatory overtime, or replacement of RNs with LVNs–LPNs or unlicensed assistive personnel), the first question the nurse asks and answers should be, "Is this legal?"

California became the first state, and remains the only state, to enact a nurse-to-patient ratio law (California Assembly Bill 394). The law mandates the establishment of minimum ratios in acute care facilities including critical care, step-down and medical-surgical units, and maternity departments. No other state has followed California's lead with the exception of Massachusetts, which mandates a 1:1 nurse-to-patient ratio, but only in the ICU. Nurses may elect to take a second patient based on their judgment and use of an acuity tool (958 CMR 8.00).

Eighteen states have enacted laws or regulations that either limit or prohibit mandatory overtime for nurses (Deering, 2022; Skinner, 2023). ANA has advocated for passage of a Federal law to establish safe nurse-to-patient ratios for more than 20 years. In 2023 a bill was reintroduced in the US Senate to establish nurse-to-patient staffing ratio requirements in hospitals (S.1113, Nurse Staffing Standards for Hospital Patient Safety and Quality Care Act of 2023). It requires hospitals that participate in Medicare—nearly all hospitals in the United States— to implement staffing plans and safe nurse-to-patient ratios, which are established by a committee composed of a majority of direct-care nurses for each nursing unit and shift. With the growing number of nurses leaving the profession, due in significant part to inadequate and unsafe staffing levels, there is greater hope that passage of the law will become a reality in the near future.

An increasing number of lawsuits against health care facilities have set forth claims of corporate negligence for inadequate staffing or "understaffing" when adverse outcomes occur. A jury awarded a $1.7 million verdict against a nursing home for the death of a resident who fell from her wheelchair. Evidence revealed that there was a widespread pattern of understaffing at the nursing home (*Sunbridge Healthcare Corp. v. Penny*, 2005). In 2006 another jury awarded $240,000 in punitive damages (out of a total award of $400,000) against a nursing home because understaffing at the facility was considered an aggravating factor in a patient's death (*Miller v. Levering Regional Healthcare Center*, 2006). The patient was 91 years of age and suffered from Alzheimer's disease. The resident (patient) was left unattended and fell, hitting her head, and subsequently died of her injuries. The court records contained adequate evidence that the facility knew it had a chronic understaffing problem and that the problem directly led to the woman's death (Snyder, 2006). The director of nursing was also found negligent for failing to comply with Medicare guidelines that required the facility to provide sufficient staffing. In *Lavender v. Skilled Healthcare Group* (2010) a class-action suit was filed on behalf of 32,000 current and former residents claiming that the company violated the residents' rights because the facilities were inadequately staffed. A jury awarded $619 million to the plaintiffs.

Reporting Statutes

The federal government and states seek to protect at-risk individuals (children and older adults) by requiring nurses and other health care providers to report specific types of suspected or actual patient–client injury, abuse, or neglect. Boards of nursing are created to protect the public from unethical, incompetent, or impaired nursing practice. Some states have enacted statutes that *mandate* nurses to report unsafe, illegal, or unethical practices by nursing colleagues or physicians (Jenkins et al., 2023; Cole et al., 2019) or by administrators of health care facilities that place patients in jeopardy. With these mandates and protections in mind, the following case illustrates the adverse consequences that nurses may still face when reporting and/or whistleblowing.

A nurse practitioner was contracted to provide health care services to inmates at a county jail in the state of Nevada. During the course of her work she collaborated with a physician who also treated those incarcerated in the jail. The nurse practitioner, as well as other health care workers providing services in the facility, objected when the physician did not at all times write progress notes as he evaluated and treated the inmates. The primary concern was one of patient well-being because the nurse and other health care workers relied on the physician's notes to provide safe and effective care. Additionally, the nurse practitioner feared for the health and safety of patients because another physician, the prison's staff psychiatrist, failed to perform timely assessments of inmates with psychiatric disorders. The nurse practitioner lodged complaints about the two physicians through the facility's formal chain of command and was terminated by prison management.

The nurse sued her employer, claiming wrongful termination under Nevada's whistleblower protection statute. The nurse's former employer claimed she could not sue for wrongful termination because she did not comply with the state's "generic" whistleblower law, requiring her to report patient safety concerns directly to a public agency (Nevada State Department of Health). However, the US District Court for the District of Nevada ruled that the fired nurse practitioner had the right to sue her former employer for retaliating against her. The court based its opinion on the state of Nevada's "special" whistleblower law for health care workers. That special law protected nurses from retaliation (including termination) for internally reporting a situation that could compromise patient safety (*Scott v. Corizon Health*, 2014). The Court supported the nurse's claim that her employer violated the Nevada Revised Statute 449.207 regarding retaliation. The outcome of the nurse's suit against her former employer has not been reported in the legal literature.

Nursing publications provide recommendations and guidelines to any nurse considering the duty to report and its consequences (Kakacek, 2022; Lachman et al., 2012; Philipsen & Soeken, 2011). Nurses should be extremely careful to clarify their state's whistleblower protection law for health care workers before engaging in whistleblower activities. States vary widely in the requirements that must be met in order for a nurse to claim protection against retaliation for whistleblowing. A first step requires the nurse to contact the state's board of nursing to determine whistleblowing requirements established by the licensing board and/or formalized in that state's whistleblowing protection statute. An increasing number of legal experts advise the nurse to seek the services of an attorney who specializes in reporting and whistleblowing activities for nurses before making a decision to report (Delk, 2013; Snyder, 2014).

The types of conduct that the boards of nursing require nurses to report vary from state to state. Nurses can access the specific requirements for reporting nurse coworkers at their board of nursing website. Some states require nurses and providers to report victims of domestic or interpersonal violence, whether or not the victim (patient) consents. Nurses can access current information regarding federal and state reporting requirements under family or domestic violence statutes. For a list of family violence statutes compiled by The Pace Law

School Library (2021) visit https://libraryguides.law.pace.edu/c.php?g=319385&p=2134679. Certain specifiable communicable diseases, such as bubonic plague, Ebola, anthrax, and botulism, must also be reported to the Centers for Disease Control and Prevention (CDC). (For the list of reportable diseases visit https://www.cdc.gov/nchs/fastats/infectious-disease.htm.) State law may also require nurses to report injuries resulting from the use of weapons, attempts to harm the self, or impaired driving (Starr, 2019). Nurse managers and administrators are responsible for ensuring that reports made by direct-care nurses are forwarded to the appropriate legal authorities. Nurse leaders who fail in this duty may face criminal charges, claims of negligence, and disciplinary action by the nursing board (NSO/CNA, 2022).

Child Abuse Reporting Statutes. In 1974 the US Congress enacted the Child Abuse Prevention and Treatment Act, which mandates all states to meet specific uniform guidelines to qualify for federal funding of child abuse programs. All 50 states and the District of Columbia have created laws that require reporting of specific health problems and the *suspected* or confirmed abuse of infants or children. Nurses often are explicitly named within the context of these statutes as one of the groups of designated health professionals who must report the specified problems under penalty of fine or imprisonment. Nurses need not fear legal reprisal from individuals or families who are reported to authorities in suspected cases of abuse. Most legislatures have granted immunity from suit within the context of the mandatory reporting statute. There is also a long history of court decisions shielding the nurse from civil claims by parents or guardians when that report is made in good faith and in compliance with federal and state laws. The case of *Heinrich v. Conemaugh Valley Memorial Hospital* (1994) upheld this doctrine of immunity. The family of an injured child initiated a lawsuit against a hospital that reported suspected child abuse after a state investigation found them innocent of the charge. The court ruled that the hospital and the physician who made the report in "good faith" were immune from litigation under the Pennsylvania Child Protective Service Law that required reports of suspected child abuse.

It is crucial that nurses understand the requirements of abuse reporting statutes as they apply to their practice setting. For example, ED and pediatric nurses must have in-depth knowledge regarding child abuse reporting laws. Agency policies and procedures in the work setting may provide guidance in regard to reporting duties. If in doubt the nurse should immediately contact their supervisor, an administrator, or the agency's compliance officer (the individual responsible for understanding and ensuring adherence to federal and state statutes) for additional guidance in the matter. In rare situations, when information is not available within the institution, the nurse may consult with the state Department of Health and Human Services or the state nurses' licensing board for guidance and to obtain the reporting statutes. There are serious ramifications for failing to report as required by the state's specific statute, which could result in criminal charges and claims of negligence.

Institutional Licensing Laws

All facilities (e.g., hospitals, nursing homes, rehabilitation centers) providing health care services must comply with licensing laws promulgated by state legislatures. These laws are created to protect the public and ensure the safe and effective provision of health care services. Specific language usually is contained within health facility licensing statutes regarding the following issues:

- Minimal standards for the maintenance of the physical plant
- Basic operational aspects of major departments (nursing, dietary, clinical laboratories, and pharmacy)
- Essential aspects of patients' rights and the informed-consent process

Many state licensing laws mandate minimal levels of education, experience, or credentialing for department administrators, such as nurses, anesthesia personnel, pediatricians, and obstetricians. Several states also require minimum nurse–patient ratios in critical care units and other specialty departments, such as the operating room, nursery, and ED.

Health care redesign and cost-reduction efforts have led to many changes in the way health care services are provided and the settings in which care is rendered. Not all change has been positive, and some redesign schemes have resulted in adverse outcomes for patients (Mahlmeister, 2009). Investigations by state authorities on reports of patient injuries or death have discovered that in some cases health care facilities have operated in violation of existing licensing laws. In the past direct-care RNs generally could rely on their nurse managers to have a comprehensive knowledge of health facility licensing law and to create policies and procedures that implement and enforce applicable aspects of the law. The trend toward flattened management and reduction in role development for leaders has altered this picture. In an increasing number of settings nurse managers have been replaced with nonnurse administrators who may have minimal knowledge of the CoPs for Medicare and the state health facility licensing laws (Mahlmeister, 2015).

In light of these changes, direct-care nurses should have a working knowledge of current licensing laws as they relate to nursing care and patient care services. The nurse also is guided by the ANA's *Nursing: Scope and Standards of Practice*, which states: "The registered nurse systematically enhances the quality and effectiveness of nursing practice" (ANA, 2021). In many instances, nurses who have serious questions regarding quality of care in their employment setting have been able to resolve these concerns once they have read applicable sections of the health facility licensing law relevant to their setting. Bringing the pertinent section of the law to the attention of managers, administrators, a compliance officer, or the risk management department is often the most effective strategy to resolve problems. In settings in which nurses are represented by union contracts potential violations of health facility licensing laws may be most effectively addressed through union representatives.

Internet access has allowed nurses to obtain information about current institutional licensing laws easily. Information can be downloaded and printed quickly. Nurses also can obtain a copy of the health facility's licensing law for their employment setting through the state department or health division of licensing and certification. Other states provide the statute and address questions through the state department of health's divisions of facilities regulations, health facilities inspection, or health quality assurance. The telephone number for this agency can be found in the white pages of the local telephone directory under the heading "State of" (e.g., Michigan). Nurses can call their licensing board or the state nursing association for guidance in reaching the appropriate authority to obtain a copy of the licensing law and to speak to a consultant about concerns.

COMMON LAW

In addition to statutory law nursing practice is guided by common law, also known as decisional or *judge-made law*. Common law is created through cases heard and decided in federal and state appellate courts. Throughout the years judge-made law regarding nursing practice has accumulated in the form of written opinions. These opinions eventually contribute to the expected standard of nursing conduct. The body of written opinions about nurses also is known as nursing case law. The importance of nursing case law in establishing the current standard of practice cannot be overstated.

One of the most important cases to establish the expected conduct of nurses was *Utter v. United Hospital Center, Inc.* (1977). This West Virginia case affirmed that nurses were required to exercise independent judgment to prevent harm when caring for patients. Before the 1970s the issue of whether nurses were licensed professionals who made independent judgments was not clearly established. In the Utter case a patient whose arm was casted had signs and symptoms of compartment syndrome. The affected limb became progressively more edematous and eventually turned black. The nurses failed to activate the chain of command when the primary providers did not respond to their reports and requests for medical reevaluation. The patient's arm eventually had to be amputated. The court wrote:

> "Nurses are specialists in hospital care who, in the final analysis, hold the well-being, in fact in some instances, the very lives of patients in their hands. In the dim hours of the night, as well as in the light of day, nurses are frequently charged with the duty to observe the condition of the ill and infirm in their care. If the patient, helpless and wholly dependent, shows signs of worsening, the nurse is charged with the obligation of taking some positive action ... [T]here was evidence that certain nurses did not fulfill their obligation."

The duty to prevent harm, known as the nurse's "affirmative duty," has been supported in numerous court decisions. In *Rowe v. Sisters of Pallottine Missionary Society* (2001) a hospital and its ED nurses were found negligent for failing to question a physician's discharge order. A 17-year-old motorcyclist was admitted to the ED for an injury to his left leg. He complained of severe pain in his left knee and numbness in his left foot.

The nurses were unable to find a pulse in the left leg or foot. The physician issued a discharge order and gave instructions that included the application of ice and elevation of the affected leg. The next day the man sought emergency care at another hospital for worsening pain and swelling of his leg. An examination revealed a lacerated popliteal artery and dislocated knee. He underwent extensive surgery and suffered permanent impairment of the affected limb. The physician settled the suit against him for $275,000. The jury returned a verdict for the patient in excess of $880,000 and found the nurses negligent for failing to question the discharge order and to invoke the chain of command to obtain additional medical consultation and advice.

Every nurse should understand the effect that nursing case law has on their current practice. Case law made in appellate court decisions has addressed a range of vital issues related to professional nursing, including:

- Nursing malpractice cases
- Questions concerning labor law and collective bargaining
- Lawsuits alleging wrongful termination
- Legal challenges to state board of nursing disciplinary action against a nurse's license
- Legal actions against the nurse instituted by medical licensing boards
- "Practicing medicine without a license" claims
- Lawsuits claiming violation of the nurse's civil rights, including free speech issues and reasonable accommodation for nurses with disabilities

Efforts should be made by professional nurses to review case law as it is published and discussed in nursing journals. There has been a trend to incorporate "legal advice" columns into many practice journals, and journals often include discussions about nursing case law. There also has been a proliferation of nursing journals dedicated solely to legal issues in nursing practice.

Nurse managers, in particular, should have knowledge regarding the disposition of cases in their jurisdiction. A risk manager or agency attorney may help any nurse understand how judge-made law in their state relates to expectations for nursing practice in the local community. Many medical libraries also subscribe to publications that review federal or appellate court decisions in health care law that are relevant to the local community. Although local jury verdicts do not contribute to common law, it is useful for managers and interested nurses to periodically review published reports of malpractice cases in the state and their immediate community. Medical libraries also often subscribe to a local "jury verdicts" publication. (More information on finding nursing case law is available on the Evolve site at http://evolve.elsevier.com/Cherry/.)

CIVIL LAW

Two major categories of law have been created to deal with conduct that is considered unacceptable—criminal law and civil law. Nurses generally are more familiar with civil law and, in particular, the branch of civil law that deals with torts. Tort law is discussed first, with a discussion of criminal law following.

A *tort* is a civil wrong or injury committed by one person against another person or a property. The wrong results from a breach in one's legal duty regarding interpersonal relationships between private persons. This duty is established through societal expectations regarding interpersonal conduct (Butts & Rich, 2019). Civil suits are almost always brought by one person against another and generally are based on the concept of "fault." The person who initiates the civil lawsuit, the plaintiff, seeks damages for the wrongful behavior from the offending person, known as the defendant. The determination whether wrongful behavior has occurred usually is made by a jury, although in certain cases the right to a trial by jury can be waived by the private parties in the suit; in that case the judge considers the facts and determines the outcome. If the plaintiff succeeds in the civil lawsuit (plaintiff verdict) damages are generally awarded in the form of monetary compensation. Damages may include "hard" damages—financial reimbursement for treatment of injuries, loss of wages, rehabilitation services, or special equipment—and "soft" damages—monetary compensation for pain and suffering, loss of companionship, or mental anguish, among others (DeMarco et al., 2019).

Negligence and Malpractice

There are two types of torts: an unintentional tort (or wrong) and an intentional tort. An unintentional tort is an unintended wrong against another person. The two most common unintentional torts are negligence and malpractice.

Negligence is defined as the failure to act in a reasonable and prudent manner. The claim of negligence is based on the accepted principle that everyone is expected to conduct themselves in a reasonable and prudent fashion. This is true of laypersons, student nurses, and licensed professionals. A more formal definition of negligence is the failure of a person to use the care that a reasonably prudent and careful person would use under similar circumstances (DeMarco et al., 2019).

Malpractice is a special type of negligence (i.e., the failure of a professional, a person with specialized education and training, to act in a reasonable and prudent manner). As state NPAs have evolved to reflect the growing professionalism of RNs, courts have begun to recognize the negligent acts of nurses as malpractice. Evidence of this change in perceptions is apparent in the increasing use of RNs as expert witnesses in malpractice cases.

In general expert testimony is not needed in cases of "simple negligence" if the actions of the defendant are so obviously careless that even a layperson would recognize the conduct as negligent. In contrast, if the jury does not possess the special knowledge and information that professionals ordinarily have, an expert witness is required to establish whether the person breached the expected standard of care. In this case the breach of duty is not simple negligence but malpractice.

Elements Essential to Prove Negligence or Malpractice. Although any patient (or surviving family member, in the case of a patient death) may sue the nurse and their employer, the following elements must be proved for the plaintiff to succeed in the case.

1. The nurse owed the patient or client a special duty of care based on the establishment of a nurse–patient relationship. The nurse's acceptance of a patient assignment establishes the relationship and requires the nurse to meet their duty to the patient. The duty of the nurse is to possess the knowledge and skill that a reasonable and prudent nurse would possess and exercise in the same or similar patient care situation. The duty of the nurse as described is the standard of care. A nurse–patient relationship also may be established through telephone communication in the case of a nurse who performs telephone triage and advice or via computer or audiovisual systems that are being introduced in many health care settings (American Academy of Ambulatory Care Nursing, 2018). The COVID-19 pandemic has significantly accelerated the number of nurses engaged in telehealth and virtual care and will require enhanced guidelines and standards of practice that clearly articulate the nurse–patient relationship in this field of evolving nursing practice (Rutledge & Gustin, 2021; American Hospital Association, 2020).

2. The nurse has breached their duty to the patient or client. Evidence is presented that proves the nurse breached the standard of care. The standard of care is derived from a multiplicity of sources; these are described in Box 8.3.

3. Actual harm or damage is suffered by the patient.

4. There is proximate cause or a causal connection between the breach in the standard of care by the nurse and the patient's injury:
   - No intervening event is responsible for the injury.
   - A direct cause and effect can be demonstrated.
   - In some jurisdictions the nurse's breach of duty must only be proven to be a substantial cause of the patient's injury.

This last element merits further discussion. The relationship between the nurse's breach in the standard of care and the patient's injury must be established by the plaintiff. To prove proximate cause there must be a direct causal link. For example, a patient reports that he has an allergy to penicillin and wears a MedicAlert bracelet to that effect. A physician orders penicillin to treat the patient's infection. The nurse fails to check or to ask the patient about allergies. The nurse administers the penicillin, and the patient suffers an anaphylactic reaction and dies. There is a direct connection between the nurse's actions and the patient's death. Proximate cause has been established.

One may ask what the physician's liability is in this case. The physician also owes a duty to the patient and may be found negligent for ordering penicillin if they had knowledge of or should have had knowledge of the allergy. However, even in the case of a physician's negligence—"I knew about the penicillin allergy, but forgot"—the nurse has a separate and independent duty to the patient to prevent harm. The nurse must review the patient's medical record for information about allergies, ask the patient about allergies, and check the patient's identification band before administering a drug.

In some jurisdictions it is necessary only to prove that the nurse's actions were a substantial cause of the injury or harm to prove negligence. For example, in a large teaching hospital a nurse notes a significant change in a patient's vital signs, suggesting deterioration in his condition. A first-year resident is called to the bedside

---

BOX 8.3   Sources That Contribute to the Standard of Nursing Care

Federal Laws
Emergency Medical Treatment and Active Labor Law
Americans with Disabilities Act
Patient Self-Determination Act
Occupational Health and Safety Act
The Patient Safety and Quality Improvement Act

Federal Administrative Rules and Regulations
Rules and regulations for participation in Medicare

Federal Agencies
US Food and Drug Administration
Agency for Healthcare Research and Quality clinical
    guidelines
National Institutes of Health publications
Centers for Disease Control and Prevention publications
    (*Morbidity and Mortality Weekly Report*)
State Statutes
Nurse practice acts
State reporting statutes:
• Child abuse/elder abuse reporting statutes
• Domestic violence reporting statutes
• Health facility licensing laws

State Administrative Rules and Regulations
Licensing board rules

Board of Nursing
Position statements and advisories

Nursing Case Law
Appellate court decisions

Professional Organizations
Standards and guidelines for practice
Nursing journals
Position statements
Technical bulletins and practice resources
Code of Ethics

Manufacturer Guidelines
Durable medical equipment
Drugs and solutions
Disposable equipment and supplies

Agency Policies and Procedures
Job descriptions
Agency-specific documents
Nursing care plans
Care maps or critical pathways
Unit- or department-based standards of practice
Medical staff bylaws

---

and made aware of the patient's status. The resident orders the nurse to simply continue observing the patient. The first-year resident remains immediately available in the unit and receives repeated reports of a continued decline in the patient's condition. A clear chain-of-command policy is established in the hospital, which takes into account varying levels of skill and expertise of the residents in training. There is also a chain-of-command policy to deal with unresolved disagreements between health care professionals and nonresponsive providers. Despite the existence of these policies the nurse does not activate the chain of command.

The patient suffers hypovolemic shock caused by internal bleeding, leading to permanent anoxic brain damage. In this case the nurse's failure to obtain additional medical advice and consultation (a senior resident was physically present and available in the hospital) was a substantial cause of the patient's injury. These two examples illustrate that negligence may constitute a commission (inappropriate penicillin administration) or an omission (failure to activate the chain of command) in care.

Negligence and the Doctrine of *Res Ipsa Loquitur.*

In the majority of cases a plaintiff must retain a nurse expert witness because the jury does not ordinarily possess the scientific and technologic knowledge necessary to determine the required standard of care. When the negligent act clearly lies within the range of a jury's common knowledge and experience the doctrine of *res ipsa loquitur* ("the thing speaks for itself") may be applied. For instance, studies have reported close to 5000 foreign objects (instruments, needles, surgical sponges) inadvertently left in patients' bodies following surgery each year. Retained foreign bodies were associated with a higher average cost of health services than uncomplicated postsurgical care ($26,678 vs $12,648) (Al-Qurayshi et al., 2015).

Leaving a surgical instrument in the patient's body after an operation is one case in which the doctrine of *res ipsa loquitur* may apply. It would be obvious to any layperson that failure to remove a surgical instrument is below the standard of care.

Dickerson v. Fatehi (1997) illustrates this point. A woman who underwent neck surgery experienced severe pain in her right arm, hand, and neck after the procedure. Approximately 20 months later a second procedure was performed to determine the cause of the patient's continued pain. An 18-gauge hypodermic needle with a plastic attachment for a syringe was discovered in her neck and removed. The woman sued the surgeon and nurses involved in the original surgical procedure. The claims against the nurses included a failure to maintain a proper needle count and a failure to ensure the removal of the needle after surgery. The court hearing this case dismissed the suit. On appeal the Supreme Court of Virginia reversed the lower court's decision and directed the case for trial. The Supreme Court held that in this particular case expert testimony was not necessary to establish the applicable standard of care and that the doctrine of *res ipsa loquitur* applied. A jury would be able to determine whether a reasonably prudent circulating nurse and scrub nurse should have made and reported an accurate needle count.

Gross Negligence. In some cases the negligent act of the nurse is so reckless and reflects such a conscious disregard for the patient's welfare that it represents gross negligence. When the nurse acts with complete indifference to the consequences for their patient the court may award special damages meant to punish the nurse for the outrageous conduct. These damages are referred to as *punitive damages*. Each state has established standards to determine when punitive damages may be awarded. In *Mobile Infirmary Medical Center v. Hodgen* (2003) the jury awarded $2.5 million in punitive damages (later reduced to $1.5 million) when a new graduate, not yet licensed, administered five times the ordered dose of digoxin. The jury found that the new graduate had been improperly supervised by the novice nurse assigned as her preceptor by the shift charge nurse. The charge nurse was also found liable for failing to properly direct the preceptor in her role responsibilities. The Supreme Court of Alabama found that the nurses acted callously and wantonly, the legal threshold that must be crossed before punitive damages can be awarded (Snyder, 2003).

Claims of Negligence and Student Nurses

Claims of negligence may arise when student nurses provide care. The emphasis on patient safety and reporting preventable adverse outcomes has brought an increasing number of student errors to light (Silvestre et al., 2023; Willey, 2018). In a 2020 report of claims paid by a large indemnifier, allegations of negligence arising from care provided by student nurses resulted in the highest average total damages paid of all health care licensure types (NSO/CNA, 2022). Because the student is not yet a licensed professional the faculty member or licensed nurse who is supervising the student is also often named in the lawsuit. The state board of nursing may have an advisory or position statement regarding the scope of practice of nursing students, and the duty of the registered nurse supervising the student, to maintain the appropriate level of oversight. Such is the case in California, where the Board of Nursing has promulgated a position statement, "Clinical Learning Experiences: Nursing Students," to guide the supervising nurse in her duty (California Department of Consumer Affairs, 2008). The agency or hospital in which the student is practicing also may be named under the legal doctrine of vicarious liability. *Dimora v. Cleveland Clinic Foundation* (1996) is a case in point. A student nurse was assigned to care for a patient who had serious difficulty maintaining her balance and required close supervision when standing, walking, and transferring. The student nurse testified that she knew the patient had an unsteady gait but still left her unattended on a commode. The patient fell and was injured. The hospital was named in the lawsuit and appealed, claiming the student was not an employee. The Ohio Court of Appeals ruled that a hospital was held to the same legal standard of care for a student nurse's error as for the same error committed by a licensed professional nurse.

Several other cases reinforce the importance of informing the patient that a student is providing the care and of documenting that the patient agrees to the care. In *Lovett v. Lorain Community Hospital* (2004) a student nurse, under the direct supervision of an instructor, administered Demerol and Vistaril by the intramuscular route and punctured the patient's sciatic nerve. The patient sued the hospital for negligence. A lower court dismissed the initial lawsuit because the student and the instructor were not employees of the hospital. The Ohio Court of Appeals reversed the lower court's decision.

The higher court affirmed that a patient may assume that the care they receive in a hospital is provided by that institution. The patient can assume that the student and instructor are agents of the hospital, unless the patient has been specifically informed and has agreed to receive care from the student (Snyder, 2004). Because a student nurse is not yet a licensed professional, if a lawsuit is filed the alleged claim is usually "ordinary negligence" rather than "professional malpractice."

Criminal Negligence

Criminal negligence applies when the negligent acts of the nurse (normally an unintentional civil wrong) also constitute a crime. In most states a nurse can be prosecuted when the conduct is deemed so reckless that the action results in serious harm to or death of the patient. Nurses with criminal convictions accounted for approximately 10% of the disciplinary actions taken by state boards of nursing (BONs) between 2003 and 2013 (Zhong et al., 2016).

In 1997 two RNs and an advanced practice nurse licensed in Colorado were charged with criminal negligent homicide in the death of a newborn resulting from a medication error (Kowalski & Horner, 1998). In this case an oil-based form of penicillin was erroneously administered to the infant. The drug was administered at 10 times the physician's prescribed dose. This case, first discussed in the nursing literature in 1998, describes medication dispensing and administration practices that still exist in many US hospitals, placing patients in immediate jeopardy and exposing nurses to claims of criminal negligence. A case that occurred in Wisconsin in 2006 illustrates the ongoing risks for catastrophic medication errors (Medical Ethics Advisor, 2007). A labor and delivery nurse inadvertently administered a piggyback solution bag of epidural anesthesia through a peripheral intravenous line. The patient, a 16-year-old female, experienced cardiovascular collapse and died. The error was compounded by failures to place an identification band on the patient and to use the available point-of-care barcode system. In the root cause analysis of this sentinel event conducted at a later date "multiple latent systems failures" were also identified (Smetzer et al., 2010). The Wisconsin Department of Justice charged the nurse with a felony criminal offense. The charge was eventually reduced to a misdemeanor count of illegally administering prescription medications. The Wisconsin Department of Health

and Human Services imposed restriction on the nurse's ability to participate in any capacity in a facility funded by Medicare and Medicare programs for 5 years. The Wisconsin Department of Regulation and Licensing suspended the nurse's license for 9 months, and the hospital terminated her employment. In response to the Wisconsin case the ANA released a statement opposing charges of criminal misconduct against a registered nurse who did not intentionally mean to harm the patient (ANA, 2007). The American Association of Nurse Attorneys (TAANA) in collaboration with the American Association of Legal Nurse Consultants (AALNC) also published a Position Paper, "Criminal Prosecution of Health Care Providers for Unintentional Human Error" (TAANA, 2011).

Despite the opposition to criminalization of errors serious concerns persist. In 2022 a Tennessee jury found a nurse guilty of criminally negligent homicide and gross neglect of an impaired adult patient. The charges and subsequent verdict resulted from the death of a patient in 2017, after the nurse administered the wrong medication. Although the nurse could have been sentenced to up to 8 years in prison, the judge granted leniency. The nurse was sentenced to 3 years of supervised probation. The case was reported widely by news media and in health care publications. Both nursing organizations and individual nurses once again spoke out against the criminalization of nursing errors. When the incident was evaluated by experts in the field of patient safety significant systems flaws were identified that contributed to the medication error (ISMP, 2022). In 2019 the ANA again released a statement in opposition to the criminalization of errors (ANA, 2019). The Colorado, Wisconsin, and Tennessee cases should be read by every student nurse and licensed nurse for full appreciation of the change in the legal climate in the United States. They reflect the changing perspective of our justice system when negligent acts of health care professionals result in patient death.

Conservative estimates published in 2020 (Brittain & Carrington, 2021) suggested that as many as 225,000 patients die each year as a result of the negligence and malpractice of health care providers and another 90,000 deaths per year are attributed to hospital-acquired infections (CMS, 2020c). National data regarding hospital-acquired infections may be accessed at the CDC's National Healthcare Safety Network (http://www.cdc.gov/nhsn/). Later data derived from surveillance activities conducted by the Institute for Healthcare Improvement (IHI) using a new tracking tool, the "Global Trigger Tool," found that the number of adverse events in hospitals may *be 10 times greater than previously measured* (Classen et al., 2011). There is still uncertainty regarding the actual number of deaths occurring each year from error. However, based on statistical analyses of closed medical records, and data reported to the CDC and the CMS, there are an estimated 250,000 deaths each year attributed to medical error (Clark, 2020).

Other negative consequences that a nurse faces when criminal charges are filed include the loss of their job and disciplinary action by the state licensing board. Even when the criminal charges are not supported the nurse's license can be suspended or revoked, and out-of-pocket fines may be levied by the board if there is evidence of violation of the NPA. An attorney may have to be retained to represent the nurse when criminal charges are filed, and the nurse's malpractice insurance generally does not cover the attorney's fees in these cases (CNA/NSO, 2020a). Neither is the nurse's employer obligated to pay the legal fees of a nurse charged with a felony. In the Colorado case the nurse practitioner was immediately terminated. The two direct-care nurses were permitted to work in nonpatient care areas. The costs of the criminal defense of all three nurses were paid by the hospital.

Nursing care that is deemed "deplorable" by the courts may result in disqualification of the nurse's employer from participation in the federal government's Medicare or Medicaid programs. Essentially the facility will be without adequate funding to continue operating. A case in point is *Barbourville Nursinghome v. U.S. Department of Health and Human Services* (2006). During a compliance survey visit to the facility by the US Department of Health and Human Services (USDHHS) major infractions of nursing home regulations were discovered. The federal government levied a fine in excess of $24,000 and, because the actions of the nurses placed the patients in immediate jeopardy (e.g., contaminating wounds with feces during dressing changes and inadequate skin care resulting in severe pressure sores), the nursing home was disqualified from participating in Medicare.

Defenses Against Claims of Negligence

In some cases a nurse can use certain legal doctrines as a defense against a claim of negligence. These standard defenses are discussed in the next section. In no case may a nurse provide a defense of "only following the provider's orders" against allegations of negligence (Clanton, 2022; ANA, 2015a; Greenberg, 2017). The NPA, licensing board rules and regulations, and nursing case law have delineated the nurse's independent duty to evaluate all provider orders before implementing them. In doing so the nurse must consider two points: (1) is the order lawful and (2) is the order in this particular patient's best interest?

Each nurse has an absolute duty to take some positive action to prevent harm when orders are inappropriate or incomplete or when the actions of another health care provider endanger the patient's well-being. This principle of affirmative duty is well recognized in law and in ethics. The ANA *Code of Ethics for Nurses* (2015a) and the American Medical Association's *Code of Medical Ethics* (2016) recognize the central role of nurses in preventing patient harm. A second principle underlying the nurse's legal and professional obligation to address questionable physician's orders or plan of care is patient advocacy (Ramsay et al., 2022; ANA, 2015a). The nurse's duty to "speak out" to support and protect patients has been reaffirmed by The Joint Commission in its "Speak Up" initiative (TJC, 2014). An identified barrier to speaking up is the nurse's cultural and ethnic background as well as gender (Lee et al., 2021).

In *Columbia Medical Center of Las Colinas v. Bush* (2003) a jury awarded $13.1 million to a patient who suffered permanent brain damage and had no independent motor function or capacity for speech after receiving the wrong medication for a cardiac dysrhythmia. After consulting with a cardiologist the ED physician had ordered verapamil for treatment of the patient's ventricular tachycardia. The ED nurse, who was certified in advanced life support, and her nursing supervisor, who was present, knew the drug was contraindicated for ventricular tachycardia. The two nurses did not question the order and permitted an emergency medical technician (EMT) to give the drug. The patient suffered profound hypotension and cardiopulmonary arrest. The Texas Court of Appeals opined that the nurse and her supervisor had a duty, when they had serious questions about a medication involving extreme risk to the patient, to activate the chain of command to obtain additional medical consultation and advice (Tammelleo, 2003).

Emergency Situations

Nursing care rendered in a life-threatening emergency may breach the standard of care required under ordinary circumstances. For instance, a woman who is 8 months pregnant arrives in the labor and delivery suite. She is hemorrhaging because of a premature separation of the placenta (abruptio placentae). An emergency cesarean delivery is ordered by the physician. The woman is near death as a result of blood loss. There also are clear signs of fetal distress. To expedite the surgical delivery the operating room team does not observe the strict aseptic technique normally required during insertion of a Foley catheter into the woman's bladder and forgoes the lengthy abdominal scrub normally performed with an iodine solution.

The mother and infant are brought through the crisis safely, although a skin infection develops at the site of the woman's abdominal incision, which causes noticeable scarring. She also must be treated for a bladder infection, which resolves by discharge on the fourth postpartum day. She sues the nurses and physician. In this case the defense could argue that the methods used were reasonable and prudent to save the life of the mother and baby. Even a delay of seconds could have resulted in the death of the woman or her infant. Expert witnesses are produced to support the defense assertion that in this particular situation following customary procedures in preparing this woman for surgery would have breached the standard of care.

Governmental Immunity

For nurses working in federal or state health care facilities a defense of governmental immunity may be used. Laws have been enacted that shield individual health care workers employed in federal or (some) state facilities from personal responsibility for damages awarded in malpractice cases. Nurses employed by the Department of Veterans Affairs, the US Public Health Service, the National Aeronautics and Space Administration, and the Department of Defense are shielded from civil suits when in the performance of professional duties. This immunity was granted through enactment of specific federal statutes, including the Federal Tort Claims Act of 1946 and the Federal Employees Liability Reform and Tort Compensation Act of 1988. The intent of these laws was to substitute the US government as the defendant in a malpractice suit. The government has waived its sovereign immunity against suit and pays the damages for injuries caused by the negligent acts of health care professionals employed in the aforementioned federal agencies.

State immunity statutes vary. In some instances, individual states have not waived their sovereign immunity from lawsuits. In these cases, the state is *not* substituted for the individual health care provider in malpractice cases. Nurses and physicians are liable for their negligent acts in these states and are personally responsible for damages awarded. It may be imperative in this circumstance for the health care professional to have individual malpractice insurance (O'Neill, 2021; Pohlman, 2015). The nurse should seek the advice of an attorney to determine whether it would be prudent to purchase malpractice insurance. The state affiliate of the ANA may also be helpful in this regard.

Good Samaritan Immunity

Good Samaritan laws may limit a nurse's liability or shield the nurse from a malpractice claim if the nurse renders assistance in an emergency that occurs outside the employment setting. Although in most states the nurse owes no legal duty to an accident victim, once the nurse makes a decision to stop and render aid (an ethical decision) a nurse–patient relationship is established. (Some states, including Vermont, Minnesota, and Wisconsin, have enacted "duty to rescue" or "compulsory assistance" laws.) Nurses should contact the state licensing board or the state association of the ANA to determine whether the state in which they are licensed has a "duty to rescue" law.

When the nurse renders care at the scene of an accident they are required to render the standard of care that any reasonable and prudent nurse would render in a similar situation. To prevail in a malpractice suit under the Good Samaritan laws the injured plaintiff must prove that the nurse intentionally caused the injury or was grossly negligent (Varacallo, 2020). Therefore each nurse should be familiar with their state-specific Good Samaritan statute. Nurses also should be reassured by the fact that the preponderance of malpractice cases that invoke the Good Samaritan defense are settled in favor of the nurse.

Statutes of Limitation in Malpractice Cases

Each state has established a time limit in which a person may initiate a lawsuit. Although many states have established a time limit of 2 or 3 years from the date of the patient's injury or death in which the plaintiff must sue, statutes of limitation vary widely from state to state. In some jurisdictions a "termination of treatment" rule exists. It is predicated on the assumption that some injuries result from a series of treatments over time. In this case the statute of limitation does not begin to run until the treatment ends.

Other rules and regulations govern the "tolling" or running of the statutes of limitation. The court recognizes that an injured party cannot initiate a malpractice case until they discover that some harm was done (discovery rule). This can occur when health care providers actually hide the facts in the case of an injury through fraud, deceit, or concealment, such as through:

- Fraudulent or misleading entries in the medical record
- Destruction of evidence
- Destruction of the medical record

An Iowa case provides an example of a situation in which the statute of limitations may be extended (*Hanssen v. Genesis Health*, 2011). An orthopedic nurse erroneously gave a patient twice the dose of narcotic pain medication ordered by the physician. The patient became lethargic, experienced breathing problems, and fell twice in the bathroom. After the patient was discharged from the hospital the orthopedic unit nurse manager wrote a letter to him. In the letter the manager falsely stated that upon review of his chart it was discovered that he had not received an incorrect dose of medication, but that he had a sensitivity reaction to the drug. The patient subsequently requested a copy of his complete medical record and decided to file a lawsuit against the nurse and hospital. The suit was filed more than 2 years after the alleged malpractice, which exceeded Iowa's 2-year statute of limitations. The hospital petitioned the court to dismiss the case on the basis of the tolling of the statute. The court ruled that there were legal grounds for extending the statute because the patient was not aware of the medication error until he received a complete copy of the medical record, at which time he filed a claim.

The statute of limitation also is altered when a foreign object is left in the patient's body. Until the foreign object is discovered the statute of limitation does not begin to run. States have rules that regulate the tolling of the statute of limitation in cases involving mentally incompetent adults and minors. In the case of an adult patient who is so severely injured that there is a loss of

mental capacity the statute of limitation may not begin to toll until the patient regains mental competence. The statute of limitation varies in the case of minors and may expire only when the child reaches the age of majority (18 or 21 years of age) (DeMarco et al., 2019).

Each nurse should be familiar with the statute of limitation for their state. If the nurse suspects that some form of fraud or deceit has occurred relative to a patient's injury the agency's risk manager or attorney should be contacted immediately. Major penalties and fines are applicable in cases in which health care providers deliberately deceive the patient or destroy evidence. These acts rise to the level of criminal misconduct and can result in loss of one's professional license and possible incarceration.

Transparency and Disclosure of Error. When errors occur in practice studies repeatedly confirm that telling the patient (and family) about the mistake (voluntary disclosure) results in far less severe ramifications for the clinicians and health care facility (Kaldjian, 2021; Hannawa et al., 2016). In 2001 TJC established a new patient safety care standard requiring that institutions have a process in place to disclose unanticipated outcomes to patients. Disclosure of errors and unanticipated adverse outcomes is a key element of the national patient safety movement (PS Net 2019b). The process of disclosure has been delineated by the National Quality Forum (NQF) in its publication, "Safe Practices for Better Healthcare" (2010). Safe Practice Number 7 states:

Following serious unanticipated outcomes, including those that are clearly caused by systems failures, the patient, and as appropriate, the family should receive timely, transparent, and clear communication concerning what is known about the event (Welsh, 2021) (p. v).

When an unanticipated outcome occurs the provider is generally responsible for discussing the situation with the patient and/or family members. Other agency representatives may be involved in the disclosure process, including administrators, risk managers, and attorneys. The nurse should not assume responsibility for disclosure before speaking to the provider and agency leaders (Shannon, 2009). It should be determined in advance who will speak with the patient (or family) and how questions and concerns about the patient's condition, subsequent treatment, and the cost of any required care will be addressed. Fear that disclosure will lead to a malpractice claim is a significant barrier to voluntary disclosure, despite research findings to the contrary (PS Net, 2019c). In fact, patients sue for many reasons, including withdrawal of health team members after the event, silence, mishandling of information about unanticipated outcomes, delayed communication about adverse events, and anger when they believe they have not been told the truth about events (Bell et al., 2017).

If a nurse believes that the patient has not received essential information the nurse discusses such concerns first with the provider. If further clarification is required the nurse refers to the facility's chain of command or unresolved dispute policy. Research conducted (Choi et al., 2021) on nurses' perceptions regarding disclosure found that nurses conceived of disclosure as a team event rather than a physician–patient discussion. Nurses believed they were excluded from the disclosure process. Furthermore, nurses in the study focus groups admitted to routinely and independently disclosing nursing errors that did not involve serious injury, but believed that when systems flaws or team mistakes contributed to the error and injury the physician should serve as the team leader in the disclosure discussion.

Nursing Malpractice Insurance

With more states recognizing nursing malpractice as a legitimate claim in a civil suit the question of whether nurses should carry malpractice insurance has become increasingly important. Nursing journals have published a number of articles that either address this question or describe the types of malpractice coverage the nurse should consider (O'Neill, 2021); textbooks also discuss the issue of liability insurance. A growing consensus appears to recommend that because of changes in the health care system, civil law, and insurance company policies, all nurses purchase malpractice insurance. Legal writers also are quick to note the fallacy of the assumption that having malpractice insurance increases the risk that the nurse will be targeted in a malpractice case. Lack of coverage will not discourage a lawsuit when there is a legitimate claim. Reasons given for the purchase of malpractice insurance by RNs include:

- Expanding functions of RNs and advanced practice nurses
- Floating and cross-training mandates
- Increasing responsibility for supervising subordinate staff
- Failure of some employers to initiate an adequate defense for nurses

- Work liability (insurance) coverage limits that are lower than the actual judgment made against the nurse in a lawsuit

Other considerations that the nurse must take into account when considering malpractice insurance include whether they are employed by the federal government. In this case the nurse may be shielded from personal liability by federal tort statutes, although some states still uphold the doctrine of "sovereign immunity," making it impossible to sue a state-run medical facility for negligence. In these states it is a virtual necessity for nurses to purchase malpractice insurance because health care workers become the only available targets in a malpractice case.

Liability

Closely tied to the concepts of negligence and malpractice is liability. Liability asserts that every person is responsible for the wrong or injury done to another resulting from carelessness.

Personal Liability

Within the context of nursing practice the nurse is always accountable for the outcomes of their actions in carrying out nursing duties. The rule of personal liability requires the professional nurse to assume responsibility for patient harm or injury that is a result of their negligent acts. The nurse cannot be relieved of personal liability by another professional, such as a provider or nurse manager, who asserts, "Don't worry; I'll take responsibility for the consequences."

The principle of personal liability is illustrated in a Connecticut case, *Osiecki v. Bridgeport Health Care Center, Inc.* (2005). A jury found that a nurse caring for a patient with a tracheostomy failed to provide proper tracheostomy care, assessment of breath sounds, and reevaluation of the patient's pulmonary status at appropriate intervals. The patient died secondary to a pulmonary hemorrhage, and the breaches in the standard of nursing care were found to be a substantial factor contributing to the patient's death. Had the nurse properly assessed the patient and at frequent intervals, early identification of pulmonary congestion would have permitted timely treatment. The surviving spouse was awarded $827,000 for the nurse's negligent actions. In another case, *Janga v. Colombrito* (2011), the nurses caring for a patient receiving anticoagulants were sued individually for his death, which was due to complications of bleeding. The nurses were found negligent for failing to question the order for anticoagulants before a patient underwent a lumbar puncture. There was conflicting testimony about whether or not a physician had issued an order to discontinue the anticoagulants. However, even if the physician did not direct the nurses to stop the medications, the plaintiff's expert witness nurse asserted that they had a duty to recognize that anticoagulants should not be given prior to a lumbar puncture and to advise the physician that they had nevertheless been administered. The court directed the jury to weigh the extent to which the nurses' negligence contributed to the unfortunate outcome (comparative negligence). The jury directed the nurses to pay 15% of the monetary award.

In 1989 the ANA summarized the most frequent allegations of negligence leveled against nurses in malpractice cases (Box 8.4). These charges have not substantially changed in the ensuing decades (CNA/NSO, 2020b). As nurses assume more and more responsibility for the monitoring and care of patients with complex health problems, the claim of "failure to rescue" is made with increasing frequency (Kendall et al., 2020; The Joint Commission, 2018; Garvey, 2015). Nurses may be educated to implement effective risk-control strategies

---

BOX 8.4 Most Frequent Allegations of Nursing Negligence

- Failure to communicate and report*
- Failure to monitor the patient and report significant findings
- Failure to ensure patient safety
- Failure to rescue
- Improper treatment or negligent performance of the treatment
- Medication errors
- Failure to follow the agency's policies and procedures
- Failure to invoke the chain of command/access the line of authority

*The Joint Commission found that communication failures (i.e., reporting, situation-background-assessment-recommendation [SBAR] communication, and shift handoffs) were the number-one contributing cause of medical error and preventable adverse outcomes.
From The Joint Commission (TJC). (2005). *Joint Commission guide to improving staff communication.* TJC; and The Joint Commission (TJC). (2017). *Inadequate handoff communication.* Sentinel Event Alert Issue 58. TJC.
Adapted from McGuire, C., & Mroczek, J.M. (2023). *Nursing malpractice.* Course 125. The National Center of Continuing Education. https://www.nursece.com/pdf/125_NurseMalpractice.pdf

---

that reduce these claims. These personal and system-wide strategies are discussed in the next section.

Many nurses practice under the misconception that they are protected from personal liability when employed by a health care entity such as a hospital. I have heard nurses say, "Why would a patient sue me personally? I don't have the financial resources of this (hospital, nursing home, home health care agency)!" Nurses can and have been individually named in lawsuits and found negligent. Damages can be levied against the nurse's current assets and future earnings for negligent acts. Furthermore as Snyder (2003) reports, hospitals have sued nurses to recoup financial losses suffered when they were required to pay damages for the alleged negligence of the nurses named in the malpractice case. Personal liability is illustrated in the case of *Siegel v. Long Island Jewish Medical Center* (2003).

Personal Liability with Floating and Cross-Training

New models of patient care often mandate floating and cross-training of patient care staff to enhance efficiency and reduce staffing costs. These models of care have increased the personal liability of nurses. Professional nurses must be cognizant of state statutes and case law when asked to perform services outside of their usual area of practice. Many State Boards of Nursing have also published Advisories or Position Statements regarding floating. The New York State Nursing Association has posted online its "Position Statement on Floating" which can be accessed at: https://www.nysna.org/search/node/position%20statement%20on%20floating.

In no case is a nurse permitted to perform tasks or render services for which they lack the requisite knowledge and skill to do so competently.

The NPA and the administrative rules and regulations of the licensing board provide explicit statutory language regarding a nurse's duty to provide safe and competent care. For example, the Administrative Rules of the Tennessee Board of Nursing (revised, 2019) state:

The Board believes that the individual nurse is responsible for maintaining and demonstrating competence in the practice role whether the recipient of the nursing intervention is the individual, family, community, nursing staff, nursing student body, or other.

Tennessee Rules and Regulations of Registered Nurses Rule 1000-01-14: Standards of Nursing Competence

In addition to the laws governing practice in floating and cross-training situations, an increasing body of nursing case law also defines the limitation of assignments. Appellate court decisions have addressed the issue of when a nurse may safely refuse an assignment to float without the risk of job termination. A landmark case, *Winkelman v. Beloit Memorial Hospital* (1992), addressed the legal issues surrounding floating. The Supreme Court of Wisconsin ruled in this case that under certain circumstances a nurse had a right to refuse floating assignments without fear of reprisal.

Nurse Winkelman was a skilled maternity nurse who was employed for 16 years at Beloit Memorial Hospital, working exclusively in the nursery. In 1987 the hospital created a policy that required nurses in the maternity setting to float when the patient census was low in their unit. Nurse Winkelman was asked to float to an adult floor dedicated to the care of postoperative and geriatric patients. She notified her immediate supervisor that she did not feel qualified to float to that unit and that attempting to provide care in that setting would place the patients at risk. In her testimony the nurse said that she was given three choices: float, find another nurse who would float in her place, or take an unexcused absence day. She subsequently went home, and her employer construed her actions as "voluntary resignation of her employment." Nurse Winkelman then filed a complaint for wrongful discharge and breach of contract. A jury verdict was rendered in favor of Nurse Winkelman on the charge of wrongful discharge. The case was appealed and affirmed by the Supreme Court of Wisconsin. The court found that the nurse had identified a fundamental and well-defined public policy in the Wisconsin Administrative Code, which stated that a nurse should not offer or perform services for which they are not qualified by education, training, or experience.

The nurse's right to refuse a floating assignment has not been supported in all cases. Courts have affirmed the right of a health care facility to redirect staff to meet the needs of patients. The New Mexico Supreme Court, in *Francis v. Memorial General Hospital* (1986), held that the hospital was not prohibited from discharging a nurse who refused to float when the employer had made a reasonable offer to train the nurse for new responsibilities. Nurse Francis, a critical care nurse, refused to float to an orthopedic unit, stating he did not feel qualified to care for orthopedic patients. The hospital then offered to provide him with an orientation to the floors where he might float in the future. When he refused the opportunity for orientation he was terminated. The court upheld his discharge.

Although it is clear that nurses have a legal duty to refuse specific tasks that they cannot perform safely and competently, the prudent nurse should carefully consider the consequences of not floating. Careful negotiation with the nursing supervisor and the team leader making the actual assignment often results in a satisfactory compromise. The floated nurse should clarify which aspects of professional nursing care they can safely carry out and which tasks are beyond their current capabilities. A reasonable supervisor will not insist that a nurse attempt to perform a task that they have no education, training, or current expertise to implement.

Another important strategy that may reduce the nurse's personal liability is to request that the team leader appoint a resource nurse who is skilled in the care of the patients on the unit. The resource nurse can assist the floated nurse as needed. It also is prudent practice for the floated nurse to enter a note in the medical record naming the resource or support nurse who will be available and responsible to assist with planning and evaluating care. For instance:

Assumed care of Mrs. Jones after report completed. L. Doe, RN, will co-manage patient and assist with procedures, planning, and evaluation of care as needed.

J. Smith, RN (Floater)

An NPA affirms that an RN ultimately is responsible for the quality of care provided to each patient, regardless of who actually is delegated the responsibility of carrying out the task. A claim of negligence may be leveled against the team leader who does not assign a competent "backup" or resource nurse to assist the floater. Only a nurse who is competent in the care of the patients normally treated in the setting (hospital, clinic, or home) can properly supervise a lesser-skilled worker and evaluate the outcomes of care.

Furthermore, TJC requires accredited organizations to ensure that all staff providing patient care, including float staff and agency or registry nurses, are properly oriented to their jobs and the work environment before providing care (2023). Chapter 13 provides additional information about floating and accepting assignments.

Personal Liability for Charge Nurses and Team Leaders and Managers

The concept of personal liability extends to nurses who function as team leaders, supervisors, and upper-level managers. Team leaders, charge nurses, and managers are held to the standard of care of the reasonably prudent nurse employed in that role (CNA/NSO, 2020b). Claims of negligence leveled against charge nurses generally surround the following situations:

- Functioning as a first responder in emergencies
- Triage of patients and allocation of staff and equipment
- Delegation of patient care tasks
- Supervision of orientees, float staff, and subordinates
- Reporting performance deficits in team members
- Supporting or invoking the chain-of-command process when indicated

Nurse managers and administrators at the upper end of the management ladder also may be held liable for the following scenarios:

- Inadequate training
- Failure to periodically reevaluate staff competencies
- Failure to discipline or terminate unsafe workers
- Negligence in developing appropriate policies and procedures
- Failure to uphold institutional licensing laws and state and federal statutes

The critical role of the charge nurse in promoting positive patient outcomes and reducing error is reflected in an Ohio Nurses Association Nursing Practice Statement (NP 21) regarding charge nurse responsibilities. The Practice Statement identifies 18 essential duties of the charge nurse (ONA, 2016). The many and varied role responsibilities of the charge nurse or team leader increases the risk for claims of malpractice.

The implementation of new models of care that alter staffing patterns and mixes may place managers at the same risk for liability as the health care providers delivering the actual bedside care (CNA/NSO, 2020b). The ANA affirms this view in the *Code of Ethics for Nurses* (2015a): "Although nurses in administration, education, and research have relationships with patients that are less direct, in assuming the responsibilities of a particular role, they share responsibility for the care provided by those whom they supervise and instruct" (p. 17).

The appropriate standard of care is established in the case of team leaders, charge nurses, managers, and leaders by expert nurse witnesses who function in those positions. An increasing body of case law in malpractice suits also is contributing to expectations about team leader and manager conduct. Although nurse managers and administrators generally are well aware of their particular liability risks, direct-care nurses who are relatively unfamiliar with the expanding role of team leaders or charge nurses may be particularly vulnerable to claims of negligence. Health care redesign has resulted in considerable flattening of the chain of command for nursing departments.

In September 2003 the American Organization of Nurse Executives, the American Hospital Association, and other health-related organizations submitted an *amicus curiae* (friend of the court) brief in support of the unique role of the charge nurse (Oakwood Healthcare, Inc., 348 J.L.R.B., No. 37, 2006). These associations responded to a National Labor Relations Board invitation to file briefs to provide guidance on the meaning of the term independent judgment and the scope of discretion required for independent judgment with respect to the charge nurse. The brief asserts: "The charge nurse's background in the hospital's organization and in nursing practice enables him or her to step in when there is crisis or conflict, quickly to assess the situation and identify needed resources. Charge nurses also direct other employees, sometimes making split-second decisions that can literally be a matter of life or death" (pp. 6–7).

Team leaders, regardless of their title or designation, have assumed greater responsibility for unit- or department-based functions American Nursing Association (ANA) (May 19, 2023).

Any RN functioning in the role of team leader or charge nurse should review the following documents from administration:

- Detailed job description for the role, including how responsibilities are limited when the nurse is asked to lead a team or serve as a charge nurse on an unfamiliar floor or department
- Job descriptions for the team members assigned delegated tasks
- Formal period of training and mentoring in the role
- Validated proof of competence before leading a team independently
- Guidelines regarding personal patient care assignment when also serving as team leader
- Chain-of-command model for the facility, department, or unit

Administrators and nurse managers should be aware of landmark case laws regarding incompetent charge nurses and team leaders. A jury directed a verdict in excess of $7 million against a hospital in a 1995 Illinois case, *Holston v. Sisters of the Third Order* (1995). A charge nurse repeatedly refused a direct-care nurse's requests to personally evaluate a patient whose vital signs were rapidly deteriorating after gastric bypass surgery. The charge nurse also refused to call the patient's physician until the patient experienced cardiopulmonary collapse. Emergency surgery revealed that a central venous pressure catheter had migrated and perforated the cardiac muscle. The patient experienced cardiac tamponade and died approximately 1 week after this critical incident.

This case illustrates the necessity of validating the strong clinical skill of all RNs who are being considered for a leadership role that includes clinical supervision and consultation. Effective risk management of an unresolved clinical problem requires direct-care nurses to consult early and frequently with team leaders or managers. Each consultation with the team leader or manager should be carefully documented in the patient's medical record to demonstrate that appropriate chain-of-command process has occurred. The employer will likely be named in any lawsuit under the rule of vicarious liability if the team leader or manager offers negligent advice. Vicarious liability is discussed later in this chapter.

Personal Liability in Delegation and Supervision of Team Members

Team leaders and charge nurses who are responsible for delegation and supervision of team members must be absolutely clear about the legality of patient care assignments. In 2019 the American Nurses Association and the National Council of State Boards of Nursing (NCSBN) jointly published the "National Guidelines for Nursing Delegation." This resource delineates in detail the legal and professional duties of the RN when delegating care. The RN must determine whether it is reasonable and prudent to delegate a particular task on the basis of their knowledge of the worker, scope of practice, the patient's status and complexity of care, and the current conditions in the work setting. The duty to safely and lawfully delegate tasks and activities is integral to the professional role of the RN, whether a direct care provider, a charge nurse/team leader or a nurse who is a member of the leadership team. The determination whether a nurse has been negligent in

delegating any particular patient care task or supervising subordinates is based on these aforementioned considerations.

Mobile Infirmary Medical Center v. Hodgen (2003) is a case in point. A patient with cardiac problems sued after suffering catastrophic physical and mental disabilities when a graduate nurse, not yet licensed, administered five times the ordered dose of digoxin. The shift charge nurse assigned another nurse with only 7 months' experience to act as the graduate nurse's preceptor. The preceptor did not supervise the new graduate when she administered the drug. The jury found all three nurses negligent. The court criticized the shift charge nurse for assigning a novice nurse as a preceptor and for failing to give her explicit directions regarding the level of supervision required in the circumstances. The court also faulted the preceptor, who had never worked with the new graduate, for inadequate supervision. The jury awarded $2.5 million in punitive damages.

In *Williams v. West Virginia Board of Examiners* (2004) the Supreme Court of Appeals of West Virginia upheld the Kentucky Board of Nursing's disciplinary action of an RN. The nurse was responsible for supervising the care of home health aides. Inspectors found numerous violations of the nurse's duty to delegate and supervise care given by the aides. Furthermore, there was evidence that the nurse falsified patients' records, indicating that home health aides were present when in fact they were absent from the home. The nursing board suspended the nurse's license for 1 year.

Employer Liability

Although a nurse is never relieved of personal liability, the doctrine of vicarious or substituted liability permits a person to also sue the employer for the negligent conduct of nurses within the scope of their employment. Vicarious liability is based on the legal principle of *respondeat superior*, a Latin term that means "let the master answer" (for the actions of subordinates or servants). Because the employer has some control over the worker, the courts have affirmed that the employer may be held responsible for the employee's negligent acts when injury occurs.

In a New York case, *Pedraza v. Wyckoff Heights Medical Center* (2002), a hospital was found liable for the negligence of its nurses when they failed to adhere to the explicit policy it had established that bedrails were to be raised at all times for a particular category of high-risk patients. An 86-year-old patient with Alzheimer's disease was admitted to the hospital for pulmonary problems. Because the woman had Alzheimer's disease she was classified as high risk for falling and a fall-injury prevention protocol was to be implemented per hospital policy. A safety alert sign was to be posted above the bed, the patient was to be checked every 2 hours, the bed was to be kept in the lowest position, and all bedrails were to be up at all times. This protocol was not followed. A nurse found the patient face down on the floor in the hallway. One bedrail had been left down when the nurse put the patient to bed after ambulating her. The hospital argued, in its defense, that keeping all four bedrails raised amounted to physical restraints and that restraints could not be applied without a physician's order. The court ruled in favor of the injured patient. The court opined that express violation of the institution's own internal policy by a hospital employee is evidence of negligence. A further discussion about the legal aspects related to the use of restraints is presented later in this chapter.

Corporate Liability

Hospitals and other health care facilities have evolved into dynamic systems that coordinate the care provided by a range of health care professionals. As a consequence of these changes the courts have expanded the concept of corporate negligence in verdicts rendered against health care giants. In *Brodowski v. Ryave* (2005) the Pennsylvania Superior Court ruled that there was sufficient evidence that a systematic breakdown in communication caused an improper diagnosis and led to the patient's admission to a psychiatric unit before a stroke had been ruled out (Passarella, 2005). The patient was not properly treated, is now partially paralyzed, and has brain damage. The "standard of care" required of a health care corporation has been established through these cases but varies from state to state. Some jurisdictions have permitted TJC standards or state department of health licensing laws to define the "corporate standard of care." An agency's own medical bylaws or policies and procedures have been admitted as evidence of the appropriate corporate standard of care. In an earlier case, *Thompson v. Nason Hospital* (1991), the court elaborated four duties of a health care corporation:

1. Maintain safe and adequate physical facilities and equipment.

2. Select and retain competent physicians.
3. Oversee the acts of all persons who practice medicine within the facility as they relate to patient care.
4. Formulate, adopt, and enforce rules and policies to ensure quality of care.

The court in the *Brodowski* case based its ruling on the doctrine of corporate liability outlined in the *Thompson* case.

Health care facilities also have been found corporately liable for failing to have adequate numbers of qualified nursing staff assigned on each shift to meet the needs of patients. In a landmark case, *HCA Health Services v. National Bank* (1988), an unattended infant experienced respiratory arrest and suffered permanent anoxic brain damage. The jury rendered a verdict for the plaintiff and awarded $2 million in compensatory damages (for the cost of ongoing care) and $2 million in punitive damages for failing to provide an adequate number of qualified staff.

Nurses must develop a clear understanding of the principles of safe staffing and must advocate for appropriate staffing levels. Guidelines published by the ANA (2020a) can assist nurses to ensure the efficient use of human resources. Nurses should review position statements published by the board of nursing as well as their specialty nursing organizations (e.g., Association of Perioperative Registered Nurses [AORN] or the Association of Women's Health, Obstetric and Neonatal Nurses [AWHONN]). Staffing guidelines promulgated by these organizations may assist the nurse in articulating concerns and formulating recommendations for improved staffing levels.

As more nurses become independent contractors working for temporary staffing agencies courts have been asked to determine whether a hospital using temporary nursing staff is liable for the acts of an agency nurse. In *Ruelas v. Staff Builders Personnel Services, Inc.* (2001) an agency nurse was alleged to have abused a patient during administration of an enema. (The precise nature of the abuse was not delineated.) The court affirmed that as a general rule, the employer (in this case, Staff Builders) is legally liable for an employee's wrongful conduct. However, in this case, the agency had no practical or even theoretical right to control how its nurses carried out their clinical responsibilities in a particular setting. Although the agency is responsible for ensuring that the nurse has the requisite license, education, experience, and certifications, the hospital has direct control and supervision of the nurse's actions. Staff Builders was dismissed from the lawsuit.

TJC has developed detailed standards related to the orientation, training, and education of agency (contracted) staff (TJC, 2024). Courts have affirmed that facilities have a duty to provide a targeted orientation for agency nurses. A job-based or unit-based handout, if readily available, can be a useful reference for the agency nurse. A mentor or resource nurse should be provided during the targeted orientation and thereafter as needed when a new task or problem is encountered. Team members should have an opportunity to evaluate the agency nurse and provide written feedback about performance.

REDUCING LEGAL LIABILITY

Risk Management Systems: Risk Manager, Patient Safety, and Corporate Compliance Officers

One of the most powerful allies the nurse has in any health care setting to facilitate positive change and reduce personal and corporate liability is the risk manager. The risk manager is a professional who tracks accidents and injuries that occur in the facility. The job of the risk manager is to establish and strengthen systems within the agency to reduce preventable patient injuries or deaths and to eliminate the loss of revenues as fines or the payment of damages through the insurance carrier. The patient safety and compliance officers are relatively new members of the team dedicated to reducing preventable adverse events and responding to them when they occur. The patient safety officer collaborates with clinical staff to identify potential barriers to the provision of safe and effective care, develops policies and procedures that reflect best practices, and may be a part of the debriefing team after a near-miss or adverse event occurs (The Joint Commission, 2013; McDonough, 2018). The compliance officer is generally the most knowledgeable about federal and state administrative rules and regulations affecting health care systems, health care licensing laws, and health care case law (Ratcliffe, 2023). This knowledge is essential to prevent inadvertent violation of health care laws and to reduce claims of negligence and malpractice within the institution. These three professionals may assist nurse managers and educators in the development of continuing education programs and policies and procedures to enhance patient safety and reduce adverse events.

The landmark report from the Institute of Medicine (2000), *To Err Is Human: Building a Safer Health System*, recommended a proactive approach to risk management. Nurses are encouraged to anticipate the potential for errors, report "near misses," and work closely with the risk manager to reduce preventable adverse events. All health care providers are urged to develop high-reliability operating systems. This concept is derived from the airline and nuclear energy industries. Both have established excellent safety records despite the highly complex and dangerous nature of their operations. The IOM report recommends creation of a nationwide mandatory reporting system for collection of information about adverse events and the development of performance standards that focus on patient safety.

Incident Reports or Unusual Occurrence Reports

Nurses are legally bound to report critical incidents to their nurse managers, agency administration, and the risk manager through a formal intraagency document titled the "Unusual Occurrence Report" or "Incident Report" (Sergi & Davis, 2023). Emphasis on patient safety and quality has resulted in renaming of the Incident Report in many health care settings. The document is frequently referred to as the "Unusual Occurrence Form" but is also known by other titles, such as the "Quality Variance Report." This form often is directed to the risk management department through the nurse's immediate manager. The nurse manager has an opportunity to review the written report and begin the process of collecting information and mitigating any identified systems flaws in a timely fashion, depending on the nature of the incident. The report then is forwarded (usually within 24 hours) to the risk manager. If an ongoing problem does not appear to be any closer to resolution as the nurse works through the formal chain of command, beginning with the charge nurse and/or immediate nurse manager, the nurse may speak directly to the risk manager for guidance and advice.

Unfortunately, studies indicate that the rate of incident reporting still remains relatively low, particularly among physician providers (Macrea, 2016; PS Net, 2019c; USDHHS, 2012). As a condition of participation in the Medicare program federal regulations require that hospitals develop and maintain Quality Assessment and Performance Improvement (QAPI) programs. To satisfy these requirements hospitals must "track medical errors and adverse patient events, analyze their causes, and implement preventive actions and mechanisms that include feedback and learning throughout the hospital" (USDHHS, 2012). Unfortunately, a report released by the Office of Inspector General (OIG) found that hospital incident reporting systems captured only an estimated 14% of the patient harm events experienced by Medicare beneficiaries. Hospital risk managers, clinical managers, and administrators investigated only those reported events that they considered most likely to lead to quality and safety improvements. Few policy or practice changes were implemented as a result of reported events. Hospital administrators classified the remaining events (86% of all incident reports) as either events that staff did not perceive as reportable (61%) or as events that staff commonly report but did not report in this case (25%). The OIG recommended that (1) the CMS and AHRQ collaborate to create and promote a list of potentially reportable events for hospitals to use and (2) the CMS provide guidance to accreditors regarding their assessments of hospital efforts to track and analyze events.

Critical incidents that result in patient injury or death eventually may lead to a malpractice claim. Because state laws vary as to whether the incident report may be "discovered" by the plaintiff's attorney in a lawsuit, it is essential that the nurse follow appropriate procedures when completing and filing this document:

1. The nurse should describe all events objectively and should avoid subjective comments, personal opinions about why the incident occurred, and assumptions about events that were not witnessed. For example, if a patient was found lying on the floor at the foot of the bed the nurse should avoid the statement, "Patient fell out of bed—found on floor." That the patient fell out of bed is an unfounded assumption. The nurse should instead state, "Entered room. Patient discovered lying prone at the foot of the bed. Both upper and lower side rails were raised."

2. The nurse should never note in the patient's medical record that an incident report has been completed and filed. This notation might alter the protection from discovery normally provided by the document in some states. The jury also would be made aware that an incident report has been filed because they

have access to nurses' notes submitted in evidence during the trial.

3. The nurse should never photocopy or print a copy of an incident report for personal use and retention. Keeping a copy of the incident report generally is prohibited by agency policy and may be expressly prohibited in writing on the incident report itself. Taking a copy of the incident report out of the agency violates patient confidentiality. It may fall into the hands of individuals who are not authorized to read any information about the patient. It may fall into the hands of the plaintiff's attorney, should a lawsuit be filed, with damaging effects on the agency's ability to defend against the claims of negligence.

4. Physicians and advanced practice nurses should not write or enter an order for an incident report in the medical record. Doing so would bring the existence of an incident report to the attention of the plaintiff's attorney and may be discoverable in some states.

5. The nurse should report every "near miss," unusual occurrence, or incident. The nurse should not assume that "everyone knows about the problem or event." Box 8.5 lists circumstances under which an incident report should be filed.

INTENTIONAL TORTS IN NURSING PRACTICE

Ordinarily, in the course of carrying out one's nursing duties breaches in the applicable standard of care are assumed to be unintentional acts McGuire & Mroczek, 2017. In other words the nurse did not intend to harm the patient. As noted, this civil wrong is referred to as an *unintentional tort*. An intentional tort is a second category of civil wrong. It involves the direct violation of a person's legal rights. In this case the nurse intends to perform the offensive act, although normally most nurses do not mean to harm the patient. The following acts are intentional torts:

- Assault
- Battery
- Defamation of character
- False imprisonment
- Invasion of privacy
- Intentional infliction of emotional distress

In the case of intentional torts the plaintiff does not have to prove that the nurse breached a special duty or was negligent. The duty is implied in law (e.g., the duty to respect a patient's right to privacy). In general legal

BOX 8.5 Circumstances Under Which an Incident Report Should Be Filed*

- Patient or client injury
- Unanticipated patient death
- Malfunction or failure of durable medical equipment
- Significant or unanticipated adverse reactions to ordered therapy or care
- Inability to meet a patient's need(s), ordered therapy, medications, or treatments after consultation with appropriate nurse mangers or providers. This may be related to:
- System problems (e.g., pharmacy closed, drug not available)
- Unresolved problem with order (e.g., incomplete or illegible order)
- Lack of qualified staff to implement order to provide needed care (e.g., registered nurse [RN] not available to perform task that law stipulates only an RN may perform)
- Patient or family refusal of care (e.g., request for do-not-resuscitate [DNR] orders)
- Unresolved problems with physical plant that jeopardize patient well-being (e.g., electrical hazard, loose carpet section, delay in repair of essential equipment)
- Unethical, illegal, or incompetent practice that is witnessed or reported
- Patient complaint about provider or health care worker
- Toxic spills, fires, other environmental emergencies
- Violent behavior or verbal abuse/threats on the part of family or patient
- Near-misses that could potentially result in patient injury

*This list is not comprehensive but is a representative list of occurrences that should be reported.

remedies for intentional torts include fines and punitive damages, although some intentional torts rise to the level of a criminal act (such as battery) and may result in a jail sentence. Some states, such as California, also have enacted penalties that include a term of imprisonment for willful and malicious breach of confidentiality in releasing information about a patient's human immunodeficiency virus (HIV) status.

Assault and Battery

Patients who agree to treatment or nursing care do not surrender their rights to determine who touches them. Assault is causing the person to fear that they will be touched without consent. Battery is the unauthorized or the actual harmful or offensive touching of a person. It is important to note that a charge of battery does not require proof of harm or injury. Nurses engaged in drawing blood samples or in therapeutic procedures may face charges of battery if they touch a patient without consent. In *O'Brien v. Synnott* (2013) a man was admitted to a hospital for surgery. He had suffered a gunshot wound after ramming a police cruiser. A police officer attempted to obtain a blood sample from the patient in the postanesthesia care unit (PACU) for the purposes of alcohol screening. The patient, who objected to the blood draw, was uncooperative and resisted the officer's efforts. After the police officer was unsuccessful a PACU nurse drew the blood sample, "implicitly leading the patient to believe that she was acting" in her capacity as a care provider. The patient believed the nurse was obtaining the sample for medical purposes, not for drug testing. The Supreme Court of Vermont ruled that the patient could sue the nurse and her employer for medical battery.

It is essential that the nurse ask the patient's permission to proceed before drawing blood samples or initiating any procedure, particularly those of an invasive nature. The nurse must be truthful regarding the reason for performing the procedure. Nurses also should document that the patient has given permission for the treatment or procedure. Consider the following situation:

A woman in active labor cries out through each contraction. The nurse has a standing order from the obstetrician for administration of an intravenous narcotic should the woman request pain relief. However, the woman refuses, being determined to experience a medication-free birth. As labor progresses the woman's cries become so loud that other laboring women and visitors in the unit express concern and anxiety. Repeated efforts to assist the woman with breathing and relaxation exercises to reduce her vocalization have failed.

The nurse finally says to the patient, "Look, if you don't stop screaming and making those horrible noises I'm going to give you the pain medication your doctor has ordered, whether you want it or not. You're frightening the other patients!" She repeats this threat several times and in the presence of the woman's family.

Although the woman continues to cry out, the nurse does not give the medication. The delivery of the infant is uneventful and without problems.

After discharge from the hospital the patient retains a lawyer, claiming she was threatened with being sedated against her will. She further asserts that the nurse's repeated threats to inject her with a narcotic created an unbearable level of anxiety that interfered with her ability to cooperate with other necessary procedures during the birth. This assertion could result in a charge of negligence or intentional infliction of emotional distress.

In this case the nurse is charged with assault (i.e., threatening the patient with unauthorized touching). Had the nurse actually carried out her threat of giving the medication the charge could be expanded to assault and battery. Consequences for the nurse charged with assault may include:

- Imposition of fines and punitive damages
- State board of nursing disciplinary action
- Termination by the employer

When battery occurs the nature of the touching may raise the offense to the level of a crime. In the aforementioned scenario assume that the nurse decides to give the narcotic against the woman's will. She engages the assistance of a scrub technician to physically restrain the woman so that she can access a vein for the injection.

The technician, becoming frustrated with the woman's resistance to the procedure, says, "You're going to be sorry if you don't stop struggling." The technician purposefully hyperextends the woman's arm and says, "There, maybe if it hurts enough you'll stop this nonsense."

A loud snapping sound is heard, and tests indicate that the technician has fractured the woman's arm. The charge of battery in this case may result in more serious ramifications, including punitive damages and a term of imprisonment.

Defamation of Character

A person has a right to be free from attacks on their reputation (defamation of character). *Libel* is a form of defamation caused by written work. *Slander* refers to an injury to one's reputation caused by the spoken word. Nurses may be subject to a charge of libel for subjective comments meant to denigrate the patient that are placed in the medical record or in other written materials read by others.

For example, a patient suffering from extreme pain who requests narcotics frequently is labeled as a "whiner," a "liar," and a "drug seeker" with an "addictive personality." These comments are noted on the medical

record, on the nursing Kardex, and in the nurses' notes attached to a clipboard, which is kept on a wall peg outside the patient's room. The patient subsequently is found to have a severe intraabdominal infection that accounts for the intense pain he experiences.

The patient sues for failure of the medical staff to identify and treat the infection. In the process of discovery the patient, his family, and the attorney he has retained read the defamatory comments about his character. It is a distinct possibility that other family members, coworkers, and the patient's employer who visited may have read these subjective comments on the clipboard. A charge of libel is leveled against the nursing staff.

Nurses also may face charges of slander when they repeat similar types of subjective comments about patients in public places, such as elevators and hospital cafeterias. All patient care staff must be extremely cautious about discussing a patient or their opinions about a patient in public places. Even in report rooms or conference rooms, nurses should consider who in the immediate vicinity could inadvertently overhear the conversation. In all circumstances, only objective, professional language should be used in discussing patients.

False Imprisonment

False imprisonment is defined as the unlawful restraint or detention of another person against their wishes. Actual force is not necessary to support a charge of false imprisonment. An adult of sound mind (mentally competent) has a right to refuse any treatment that has previously been agreed. If they refuse the person may leave the facility (e.g., hospital, rehabilitation center, long-term care facility) whenever they choose. The nurse has no authority to detain the patient, even if discontinuing therapy may result in harm or injury.

The nurse has a duty to immediately notify the provider and appropriate nursing supervisors when a competent patient intends to leave "against medical advice" (AMA) but may not in any way prevent the individual from leaving the facility. Many agencies request that a patient sign an AMA form when they intend to leave in contradiction to the plan of care and despite the absence of a discharge order. The form may provide the facility with a reasonable defense against a malpractice claim if the patient's condition worsens or an injury is sustained and a malpractice claim is filed.

Intentional Infliction of Emotional Distress

When the nurse's behavior is so outrageous that it leads to emotional shock in a patient the court can compensate the patient for emotional distress. A case in the area of maternity nursing illustrates the potential for a claim of intentional infliction of emotional distress.

In *Roddy v. Tanner Medical Center* (2003) a woman brought suit against the hospital after she was treated in the ED for a miscarriage at approximately 10 weeks' gestation. While en route to the hospital Ms. Roddy felt something large extrude from her vagina, and she bled heavily. She reported to the ED nurse that whatever she had passed was still in her underpants with a great deal of blood. Ms. Roddy indicated that the nurse told her she would take whatever she could out of her clothes, and then the nurse placed the soiled clothes in a plastic bag.

Ms. Roddy was subsequently discharged home in stable condition after a gynecologic examination confirmed that she had passed the products of conception. When she returned home and began to remove her clothes from the plastic bag to launder them the intact fetus dropped to the floor. Ms. Roddy claimed intentional infliction of emotional distress. The court permitted the case to go forward, indicating that there was evidence of "reckless disregard" of the rights of the patient.

Invasion of Privacy

Another basic right is to be free from interference with one's personal life. An invasion of privacy occurs when a person's private affairs (including health history and status) are made known to hospital staff who are not involved in the patient's care or to the public without consent. The nurse has a legal and ethical duty to maintain patient confidentiality, and there may be serious repercussions when the nurse breaches this duty and violates this fundamental patient right.

With the growing use of electronic information systems, issues related to patient confidentiality and invasion of privacy are now being addressed by federal and state legislatures. Statutes, including HIPAA, have been enacted to control access to electronic health data. Nurses are given passwords to access patients' electronic medical records. Nurses should never share passwords with colleagues because doing so increases the risk of unauthorized access to patients' records. Discussion of patients on social media Internet sites and taking unauthorized pictures of patients with personal electronic devices is a growing area for claims of HIPAA violation and invasion of privacy. The ANA (2011) and the NCSBN (2018a) have both published guidelines regarding use of social media for nurses, along with precautionary advice.

In certain circumstances the law permits or requires divulging information contained in a patient's medical record or that has been reported by the patient, family, or significant other. These situations include reporting certain communicable diseases, child abuse, partnter or domestic violence, and gunshot wounds to the proper authorities.

If a nurse is asked to provide information to any sources the matter should immediately be referred to the agency's administrator or risk manager. In no case should the nurse personally divulge the information or provide copies of the patient's record to another person or agency. Another fact-based case known to this author illustrates the intentional torts of invasion of privacy and intentional infliction of emotional distress. Consider the following situation:

A nurse works in a physician's office in a small, semirural community. The majority of the town's residents know one another. A patient being treated for several opportunistic infections is tested for HIV. The nurse also is aware that the patient has been questioned by the physician about his sexual activities and that he has divulged that he is gay and has had unprotected sex with several male partners. When the test results are reported as positive the nurse calls several close friends (who also know the patient) and reports the finding and information about the patient's sexual conduct. Before the physician informs the patient about his diagnosis the patient encounters two of the people who have been told about the HIV test result. They tell him that they know he is gay and infected with the HIV virus. He then discovers that the nurse has informed them about his condition. Suffering from intense shock and emotional pain, the man unsuccessfully attempts suicide.

In this case the nurse's actions rose to the level of willful, malicious, and intentional infliction of emotional distress. The nurse faces serious charges and, in some states with HIV confidentiality laws, could face a prison sentence for intentionally violating the patient's confidentiality in a manner meant to harm the patient. It is likely that the nurse's license also will be revoked for her actions, and the board may impose a significant fine.

New issues related to invasion of privacy have arisen since the US Supreme Court overturned Roe v. Wade in

2022. Some states that prohibit or strictly limit a woman's right to abortion are now attempting to obtain the out-of-state medical records of women suspected of or known to have obtained an abortion in another state. Many of these states have established mandatory reporting laws, requiring health care workers to notify state authorities if they suspect or know that a woman has self-aborted or obtained an abortion in another state. Legal challenges are ongoing to prevent states from obtaining the woman's confidential medical records and the resolution is uncetain. Many nurses are experiencing a crisis of conscience, finding it difficult or impossible to comply with a law that requires violation of patient confidentiality. Professional nursing organizations are developing resources and support systems for nurses who are struggling with, or are opposed to, invading the person's privacy and violating patient confidentiality. Nurses are strongly advised to review the ANA Code of Ethics (2015a) and to seek the assistance of an attorney skilled in health care statutes before making a decision about complying with these laws.

The Nurse and Criminal Law

A crime is an offense against society, defined through written criminal statutes or codes. A criminal act is deemed to be conduct so offensive that the state is responsible for prosecuting the offending individual on behalf of society. Legal remedies for crimes include fines, imprisonment, and, in some states, execution (death penalty). Criminal acts are classified as either minor offenses (misdemeanors) or major offenses (felonies). Misdemeanors that nurses are commonly charged with include:

- Illegal practice of medicine
- Failing to report child or elder abuse
- Falsification of a patient's medical record
- Assault and battery and physical abuse of patients

Felony acts may be committed against the federal government and generally involve drug trafficking offenses and, increasingly, fraud in billing for services of Medicare patients. Other serious criminal acts include theft, rape, and murder. A nurse found guilty of a felony generally serves time in prison and usually suffers the permanent revocation of their nursing license. For example, in the death of a 97-year-old nursing home patient five RNs were indicted on 21 counts, including falsification of records, alteration of forms filed with the state department of health, and tampering with physical

evidence (Kelley, 2000). The patient died after being fed through a stomach tube attached to an enema bag. The nurses used the enema bag in lieu of the appropriate feeding equipment, which was not available. The nursing director was found guilty on three counts and also surrendered her nursing license.

THE LAW AND PATIENT RIGHTS

Advance Directives

Society now recognizes the individual's right to die with dignity rather than be kept alive indefinitely by artificial life support. As a consequence, the majority of states have enacted "right-to-die" laws. These statutes grant competent adults the right to refuse extraordinary medical treatment when there is no hope of recovery. The term advance directive refers to an individual's desires regarding end-of-life care. These wishes generally are made through the execution of a formal document known as a living will. Right-to-die statutes vary from state to state; therefore, the nurse must become familiar with the state-specific statute. Agency policies and procedures in the nurse's employment setting also guide the nurse in an understanding of the patient's rights in this matter.

Living Wills

A living will is a legal document, a type of advance directive, in which a competent adult makes known their wishes regarding care that will be provided in the final stages of a terminal illness. A living will generally contains the following directives:

- Designation of the individual (proxy or surrogate) who is permitted to make decisions once the patient is incapacitated and no longer able to make decisions (often referred to as "decisionally incompetent" or "decisionally incapacitated")
- Specific stipulations regarding what care is acceptable and which procedures or treatments are not to be implemented
- Authorization of the patient's physician to withhold or discontinue certain life-sustaining procedures under specific conditions

Although living wills are legal in every state they may not be legally binding. In some cases a proxy is not recognized or sanctioned by the state statute. Living wills have been overturned, particularly if disputes arise among family members or significant others when the terminally ill patient is no longer able to make decisions. A living will may be revoked under any of the following conditions:

- There is evidence that the patient was not competent when the living will was executed.
- The patient's condition is not terminal.
- A state-imposed time for enforcement of the will has expired, and a new living will must be executed.
- The patient's condition has changed substantially, and the stipulations of the will no longer apply.

A living will must be written (in some cases, using a state-specific document), dated, signed, and witnessed. If asked to witness a patient's living will the nurse should refer the matter to the agency's risk manager. It may not be lawful in a particular state for the nurse to witness this document.

Medical or Physician Directives and DNR Orders. A more specific type of living will that the patient may execute is known as the medical or physician directive. This document lists the desire of the patient in a particular scenario, such as whether they would want to be resuscitated if cardiopulmonary arrest occurs. The physician writes DNR orders on the basis of written medical directives dictated by the patient. This medical directive, when properly executed, provides the physician with immunity from claims of negligence or intentional wrongdoing in the patient's death. The physician must also follow any state-specific statute and the agency's policies and procedures before writing a DNR order. Research has discovered a serious lack of uniformity among and within health care facilities in making certain that direct-care nurses and providers are aware of a patient's DNR status. The lack of awareness can result in a significant risk for confusion and error and contribute to claims of negligence.

The nurse has an absolute duty to respect the patient's wishes in the case of DNR orders. A lawfully executed DNR order must be followed. Nurses have been sued for failure to observe DNR orders. Claims against the nurse include battery, negligent infliction of pain and suffering, and "wrongful life" (*Anderson v. St. Francis–St. George Hospital*, 1992). Three problems may arise regarding a DNR order: (1) a physician refuses to comply with the patient's wishes and initiates resuscitation; (2) the patient revokes consent to the DNR order; and (3) a family member demands that the DNR order be rescinded despite the patient's continued objection to

resuscitation (Teno, 2008). If one of these issues arises the nurse must act promptly to enlist the assistance of the nursing supervisor or a hospital administrator. One must remember that a patient may revoke a living will, including a DNR order, at any time. The ANA published a position statement in 2020: "ANA Position Statement: Nursing Care and Do-Not-Resuscitate (DNR) Decision" (Stokes, 2020). This document clarifies the nurse's roles and responsibilities related to end-of-life decisions and DNR orders. https://search.yahoo.com/yhs/search?hspart=mnet&hsimp=yhs-001&type=type9097303-spa-4056-84481&param1=4056&param2=84481&p=ANA+Position+Statement%3A+Nursing+Care+and+Do-Not-Resuscitate+%28DNR%29+Decision

Durable Power of Attorney for Health Care. In 1993 the Uniform Health-Care Decisions Act was approved. The Act recognizes an individual's right to make decisions about health care and enables a patient to accept or refuse treatment. The act is also designed to give the patient autonomy to make end-of-life decisions. Durable power of attorney is a legal document that authorizes the patient to name the person (the health care proxy) who will make the day-to-day and final end-of-life decisions once they are decisionally incompetent. Naming a proxy who is intimately knowledgeable about the person's true wishes is important to ensure that the patient's desires will be carried out when they are no longer able to make decisions. Health care law experts recommend that individuals interested in naming a proxy seek legal assistance with executing a durable power of attorney for health care.

Nurses may be asked questions about living wills and durable power of attorney for health care by patients and their families. An important aspect of speaking to the patient about these issues is to provide the written materials about advance directives that are required under the federal statute the Patient Self-Determination Act, which was passed in 1990.

Informed Consent

For any patient to make meaningful choices about a particular procedure or treatment the provider must convey certain material information. Under the doctrine of informed consent the physician or advanced practice nurse has a duty to disclose information so that the patient can make intelligent decisions (Farmer & Lundy, 2017). This duty is mandated by federal statute (in the case of Medicare and Medicaid patients) and state law and is grounded as well in common law. In the case of routine as well as specialized care the primary provider must disclose the following information:

- Nature of the therapy or procedure
- Expected benefits and outcomes of the therapy or procedure
- Potential risks of the therapy or procedure
- Alternative therapies to the intended procedure and their risks and benefits
- Risks of not having the procedure

This duty to disclose rests with the provider and cannot be delegated to the RN (Dowie, 2021). When the nurse has reason to believe that the patient has not given informed consent for a procedure the provider should be immediately notified. In no case should the nurse proceed with initiating any part of the therapy that they are responsible for implementing. The patient's questions or concerns should be documented in the medical record to indicate why there has been a delay in carrying out the procedure (Axson et al., 2017). If the nurse is responsible for witnessing the patient's signature on a consent form for the specified procedure this process also should be deferred until the provider has had an opportunity to clarify the patient's questions.

A variety of negligence claims arise out of the informed consent process. The provider may be alleged negligent for failure to obtain informed consent. With adoption in some states of the corporate negligence doctrine an increasing number of appellate courts have ruled that hospitals and nurses may be liable for failure to ensure that informed consent was given to the provider (*Doctors Hospital of Augusta v. Alicea*, 2016; *William McDougald et al. v. St. Francis North Hospital Inc.*, 2014). Nurses have a duty to discuss concerns about informed consent with the primary provider. Should the nurse be unable to resolve the issue the chain of command should be invoked to clarify questions or concerns.

In some cases timely notification of a nursing manager may be essential to prevent violation of the patient's right to give consent. The following scenario provides a case in point. An RN is circulating in a surgical procedure intended to clean a severe leg wound. The consent form signed by the patient explicitly lists "wound debridement" as the procedure to be performed. On beginning the procedure the surgeon asks for additional instruments, indicating that the wound is so infected

that the leg will have to be amputated below the knee. Because the patient has received general anesthesia and is unable to give consent, and the consent form itself does not authorize an amputation procedure, the nurse must question the surgeon's intention to remove the leg. If the surgeon refuses to discuss the matter, or again requests the instruments necessary for the procedure, the nurse must obtain immediate assistance from her supervisor and, if possible, the medical administrator (chief of surgery). The instruments for surgical amputation should not be placed on the sterile table, and in compliance with intraoperative communication standards, all other team members should be alerted that there is an unresolved question about the procedure and that a manager or administrator is on the way to evaluate the surgical plan.

Communication Barriers and Informed Consent. Health care organizations that receive federal funds are required to meet the language access provision of the Culturally and Linguistically Appropriate Services (CLAS) Standards for Health. The standards were issued in 2001 by USDHHS and were substantially enhanced in 2011 through a collaboration of the USDHHS Office of Minority Health (OMH) (USDHHSOMH, 2011) and the National Partnership for Action to End Health Disparities.

The standards require that the hospital or health facility must:

- Offer and provide free and timely language assistance services, including bilingual staff and interpreter services, at all points of contact at all hours of operation.
- Provide verbal and written notices (in the individual's preferred language) of the right to receive language assistance services.
- Ensure competence of language assistance provided by interpreters and bilingual staff.

Family and friends should *not* be used as interpreters except at the care recipient's request (USDHHSOMH, 2011). The duty to ensure appropriate communication is also established by the ADA (discussed previously). When an interpreter is used to facilitate communication the nurse should document this process. The medical record should contain the name of the interpreter, the topic of the educational session or substance of the informed consent discussion, and the patient's questions and consent, if given.

TJC's *Comprehensive Accreditation Manual for Hospitals* requires the facility to respect a patient's right to and need for effective communication (TJC, 2024). Written materials, including consent forms and discharge instructions, should be available in the patient's preferred language. Educational materials should be culturally sensitive, and at a reading level that recognizes literacy limitations. TJC provides detailed information and guidance for development of a central office to coordinate all communication services, including the availability of interpreters fluent in medical terminology, for informed consent discussions between the provider and patient. Language access also includes access to interpreters skilled in signing for hearing-impaired patients and materials in Braille for vision-impaired individuals.

A New Jersey case (*Borngesser v. Jersey Shore Medical Center*, 2001) illustrates the duty to provide an interpreter before informed consent is given for an invasive procedure. A female patient was admitted to the hospital with severe cardiac disease. She was also completely deaf and mute. Notes in the medical record stated, "Patient deaf and dumb and difficult to assess." The nurses established a diagnosis of "Sensory deficit: hearing impaired" and recorded that it was difficult to communicate with the patient. Providers and nurses documented continued difficulty with assessments, patient education, and obtaining informed consent. The patient's 17-year-old daughter was not deaf and could sign but was not a trained medical interpreter. Ms. Borngesser subsequently died from severe cardiac disease and associated complications. Her daughter sued the hospital, claiming that the facility failed to make reasonable accommodation for her deaf and mute mother. *There were no claims of medical or nursing negligence.* The Superior Appellate Court of New Jersey affirmed that the case against the hospital could go forward. The court stated, among other things, that when a hearing-impaired patient is asked to give informed consent the hospital has a duty to ensure that communication is effective by providing an interpreter fluent in American Sign Language (ASL).

The unique legal requirements related to informed consent in minors is a complex issue. The American Academy of Pediatrics (AAP) published a *Technical Report*, delineating important aspects of informed consent for pediatric patients (AAP, 2016). All 50 states and the District of Columbia explicitly allow a minor to consent to testing and treatments for sexually transmitted diseases, except HIV testing and treatment. All other statutes regarding informed consent in adolescents vary widely from state to state. As noted earlier, when dealing with minors the nurse must use agency resources, including social workers, managers, administrators, and risk managers, when facilitating an appropriate informed consent process between the provider and adolescent or older child.

The Right to Refuse Diagnostic Testing, Treatment, and Care

As noted, an adult of sound mind has a right to refuse any treatment that has previously been agreed to (Colwell, 2016; Oshodi et al., 2019). A Connecticut Supreme Court decision affirmed the fundamental right of adults to refuse medical treatment. In the case of *Stamford Hospital v. Vega* (1996) a woman who hemorrhaged after the birth of her infant refused blood on the grounds that it violated her beliefs as a Jehovah's Witness. The hospital obtained an emergency court order authorizing the facility to administer blood. The woman survived and was discharged in good health. Although it was a moot point (the blood already had been given) the family appealed the initial court decision authorizing the blood transfusion. The Supreme Court decided to hear the case and reversed the lower court's decision, stating the hospital did not have a right to substitute its decision for that of the patient.

If a patient who is under the nurse's care refuses treatment the nurse has a duty to notify the primary provider. The same principles pertaining to the informed consent process apply to situations in which the patient refuses care (Pirotte & Benson, 2023). The physician or advanced practice nurse should provide the patient with information about the consequences, risks, and benefits of refusing therapy. The provider also must explore any alternative treatments that may be available to the patient.

Leaving Against Medical Advice

A common allegation made when a patient self-discharges against medical advice and is subsequently injured is that the patient was not fully apprised of the risks inherent in leaving the facility. If a patient intends to leave the facility without a written order the nurse must act promptly to notify the provider. When circumstances suggest that the person may suffer immediate physical harm the nurse must clearly articulate the dangers inherent in leaving. This precautionary statement is reserved for situations in which the life and limb of the patient are at risk and the appropriate providers (physicians or advanced practice nurses) are not available to address the direct and indirect consequences with the patient. The nurse should document all of these actions and any communication with the aforementioned parties.

If the primary provider has not arrived before the patient leaves the nurses' notes should reflect the specific advice given the patient, which should include the fact that leaving the facility could:

- Aggravate the current condition and complicate future care.
- Result in permanent physical or mental impairment or disability.
- Result in complications leading to death.

In the case of a competent elder prompt notification of the immediate family would also be a reasonable and prudent action.

Lyons v. Walker Regional Medical Center (2000) is a case in point. An ED nurse was found negligent for failing to warn a patient who was leaving AMA that his laboratory results indicated a state of diabetic ketoacidosis, a condition that could be lethal. When the "panic" value laboratory findings were displayed on the computer the nurse did not bring the results to the physician's or patient's attention. Instead she directed the unit secretary to complete the patient's discharge paperwork. The patient left, and he died 3 days later.

In a study of patient characteristics associated with discharge AMA has found that low socioeconomic status, substance abuse, sickness within the family, underlying (and often untreated) psychiatric disorders, anger and anxiety about the admission diagnosis, and lack of effective communication with team members correlate with self-discharge (Radziewicz et al., 2014). Nurses and providers should collaborate to address immediate patient concerns, communicate a time-limited plan of care, and advocate for appropriate consultations (e.g., psychiatry, social work, pastoral services, pain management) to reduce the likelihood of patient self-discharge.

Almost all health care facilities have an AMA form that patients are asked to sign when they decide to refuse or discontinue ordered therapy or intend to leave the facility. The value of the document in countering a claim of negligence should the patient or family later sue will depend in great part on the quality of the nurse's charting.

Nurses have also been charged with a variety of offenses when unlawfully detaining patients, including assault, battery, and false imprisonment (Rege, 2016). These charges generally arise when well-meaning nurses try to prevent the patient from carrying out their intent. Actions that lead to a claim of false imprisonment include applying restraints, refusing to give the patient their clothes or access to a telephone, intimidating the patient by assigning a security person to guard their room, and sedating the patient against their will.

Use of Physical Restraints

One last but equally important area of patient rights is the right of a competent adult to be free of restraint. Even patients with mental illness cannot be incarcerated or restrained without due process, and the institution must have the treatment and rehabilitation services necessary to reintegrate the individual into society (Bellenger et al., 2017). Restraint of any kind is a form of imprisonment, and the reasonable and prudent nurse will closely adhere to all laws, rules, and policies pertaining to the use of restraints. The goal when restraints are clinically indicated is to use the least restrictive restraint and only when all other strategies to ensure patient safety have been exhausted. Patients may never be restrained physically or chemically because there is not enough staff to properly monitor them. Nurses have a legal and ethical duty to report institutions or individuals who violate patient rights through unlawful restraint.

As noted, one of the most common allegations leveled against nurses is a failure to ensure patient safety. Nurses in many practice settings must balance the right of patients to unrestricted control of their bodies and movements against the need to keep vulnerable patients safe from harm. The use of seclusion, chemical restraints, and physical restraints, including vests, mittens, belts, and wrist restraints, is governed by federal and state statutes and accrediting bodies, such as TJC. Many nurses do not realize that even bedrails and chair trays fall under the category of physical restraints; these articles may not be used indiscriminately.

Violation of restraint statutes and the administrative rules and regulations promulgated to enact these laws can result in stiff penalties. The institution can lose its Medicare contract (decertification) and TJC accreditation, effectively putting it out of business. Patients and family members may initiate civil suits for unlawful restraints, resulting in monetary damages if the plaintiff succeeds in the suit. Charges of assault, battery, and/or false imprisonment may be leveled against nurses who use restraints improperly. Claims of negligence may arise from improper monitoring of the patient who has been appropriately placed in restraints in compliance with applicable laws and hospital policy.

Careful nursing documentation is essential when restraints are applied. The patient's mental and physical status must be assessed at regular and frequent intervals, as prescribed by law and the agency's policies. The chart must reflect these assessments and the frequency with which restraints are removed. Neurovascular and skin assessments of limbs or other body parts covered by the restraints also must be entered in the medical record. Written physician orders for restraints must be timed and dated, and renewal of orders must be accompanied by evidence of medical evaluations and nursing reassessments.

On the basis of the aforementioned information some nurses are under the misconception that current law prohibits restraining patients until a written order is obtained. Nurses may lawfully apply restraints in an emergency, when in their independent judgment no other strategies are effective in protecting the patient from harm. The physician must be contacted promptly to discuss the patient's condition and the need to restrain and to obtain an order for temporary continuance of restraints. The nurse is guided in the decision to restrain by knowledge of the laws, the agency's policies and procedures, qualifications of the staff, and conditions on the unit or in the department. The nurse also refers to the "ANA Position Statement: The ethical use of restraints: Balancing dual nursing duties of patient safety and personal safety" (ANA, 2020b) for additional information and decision support.

VIGNETTE

On July 26, 2017, an unconscious man injured in a motor vehicle accident was conveyed to the University of Utah Hospital in Salt Lake City (Smart, 2017). A registered nurse was directed by a police officer, who had entered the emergency department (ED), to draw blood from the man who was still unresponsive. The blood sample would be tested for alcohol, drugs, and illicit substances that could alter mentation. A charge nurse explained to the officer that neither she nor the police were permitted to obtain the sample because the patient had not given consent. The police officer telephoned his supervisor, who supported the officer's directive to draw the blood sample. The nurse had alerted a hospital supervisor about the unresolved disagreement, but that person had not yet arrived in the ED.

A videotape captured the encounter between the nurse and officer. It was released in September of 2017 to the media (*The Salt Lake Tribune*, 2017). The nurse was able to contact a hospital representative to speak telephonically with the police officer. When the nurse continued to respectfully refuse the order the officer arrested her, forcefully removed her from the ED, handcuffed her, and conveyed her to the police department.

SUMMARY

To summarize the chapter let's review the questions posed at the beginning of the chapter and see what you have learned.

1. What was the nurse's legal duty?

The nurse is required to comply with federal and state laws, rules, and regulations in all situations when the nurse is performing invasive procedures. Invasive procedures carrying risks (physical, mental, and legal) ordinarily require the person's "informed" consent. The concept of informed consent is discussed in this chapter.

All health care systems have written policies and procedures that address informed consent and delineate the nurse's legal duty to comply with the health facility's requirements for performing invasive procedures, such as drawing blood for drug testing. In this vignette the patient was brought into the emergency department in an unconscious state and was incapable of giving consent to the blood draw. The nurse had a legal duty to strictly comply with the hospital's policies and procedures related to consent and blood draws and those policies are predicated on federal and state laws.

In addition, in this case drawing blood for a drug test without consent would allow unlawful access to the patient's health information to unauthorized persons (the police). This would violate provisions of the Health Insurance Portability and Accountability Act of 1996 (HIPAA) (Pub. L. 104–191). These laws are discussed in the chapter.

2. What legal principles underlie the nurse's obligations to the patient?

The patient's right to self-determination and autonomy underpin the legal principle of "informed" consent. As a patient advocate the nurse has a duty to uphold a patient's right to accept or refuse treatment. A competent patient makes an informed decision based on a discussion with the providers about the risks and benefits of the procedure. When the patient is incapacitated the nurse must follow the hospital's policies and procedures related to consent and blood draws for drug (toxicology) tests. When a law enforcement officer directs a nurse to draw blood the specific legal risks of complying must be considered. In this case the patient was unconscious and unable to give informed consent. Therefore the nurse had a legal duty to comply with hospital policies and procedures. The nurse is also obligated to request the assistance of a nursing manager and/or a hospital compliance officer if there is an unresolved issue with the police officers demanding the blood draw.

3. What laws, if any, would govern the nurse's decision-making process in this case?

Federal law governs the requirements for ensuring that the patient's right to informed consent is upheld. The Patient Self Determination Act 1991 (§§ 4206, 4751, 104 Stat. at 1388–115, 1388–205) empowers patients to play a central role in the decision-making process of their health care. Nurses have a legal and ethical duty to ensure patients know and understand their health care-related rights. When a patient is unconscious the law provides for remedies to protect the patient's rights and limits access to health care information. These are spelled out in hospital policies and procedures.

The Patient Bill of Rights was enacted as part of the Patient Protection and Affordable Care Act 2010 (Pub L. No. 111–148, 124 Stat 119, 2010). It also mandates the confidentiality of the patient's health information and protects unauthorized persons access to that information.

State laws also establish the patient's absolute right to give informed consent or informed refusal for any procedure. In the Utah case if a patient was incapacitated one of two legal requirements had to be met to draw a blood sample:

1. A warrant had to be issued by a court for the blood draw or
2. The person was under arrest for a violation of law, permitting a blood draw.

Neither of these conditions were met. The patient was neither under arrest nor had a court authorized order for the blood draw. While these requirements are almost universal among states, prerequisites for lawful drug testing may vary slightly. When the patient cannot give consent the nurse has a duty to refer to the hospital's specific policies and procedures for guidance in obtaining a blood sample (or for any invasive procedure) when the patient is incapacitated.

4. In this situation does the police officer's order to draw the blood supersede the nurse's right to refuse the order?

No, the police officer's order to draw blood does not supersede the nurse's right to refuse the order. The nurse has a duty to comply with federal and state law as delineated in the hospital's consent policy and procedure. The nurse must understand that federal and state laws supersede a police officer's request or demand for a blood draw. In this case the nurse's actions were correct. She complied with the consent policy and she notified her manager about the disagreement between the police officer's repeated directive to draw the blood specimen and the hospital's policy. Ultimately, in this case legal authorities confirmed that the nurse was correct in carrying out her duty to the patient. The nurse was released from jail and was compensated by Salt Lake City for the wrongful arrest and the attendant distress experienced.

5. Could the patient sue the charge nurse if she had drawn the blood sample and given it to the police officer?

Yes, the charge nurse could be sued if she had drawn the blood sample because the hospital policy and procedure did not permit it in this situation. A growing consensus appears to recommend that because of changes in the health care system, civil law, and insurance company policies, all nurses purchase malpractice insurance.

6. What would the likely claims of nursing negligence be if a lawsuit had been filed on behalf of the patient? Claims of negligence, which could be asserted in this case and discussed in the chapter, include:
1. Assault and battery;
2. Violation of the hospital's informed consent/blood draw policies and procedures;
3. Violation of the patient's right to give consent in this situation, because there was neither a court order nor an arrest warrant issued permitting the blood draw;
4. Infliction of emotional pain and distress experienced when consciousness was regained and the patient discovered:
   • there was a violation of the basic human right to consent
   • blood was drawn for a drug test not authorized by hospital policy;
5. Willful disregard for the patient's right to autonomy and self-determination when inserting a needle into the patient's body and drawing blood without explicit consent.

This last potential claim of "willful" disregard could open the nurse to an assertion of "gross negligence" because the nurse violated the fundamental human right to consent or refusal of an invasive procedure. The procedure had inherent risks associated with venipuncture including inadvertent puncture of an artery or nerve or infection at the needle insertion site. Although these are rare events they do happen and lawsuits have been filed for actual injuries suffered by patients during venipuncture.

In this case the nurse performed a procedure that resulted in unwarranted access to the patient's body when there were attendant risks not explained to the patient and there was no arrest or court order for the blood draw. A claim of "gross" negligence can result in punitive damages with significant monetary awards not covered by a malpractice insurance policy, fines, and disciplinary actions by the state licensing board for nurses.

REFERENCES

Abernathy v. Valley Medical Center, WL 3754792 (W.D. Wash., 2006).

Al-Qurayshi, Z.H., et al. (2015). Retained foreign bodies: Risks and outcomes at the national level. *Journal of the American College of Surgeons, 220*(4), 749–759. https://doi.org/10.1016/j.jamcollsurg.2014.12.015

American Academy of Ambulatory Care Nursing (2018). *Scope and standards of practice for professional telehealth nursing* (6th ed.) American Academy of Ambulatory Care Nursing.

American Academy of Pediatrics (AAP) (2016). Informed consent in decision-making in pediatric practice. Technical Report. *Pediatrics, 138*(2), e1–e16. http://pediatrics.aappublications.org/content/pediatrics/early/2016/07/21/peds.2016-1485.full.pdf

American Hospital Association. (2020). *Telehealth and virtual care: Best practices*. https://www.aha.org/system/files/media/file/2020/04/COVID-19-Telehealth-Best-Practices_final.pdf

American Hospital Association. (February 7, 2023). *Special Bulletin. Public health emergency to end May 11*. https://www.aha.org/system/files/media/file/2023/02/Special-Bulletin-Public-Health-Emergency-to-End-May-11.pdf

American Medical Association (2016). *Code of medical ethics*. American Medical Association.

American Nurses Association (ANA). (2007). *Comments on the WI Department of Justice Decision to pursue criminal charges against an RN in Wisconsin*. https://go.gale.com/ps/i.do?id=GALE%7CA166945694&sid=sitemap&v=2.1&it=r&p=HRCA&sw=w&userGroupName=anon%7E505e8d7d&aty=open-web-entry

American Nurses Association (ANA) (2009). *Safe staffing saves lives*. ANA. http://www.safestaffingsaveslives.org/WhatIsANADoing/StateLegislation/StaffingPlansandRatios.GM5Editor.html

American Nurses Association (ANA) (2011). *Social networking principles toolkit*. ANA. https://search.yahoo.com/yhs/search?hspart=mnet&hsimp=yhs-001&type=type9097303-spa-4056-84481&param1=4056&param2=84481&p=ANA+social+networlking *ethics for nurses*. ANA

American Nurses Association (ANA). (2015a). *Code of Ethics for Nurses with Interpretive Statements*. https://www.nursingworld.org/practice-policy/nursing-excellence/ethics/code-of-ethics-for-nurses/

American Nurses Association (ANA) (2015b). Understanding the charge nurse's role in staffing. *American Nurse*, September 10, 2015. https://www.myamericannurse.com/understanding-charge-nurses-role-staffing/

American Nurses Association and National Council of State Boards of Nursing (ANA & NCSBN). (2019). National Guidelines for Nursing Delegation. https://www.nursingworld.org/;4962ca/globalassets/practiceandpolicy/nursing-

excellence/ana-position-statements/nursing-practice/
ana-ncsbn-joint-statement-on-delegation.pdf

American Nurses Association (ANA). (2020a). *ANA's principles for nurse staffing*. https://www.nursingworld.org/practice-policy/nurse-staffing/staffing-principles/

American Nurses Association (ANA). (2020b) *Position Statement: The ethical use of restraints: Balancing dual nursing duties of patient safety and personal safety*. https://www.nursingworld.org/,48f80d/globalassets/practiceandpolicy/nursing-excellence/ana-position-statements/nursing-practice/restraints-position-statement.pdf

American Nurses Association (ANA). (2021). *Nursing: Scope and standards of practice* (4th ed.) ANA.

American Nurses Association (ANA). (2014). *Mandatory overtime. Policy and advocacy*. ANA. https://www.nursingworld.org/~49de63/globalassets/practiceandpolicy/health-and-safety/nurse-fatigue-position-statement-final.pdf

Anderson v. St. Francis–St. George Hospital, 614 NE 2d 841 (OH, 1992).

Axson, S.A. (2017). Evaluating nurse understanding and participation in the informed consent process. *Nursing Ethics, 26*(4), 1050–1061.

Barbourville Nursing Home v. USDHHS, No 05-3421, 6 Cir 04/06/2006 (F3d-KY).

Basen, R. (2021). Is nursing board discipline getting more aggressive? *Medpage Today*. February 23, 2021.

Bell, S.K., et al. (2017). Transparency when things go wrong: Physician attitudes about reporting medical errors to patients, peers and institutions. *Journal of Patient Safety, 13*(4), 243–248.

Bellenger, E.N., et al. (2018). The nature and extent of physical restraint-related deaths in nursing homes: A systematic review. *Journal of Aging and Health, 30*(7), 1042–1061.

Berglund, C. (2019). *Integrating law, ethics and regulation: A guide for nursing and health care students*. Oxford University Press.

Borngesser v. Jersey Shore Medical Center, 774 A. 2d 615 (N.J. App. Ct., 2001).

Boyer v. Tift County Hospital, WL 2986283 (M.D. Ga., 2008).

Brent, N. (2017). Nurse.com on Course Learning. *Court case highlights nurses' duty to follow EMTALA*. https://www.nurse.com/blog/.../court-case-highlights-nurses-duty-to-follow-emtala/

Brief amici curiae American Hospital Association. American Organization of Nurse Executives, American Society for Healthcare Human Resources Administration, Michigan Health and Hospital Association in response to the National Labor Relations Board's July 24, 2003. Notice and Invitation to File Briefs, Filed Sept 22, 2003, United States of America before the National Labor Relations Board.

Brittain, A., & Carrington, J. (2021). Organizational health and patient safety: a systematic review. *Journal of Hospital Management and Health Policy, 5*(2). https://jhmhp.amegroups.org/article/view/6544/html

Brodowski v. Ryave, 885 A.2d 1045 (PA Supr Ct. 2005).

Butts, J., & Rich, K. (2019). *Nursing ethics*. Jones & Bartlett Learning.

California Department of Consumer Affairs (2008). *Clinical learning experiences of nursing students*. California Board of Registered Nursing, http://www.rn.ca.gov/pdfs/regulations/npr-b-66.pdf

Cares, A., et al. (2015). Substance use and mental illness among nurses: Workplace warning signs and barriers to seeking assistance. *Substance Abuse, 36*, 59–66. https://doi.org/10.1080/08897077.2014.933725

Centers for Medicare & Medicaid Services. (2008). Roadmap for Implementing Value Driven Healthcare in the Traditional Medicare Fee-for-Service Program 2008. https://search.yahoo.com/yhs/search?hspart=mnet&hsimp=yhs-001&type=type9097303-spa-4056-84481&param1=4056&param2=84481&p=Centers+for+Medicare+%26+Medicaid+Services.+%282008%29.+Roadmap+for+Implementing+Value+Driven+Healthcare+in+the+Tradi-tional+Medicare+Fee-for-Service+Program+2008

Centers for Medicare and Medicaid Services. (2020a). *Frequently asked questions hospitals and critical access hospitals regarding EMTALA*. https://search.yahoo.com/yhs/search?hspart=mnet&hsimp=yhs-001&type=type9097303-spa-4056-84481&param1=4056&param2=84481&p=.++https%3A%2F%2Fwww.cms.gov%2Ffiles%2Fdocument%2Ffrequently-asked-questions-and-answers-emtala-part-ii.pdf

Centers for Medicare and Medicaid Services. (2020b). *COVID-19 emergency declaration blanket waivers for health care providers*. https://www.cms.gov/files/document/covid19-emergency-declaration-health-care-providers-fact-sheet.pdf

Centers for Medicare & Medicaid Services (CMS). (2020c). Hospital-acquired infections. https://www.cdc.gov/hai/index.html

Choi, E., et al. (2021). Perception gaps in disclosure of patient safety events between nurses and the general public in Korea. *Journal of Patient Safety, 17*(8), e971–e975. https://www.ncbi.nlm.nih.gov/pmc/articles/PMC8612886/#:,:text=a%20previous%20study.-,Results,the%20incidence%20of%20medical%20lawsuits

Clanton, N. (2022). Nurses can be sued for following doctors' order court rules. *The Atlanta Journal-Constitution.* (September 12, 2022).

Clark, M. (2020). Medical error statistics: When healthcare can kill you. *Etatics*. [Internet]. (September 24, 2020). https://etactics.com/blog/medical-error-statistics

Classen, D.C., et al. (2011). 'Global Trigger Tool' shows that adverse events in hospitals may be ten times greater than previously measured. *Health Affairs, 30*(4), 581–589. https://doi.org/10.1377/hlthaff.2011.0190

Cole, D., et al. (2019). The courage to speak out: A study describing nurses' attitudes to report unsafe practices in patient care. *Journal of Nursing Management, 27*(6), 1176–1181. https://doi.org/10.1111/jonm.12789

Columbia Medical Center of Las Colinas v. Bush, WL 22725001 WW3d (Tex., 2003).

Colwell, C. (2016). Know when uncooperative patients can refuse care and transport. *Journal of Emergency Medical Services, 41*(8), 45–47.

CNA/NSO. (2020a). *Nurse professional liability exposure claims report: 4th edition.* www.nso.com/nurseclaimreport

CNA/NSO. (2020b). Nurse spotlight: Nurse leadership liability. *Excerpted from: Nurse professional liability exposure claims report: 4th edition, 2020.* At: www.nso.com/nurseclaimreport

Deering, M. (August 29, 2022). Understanding mandatory overtime for nurses: Which states enforce mandatory overtime? *Nurse Journal.* https://search.yahoo.com/yhs/search?hspart=mnet&hsimp=yhs-001&type=type9097303-spa-4056-84481&param1=4056&param2=84481&p=Deering%2C+M.+%28August+29%2C+2022%29.+Understanding+mandatory+overtime+for+nurses%3A+Which+states+enforce+mandatory+over-time%3F+%5BInternet%5D.+Nurse+Journal

Delk, K. (2013). Whistleblowing – is it worth it?. *Workplace Health and Safety, 61*(2), 61–64.

DeMarco, J., Jones, G.E., & Daly, B.J. (2019). *Ethical and legal issues in nursing.* Broadview Press.

Dickerson v. Fatehi, 84 SE 2d 880 (Va., 1997).

Dimora v. Cleveland Clinic Foundation, 683 NE 2d 1175 (Ohio App, 1996).

Doctors Hospital of Augusta v. Alicea (Administrator), 2016 Ga. LEXIS 448 (2016).

Dowie, I. (2021). Understanding the legal considerations of consent in nursing practice. *Nursing Standard, 36*(12), 29–34. https://www.researchgate.net/publication/356441236_Understanding_the_legal_considerations_of_consent_in_nursing_practice#fullTextFileContent

Farmer, L., & Lundy, A. (2017). Informed consent: Ethical and legal considerations for advanced practice nurses. *The Journal for Nurse Practitioner, 13*(2), 124–130.

Francis v. Memorial General Hospital, 726 P 2d 852 (N.M., 1986).

Garvey, P.K. (2015). Failure to rescue: The nurse's impact. *Medsurg Nursing, 24*(3), 145–149.

Greenberg, P. (2017). *Medication-related malpractice claims. CRICO 2016 CBS Benchmarking Report.* Boston, CRICO Strategies.

Griffiths, P., et al. (2018). The association between nurse staffing and omissions in nursing care: A systematic review. *Journal of Advanced Nursing, 74*, 1474–1487. https://doi.org/10.1111/jan.13564

Hannawa, A.F. (2016). Medical errors: Disclosure styles, interpersonal forgiveness, and outcomes. *Social Science and Medicine, 156*, 29–38. https://doi.org/10.1016/j.socscimed.2016.03.026

Hanssen v. Genesis Health, WL 665318 (Iowa Appel. Ct., 2011). Preventable-hospital-deaths-are-too-high-new-study-shows.

HCA Health Services v. National Bank, 745 SW 2d 120 (Ark., 1988).

Heinrich v. Conemaugh Valley Memorial Hospital, 648 A 2d 53 (Pa., 1994).

Holston v. Sisters of the Third Order, 650 NE 2d 985 (Ill., 1995).

Institute for Safe Medication Practices (ISMP). (2022). ISMP speaks out against criminalization of medication errors. https://www.ismp.org/news/ismp-speaks-out-against-criminalization-medication-errors

Institute of Medicine (IOM)(2000). *To err is human: Building a safer health system.* National Academies Press.

Janga v. Colombrito, S.W, 3d WL6146197 (Tx. Appel. Ct. 2011).

Jenkins, D., et al. (May, 2023). Nurses as disciplinary agents of the state: Ethical practice and mandatory reporting in the United States. *Advances in Nursing Science.* (Published ahead of print).

Kakacek, B. (2022). Whistleblower rights and protection for nurses. *Nurse.org.* https://nurse.org/articles/whistleblower-protection-for-nurses/

Kaldjian, L. (2021) Communication about medical errors. *Patient Education and Counseling, 10*(5), 989–993.

Kalisch, B., & Lee, K. (2012). Missed nursing care: Magnet versus non-magnet hospitals. *Nursing Outlook, 60*(5), 32–39.

Kelley, T. (2000). Death at a nursing home leads to indictment of five. *New York Times*, B–1.

Kendall, K., et al. (2020). Failure to rescue. In: Hall, K.K., et al. Making healthcare safe III: A critical analysis of existing and emerging patient safety practices. Agency for Healthcare Research and Quality. Rockville, MD. https://www.ahrq.gov/sites/default/files/wysiwyg/research/findings/making-healthcare-safer/mhs3/failure-to-rescue-1.pdf

Khoshmehr, et al. (2020) Moral courage and psychological empowerment among nurses. *BMC Nursing, 19*(43), 1–7. https://www.researchgate.net/publication/341614217_Moral_courage_and_psychological_empowerment_among_nurses/citations#fullTextFileContent

Kowalski, K., & Horner, M.D. (1998). A legal nightmare: Denver nurses indicted. MCN. *The American Journal of Maternal Child Nursing, 23*(3), 125–129. https://doi.org/10.1097/00005721-199805000-00004

Lachman, V.D., et al. (2012). Doing the right thing: Pathways to moral courage. *The American Nurse, 7*(5), 1–3.

Lasater K.B., Aiken L.H., Sloane, D.M., et al. (2021) Is hospital nurse staffing legislation in the public's interest? An observational study in New York State. *Medical Care, 1;59*(5): 444–450.

Lavender v. Skilled Healthcare Group, No DR060264 (CA Super. Ct., Humboldt Co. 2010. WL 4926747.

Lee, S., et al. (2021). Factors affecting nurse's willingness to speak up regarding patient safety in East Asia: A systematic review. Risk Management and Healthcare Policy, 14, 1053–1063. https://www.ncbi.nlm.nih.gov/pmc/articles/PMC7966392/#:,:text=Speaking%20up%20for%20patient%20safety,procedures%2C%20and%20other%20sentinel%20events

Love v. Rancocas Hospital, WL1541052 (Distr Ct New Jersey, 2006).

Lovett v. Lorain Community Hospital, WL239927 N.E. 2d. (Ohio, 2004).

Lyons v. Walker Regional Medical Center, 791 So. 2d 937 (Ala., 2000).

Macrea, C. (2016). The problem with incident reporting. *BMJ Quality & Safety*, 25:71–75.

Mahlmeister, L. (2015). Crosswalk: The joint commission and centers for medicare and medicaid services pathways to patient safety and quality. *The Journal of Perinatal & Neonatal Nursing*, 29(2), 107–115. https://doi.org/10.1097/JPN.0000000000000093

Mahlmeister, L.R. (2009). Best practices in perinatal care: Maintaining safe and cost-effective staffing models during the current economic downturn. *The Journal of Perinatal & Neonatal Nursing*, 23(2), 111–114. https://doi.org/10.1097/JPN.0b013e3181a7282c

McDonough, W. (2018). Designate a patient safety officer. Institute for Healthcare Improvement (IHI). https://www.ihi.org/resources/Pages/Changes/DesignateaPatientSafetyOfficer.aspx

McGuire, C., & Mroczek, J. (2017). Nurse Malpractice. National Center of Continuing Education, Inc.

Medical Ethics Advisor. (2007). Nurse charged with felony in fatal medical error. *Online Nursing Papers*. https://onlinenursingpapers.com/nurse-charged-felony-fatal-medical-error/

Miller v. Levering Regional Healthcare Center, S.W. 3d. WL1889883 (Mo. App. Ct., 2006).

Mobile Infirmary Medical Center v. Hodgen, So 2d, WL 22463340 (Ala., 2003).

Moffat, J. (2023). *EMTALA answer book*. Wolters Kluwer.

National Council of State Boards of Nursing (NCSBN). (2018a). *A nurse's guide to the use of social media*. https://search.yahoo.com/yhs/search?hspart=mnet&hsimp=yhs-001&type=type9097303-spa-4056-84481&param1=4056&param2=84481&p=National+Council+of+State+Boards+of+Nursing+%28NCSBN%29.+%282018a%29.+A+nurse%E2%80%99s+guide+to+the+use+of+social+me-dia

National Council of State Boards of Nursing (NCSBN). (2018b). *Substance use disorder in nursing*. https://ncsbn.org/nursing-regulation/practice/substance-use-disorder/substance-use-in-nursing.page

National Council of State Boards of Nursing (NCSBN). (2023a). *Nursing Regulation: Nurse Licensure Guidance*. https://www.ncsbn.org/nursing-regulation/licensure/nurse-licensure-guidance.page

National Council of State Boards of Nursing (NCSBN). (2023b). *NCSBN research projects significant nursing workforce shortages and crisis*. https://www.ncsbn.org/news/ncsbn-research-projects-significant-nursing-workforce-shortages-and-crisis

National Quality Forum (NQF)(2010). *Safe practices for better healthcare—2010 update. Executive summary*. National Quality Forum, http://www.qualityforum.org/Publications/2010/04/Safe_Practices_for_Better_Healthcare_%E2.

NSO/CNA. (2022). *Nurse Professional Liability Exposure Report* (5th ed.). Nursing Service Organization. https://www.nso.com/Learning/Artifacts/Claim-Reports/Minimizing-Risk-Achieving-Excellence

Nursing Service Organization NSO. (2021). Nurse case study: ICU charge nurse allegedly failed to monitor a critical patient and escalate treatment. https://www.nso.com/Learning/Artifacts/Legal-Cases/ICU-Charge-Nurse-allegedly-failed-to-monitor-a-critical-patient

Oakwood Healthcare, Inc., 348 J.L.R.B.., No. 37, September 29, 2006.

O'Brien v. Synnott, ___A 3d___2012 WL 2124161 (Vt. May 17, 2013).

Ohio Nurses Association (ONA) (2016). The role of the registered nurse as charge nurse. *Nursing Practice Statement, 21*, 2016.

O'Neill, S. (2021). Individual nurse liability insurance. *American Nurse Journal*, 16(5), 54–58

Oshodi, T. (2019). Registered nurses' perceptions and experiences of autonomy: A descriptive, phenomenological study. *BMC Nursing, 18*, 51. https://doi.org/10.1186/s12912-019-0378-3.

Osiecki v. Bridgeport Health Care Center, Inc., 2005 WL 1331225 (Conn. Super, May 12, 2005).

Parco v. Pacifica Hospital, WL 2491516 (Supr Ct. Los Angeles County, Calif., 2007).

Passarella, G. (2005). Hospital faces trial on corporate negligence claim. *The Legal Intelligencer*. https://thelegalintelligencer.typepad.com/tli/gina-passarella/.

Pedraza v. Wyckoff Heights Medical Center, NYS2d, 2002 NY Slip Op 22094, 2002 WL 1364153 (N.Y. Sup, June 4, 2002).

Philipsen, N.C., & Soeken, D. (2011). Preparing to blow the whistle: A survival guide for nurses. *Journal of Nurse Practitioner, 7*(9), 740–746.

Pirotte, D., & Benson, S. (2023). Refusal of care. [Updated 2023 July 24]. In: *StatPearls*. Treasure Island, FL: StatPearls Publishing. https://www.ncbi.nlm.nih.gov/books/NBK560886

Pohlman, K. (2015). Why you need your own malpractice insurance. *American Nurse Today, 10*(1). https://www.americannursetoday.com/need-malpractice-insurance/.

PS Net (2019a). *Missed nursing care.* Agency for Healthcare Research and Quality. https://psnet.ahrq.gov/primer/missed-nursing-care.

PS Net (2019b). *Disclosure of errors.* Agency for Healthcare Research and Quality. https://psnet.ahrq.gov/primer/disclosure-errors

PS Net (2019c). *Reporting patient safety events.* Agency for Healthcare Research and Quality. https://psnet.ahrq.gov/primer/reporting-patient-safety-events

Radziewicz, R., et al. (2014). Assessment and management of patients who lack decision-making capacity. *Nurse Practitioner, 39*(3), 11–15. https://doi.org/10.1097/01.NPR.0000443234.97013.ff

Ramsay, A., Birks, M., & Hartin, P. (2022). Advocacy in nursing: Speaking truth to power. *Collegian, 29*(5), 549–550. https://www.ncbi.nlm.nih.gov/pmc/articles/PMC9529361/

Ratcliffe, A. (2023). The vital role of compliance officers in healthcare organizations. *MedTrainer.* https://medtrainer.com/blog/compliance-officer/

Rege, A. (2016). UIC nurse charged with aggravated battery to 8-month old patient. *Becker's Hospital Review.*

Roberts v. Galen of Virginia, Inc, 111 F 3d 405 (6 Cir, 1997).

Roddy v. Tanner Medical Center, 585 SE 2d 175 (Ga., 2003).

Roussel, L. (2011). *Management and leadership for nurse administration.* Jones & Bartlett.

Rowe v. Sisters of Pallottine Missionary Society, WL 1585453 SE 2d (W.Va., 2001).

Ruelas v. Staff Builders Personnel Services, Inc., 18 P 3d 138 (Ariz. App, 2001).

Russell, K. Nurse Practice Acts guide and govern: Update 2017. *Journal* of *Nursing Regulation, 8*(3), 18–25. https://www.ncsbn.org/public-files/2017_NPA_Guide_and_govern.pdf

Rutledge, C., & Gustin, T. (2021). Preparing nurses for roles in telehealth: Now is the time. *OJIN: The Online Journal of Issues in Nursing, 26*(1), Manuscript 3. DOI: 10.3912/OJIN.Vol26No01Man03 https://doi.org/10.3912/OJIN.Vol26No01Man03

Scott v. Corizon Health, 2014 WL 1877431 (D. Nevada, May 9, 2014).

Sergi, C., & Davis, D.D. (2023). Incident Reporting. [Updated 2023 July 25]. *StatPearls.* https://www.ncbi.nlm.nih.gov/books/NBK560498

Shannon, S.E. (2009). Disclosing errors to patients: Perspectives of registered nurses. *Joint Commission Journal on Quality and Patient Safety, 35*(1), 5–12. https://doi.org/10.1016/s1553-7250(09)35002-3

Siegel v. Long Island Jewish Medical Center, NYS 2d NY Slip Op 17790 WL 22439814 (N.Y., NY, 2003).

Silber, J.H., et al. (2016). Comparison of the value of nursing work environments in hospitals across different levels of patient risk. *JAMA Surgery, 151*, 527–536. https://doi.org/10.1001/jamasurg.2015.4908

Silvestre, J., & Spector N. (2023). Nursing student errors and near misses: Three years of data. *The Journal of Nursing Education, 62*(1), 12–19.

Skinner, M. (2023). A guide to mandatory overtime for nurses. *IntelyCare.* https://www.intelycare.com/career-advice/a-guide-to-mandatory-overtime-for-nurses/

Smart, C. (2017). University Hospital boss talks changes after nurse arrest, says 'this will not happen again.'. *The Salt Lake Tribune.* http://www.sltrib.com/news/health/2017/09/04/live-university-hospital-officials-discuss-arrest-of-nurse-who-refused-to-draw-blood

Smetzer, J., et al. (2010). Shaping systems for better behavioral choices: Lessons learned from a fatal medication error. *Joint Commission Journal on Quality and Patient Safety, 36*(4), 152–163. https://doi.org/10.1016/s1553-7250(10)36027-2

Snyder, E. (2003). Digoxin overdose: $1.5 million punitive damages. *Legal Eagle Eye Newsletter for the Nursing Profession, 11*(12), 4–5.

Snyder, E. (2004). Student nurse/instructor: Court discusses host hospital's legal liability. *Legal Eagle Eye Newsletter for the Nursing Profession, 14*(3), 4.

Snyder, E. (2006). Understaffing, fall, no neuro assessment, epidural hemorrhage, death: Nurses faulted. *Legal Eagle Eye Newsletter for the Nursing Profession, 14*(8), 6.

Snyder, E. (2007). Disability discrimination: Quad on ventilator could not communicate with his caregivers. *Legal Eagle Eye Newsletter for the Nursing Profession, 15*(10), 1.

Snyder, E. (2014). Whistleblower: Court upholds nurse's rights. *Legal Eagle Eye Newsletter for the Nursing Profession, 23*(2), 6.

Stamford Hospital v. Vega, 674 A 2d 821 (Conn., 1996).

Starr, K.T. (2019). After a physical assault by a patient: What are your options?. *Nursing, 49*(6), 12–13. https://doi.org/10.1097/01.NURSE.0000554611.25772.c1

Stokes, L. (2020). ANA Position statement; Nursing care and Do-Not-Resuscitate (DNR) decisions. *The Online Journal of Issues in Nursing OJIN, 26*(1). https://ojin.nursingworld.org/MainMenuCategories/ANAMarketplace/ANAPeriodicals/OJIN/TableofContents/Vol-26-2021/No1-Jan-2021/Nursing-Care-and-DNR-Decisions.html

Sunbridge Healthcare Corp. v. Penny, SW3d, 2005 WL 562763 (Tex. App, March 11, 2005).

Tammelleo, D. (2003). Failure to act when you know error on meds risk lives. *Nursing Law's Regan Report, 44*(11), 1.

Toney-Butler, T., & Siela, D. (2022). Recognizing alcohol and drug impairment in the workplace in Florida. [Updated 2022, Dec. 9]. In: *StatPearls.* Treasure Island (FL): StatPearls Publishing. https://www.ncbi.nlm.nih.gov/books/NBK507774/

Teno, J. (2008). The wrongful resuscitation. *Patient Safety Network. Agency for Healthcare Research and Quality.* https://psnet.ahrq.gov/webmm/case/175/the-wrongful-resuscitation

The American Association of Nurse Attorneys and the American Association of Legal Nurse Consultants (TAANA & AALNC). (2011, August). Criminal Prosecution of Health Care Providers for Unintentional Human Error. TAANA – AALNC Position Paper. August, 2011. http://www.taana.org/position_papers#cphcpuhe

The Joint Commission (TJC) (2014). *Speak up initiatives.* The Joint Commission, Oakbrook Terrace, IL. http://www.jointcommission.org/speakup.aspx

The Joint Commission (TJC) (2013). *The essential guide for patient safety officers.* The Joint Commission, Oakbrook Terrace, IL. https://store.jointcommissioninternational.org/assets/1/14/ebpsoh12sample.pdf

The Joint Commission (TJC). (2018). Case Example # 1: A death resulting from failure to rescue. Department of Corporate Communication. The Joint Commission, Oakbrook Terrace, IL. https://search.yahoo.com/yhs/search?hspart=mnet&hsimp=yhs-001&type=type9097303-spa-4056-84481&param1=4056&param2=84481&p=.+https%3A%2F%2Fwww.jointcommission.org%2F-%2Fmedia%2Ftjc%2Fdocuments%2Flwz%2Flwz_case_study_failure_to_rescue.pdf

The Joint Commission (TJC). (2024). *Comprehensive accreditation manual for hospitals.* The Joint Commission, Oakbrook Terrace, IL.

The Salt Lake Tribune. (2017, August 31). Arrest of university hospital nurse Wubbels. https://youtu.be/ihQ1-LQOkns

Thompson v. Nason Hospital, 591 A 2d 703, 707 (Pa., 1991).

US Department of Health and Human Services Office of Minority Health (USDHHSOMH). (2011). *National partnership for action to end health disparities.* US Office of Inspector General (OIG). http://minorityhealth.hhs.gov/npa

US Department of Health and Human Services, Office of Inspector General (USDHHS). (2012). *Hospital incident reporting systems do not capture most patient harm: Summary.* Report OEI-06-09-00091. http://oig.hhs.gov/oei/reports/oei-06-09-00091.pdf

US Department of Justice. (February 7, 2023*). False Claims Act settlements and judgments exceed $2 billion in fiscal year 2022.* Office of Public Affairs. https://www.justice.gov/opa/pr/false-claims-act-settlements-and-judgments-exceed-2-billion-fiscal-year-2022

Utter v. United Hospital Center, Inc., 236 SE 2d 213 (W.Va, 1977).

Varacallo, M. (2020). *Good Samaritan laws. StatPearls.* https://www.ncbi.nlm.nih.gov/books/NBK542176/

Welsh, D., et al. (2021). Development of the Barriers to Error Disclosure Assessment Tool. *Journal of Patient Safety,* 17(5), 363–374. doi: 10.1097/PTS.0000000000000331. PMID: 28671908; PMCID: PMC5748022

https://journals.lww.com/journalpatientsafety/abstract/2021/08000/development_of_the_barriers_to_error_disclosure.5.aspx

William McDougald et al. v. St. Francis North Hospital Inc. No. 48,955 (L. App. 2nd Cir. April 9, 2014).

Williams v. West Virginia Board of Examiners, S.E. 2d WL1432298 (W.Va., 2004).

Willey, J. (2018). Legal implications for student nurses and preceptors. *Delaware Nurses Association: DNA Reporter,* 43(2), 5

Winkelman v. Beloit Memorial Hospital, 483 NW 2d 211 (Wis., 1992).

Yaboah-Samponng, et al. (2021). Emergency: Hospitals are violating federal law by denying required care for substance use disorders in emergency department. *Legal Action Center.* New York. https://www.lac.org/work/priorities/fighting-discrimination/health-care-discrimination

Zhong, E., et al. (2016). A review of criminal convictions among nurses 2012–2013. *Journal of Nursing Regulation,* 7(1), 27–33. https://doi.org/10.1016/S2155-8256(16)31038-9

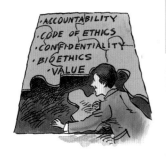

Ethical and Bioethical Issues in Nursing and Health Care

Carla D. Sanderson, PhD, RN, FAAN

...hical dilemmas are the great challenges of life.

Additional resources are available online at: http://evolve.elsevier.com/Cherry/

LEARNING OUTCOMES

After studying this chapter, the reader will be able to:

1. Integrate basic concepts of human values that are essential for ethical decision-making.
2. Analyze selected ethical theories and principles as a basis for ethical decision-making.
3. Analyze the relationship between ethics, morality, and mortality in relation to nursing practice.
4. Use an ethical decision-making framework for resolving ethical problems in health care.
5. Apply the ethical decision-making process to specific ethical issues encountered in clinical practice.

KEY TERMS

Accountability An ethical duty stating that one should be answerable legally, morally, ethically, or socially for one's activities.

Autonomy Personal freedom and the right of competent people to make choices.

Beneficence An ethical principle of compassion and patient advocacy stating that one should do good and prevent or avoid doing harm.

Bioethics The study of ethical problems resulting from scientific advances.

Code of ethics A set of statements encompassing rules that apply to people in professional roles.

Deontology An ethical theory stating that moral rule is binding.

Ethics Science or study of moral values.

Ethics acculturation The didactic and experiential process of developing ethical reasoning abilities as a part of ongoing professional preparation.

Fidelity The agreement to keep promises and commitments, based on the virtue of caring.

Justice The equal and fair distribution of resources, regardless of other factors.

Moral courage Standing up and taking action for what is right based on ethical principles.

Moral distress An emotional state that may arise when an ethically correct action differs from a given task or responsibility.

Moral resiliency Being morally responsible to navigate ethically challenging situations and deepening the commitment to mature in ethical decision-making over time.

Nonmaleficence An ethical principle stating the duty to not inflict harm.

Paternalism On the basis of the health care provider's belief about what is in the best interest of the patient, they choose to reveal or withhold patient information such as diagnosis, treatment, or prognosis.

Rights of conscience The civil right that protects conscientious health care providers against discrimination, allowing them the right to act according to the dictates of their consciences.

Utilitarianism An ethical theory stating that the best decision is one that brings about the greatest good for the most people.

Values Customs, ideas of life, and ways of behaving that society regards as desirable.

Veracity An ethical duty to tell the truth.

PROFESSIONAL/ETHICAL ISSUE

Nursing students are introduced to the ethical and legal implications of the profession of nursing during the foundational nursing course offered early in their nursing program.

The most dreaded course in the entire nursing curriculum is Adult Health Nursing. For the first time in your nursing program, your grade point average in the course is only two points above passing. There is so much to learn, so many concepts to put together, so many possible ways to think through test questions, and, in fact, your professor has told you that you are over-thinking the answers.

The last unit test is in 5 days: the Unit 4 examination. So much is riding on your ability to do well. You need to score higher than you have on any Adult Health unit examination to date, yet the Unit 4 examination has the reputation for being the hardest of all, with the lowest scores of the semester.

As you begin to organize your study plan for the test, a friend sends a text to tell you that his friend has a copy of an old Adult Health–Unit 4 examination. He invites you to his apartment that evening, where a group of six to eight students will be reviewing for the examination with the copy in hand.

Your nursing program has made it very clear that no copies of prior exams are available or appropriate for use. You know how important it is to be competent in Unit 4 materials, to possess the independent reasoning ability to pass the examination unaided. In fact, you know that knowing the Unit 4 material could easily be a matter of life and death for a patient who will someday soon be in your care.

And what about those six to eight other nursing students? What if they are able to pass the test without developing the knowledge needed to give safe, competent care?

What are you to do? Do you attend the review with your classmates? Do you determine that it is more important to pass this test and get through nursing school,

thinking you can worry about truly learning the material later? Do you have any responsibility over the actions of your classmates? What is your moral and ethical responsibility for the wrongdoing of others?

VIGNETTE

Joe Smith accepted a position as the nurse manager in a very busy urban emergency department, which serves patients from diverse cultures. Among Joe's many responsibilities is developing the 24-hour, 7-day/week work schedules of the department's nursing workforce in which he has 10 unfilled positions. Another responsibility is implementing the hospital's policy of offering all patients, regardless of cultural beliefs, the right to an advance directive for end-of-life care. At the same time Joe must ensure that each patient who enters the emergency department receives appropriate high-quality care from competent professional care providers who respect and respond to patients' individual needs and desires. With these responsibilities come challenges, sometimes so significant that the nurse manager is faced with an ethical dilemma.

Questions to Consider While Reading This Chapter

1. How will ethical and bioethical issues in nursing and health care affect my professional nursing practice?
2. What ethical theories and principles serve as a basis for nursing practice?
3. How am I to think about ethical dilemmas with moral integrity and consistency within my belief system?
4. How do I prepare to guard against moral distress in my own nursing practice?
5. What goals can I establish to move me toward excellence in moral and ethical reasoning?
6. How can I assist patients and families who face difficult ethical decisions?

CHAPTER OVERVIEW

In a nursing education program, nursing students begin to embrace the complexities and profound opportunities that are characteristic of the profession of nursing. Prelicensure nursing education is only an introduction to a discipline in which there are no knowledge boundaries. The abundance of nursing practice information is evident from a quick glance across the nursing textbook selections in the campus or online bookstore.

Most of that information addresses the "how-to" aspects of nursing care. The scientific aspects of nursing care are rapidly evolving as a host of nurse researchers delve into questions about the safe, competent, and therapeutic aspects of professional nursing care. As quickly as nursing science produces new knowledge, "how-to" information is shared through journals, textbooks, and Internet resources. The scientific aspects of care evolve constantly through "how-to" research.

A myriad of potential questions surpass the "how-to" body of knowledge that is inherent in the profession of nursing. Everywhere in today's health care delivery system are potential questions of another nature—the "how-should" questions, which are challenging and sometimes evolve into ethical dilemmas. The "how-should" questions that the emergency department nurse manager faces may sound something like the following:

- How should I determine the competency of an acutely ill 80-year-old patient who comes to the emergency department without an advance directive? Is her competency intact? How should I determine whether she is capable of giving an informed advance directive?
- How should I act if her decision for her own end-of-life care is not consistent with what her family wants for her? Or how should I respond if the family, because of cultural beliefs, will not even allow information about end-of-life care to be shared with their loved one?
- How should I view the care of this 80-year-old patient? Is an emergency resuscitation effort for such a patient considered ordinary and routine, or is it considered extraordinary and heroic?
- How should I respond to her if, in the course of efforts to stabilize her, she calls me in to ask me whether she is dying?
- How much of the truth is warranted?

- How should I decide when the availability of one-on-one trauma care beds becomes threatened and the decision must be made to move someone out of one bed to make room for this 80-year-old woman whose condition is rapidly deteriorating?
- Is the life of this 80-year-old woman any less significant than that of the 40-year-old father of four who has just been admitted after a tragic car accident?
- How should I react when another health care provider on duty devalues the significance of this patient's life?
- How should I feel when this 80-year-old patient is entered into a research study designed to test a new drug for flash pulmonary edema from congestive heart failure that has previously been tested only on a younger population?
- How should I make staffing assignments when the number of nurses on a given shift is insufficient to provide effective and adequate emergency department care to all?
- How should I respond when one of the few nurses reporting to work on a given day refuses to accept the care of patients because of inadequate staffing?
- How should I react when presented with situations that test my own sense of conscience and moral integrity?

This chapter introduces the nursing student to a different aspect of nursing care—the "how-should" aspect or, as it is more appropriately called, the ethical aspect. Ethics is a system for deciding, on the basis of principles, how one should think and what one should do. With the goal of developing excellence in moral and reasoning ability, the nursing student begins a career-long process of ethics acculturation. Just as in language acculturation, where you learn a second language while immersing yourself in it, students of ethics learn to practice ethically by reading about ethical dilemmas, discussing ethical dilemma case studies with others, and listening to patients talk about dilemmas they face.

This process allows the professional nurse to practice with an increasing level of understanding that goes beyond the scientific and moves toward a more complete and whole understanding of human existence and the nurse's role in sustaining (or upholding) it.

NURSING ETHICS

Nursing ethics is a system of principles concerning the actions of the nurse in their relationships with patients,

patients' family members, other health care providers, employers, policymakers, and society as a whole. A profession is characterized by its relationship to society. The results of a 2023 Gallup poll on professional honesty and ethics indicate that the public ranks nursing as the most ethical of all professions and has for almost two decades (Gallup News, 2023).

https://news.gallup.com/poll/467804/nurses-retain-top-ethics-rating-below-2020-high.aspx

Codes of ethics provide implicit standards and values for the professions. A nursing code of ethics was first introduced in the late 19th century and has evolved through the years as the profession has evolved and as changes in society and health care have come about. Current dynamics, such as the ethical climate of the workplace given staffing and supply shortages during the COVID-19 pandemic, the Patient Protection and Affordable Care Act, the emerging genetic interventions associated with therapeutic and reproductive cloning, debates about securing stem cells for research and treatment, and ongoing questions about euthanasia and assisted suicide now bring nursing's code of ethics to the forefront (Boxes 9.1 and 9.2).

BIOETHICS

Nursing ethics is part of a broader system known as bioethics. Bioethics is an interdisciplinary field within the health care organization that has developed only in the past 75 years. Whereas ethics has been discussed since there was written language, bioethics has developed with the age of modern medicine, specifically with the development of hemodialysis and organ transplantation. New questions surface as science and technology produce new ways of knowing. Think of the questions that come from stem cell research, sexual reassignment, organ transplantation, funding for end-of-life care, and reproductive-assisting technologies such as donor insemination, in vitro fertilization, removal of unused zygotes, and surrogate parenting. Bioethics is a response to these and other contemporary advances and challenges in health care. It is difficult to imagine a time when answers will be more plentiful than bioethical questions.

Dilemmas for Health Professionals

Physicians, nurses, social workers, psychiatrists, epidemiologists, clergy, philosophers, theologians, researchers,

---

BOX 9.1 American Nurses Association Code of Ethics for Nurses

- The nurse practices with compassion and respect for the inherent dignity, worth, and unique attributes of every person.
- The nurse's primary commitment is to the patient, whether an individual, family, group, community, or population.
- The nurse promotes, advocates for, and protects the rights, health, and safety of the patient.
- The nurse has authority, accountability, and responsibility for nursing practice; makes decisions; and takes action consistent with the obligation to promote health and to provide optimal care.
- The nurse owes the same duties to self as to others, including the responsibility to promote health and safety, preserve wholeness of character and integrity, maintain competence, and continue personal and professional growth.
- The nurse, through individual and collective effort, establishes, maintains, and improves the ethical environment of the work setting and conditions of employment that are conducive to safe, quality health care.
- The nurse, in all roles and settings, advances the profession through research and scholarly inquiry, professional standards development, and the generation of both nursing and health policy.
- The nurse collaborates with other health professionals and the public to protect human rights, promote health diplomacy, and reduce health disparities.
- The profession of nursing, collectively through its professional organizations, must articulate nursing values, maintain the integrity of the profession, and integrate principles of social justice into nursing and health policy.

Reprinted with permission from American Nurses Association (ANA). (2015). *Code of ethics for nurses with interpretive statements*. Nursebooks.org, American Nurses Association. Available online at https://www.nursingworld.org/practice-policy/nursing-excellence/ethics/code-of-ethics-for-nurses/coe-view-only/.

---

and policymakers are joining through interprofessional initiatives to address ethical questions, difficult right-versus-wrong questions. As they seek to deliver quality health care, these professionals debate situations that pose dilemmas. They are confronting situations for which there are no clear right or wrong answers. Because of the diverse society in which health care is practiced, there are at least two sides to almost every issue faced.

BOX 9.2   International Council of Nurses Code of Ethics for Nurses

1. Nurses and People

The nurse's primary professional responsibility is to people requiring nursing care.

In providing care, the nurse promotes an environment in which the human rights, values, customs, and spiritual beliefs of the individual, family, and community are respected.

The nurse ensures that the individual receives accurate, sufficient, and timely information in a culturally appropriate manner on which to base consent for care and related treatment.

The nurse holds in confidence personal information and uses judgment in sharing this information.

The nurse shares with society the responsibility for initiating and supporting action to meet the health and social needs of the public, in particular those of vulnerable populations.

The nurse advocates for equity and social justice in resource allocation, access to health care, and other social and economic services.

The nurse demonstrates professional values such as respectfulness, responsiveness, compassion, trustworthiness, and integrity.

2. Nurses and Practice

The nurse carries personal responsibility and accountability for nursing practice and for maintaining competence by continual learning.

The nurse maintains a standard of personal health such that the ability to provide care is not compromised.

The nurse uses judgment regarding individual competence when accepting and delegating responsibility.

The nurse at all times maintains standards of personal conduct that reflect well on the profession and enhance its image and public confidence.

The nurse, in providing care, ensures that use of technology and scientific advances are compatible with the safety, dignity, and rights of people.

The nurse strives to foster and maintain a practice culture promoting ethical behavior and open dialogue.

3. Nurses and the Profession

The nurse assumes the major role in determining and implementing acceptable standards of clinical nursing practice, management, research, and education.

The nurse is active in developing a core of research-based professional knowledge that supports evidence-based practice.

The nurse is active in developing and sustaining a core of professional values.

The nurse, acting through the professional organization, participates in creating a positive practice environment and maintaining safe, equitable social and economic working conditions in nursing.

The nurse practices to sustain and protect the natural environment and is aware of its consequences on health.

The nurse contributes to an ethical organizational environment and challenges unethical practices and settings.

4. Nurses and Coworkers

The nurse sustains a collaborative and respectful relationship with coworkers in nursing and other fields.

The nurse takes appropriate action to safeguard individuals, families, and communities when their health is endangered by a coworker or any other person.

The nurse takes appropriate action to support and guide coworkers to advance ethical conduct.

From International Council of Nurses. (2012). *ICN code of ethics for nurses*. Geneva: ICN.

Every specialization in health care has its own set of questions. Life and death, the margin of fetal viability, quality of life, design of life, one life offering cure for another, right to decide, informed consent, medical confidentiality, and alternative treatment issues prevail in every field of health care. Questions about the economics of nursing care and the use of technologies in the diagnosis and treatment of illness abound. In every aspect of the nursing profession lie the more subtle and intricate questions of how this care should be delivered and how one should decide when choices are in conflict.

Many nursing students do not consider health care and the practice of nursing in terms of the personal, truthful, faithful (i.e., keeping promises to patients), qualitative, and subjective side; rather, students are likely to look just at the technical, quantitative, and objective side. Yet there are distinctively subjective factors that influence the way patients are actually treated and perceive their treatment that go beyond the data-driven aspect. In many ways advanced technology has changed the face of health care and created the troubling questions that have become central in the delivery of care.

Dilemmas Created by Technology

Advances in health care through technology have created new situations for health care professionals and their patients. For the young, the old, and generations in between, illnesses once leading to death have become manageable and are classified as high-risk or chronic illnesses. Although highly fragile human lives can now be saved, they are not being saved readily or inexpensively. Care of the acutely or chronically ill person sometimes creates hard questions for which there are no easy or apparent answers. Mortality for most people is now a long, drawn-out phenomenon laced with potential conflicts about what ought to be done.

Even the nature of life itself and the technical manipulation of DNA are under investigation. Health care professionals who adhere to an exclusively scientific or technologic approach to care will be seen as insensitive and will fail to meet the genuine needs of the patient—needs that include assistance with these more subjective concerns, such as how to think about the many advanced-care choices laid before the patient.

THE ETHICS OF CARE

The very nature of the profession of nursing is the obligation and responsibility to care (Aydogdu, 2022). The ethics of care involves the nurse fulfilling the caring task by seeking the best way to care for each patient, one patient at a time, thus fulfilling a moral imperative to alleviate suffering by taking action. Caring defines nursing, as curing often defines medicine (Nicholas & Hellman, 2020).

Toward this end, nursing's Code of Ethics, first written in 1950 with ongoing revisions across the years, was updated in 2015 to provide a "definitive framework for ethical analysis and decision-making for RNs across all practice levels, roles and settings" (American Nurses Association [ANA], 2015). The Code is made up of nine provisions, which are elaborated on through interpretive statements. Each provision establishes nursing's values and commitments, its boundaries, and its duties beyond direct patient care to duties to society. The COVID-19 pandemic has brought an opportunity to discern how to hold two of the provisions in balance—the nurse's primary commitment to the patient and the duty to promote health and safety to oneself. ANA describes the Code as "the promise that nurses are doing their best to provide care for their patients and their communities and are supporting each other in the process so that all nurses can fulfill their ethical and professional obligations" (ANA, 2015).

Today's professional nurse will be deemed competent only if they can promote well-being through the scientific and technologic aspects of care *and* uphold their ethical and professional obligations. A competent nurse is an ethically sensitive nurse (Shayestehfard et al., 2020) who can deal with the human dimensions of care that include a search for what is good and right, as well as for what is accurate and efficient. The previously listed "how-should" questions are just as important as the "how-to" questions surrounding day-to-day decision-making in the emergency department or the care of the 80-year-old patient introduced previously. As the nurse seeks to understand the "how-to" aspects of nurse management and patient care, they also must seek to understand more about respecting the rights of patients.

Answering Difficult Questions

Care that combines human dimensions with scientific and technical dimensions forces some basic questions:

- What is safe care?
- What effect might a patient's cultural preferences have on safe care?
- When staffing and/or personal protective equipment is inadequate, what care should be accepted or refused?
- What are other barriers to ethical practice brought about by the workplace environment?
- What does it mean to be ill or well?
- What is the proper balance between science and technology and the good of humans?
- Where do we find balance when science will allow us to experiment with the basic origins of life?
- What happens when the proper balance is in tension?
- What happens when tension exists between personal beliefs and values and institutional policy or patient desires?

No tension is created in the effort to save the life of a dying healthy adolescent or set the broken leg of a healthy older adult. Science and the human good are not in conflict here. No conflict exists when there is a competent nursing staff, sufficient in number and well protected to provide quality care. However, what is the answer when modern medicine can save or prolong the life of an 8-year-old child but the child's parents refuse treatment for religious reasons? Or what is the answer when modern medicine has life to offer a 30-year-old mother in need of a transplanted organ but the woman is without the financial means to cover the cost of the treatment? When a family refuses to allow the physician to share news of a terminal illness with their grandmother? When new discoveries allow some would-be parents to choose biologic characteristics of children not yet conceived? When the hospital is full of acutely ill patients and there are too few nurses and too few supplies to staff the next shift? At one end of the spectrum lies the obvious; at the other there is uncertainty. Health care professionals in everyday practice are finding themselves somewhere between the two.

Balancing Science and Morality

If nursing care is to be competent, the right balance between science and morality must be sought and understood. Nurses must first attempt to understand not just what they are to do for their patients but who their patients are. They must examine life and its origins, in addition to its worth, usefulness, and importance. Nurses must determine their own values and seek to understand the values of others.

Health care decisions are seldom made independently of other people. Decisions are made with the patient, the family, other nurses and health care providers, and employers. Nurses must make a deliberate effort to recognize their own values, learn to consider and respect the values of others and discern when to speak up for what is right.

The nurse has an obligation to present himself or herself to the patient as competent. The dependent patient enters a mutual relationship with the nurse. This exchange places a patient who is vulnerable and wounded with a nurse who is educated, licensed, and knowledgeable. The patient expects nursing actions to be thorough because total caring is the defining characteristic of the patient–nurse relationship. The nurse promises to deliver holistic care to the best of their ability. The patient's expectations and the nurse's promises require a commitment to develop a reasoned thought process and sound judgment in all situations that take place within this important relationship. The more personal, subjective, and value-laden situations are deemed to be among the most difficult situations for which the nurse must prepare.

VALUES FORMATION AND MORAL DEVELOPMENT

A value is a personal belief about worth that acts as a standard to guide behavior; a value system is an entire framework on which actions are based and is the backbone to how one thinks, feels, and acts. Perhaps many nursing students come to their education with a strong backbone and an intact value system. No doubt anyone living in these times has faced many situations in which important choices had to be made. Numerous challenges have been faced in this generation and in the COVID-19 pandemic. Values have been applied to each challenging decision that has to be made.

Nursing students are well served to seriously contemplate their value system, the forces that shaped those values, and the life and worldview decisions that have been made on the basis of such values.

Examining Value Systems

To become a competent professional in every dimension of nursing care, nurses must examine and commit themselves to a virtuous value system. A clear understanding of what is right and wrong is a necessary first step to a process sometimes referred to as *values clarification,* in which people attempt to examine the values they hold and how each of those values functions as part of a whole. Nurses must acknowledge their own values by considering how they would act in a particular situation.

Diane Uustal was one of nursing's first leaders to describe the role of values clarification as a learning tool for nursing students preparing for the ethical decision-making process of the nurse (Uustal, 1992). The deliberate refinement of one's own value system leads to a clearer lens through which the nurse can view ethical questions in the practice of the profession. A refined value system and worldview can serve the professional as they deal with the meaning of life and its many choices. A worldview provides a cohesive model for life; it encourages personal responsibility for the living of that life, and it prepares one for making ethical choices encountered throughout life. Tools to assist the reader in values clarification can be found online (http://evolve. elsevier.com/Cherry/).

Forming a worldview and a value system is an evolving, continuous, dynamic process that moves along a continuum of development often referred to as *moral development*. Just as there is an orderly sequence of physical and psychologic development, there is an orderly sequence of right and wrong reasoning and conduct development. Consider an adult of strong physical strength and moral character. With each biologic developmental milestone, there is a more mature, more expanded physical being; likewise, with each life experience that has choices between right and wrong there is a more mature, more virtuous person.

Learning Right and Wrong

The process of learning to distinguish right and wrong is often described in pediatric textbooks. Donna Wong describes such development in children (Hockenberry & Wilson, 2018). Infants have no concept of right or wrong. Infants hold no beliefs and no convictions, although it is known that moral development begins in infancy. If the need for basic trust is met in infancy, children can begin to develop the foundation for secure moral thought. Toddlers begin to display behavior in response to the world around them. They will imitate behavior seen in others, even though they do not comprehend the meaning of the behavior that they are imitating. Furthermore, even though toddlers may not know what they are doing or why they are doing it, they incorporate the values and beliefs of those around them into their own behavioral code.

By the time children reach school age, they have learned that behavior has consequences and that good behavior is associated with rewards and bad behavior with punishment. Through their experiences and social interactions outside their home or immediate surroundings, school-age children begin to make choices about how they will act on the basis of an understanding of good and bad. Their conscience is developing, and it begins to govern the choices they make (Hockenberry & Wilson, 2018).

The adolescent questions existing moral values and their relevance to society. Adolescents understand duty and obligation, but they sometimes seriously question the moral codes on which society operates, as they become more aware of the contradictions they see in the value systems of adults.

Adults strive to make sense of the contradictions and learn to develop their own set of morals and values as autonomous people, sometimes referred to as *developing a moral compass*. They begin to make choices based on an internalized set of principles that provides them with the resources they need to evaluate situations in which they find themselves (Hockenberry & Wilson, 2018).

Understanding Moral Development Theory

Perhaps the most widely accepted theory on moral development is the now classic theory developed by Lawrence Kohlberg (1971). He theorizes a cognitive developmental process that is sequential in nature, with progression through levels and stages that vary dramatically within society. At first, morality is all about rules imposed by some source of authority. Moral decisions made at this level (preconventional) are simply in response to some threat of punishment. The good–bad, right–wrong labels have meaning, but they are defined only in reference to a self-centered reward-and-punishment system. A person who is in the preconventional level has no concept of the underlying moral code informing the decision of good or bad, or right or wrong.

At some point, people begin to internalize their view of themselves in response to something more meaningful and interpersonal (conventional level). A desire to be viewed as a good boy or nice girl develops when the person wants to find approval from others. They may want to please, help others, be dutiful, and show respect for authority. Conformity to expected social and religious mores and a sense of loyalty may emerge.

Not all people develop beyond the conventional level of moral development. A morally mature individual (postconventional level), one of the few to reach moral completeness, is an autonomous thinker who strives for a moral code beyond issues of authority and reverence. Integrative thinking is required to move toward having the critical components necessary to make moral judgments. The morally mature individual's actions are based on principles of justice and respect for the dignity of all humankind, and not just on principles of responsibility, duty, or self-edification (Kohlberg, 1971).

Moving Toward Moral Maturity

The rightness or wrongness of the complex and confounding health care decisions being made today depends on the level of moral development of those professionals entrusted with the tough decisions. Moving toward the level of moral maturity required for sound ethical decision-making requires strong commitment. The first step may be overcoming fear. Looking for patient care solutions where there are no straightforward answers can seem daunting. Fear can turn to confidence with commitment and determination.

Nurses must commit themselves to such learning, to a process called ethics acculturation across the span of their career. The issues will only get more complex and confounding as new advances are introduced. The desired outcomes of ethics acculturation are integrity, personal growth, practical wisdom, and effective problem-solving on behalf of patients and their families (Shayestehfard et al., 2020). These are the qualities characteristic of an ethically sensitive and morally mature person.

As a matter of the civil rights afforded to all members of US society, health care professionals have been afforded rights of conscience to practice their own convictions about what is right and ethical care. Rights of conscience are relevant in the debate on abortion and euthanasia. Historically, much liberty has been given to professionals in choosing to participate in care they believe in and refusing to participate in care they may find ethically unsound. The current debate on health care reform and the use of federal funding for abortion have in particular sparked discussion on threats to continued rights of conscience for practitioners. Professional nurses must be ready to take up the challenge of debating the matter of whether or not the right to act according to conscience should continue to be a part of one's civil rights. Doing so will require careful examination of right and wrong, the principles and motivations that govern actions and thoughts, and accountability for actions taken.

The development of value-based behavior is essential for professional nursing. The American Association of Colleges of Nursing (AACN, 2008) has delineated five essential values, described in Table 9.1. Students who seek to become morally mature health care providers will appraise nursing's values and strive to find a comfortable union of those values with their own.

The complexity of today's health care environment may lead to value conflicts and the potential for moral distress that comes from knowing the morally right thing to do but not being able to do it because of constraints outside one's control. The lack of protective equipment for nurses working with COVID-19 patients

TABLE 9.1   Essential Nursing Values and Behaviors

Essential Values	Attitudes and Personal Qualities	Professional Behaviors
Altruism—concern for the welfare of others	Caring, commitment, compassion, generosity, perseverance	Gives full attention to the client when giving care; assists other personnel in providing care when they are unable to do so; expresses concern about social trends and issues that have implications for health care
Autonomy—right to self-determination	Respectfulness, trust, objectivity	Provides nursing care based on respect of patients' rights to make decisions about their health care; honors individual's right to refuse treatment
Human dignity—respect for inherent worth and uniqueness of individuals and populations	Consideration, empathy, humaneness, kindness, respectfulness	Values and respects all patients and colleagues, regardless of background
Integrity—acting in accordance with an appropriate code of ethics	Moral, ethical, and legal professional behavior	Is honest and provides care based on an ethical framework that is accepted in the profession
Social justice—acting in accordance with fair treatment regardless of economic status, race, ethnicity, age, citizenship, disability, or sexual orientation	Courage, integrity, morality, objectivity	Acts as a health-care advocate; allocates resources fairly; reports incompetent, unethical, and illegal practices objectively and factually

From American Association of Colleges of Nursing. (2008). *Essentials of baccalaureate education for professional nursing*. American Association of Colleges of Nursing.

against the urgent need to shift standards of nursing care to meet the demands of patient surges has presented timely examples of moral distress (Webster, 2020). Moral courage refers to being able to stand up for what is right, speaking up and taking action based on ethical principles, and protecting ethical values such as honesty, integrity, fairness, respect, responsibility, empathy, compassion, and courage, regardless of the possible consequences taking such action might present. It is one of the fundamental values of the nursing profession that provides the basis for coping with ethical problems (Khoshmehr et al., 2020). Moral courage can be developed by simulating ethical dilemmas that students and nurses can process together. The study of ethical theory and ethical principles can guide the dialogue for processing dilemmas and give one a basis for moving forward as a morally courageous professional nurse.

Ultimately, the goal of the nurse is to develop *moral resiliency*, having the capacity "to sustain, restore and deepen" one's commitment to values-based decision-making, "recognizing their sense of moral responsibility and effectively navigating ethically complex, ambiguous, or conflicting situations" (Rushton, 2017). The development of moral resiliency begins with principled actions, which come from an understanding of ethical theory and principles themselves.

ETHICAL THEORY

Ethical theory is a system of principles by which a person can determine what should and should not be done. Although there are others, utilitarianism and deontology are the theories most frequently cited in the Western world as foundational for processing ethical dilemmas.

Utilitarianism

Utilitarianism is an approach that supports what is best for most people, rooted in the assumption that an action or practice is right if it leads to the greatest possible balance of good consequences, or to the least possible balance of bad consequences. For instance, the utilitarian approach would be at work if the government made a decision to forgo Medicare funding treatment for a particular population with terminal disease and to redistribute funding to other Medicare-eligible individuals with a greater likelihood for longevity or quality of life. Utilitarian ethics are noted to be the strongest approach used in

bioethical decision-making. An attempt is made to determine which actions will lead to the highest ratio of benefit to harm for all persons involved in the dilemma.

Deontology

Deontology is an approach that is rooted in the assumption that humans are rational and act out of principles that are consistent and objective and compel them to do what is right. Ethics are based on a sense of a universal principle to consistently act one way. For instance, the deontological approach would be at work if a decision is made to resuscitate and provide mechanical ventilation to a 23-week otherwise-viable fetus, despite ability to pay for care and availability of newborn intensive care beds. In bioethical decision-making, moral rightness is the act that is determined not by the consequences of the actions it produces but by the intentions and moral qualities intrinsic to the act itself. Deontological theory claims that a decision is right only if it conforms to an overriding moral duty and wrong only if it violates that moral duty. All decisions must be made in such a way that the decision could become universal law. Persons are to be treated as ends in themselves and never as means to the ends of others.

ETHICAL PRINCIPLES

Perhaps the most useful tool for the morally mature professional nurse is a set of principles, standards, or truths on which to base ethical actions. Common ground must be established between the nurse and the patient and family, between fellow nurses, between the nurse and other health care providers, and between the nurse and other members of society. Such common ground can be established by adhering to a set of principles that can move everyone involved toward understanding and agreement.

The practice of ethics involves applying principles to the two ethical theories described—utilitarianism and deontology—or to other theories that are described elsewhere. Principles can permit people to take a consistent position on specific or related issues. If the principles, when applied to a particular act, make the act right or wrong in one situation, it seems reasonable to assume that the same principle, when applied to a new situation, can have the same result.

Three principles have proven to be highly relevant in bioethics: (1) autonomy, (2) beneficence and nonmaleficence, and (3) veracity. These principles do not form a complete moral framework. One principle may be relevant to a particular situation but the others are not. Yet these principles are sufficiently comprehensive to provide an analytic framework by which moral problems can be evaluated.

Autonomy

Autonomy, the principle of respect for a person, is sometimes called the *primary moral principle*. This concept holds that humans have incalculable worth or moral dignity not possessed by other objects or creatures. There is unconditional intrinsic value for everyone. People are free to form their own judgments and whatever actions they choose. They are self-determining agents, entitled to determine their own destiny.

If an autonomous person's actions do not infringe on the autonomous actions of others, that person should be free to decide whatever they wish. This freedom should be applied even if the decision creates risk to their health, and even if the decision seems unwise to others. Concepts of freedom and informed consent are grounded in the principle of autonomy.

Although the principle of autonomy may seem basic and universal, there are times when this principle may be in conflict with other principles, such a familial ones. For instance, in some male-dominated or patriarchal cultures, the family leader's rights may override the individual and autonomous rights of a family member. In this situation, action based on the moral principle of autonomy may perpetuate conflict.

Beneficence and Nonmaleficence

In general terms, to be *beneficent* is to promote goodness, kindness, and charity. A different yet related principle is *nonmaleficence,* which is a duty not to inflict harm. In ethical terms nonmaleficence is abstaining from injuring others and helping others further their own well-being by removing harm and eliminating threats, whereas *beneficence* is to provide benefits to others by promoting their good. The beneficence–nonmaleficence principle is largely a balance of risk and benefit. At times, the risk for harm must be weighed against the possible benefits. The risk should never be greater than the importance of the problem to be solved.

Although it may seem natural to promote good at all times, the most common bioethical conflicts result from an imbalance between the demands of beneficence and those acts and decisions within the health care delivery system that might pose threats. For instance, it is not always clearly evident what is good and what is harmful. Is the resuscitation effort for the 80-year-old woman good or harmful to her overall sense of well-being? How much beneficence is there in supporting someone toward a peaceful death? What is the balance between beneficence and nonmaleficence in an understaffed emergency department? Is it better to do as much good as you can with the limited resources you have or to refuse to assume care in an effort to prevent harm that can come from being understaffed?

Veracity

Most contemporary professionals believe that telling the truth in personal communication is a moral and ethical requirement. If there is the belief in health care that truth-telling is always right, then the principle of veracity can itself pose some interesting challenges.

In the past, truth-telling was sometimes viewed as inconvenient, distressing, or even harmful to patients and families. In fact, the first American Medical Association Code of Ethics in 1847 contained such a message: "The life of a sick person can be shortened not only by the acts, but also by the words or the manner of a physician. It is, therefore, a sacred duty to guard himself carefully in this respect, and to avoid all things that have a tendency to discourage the patient and to depress his spirits."

The belief that the truth could at times be harmful was held for many years. With the shift over the last 30 years from a provider-driven system to a consumer-driven system, the adherence to silence began to break down. With this shift have come interesting questions. Is the provider–patient relationship generally understood by both parties to include the right of the provider to control the truth by withholding some or all of the relevant information until an appropriate time for disclosure? How much deception of patients is morally acceptable in the communication of a poor or terminal prognosis?

Difficult questions surface, but at the heart of the principle of veracity is trust. Health care consumers today expect accurate and precise information that is revealed in an honest and respectful manner. A few generations ago, the trust factor may have been such that it was acceptable for providers to share parts of the truth or to distort the truth in the name of beneficence.

Today, however, for trust to develop between providers and patients there must be truthful interaction and meaningful communication. The moral conflict that results from being less than truthful to patients is too troublesome for today's practitioner. The deontologic theory that the health care provider has a duty to tell the patient the truth has taken precedence over the fear of harm that might result if the truth is revealed.

The challenge today is to mesh the need for truthful communication with the need to protect. Health care providers must lay aside fears that the truth will be harmful to patients and come to the realization that more often than not, the truth can alleviate anxiety, increase pain tolerance, facilitate recovery, and enhance cooperation with treatment. With a pledge to human decency, health care providers must commit themselves to truth-telling in all interactions and relationships.

ETHICAL DECISION-MAKING MODEL

Theories provide a cognitive plan for considering ethical issues; principles offer guiding truths on which to base ethical decisions. With the use of these theories and principles, it seems appropriate to consider a system for moving beyond a specific ethical dilemma toward a morally mature and reasoned ethical action.

Many ethical decision-making models exist for the purpose of defining a process by which a nurse or another health care provider actually can move through an ethical dilemma toward an informed decision. Box 9.3 depicts one ethical decision-making model.

Situation Assessment Procedure

Identify the ethical issues and problems. In the first step of assessment, there is an attempt to find out the technical and scientific facts and the human dimension of the situation—the feelings, emotions, attitudes, and opinions. A nurse must make an attempt to understand what values are inherent in the situation. Finally, the nurse must deliberately state the nature of the ethical dilemma. This first step is important because the issues and problems to be addressed are often complex. Trying to understand the full picture of a situation is time-consuming and requires examination from many different perspectives, but it is worth the time and effort to understand an issue fully before moving forward in the assessment procedure. Wright (1987) poses some important questions that must be addressed in this first step:

- What is the issue here?
- What are the hidden issues?
- What exactly are the complexities of this situation?
- Is anything being overlooked?

Identify and Analyze Available Alternatives for Action. In the second step a set of alternatives for action is established. The second step is an important step to follow. Because actions are based most commonly on a nurse's personal value system, it is important to list all possible actions for a given situation, even actions that seem highly unlikely. Without a deliberate listing of possible alternatives, it is doubtful that the full consideration of all possible actions will take place. Wright's (1987) questions for the second step are:

- What are the reasonable possibilities for action, and how do the different affected parties (patient, family, physician, nurse, employer) want to resolve the problem?
- What ethical principles are required for each alternative?
- What assumptions are required for each alternative, and what are their implications for future action?
- What, if any, are the additional ethical problems that the alternatives raise?

Select One Alternative. Multiple factors come together in the third step. After identifying the issues and analyzing all possible alternatives, the skillful decision-maker steps back to consider the situation again. There is an attempt to reflect on ethical theory and to mesh that thinking with the identified ethical principles for each alternative. The decision-maker's value system is applied, along with an appraisal of the profession's values for the care of others. A reasoned and purposeful decision results from the blending of all of these factors.

Justify the Selection. The rational discourse on which the decision is based must be shared in an effort to

---

BOX 9.3   **Situation Assessment Procedure**

- Identify the ethical issues and problems.
- Identify and analyze available alternatives for action.
- Select one alternative.
- Justify the selection.

From Wright, R.A. (1987). *The practice of ethics: Human values in health care.* McGraw-Hill.

justify the decision. The decision-maker must be prepared to communicate their thoughts through an explanation of the reasoning process used. According to Wright (1987), the justification for a resolution to an ethical issue is an argument wherein relevant and sufficient reasons for the correctness of that resolution are presented. Defending an argument is not an easy task, but it is a necessary step to communicate the reasons or premises on which the decision is based. A systematic and logical argument will show why the particular resolution chosen is the correct one. This final step is important to allow the nurse to advance ethical thought and to express sound judgment. Wright's formula for the justification process is:

1. Specify reasons for the action.
2. Clearly present the ethical basis for these reasons.
3. Understand the shortcomings of the justification.
4. Anticipate objections to the justification.

Usefulness and Application of the Situation Assessment Procedure

A procedure or model for ethical decision-making is useful for individuals and groups alike. The more subtle and tenuous issues that arise in health care often are resolved within the context of the patient–provider relationship that exists between two people. Dilemmas resulting from questions about truth-telling, acknowledging uncertainty, paternalism, privacy, and fidelity are examples of issues that may be resolved between as few as two people.

Questions that are more encompassing are often addressed in group settings. Institutional ethics committees are now common within health care agencies. The purpose of the committee is to provide ethics education, aid in ethical policy development, and serve as a consultative body when resolution of an ethical dilemma cannot be reached otherwise. Although institutional ethics committees do not make legal decisions that are the province of the patient, the family, or the health care provider, a model such as the situation assessment procedure can be a useful procedure to guide the thinking of a group that has been asked to provide counsel.

More and more nurses are finding themselves facing ethical dilemmas as members of hospital administration teams or policymaking bodies within professional organizations or governmental bodies. Nurses contribute a highly relevant perspective to discussions and decisions about safe and effective care in these times of change.

The situation assessment procedure can be applied to the decision-making process when procedures and policies are being developed to address conflicting variables.

Thus, application of the situation assessment procedure can occur on two levels. The procedure is applicable to the daily practice level of ethical decision-making, as patients and providers make choices between right and wrong actions. The procedure is equally applicable to the policymaking level, where professionals come together to consider right and wrong choices that affect society as a whole. Professional organizations including the ANA have established committees, such as the Ethics and Human Rights Committee, that allow nurses to meet to set policy for the practice of nursing. Inherent in the policy formation are questions that affect patient care. The situation assessment procedure can be applied to difficult questions that arise in any setting in which the nurse is responsible for or contributes to ethical decision-making.

BIOETHICAL DILEMMAS: LIFE, DEATH, AND DILEMMAS IN BETWEEN

Bioethical dilemmas are situations that pose a choice between perplexing alternatives in the delivery of health care because of the lack of a clear sense of right or wrong. It is imperative that every nursing student consider the potential dilemmas that might arise in a given practice setting. Concepts of life and death are central to nursing's body of knowledge, but a discussion of these concepts is incomplete unless the threats of conflict also are explored. A nursing student must not assume that conflict is rare or that it is to be dealt with primarily by other professionals on the health care team. Conflict must be addressed as the concepts of life and its origins, birth, death, and dying are addressed.

Life

Entire textbooks are written to address the potential conflict that surrounds questions about the beginning of life. The most significant conflict that will be recorded in the historical accounts of the 20th century is the debate about when life begins. The abortion conflict became central in 1973 when the Roe vs Wade decision was made by the US Supreme Court. Although the legal aspects of abortion have been resolved in courtrooms in the United States, the bioethical concerns continue to be debated 45 years later. The bioethical abortion conflict has been debated through the use of ethical theories and principles, value systems, rights issues, questions regarding the nature of choice, and so on. Answers acceptable to society as a whole have not materialized; thus the right or wrong of abortion continues to rest with each person. Nurses serving in health settings for women and children must be prepared to face this morally laden issue.

Closely akin to the abortion question are newer questions about reproduction. Genetic screening, genetic engineering, stem cell therapy, and cloning are newer, highly advanced, and sophisticated techniques that bring with them the most ethically entangled questions ever encountered; the entire Human Genome Project, with its rapidly developing advances, represents the greatest challenge to date. Definitions of family, surrogacy, and other related issues also bring ethically entangled questions. Moving beyond the question about when life begins, health care providers must now address their patients' questions about the right or wrong of designing life itself through the manipulation and engineering of DNA, or the right and wrong of new parenting models. Twenty-first-century science has created a whole new dimension of bioethics.

Genomic applications in health care, and the ethical implications surrounding them, are becoming increasingly relevant to the day-to-day delivery of care to patients. The National Institutes of Health provide a resource for understanding the ethical implications of genomics, the Genetics/Genomics Competency Center (G2C2), which can be accessed online (https://genomicseducation.net/). Nurses can use this center to learn how to apply ethical principles when deliberating genetic/genomic issues related to decision-making, privacy, confidentiality, and informed consent, as well as to process situations when patients' beliefs and values influence genomic care choices, and can find resources for resolving ethical dilemmas.

The End of Life

The second most debated conflict in health care involves the issue of death and dying. Since the development of lifesaving procedures and mechanical ventilation, questions about quality of life and the definition of death have escalated. With advances in health care, it has become unclear what is usual and what is heroic care. The purpose and quality of life of a person in a vegetative state continue to be debated. Health care providers regularly contend with questions of cerebral vs biologic death in their dealings with patients and families.

The United States is experiencing the aging of its largest segment of the population and is facing ethical dilemmas related to the limited resources available to care for them. There is growing concern in the public arena about the expenses associated with prolongation of the dying process, which often also prolongs suffering. Euthanasia and assisted suicide present the newest ethical questions surrounding the dying process, although the ANA has an official statement in opposition to these activities (ANA for Ethics and Human Rights, 2023). https://www.nursingworld.org/practice-policy/nursing-excellence/ethics/

The COVID-19 pandemic brought a new end-of-life challenge to bear on the practice of nursing—patients dying alone. Infectious disease restrictions impact the way nurses have traditionally provided dying patients with care. Nurses use video-calling technology to support their responsibilities for end-of-life discussions and emotional support for lonely, dying patients. The morally courageous nurse must be prepared to recognize their own attitudes, values, and expectations about death and step up to take ethical action for the good of the dying patient.

Dilemmas In Between

Life and death dilemmas receive the most attention through the media and in real-life drama played out in the news and on television and theater screens. However, a host of other questions make up most ethical decision-making activities for the professional nurse in the practice of today's health care. Between questions of life and death are questions of existence, reality, individual rights, responsibility, informed consent, cultural competence, equality, justice, ability to pay, and fairness. Added to these are an unlimited number of other questions that arise from the human dimension of caring.

It is in these ordinary day-to-day situations that many professionals find significant and troublesome ethical questions. Basic notions of individual and social justice are viewed in terms of fairness and what is deserved. A person has been treated justly when they have been given what is due or owed. Any denial of something to which a person has a right or entitlement is an act of injustice.

The Right to Health Care. Handling injustice has been a part of nursing since the days of Florence Nightingale. It has been at the forefront of the implementation of the Patient Protection and Affordable Care Act, as individuals, businesses, and the legislature debate providing quality health care for the many without sacrificing the basic rights of the few. What basic right to health care do people have? Is each person entitled to the same health care package? Should ability to pay affect the specific level of entitlement? Resolutions to such questions have been based largely on the doctrine of justice, which states that like cases should be treated alike and equals ought to be treated equally. Such issues grip at the core of nursing practice, wherein access to health care and a respect for human dignity are paramount. Justice becomes a bioethical issue at the point that it affects whether, when, where, and how a patient will receive health care. Americans have different values, beliefs, and priorities about how to surmount the injustices. Nurses must consider how their practice relates to injustice in health care and must address factors that work against individual well-being and societal health. The opportunity for true health care reform will challenge nurses and the entire nation to consider the important ethical issues of justice.

Allocation of Scarce Resources. The issues of organ transplantation, the allocation of scarce resources, and the reality of under-resourced people flow from the doctrine of justice. The COVID-19 pandemic has brought to light the problem of scarce medical resources. Which people in need of transplantation should receive organs when available organs are in shorter supply than the number of people who could benefit from them? Why are more under-resourced people dying of COVID-19? These justice questions are applicable to scarce resources' situations. The utilitarian view argues that the allocation decision should be framed so as to serve the greatest good for the greatest number of people affected. Should the selected transplant recipient be the man with the largest, most loving family who does the greatest work for society? Should upstream health care funding for under-resourced communities and schools be prioritized to prevent downstream poverty? Or should more universal laws be applied? Should the people in need of organ transplantation be placed on a first-come, first-served list, or should they be entered into a lottery? Distributive justice, or taking into

consideration the needs, interests, and wishes of each patient, cannot alone answer all allocation dilemmas. Who has the more meaningful life? Who has the best prognosis? Who can pay? Who pays for basic needs for food and shelter for all? These are the kinds of questions responsible parties must answer regarding the allocation of scarce resources. And what about the fact that nurses themselves are scarce resources? What about the challenge of the nurse's autonomous right to refuse to work in understaffed settings? Whose rights come first?

Ethical Challenges

What about the doctrines of justice and freedom and the need for human experimentation and biomedical research? What about animal experimentation? It is accepted that human and animal experimentation is necessary for the progression of health care knowledge, but what about the risk for harm and the moral imperative that providers should, above all, do no harm? What about specifically problematic aspects of research, such as the use in research of institutionalized or imprisoned subjects, or the practice of research on a viable fetus? Memories of harmful medical research and human experimentation, such as the Nazi atrocities and the Tuskegee syphilis study, have resulted in governmental regulations involving the use of human subjects in medical research. The Nuremberg Code is a set of provisions that researchers must follow so their research is approved by the federal government. Institutional review boards are established within research institutions for the purpose of ensuring that the degree of risk to the subject is minimized, if not eliminated. Human experimentation tests the principles of autonomy and respect for personhood.

The Challenge of Veracity

Everyday issues that test the principle of veracity are the concepts of alternative treatment and acknowledging uncertainty. It is the nature of health science that new knowledge must come forth to replace less-effective practices. However, new ignorance comes along with these new discoveries. Which treatment of two or more options is best for a patient in a specific situation? Which of the new drugs should be used? Should every patient be subjected to every possible form of diagnostic evaluation? Should a particular patient be treated with surgery, medication, or both? How do the economics of treatment costs factor into the decision? And most important, should the patient be made aware of all of these questions and various options for their care? Can patients comprehend medicine's esoteric knowledge, in general, and its accompanying certainties and uncertainties, in particular? Is disclosure of uncertainty ultimately beneficial or detrimental?

Acknowledging uncertainty is difficult for today's health care provider. As never before, it seems that providers need to present themselves as confident, knowledgeable, and sensitive to patients who may see them as arrogant, dogmatic, and insensitive. Acknowledging uncertainty was a necessity during COVID-19 treatment and may well be worth more broad use. For the diagnostician, it may lighten the burden by absolving them of the responsibility for implicitly making decisions for which there may be conflicting answers. For the patient, knowing about the uncertainty may give them a greater voice in decision-making and, in the event of treatment failure, may leave them better informed and more trustful of the caregiver. It seems that disclosure of uncertainty is ultimately beneficial to both parties. In fact, full disclosure and open communication through a commitment to veracity could prevent many everyday ethical situations. Optimal health care results from an exchange between patient and provider, with open communication about the patient's wants and needs and the provider's judgment and advice. All too often, time is not taken for open communication, and the exchange becomes one in which the patient listens to what the all-knowing and wise provider says about the patient's needs. In this scenario, it is easy for the provider to assume a paternalistic attitude in the delivery of health care.

The Challenge of Paternalism

Paternalism is an action and an attitude wherein the provider tries to act on behalf of the patient with the belief that their actions are justified because of a commitment to act in the best interest of the patient. Paternalism is a reflection of the "father knows best" way of thinking. The phenomenon of paternalism presumes, in the name of beneficence, to overlook the patient's right to autonomy. Thus, in the process of attempting to act in the best interest of the patient, paternalism involves actions not based on the patient's choices, wishes, and desires. Paternalism interferes with a patient's right to self-determination, and occurs when the provider believes that they can make a better decision than the patient.

Whereas it must be recognized that some cultures are highly paternalistic, the most common belief and value system in North America views paternalism as a threat to the patient–provider relationship. Every provider must guard against actions and attitudes that are paternalistic. Perhaps in the past paternalism was associated with the image of the white-coated physician as a sovereign god. Today paternalistic actions and attitudes can be found among nurses, pharmacists, physical therapists, occupational therapists, social workers, clergy, or anyone who assumes the image of the all-knowing in the delivery of care. A current threat to a healthy patient–provider relationship is the emergence of entrepreneurship in medicine, in which health care providers are called on to be business managers. The bottom-line financial realities can be threats to safe care.

The healthy patient–provider relationship is based on the open communication described previously, wherein patient choice and respect for personhood are deemed just as important as scientific knowledge and sound health care advice. In paternalistic cultures when the patient is denied knowing "the truth" about his diagnosis or choices for care, it is a challenge for health care providers to know when to give the patient information or have discussions with the patient in spite of the family's wishes. The provider–patient relationship is built on trust when the right to confidentiality and privacy become ethical and legal obligations.

The Challenge of Autonomy

The provider–patient relationship makes way for the crucial legal concept of informed consent, which stipulates that the patient has the right to know and make decisions about their health. These decisions take the form of consent or refusal of treatment. Based on the principle of autonomy, the consent process must be voluntary and without coercion; the fully informed patient must clearly understand the choices being offered.

Informed consent dilemmas evolve from questions about whether patients are competent to make informed decisions, and whether there are family members or surrogates to make these decisions by proxy. Difficult questions are posed for health care providers by the need for informed consent from minors, confused older adults, persons in emergency situations, and persons who are mentally compromised, imprisoned, inebriated, or unconscious. The burden of informed consent lies with the physician in most circumstances, although the nurse frequently is responsible for aspects of informing and obtaining consent.

In the latter part of the 20th century, another crucial concept of consent was introduced. Advances in technology and the potential to keep people alive for extended periods have brought about legislation aimed at giving people choices about end-of-life decisions while they are still healthy and well enough to make informed decisions. The opportunity for people to make advance directives is now common and is even a requirement for admission to hospitals and other health care agencies that receive federal dollars. People are not required to decide but must be given an opportunity to do so. Ideally the health care community will provide such an opportunity while the patient is well, perhaps in a community setting such as a public library or community center. Health care professionals, such as nurses and other health care educators, have an ethical obligation to educate the public about the use of advance directives. These opportunities can serve as excellent means of educating patients not only about advance directives but also about their rights in general, changes in health care delivery and managed care, and the role of the various health care providers. These are excellent opportunities to educate the public about the scope of practice of today's professional nurse.

The Challenge of Accountability

A host of specific ethical issues exists within the practice of nursing. Professional nursing is a complex profession that is unlike most others. The accountability factor in the practice of nursing is such that a keen sense of responsibility and personal integrity are necessary qualities for every practicing nurse. It is the nurse's ethical obligation to uphold the highest standards of practice and care, to assume full personal and professional responsibility for every action, and to commit to maintaining quality in the skill and knowledge base of the profession. Failure to meet such obligations places the patient–nurse relationship at risk.

Failure to be accountable for one's own actions damages the health care team, causing rifts, blame, and potentially shifting work/responsibilities and patient care between shifts. In other words, lack of accountability can negatively affect quality patient care and team building. In health professions in which the safety and health of society are at stake, the obligation of professionals to police the practice of their colleagues is important.

There are public and legal official policing bodies, such as the state board of nursing, for matters of public record and formal conviction. However, there are countless situations in which the official policing body will never be involved, and the obligation to denounce a harmful action or potentially threatening situation falls to a fellow member of the profession. Sometimes known as *whistleblowing*, the obligation to denounce is based on the fact that to remain silent is to consent to the action or threatening situation. Whether denouncing a chemical impairment, negligence, abusiveness, incompetence, or cruelty, the obligation is a moral one based at least in part on the principle of beneficence.

Every person bearing the title of nurse must aspire to maintain himself or herself as a professional of integrity who is willing to blow the whistle on those whose actions are irresponsible and harmful. If this is not the case, the wrong will continue, and the harm to others will escalate. In the end, the profession as a whole will suffer, and the well-being of society will be diminished.

SUMMARY

To summarize the chapter let's review the questions posed at the beginning of the chapter and see what you have learned.

1. How will ethical and bioethical issues in nursing and health care affect my professional nursing practice?

   Nurses make thousands of decisions in the course of their career that have ethical implications. A part of professional nursing care is upholding ethical standards when making nursing decisions. The nurse must develop thinking skills that ground their decisions in moral law and bring what is right and good to bear on their care for others.

2. What ethical theories and principles serve as a basis for nursing practice?

   While there are multiple ethical theories and principles, the ethical theory of utilitarianism is a common approach to guide the nurse's ethical practice. Utilitarianism supports what is best for most people and leads to the greatest possible balance of good consequences. Similarly, the ethical principle of autonomy, or respect for personhood, is referred to as the primary moral principle. Every human being has incalculable worth or moral dignity not possessed by other objects or creatures and must be treated accordingly as autonomous individuals.

3. How am I to think about ethical dilemmas with moral integrity and consistency within my belief system?

   Nurses make strong ethical decisions in the face of patient dilemmas when their personal values are consistent with the values of the nursing profession. Thinking carefully and well about one's own values through a values clarification process is a step toward strong decision-making as a professional nurse.

4. How do I prepare to guard against moral distress in my own nursing practice?

   The best guard against moral distress is to develop moral courage and resiliency. Moral courage is being able to stand up and speak up for what is right. Moral resiliency is an ultimate goal for the professional nurse, having the capacity to sustain and advance values-based decision-making in navigating the complex and sometimes conflicting situations facing the nurse.

5. What goals can I establish to move me toward excellence in moral and ethical reasoning?

   All nurses are encouraged toward ethics acculturation, the process of developing ethical reasoning abilities as a part of ongoing professional preparation. Nurses are encouraged to set both didactic and experiential learning goals to foster learning to think morally and ethically. For didactic goals, take advantage of webinars and even formal coursework in ethical reasoning. For experiential goals, get involved in ethical dilemmas occurring in the workplace by joining conversations, sharing perspectives and giving opinion on how to resolve the ethical conflicts at hand.

6. How can I assist patients and families who face difficult ethical decisions?

   Start by adopting a model for supporting patients in making ethical decisions, such as the Situation Assessment Procedure described in this chapter. Always keep in mind the worth of every human being. Commit to the moral principle of beneficence, which is to promote goodness, kindness, and charity, and to the related principle of non-maleficence, which is a duty not to inflict harm. Commit to truth telling. And then don't hold back or assume someone else is better equipped to assist patients and families. Stepping in to help resolve hard questions on behalf of others is a profound form of patient care.

NGN CASE STUDY/QUESTIONS

Clinical Judgment and Next-Generation NCLEX® Examination-Style Questions

1. A dehydrated 80-year-old client has been admitted to the surgical unit with severe bowel obstruction and requires emergency surgery. The client received prescribed narcotics for pain in the emergency department and is oriented to person and place at this time. The client does not have an advance directive but has told the family she wants "no heroic measures" to sustain her life. Her family is hesitant to sign an informed consent for surgery, not knowing if the surgery is considered "heroic." The nurse manager has been approached by the nurse working with the client for guidance on what is considered heroic. Which principles should guide the nurse manager's response?

Multiple Response: Select All That Apply

a. In the absence of an advance directive from the client, a member of the family must sign an advance directive before the surgery can be performed.

b. Moral resiliency is needed when working with the family members to navigate the confusing situation they find themselves in.

c. The decision to recommend surgery is based on utilitarian theory.

d. The decision to recommend surgery is based on the principle of maleficence.

e. The client's overall health, compliance with previously prescribed health care, and quality of life should be considered when helping the family determine the "heroic" nature of the recommended surgery.

2. Complete the following sentence by choosing from the list of options.

Cloze/Drop Down

The client's family determines that she would [want; not want] the recommended surgery because [the doctor recommends it; she has had a full and active life up until now; her pastor recommends it].

3. While awaiting preoperative orders from the surgeon, the nurse and nurse manager review potential interventions that will prepare the client and family for surgery. **For each potential intervention click to specify whether the intervention is essential, nonessential, or not applicable for the care of this client.**

Potential Intervention	Essential	Nonessential	Not Applicable
Preoperative consent signed	☐	☐	☐
Ethics Committee consultation	☐	☐	☐
Obtain copy of advance directive	☐	☐	☐
Have family assign a durable power of attorney for health care	☐	☐	☐
Provide a complete bed-bath	☐	☐	☐
Continue to monitor client's vital signs and level of pain	☐	☐	☐

4. To assure all clients on the unit receive safe and effective care while the nurse cares for this seriously ill client, the nurse manager reassigns the nurse's remaining clients to other staff. From the list below select three ethical principles that support the actions of the nurse manager when making staffing assignments.

Multiple Response: Select All That Apply

a. Autonomy
b. Beneficence
c. Fidelity
d. Justice
e. Nonmaleficence
f. Quality of life
g. Right to refuse care

5. After the client is transferred to the preoperative holding area the nurse manager takes a moment to evaluate how well the emergency involving a critically ill client was handled by the unit. From the list below drag to the drop zone the 4 statements that describe positive outcomes resulting from the staffing assignment changes.

Multiple Response: Select All That Apply

a. The original client's consent for surgery was completed and signed.
b. Medications were administered on time to all clients.
c. Nurses reported increased collaboration after staffing assignments were revised.
d. One client fell and broke their hip.
e. Client rights were respected.
f. Family members of three families voiced concern that their loved one was being ignored.
g. One nurse refused changes to their assignment.
h. Two clients were discharged to home.

REFERENCES

Aydogdu A.L.F. (2022). Ethical dilemmas experienced by nurses while caring for patients during the COVID-19 pandemic: An integrative review of qualitative studies. *Journal of Nursing Management, 30*(7), 2245–2258. doi: 10.1111/jonm.13585. Epub 2022 Mar 16. PMID: 35266597; PMCID: PMC9115168.

American Association of Colleges of Nursing (AACN). (2008). *Essentials of baccalaureate education for professional nursing.* American Association of Colleges of Nursing.

American Nurses Association (ANA) Center for Ethics and Human Rights. (2023). *Position statement– The Nurse's Role When a Patient Requests Medical Aid in Dying.* https://www.nursingworld.org/,49e869/globalassets/practiceandpolicy/nursing-excellence/ana-position-statements/social-causes-and-health-care/the-nurses-role-when-a-patient-requests-medical-aid-in-dying-web-format.pdf

American Nurses Association (ANA). (2015). *Code of ethics for nurses with interpretive statements.*

Faubion, D. (2023). *20 Common Examples of Ethical Dilemmas in Nursing + How to Deal With Them* https://www.nursingprocess.org/ethical-dilemma-in-nursing-examples.html accessed September 6, 2023.

Gallup News. (2023) *Nurses retain top ethics rating in US but below 2020 high, ethics.* news.gallup.com/poll/274673/nurses-continue-rat-highest-ethics.es

Hockenberry, M.J., & Wilson, D. (2018). *Wong's nursing care of infants and children* (11th ed.) Mosby.

Khoshmehr, Z., Barkhordari-Sharifabad, M., Nasiriani, K., & Fallahzadeh, H. (2020). Moral courage and psychological empowerment among nurses. *BMC Nursing, 19,* 43. https://doi.org/10.1186/s12912-020-00435-9

Kohlberg, L. (1971). *Stages of moral development as a basis for moral education.* Center for Moral Education, Harvard University, pp. 42–53.

Nicholson, K., & Hellman, D. (2020). Opioid prescribing and the ethical duty to do no harm. *American Journal of Law & Medicine, 46*(2–3), 297–310.

Rushton, C.H. (2017). Cultivating moral resilience: Shifting the narrative from powerlessness to possibility. *American Journal of Nursing, 117*(2), 11–15.

Shayestehfard, M., Torabizadeh, C., Gholamzadeh, S., & Ebadi, A. (2020). Ethical sensitivity in nursing students: Developing a context-based education. *Electronic Journal of General Medicine, 17*(2), 9–12. https://doi.org/10.29333/ejgm/7812. doi:10.3912/OJIN.Vol18No02EthCol01.

Uustal, D. (1992). *Values and ethics in nursing: From theory to practice* (4th ed.) Educational Resources in Nursing and Holistic Health.

Webster, L. (2020). Ethics in a pandemic. *American Nurse Today, 15*(9), 18–23.

Wright, R.A. (1987). *The practice of ethics: Human values in health care.* McGraw-Hill.

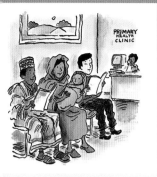

10

Patients deserve culturally competent care.

Cultural Competency, Person-Centered Care, and Social Issues in Nursing and Health Care

Susan R. Jacob, PhD, MS, RN

Ⓔ Additional resources are available online at: https://evolve.elsevier.com/Cherry

LEARNING OUTCOMES

After studying this chapter, the reader will be able to:

1. Integrate knowledge of demographic and sociocultural variations into culturally competent professional nursing care.
2. Provide culturally competent care to diverse client groups that incorporates variations in biologic characteristics, social organization, environmental control, communication, and other phenomena.
3. Critique education, practice, and research issues that influence culturally competent care.
4. Integrate respect for differences in beliefs and values of others as a critical component of nursing practice.

KEY TERMS

Cultural humility Incorporates a lifelong commitment to self-evaluation and self-critique, to redressing the power imbalances in the patient–clinician dynamic and to developing mutually beneficial and advocacy partnerships with communities on behalf of individuals and defined populations (Tervalon & Murray-Garcia, 1998).

Cultural sensitivity Experienced when neutral language, both verbal and nonverbal, is used in a way that reflects sensitivity and appreciation for the diversity of another (American Academy of Nursing Expert Panel on Cultural Competence, 2007).

Culturally competent care The process by which nurses demonstrate culturally congruent practice.

Cultural congruence Represents the process by which nurses demonstrate culturally congruent practice. Nurses design and direct culturally congruent practice and services for diverse consumers to improve access, promote positive outcomes, and reduce disparities (American Nurses Association [ANA], 2021, p. 31).

Culture Shared values, beliefs, and practices of a particular group of people that are transmitted from one generation to the next and are identified as patterns that guide thinking and action.

Diversity References a broad range of individual, population, and social characteristics, including but not limited to age; sex; race; ethnicity; sexual orientation; gender identity; family structures; geographic locations; national origin; immigrants and refugees; language; physical, functional, and learning abilities; religious beliefs; and socioeconomic status.

Equity The ability to recognize the differences in the resources or knowledge needed to allow individuals to fully participate in society, including access to higher education, with the goal of overcoming obstacles to ensure fairness.

Ethnicity Affiliation resulting from a shared linguistic, racial, or cultural background.

Ethnocentric Believing that one's own ethnic group, culture, or nation is best. Explicit biases. Conscious positive or negative feelings and/or thoughts about groups or identity characteristics. Because these attitudes are explicit in nature, they are espoused openly, through overt and deliberate thoughts and actions (Harrison et al., 2019; Wilson et al., 2000).

Health disparities A particular type of health difference that is closely linked with economic, social, or environmental disadvantage. Health disparities adversely affect groups of people who have systematically experienced greater social or economic obstacles to health based on their racial or ethnic group, religion, socioeconomic status, gender, age, or mental health; cognitive, sensory, or physical disability; sexual orientation or gender identity; geographic location; or other characteristics historically linked to discrimination or exclusion (US Department of Health and Human Services, 2010).

Implicit biases Associations that are automatically expressed and which people unknowingly hold; also known as unconscious or hidden biases. https://www.aha.org/system/files/media/file/2020/12/ifdhe_snapshot_survey_FINAL.pdf

Inclusion Inclusive environments require intentionality and embrace differences, not merely tolerate them. Everyone works to ensure the perspectives and experiences of others are invited, welcomed, acknowledged, and respected in inclusive environments.

Minority An ethnic group smaller than the majority group.

Prejudice Preconceived, deeply held, usually negative, judgment formed about other groups.

Social determinants of health The conditions in the environments in which people are born, live, learn, work, play, worship, and age that affect a wide range of health, functioning, and quality-of-life outcomes and risks.

Stereotyping Assigning certain beliefs and behaviors to groups without recognizing individuality.

Transcultural Being grounded in one's own culture but having the skills to be able to work in a multicultural environment.

PROFESSIONAL/ETHICAL ISSUE

Yei Wu, a 64-year-old Chinese female, was admitted to the emergency department (ED) with a temperature of 103°F, severe nausea and vomiting, and uterine bleeding. She was brought to the ED by her 36-year-old son, who had found her lying on the floor in her home when he went to visit her earlier in the afternoon. Because Yei speaks no English, her son provided the necessary information for her admission to the hospital. When the attending physician heard the charge nurse, Chandra, request an interpreter, he interrupted her by saying that an interpreter would not be needed because the bilingual son could provide interpretation. Chandra remembered learning in her **cultural competence** training that family members should be used for interpretation only as a last resort.

What avenues should Chandra explore for interpretation services? What are the potential risks of having family members interpret for the patient?

VIGNETTE

When my instructor taught the session on cultural differences she stressed the high alcoholism rates of American Indians. I began to fear that my instructor and fellow classmates would stereotype me because of my American Indian background. However, no one in my family drinks alcohol because we belong to the Mormon Church, where drinking is not accepted. I wish the instructor had stressed the importance of not **stereotyping**.

Questions to Consider While Reading This Chapter

1. What strategies can you implement to overcome **prejudice**?
2. How can nurses provide effective care to different cultural groups who each have a unique set of beliefs about illness?
3. How can nursing research affect the attitudes and beliefs of health professionals in regard to **minority** populations?

CHAPTER OVERVIEW

The United States has always been represented by a culturally diverse society. However, the volume of cultural groups entering the country is increasing rapidly. Professional nurses must provide care to persons of various cultures who have different values, beliefs, and perceptions about health and illness. This chapter explores cultural phenomena, including environmental control, biologic variations, social organization, communication, space, and time in relation to major cultural groups. It also examines different views about health, illness, and care. Federally defined minority groups, which include African Americans or Black people, Asians, Hispanics, and American Indians, are emphasized. The need for diversity in the health care workforce is explored, and strategies for recruiting and retaining minorities in nursing are suggested. Strategies that nurses can use to improve their own cultural competence in providing person-centered care also are given.

POPULATION TRENDS

The demographic and ethnic composition of the US population has experienced a marked change in the past 100 years. Minority groups have grown faster than the population as a whole. In some US cities, the number of persons from diverse cultural groups is increasing at such a rapid pace that minorities constitute more than half the population. The nation will be more racially and ethnically diverse, as well as much older, by midcentury, according to 2019 projections released by the US Census Bureau. Minorities, 37% of the US population, are expected to comprise 57% of the population in 2060.

*The number of Americans ages 65 years and older is **projected to nearly double** from 52 million in 2018 to 95 million by 2060, and the 65-and-older age group's share of the total population will rise from 16% to 23%. https://www.prb.org/aging-unitedstates-fact-sheet/#footnote-1. US Census Bureau, Population Projections. https://www.census.gov/programs-surveys/popproj.htm. These levels are projected to rise further by 2026, to 26% for men and 18% for women. Despite the increased diversity in the older adult population, the more rapidly changing racial/ethnic composition of the population under age 18 relative to those ages 65 and older has created a **diversity gap** between generations.*

Older adults are working longer. By 2018 some 24% of men and about 16% of women ages 65 and older were in the labor force. These levels are projected to rise further by 2026, to 26% for men and 18% for women (Vespa et al., 2020).

*Many parts of the country—especially counties in the rural Midwest—are **aging in place** because disproportionate shares of young people have moved elsewhere.*

Along with the dramatic aging of the US population during the next decades will come significant increases in racial and ethnic diversity. The older population is becoming more racially and ethnically diverse. As the population ages and grows more slowly in coming decades the United States is projected to continue becoming a more racially and ethnically pluralistic society. Non-Hispanic Whites are projected to remain the single largest race or ethnic group for the next 40 years (Vespa et al., 2020).

Language barriers, reduced access to health care, low socioeconomic status, and differing cultural norms can be major challenges to promoting health in an increasingly diverse older population. This demographic change introduces many interrelated social, economic, political, educational, and health problems. The fact that people are living longer allows more opportunity for the development of chronic illness. Social isolation and depression that result from losses of friends and family will present a challenge for mental health care providers. Primary care providers will be faced with identifying risks to independence and health for the aging population (Stanhope & Lancaster, 2024).

Health care providers must guard against issues of *ageism,* that is, assuming that health issues and levels of cognition are the same for every senior adult.

Federally Defined Minority Groups

Federally defined minority groups are:
- Asian American
- Black or African American
- Hispanic or Latino
- Native Hawaiian and other Pacific Islander
- American Indian and Alaska Native

ECONOMIC AND SOCIAL CHANGES

Changing world economics have had profound consequences, such as increased joblessness, homelessness, poverty, and limited access to health insurance and health care. Anxiety, hopelessness, depression, and despair commonly affect the individuals in our society who find themselves suddenly without jobs and sometimes even without homes as a result of economic downsizing. These conditions are often associated with increased stress-related symptoms, substance abuse, violence, and crime (Lenburg et al., 1995). Dramatic changes in technology and specialization in the health care field have made health care costs skyrocket. Therefore not everyone can afford health care services. A higher percentage of minorities lack health insurance than that of the general population (Nies & McEwen, 2022). Higher costs of living and lower wages for minority groups make it difficult to rise out of poverty (Stanhope & Lancaster, 2024).

Poverty

Most families with racially or ethnically diverse backgrounds have a lower socioeconomic status than does the population at large. Black people, Hispanics, and American Indians have much higher rates of poverty than non-Hispanic White people and Asians. The median family income of Asians is slightly higher than that of non-Hispanic White people, and it is consistent with Asians' high levels of education and the higher percentage of families with two wage earners. However, opportunities for education, occupation, income earning, and property ownership that are available to upper- and middle-class Americans often are not available to members of minority groups (Stanhope & Lancaster, 2024).

Poverty rates are important indicators of community well-being and are used by government agencies and organizations to allocate need-based resources. The American Community Survey (ACS) 5-year data allow for the analysis of poverty rates by race and Hispanic origin for many levels of geography. Poverty rates are also presented for selected detailed race and origin groups in the cities and towns with the largest populations of these groups.

The percentage of people in poverty in 2019 was 12.3%. By race the highest national poverty rates were for American Indians and Alaska Natives (23%) and Black people or African Americans (21.22%). Native Hawaiians and other Pacific Islanders had a national poverty rate of 16.5%. For the Asian population poverty rates were 9.6%. For Hispanics national poverty rates were 17.2%. https://www.census.gov/topics/income-poverty/poverty.html.

The poor also suffer more than the population as a whole for nearly every measure of health. In 2023 9.2% of people, or 29.6 million, were not covered by health insurance.

Substantial disparities remain in health insurance coverage for certain populations. In 2023 non-Hispanic White people had the lowest uninsured rate. More than half of the nation's children are part of a minority race or ethnic group. The uninsured rates for Black people and Asians were higher than for non-Hispanic White people, at 11.4% and 7.4%, respectively. Hispanics had the highest uninsured rate at 12.4%. Lack of health care coverage has major implications for health. For more information, see the US Census Bureau's web page on health insurance coverage. https://www.census.gov/content/dam/Census/newsroom/press-kits/2023/iphi/20230912-iphi-slides-health-insurance.pdf

Minority members of society often live in poverty. This social stratification leads to social inequality. For instance, it is widely known that school systems and recreational facilities vary significantly between the inner city and the suburbs (Nies & McEwen, 2022). Residential segregation, substandard housing, unemployment, poor physical and mental health, and poor self-image are part of the cycle of poverty. This inequality is especially disturbing as it relates to health care. The United States has a history of providing the highest quality health care to those with the highest socioeconomic status, and the worst health care to those with the lowest socioeconomic status. Social, economic, and health problems have led to heated debates about the philosophy, scope and costs, and sources of funding for health care and insurance programs. It is important to include all segments of society in these important debates to have a clear understanding of different perspectives.

Social Determinants of Health. Social determinants of health (SDOH) include the conditions in the environments in which people are born, live, learn, work, play, worship, and age that affect a wide range of health, functioning, and quality-of-life outcomes and risks. Conditions (e.g., social, economic, and physical) in these various environments and settings (e.g., school, church, workplace, and neighborhood) have been referred to as "place." In addition to the more material attributes of "place," the patterns of social engagement and sense of security and well-being are affected by where people live. Resources that enhance quality of life can have a significant influence on population health outcomes. Examples of these resources include safe and affordable housing, access to education, public safety, availability of healthy foods, local emergency/health services, and environments free of life-threatening toxins.

SDOHs have a major impact on people's health, well-being, and quality of life. Healthy People 2030 features objectives that highlight the importance of SDOH in improving health and reducing health disparities. https://health.gov/healthypeople/priority-areas

Violence

Changing economic and social conditions have contributed to the rising level of violence in our society. Statistics indicate that homicide is the second-leading cause of death among Americans 15 to 24 years of age (Nies & McEwen, 2022). Businesses, schools, restaurants, playgrounds, and churches have become common settings for random acts of violence. Although the increasing incidence of violence affects all segments of society, women, children, older adults, and culturally vulnerable groups are especially at risk. Unemployment rates among young minority men in the United States are consistently high (Stanhope & Lancaster, 2024).

This group also has the highest rate of violence, with homicide being a major problem for young Black males. The differing rates of violence among races are more likely a result of poverty than of race (Stanhope & Lancaster, 2024).

Intimate partner violence (IPV), formerly known as *domestic violence*, is the single greatest cause of injury to women 15 to 24 years of age. IPV crosses all ethnic, racial, socioeconomic, and educational lines. It includes battering, resulting in physical injury, psychologic abuse, and sexual assault (Nies & McEwen, 2022).

Attitudes Toward Culturally Diverse Groups

The term *cultural diversity* includes a broad spectrum of groups or categories. These include: race, ethnicity, sexual orientation, religion, language, gender, age, disability, and socioeconomic status. Health care workers must not only recognize the differences between different cultures and groups but respect and treat these groups equitably.

Lesbian, gay, bisexual, transgender, and queer (LGBTQ) patients often experience bias and discrimination while accessing care. Policies and programs to implement and monitor LGBTQ-inclusive health education and evaluate practice changes are recommended to improve professionals' knowledge, attitudes, and behavior (Coulter-Thompson, 2023). Inclusive, affirming services are critical for culturally competent, person-centered care and the achievement of the Healthy People 2030 Goal: Improve the health, safety, and well-being of lesbian, gay, bisexual, and transgender people.

Throughout our lives we form implicit associations regarding race, age, ethnicity, appearance, and behaviors. The implicit associations can be either negative or positive and they affect all of our associations with patients we encounter. Types of implicit biases include: affinity bias (a preference for those who look like us), ageism, bias based on outward appearance, gender bias, and name bias (favoring English-sounding names). Explicit biases can include biases against patients who are obese or patients who smoke (Harrison et al., 2019). Nurses must examine their biases and implement strategies to overcome biases and ultimately improve patient outcomes. Strategies include avoiding stereotypes and seeing the patient as a unique human being; seeking understanding of the patient's life rather than making quick judgments or assumptions; increasing opportunities for connection; and partnering with the patient as a co-collaborator in their care (Todt, 2023).

The range of attitudes toward culturally diverse groups can be viewed along a continuum of intensity, as illustrated in Fig. 10.1 is Lenberg et al., 1995, American Academy of Nursing (1995).

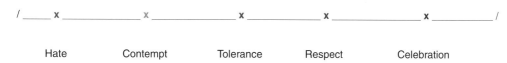

| Hate | Contempt | Tolerance | Respect | Celebration |

Fig. 10.1 A continuum of intensity of the range of attitudes toward culturally diverse groups. (From Lenburg, C.B., et al. [1995]. *Promoting cultural competence in and through nursing education: A critical review and comprehensive plan for action.* American Academy of Nursing.)

The extreme negative manifestation of prejudice is hate in its many violent and nonviolent forms. Contempt is somewhat less intense but is problematic because it is so widespread and undermines many aspects of society. Tolerance reflects a more neutral attitude that accepts differences without attempting to convert them; it is the minimal-level attitude essential in democratic societies. Respect for diversity is manifested in behaviors that integrate differences into positive interactions and relationships. Respect is a demonstration of the inherent worth of the individual regardless of differences. The most positive attitude is portrayed as a celebration (or affirmation) of the positive merits of cultural differences (e.g., the value added to life experiences by multiple perspectives, traditions, rituals, foods, and art forms). The combination of ignorance of other cultures and arrogance about one's own culture fosters disrespect and hate. The deliberate attempt to discover and apply the positive benefits of cultural variation promotes respect and a celebration of the value of diversity, whereas perpetuating prejudice fosters narrow-mindedness and contempt. By integrating these perspectives as part of professional role behavior, educators can help students prepare for culturally competent practice in communities of diversity.

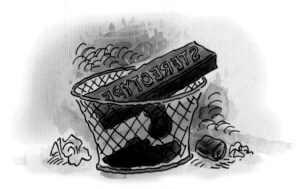

Stereotypes should be trashed.

DIVERSITY IN THE HEALTH CARE WORKFORCE

Need for Diversity in the Health Care Workforce

Members of some cultural groups are demanding culturally relevant health care that incorporates their beliefs and practices (Nies & McEwen, 2022). Consumers are becoming much more aware of what constitutes culturally sensitive and competent care and are less willing to accept incompetent care. There is a lack of diversity and ethnic representation among health care professionals, as well as limited knowledge about values, beliefs, experiences, and health care needs of certain populations, such as immigrants, older adults, and gays and lesbians. Each of these groups has a unique set of responses to health and illness.

Nurses make up the largest segment of the workforce in health care delivery. Therefore they have an opportunity to be proactive in changing health care inequities and access to health care. The changing health care system must reflect the community, and as health care moves into the community it is vital that partnerships be formed between health care providers and the community. For these partnerships to become a reality minority representation in all health professions is essential. Some factors inhibiting minority members from attaining a career in nursing include inadequate academic preparation, especially in the sciences; financial costs; inadequate career counseling; lack of valuing the role of nursing by some cultures; and better recruitment efforts by other disciplines (Minority Nurse, 2020). https://minoritynurse.com/common-barriers-for-nursing-students-how-to-overcome-them/.

Current Status of Diversity in the Health Care Workforce

The multiracial population has changed considerably since 2010. It was measured at 9 million people in 2010 and 33.8 million people in 2020, a 276% increase. https://www.census.gov/library/stories/2021/08/improved-race-ethnicity-measures-reveal-united-states-population-much-more-multiracial.html

The workforce in 2022 was more demographically diverse and representative of the country's population than in any year in which this study was previously conducted. Women continue to account for a large majority of nurses; however, the proportion of men licensed as RNs or LPNs/LVNs in the country has increased steadily since at least 2015. Currently men account for 11% of the RN workforce, an increase from 8% in 2015. Though less pronounced, the same pattern holds true for the proportion of men in the LPN/LVN workforce. RNs are more likely to report identifying as an underrepresented racial minority. Overall the RN workforce is 80% White/Caucasian, a slight decrease from 81% in 2020. In contrast 72% of the US population identifies as White/Caucasian (US Census Bureau, 2020). RNs who reported being of Hispanic or Latino ethnicity comprised 7% of the workforce in 2022, whereas in 2015 they represented 4% of the workforce. It is unclear whether this increase in diversity will continue. After years of decline, the proportion of RNs identifying as White/Caucasian in the youngest age ranges has risen back to the level of the overall population mean (Smiley et al., 2023).

Diversity within the nursing workforce—in terms of race/ethnicity and sex—is desirable because it can improve both access to and quality of care for minorities and medically underserved populations. The nursing workforce does not mirror the US population seeking care, matching for gender, ethnicity, or age. Nursing has historically been dominated by White females, and as (Table 10.1) shows, the nursing workforce is still predominantly White, out of proportion to the general population, with some minorities being more underrepresented than others. With projections pointing to minority populations becoming the majority by 2043, professional nurses must demonstrate a sensitivity to and understanding of a variety of cultures to provide high-quality care across settings. According to a 2022 survey conducted by the National Council of State Boards of Nursing (NCSBN) and the Forum of Nursing Workforce Centers, nurses from minority backgrounds represent 20% of the registered nurse (RN) workforce. In terms of racial/

TABLE 10.1 Race of Registered Nurses (RNs), 2017–2022

Race	2017		2020		2022	
	n	%	n	%	n	%
RN Survey Respondents	N = 47,966.3		N = 41,702.0		N = 272,713.6	
American Indian or Alaska Native	176.0	0.4	194.1	0.5	1209.8	0.4
Asian	3,605.6	7.5	2996.3	7.2	20,036.9	7.4
Black/African American	2,995.9	6.2	2800.7	6.7	17,273.7	6.3
Native Hawaiian or Other Pacific Islander	226.3	0.5	175.9	0.4	1136.9	0.4
Middle Eastern/North African	-	-	89.4	0.2	-	-
White/Caucasian		80.8	33,595.1	80.6	218,133.9	80.0
Other		2.9	967.7	2.3	8,133.1	3.0
More than one race category selected	828.5	1.7	882.8	2.1	6,789.3	2.5
US RN Population						
American Indian or Alaska Native	14,276	0.4	19,391	0.5	19,303	0.4
Asian	292,497	7.5	299,340	7.2	319,695	7.4
Black/African American	243,032	6.2	279,799	6.7	275,607	6.3
Native Hawaiian or Other Pacific Islander	18,362	0.5	17,573	0.4	18,139	0.4
Middle Eastern/North African	-	-	8,931	0.2	-	-
White/Caucasian	3,144,812	80.8	3,356,257	80.6	3,480,388	80.0
Other	110,960	2.9	96,676	2.3	129,766	3.0
More than one race category selected	67,214	1.7	88,195	2.1	108,325	2.5

Note. Respondents were asked to select all that apply. The responses were subsequently recoded to ensure that the race categories were mutually exclusive. Respondents selecting multiple race categories were reclassified into the "more than one race category selected" category.
Race of Registered Nurses (RNs), 2017–2022 from the NCSBN The 2022 National Nursing Workforce Survey https://www.journalofnursingregulation.com/action/showFullTableHTML?isHtml=true&tableId=t0050&pii=S2155-8256%2823%2900047-9

ethnic backgrounds the RN population is 80% White/Caucasian; 6.3% Black/African American; 7.4% Asian; 6.9% Hispanic; .4% American Indian/Alaska Native; .4% Native Hawaiian/Pacific Islander; and 3% other (NCSBN, 2022).

A 2023 Nursing Research Salary Report concludes that the average salary for nurses across the country is $82,750. https://www.rncareers.org/salary/registered-nurses/

Women in nursing receive lower pay than men. Men report making an average annual salary of $7300 more than women. https://www.rncareers.org/salary/registered-nurses/

According to the report by the American Association of Colleges of Nursing (AACN) on Enrollment and Graduations in Baccalaureate and Graduate Programs in Nursing (2022–2023), nursing students from minority backgrounds represented 38.6% of students in entry-level baccalaureate programs, 36.7% of master's students, 33.3% of students in research-focused doctoral programs, and 38.1% in practice-focused doctoral programs (Fang, et al. 2023a). In terms of gender breakdown men made up 13% of students in baccalaureate programs, 11.7% of master's students, 11.4% of research-focused doctoral students, and 14.8% of practice-focused doctoral students. Although nursing schools have made strides in recruiting and graduating nurses who reflect the patient population, more must be done before equal representation is realized. The need to attract diverse nursing students is paralleled by the need to recruit more faculty from minority populations. Few nurses from racial/ethnic minority groups with advanced nursing degrees pursue faculty careers. According to 2023 data from AACN's annual survey, only 20.6% of full-time nursing school faculty come from minority backgrounds and only 7.8% are male (Fang, et al. 2023b).

Recruitment and Retention of Minorities in Nursing

It is clear that we have been slow in preparing nurses to be reflective of our population, just as we have been unaware of the need for culturally sensitive patient care and sometimes less than welcoming to students different from the preponderant population. Recruitment and retention of students from minority populations must not be separated. In other words, recruitment programs must have retention as their primary focus because there is no point in recruiting minorities into nursing programs and then not helping them succeed.

Before World War II the only known effort to recruit minority students into nursing on a national scale was made by the National Association of Colored Graduate Nurses (NACGN), which had had recruitment of Black people into nursing as one of its objectives since its inception in 1908. During World War II the federal government set into motion a mechanism to produce additional nursing personnel by financing basic nursing education. This was done through the Cadet Nurse Corps. The corps had a number of recruiters, two of whom were Black. These two nurses confined their recruiting to 82 Black/African American colleges and universities. By the end of the war 21 Black/African American nursing schools had participated in the corps, and more than 2000 Black nurses had acquired their basic nursing education through this mechanism.

After the war national recruitment efforts for Black nurses reverted to the NACGN, an organization that voted itself out of existence in 1949 and was dissolved in 1951. However, individual Black/African American schools in the North and South continued to recruit. In the South law segregated the nursing schools, and in the North custom did so. In 1954 the unanimous Supreme Court decision *Brown v. Board of Education* asserted that "separate educational facilities were inherently unequal," making racial segregation in public schools unconstitutional. This decision was interpreted to mean that all kinds of educational discrimination would be considered, including nursing.

It was around the time of the Brown decision that schools of nursing were being accredited by national standards, and many schools, both Black/African American and White, just did not measure up to the standards. As a result many schools closed. With integration permitting Black students to be admitted to formerly all-White schools, quality Black/African American schools had difficulty attracting enough students and many of the schools closed. However, the White schools that began admitting Black students did not admit the number that would have been admitted by the Black/African American schools. For example, many White schools admitted only one or two Black students per class.

In the late 1960s many efforts were made to help the economically disadvantaged in the United States. Although not all people of minority groups are economically disadvantaged, the vast majority of disadvantaged people are members of ethnic minority groups. Nursing, too, became concerned about the disadvantaged and began concerted efforts to recruit more members of minority groups into nursing schools. The Sealantic Fund, one of the Rockefeller Brothers' funds, was one of the first foundations that helped minorities enter nursing school. Sealantic funded projects in 10 universities in different parts of the country to recruit students from minority groups and help them achieve success. The best example of an ongoing project, funded by the division of nursing since 1971, is the National Student Nurses Association's Breakthrough to Nursing, intended to accelerate the recruitment of minorities, including men.

In 1997 the American Nurses Foundation published a report of a project it had funded titled *Strategies for Recruitment, Retention and Graduation of Minority Nurses in Colleges of Nursing*. Through survey and interview analysis Hattie Bessent and a cadre of knowledgeable leaders investigated the most-effective approach to increasing the nursing profession's representation of minority nurses (Bessent, 1997). Members of Chi Eta Phi, a national Black/African American nursing society with chapters throughout the country, serve as mentors to minority nursing students. As mentors sorority members provide intellectual and inspirational stimulation along with counseling.

In 1997 the AACN published its first position statement affirming that diversity and inclusion had emerged as central issues for organizations and institutions. The AACN encouraged leadership in nursing to respond to these issues by finding ways to accelerate the inclusion of groups, cultures, and ideas that traditionally had been underrepresented in higher education.

In March 2017 the AACN endorsed a position statement entitled *Diversity, Inclusion, & Equity in Academic Nursing*, updated in 2021 with new title Diversity, Equity, and Inclusion in Academic Nursing, AACN associated with these values. They reflect the need to: (1) *improve the quality of education* by enhancing the capacity of academic nursing to maximize learning opportunities and experiences for students and faculty alike, which depend in significant ways on learning from individuals with diverse life experiences, perspectives, and backgrounds; (2) *address pervasive inequities in health care* by ensuring the preparation of nurses and other health care professionals able to meet the needs of all individuals in an increasingly diverse American society; and (3) *enhance the civic readiness and engagement potential of nursing students* who will be in positions of leadership in health care, as well as in society, more broadly.

As used in AACN's (2023) position statement diversity references a broad range of individual, population, and social characteristics, including but not limited to age; sex; race; ethnicity; sexual orientation; gender identity; family structures; geographic locations; national origin; immigrants and refugees; language; physical, functional, and learning abilities; religious beliefs; and socioeconomic status. Inclusion represents environmental and organizational cultures in which faculty, students, staff, and administrators with diverse characteristics thrive. Inclusive environments require intentionality and embrace differences, not merely tolerate them. Everyone works to ensure the perspectives and experiences of others are invited, welcomed, acknowledged, and respected in inclusive environments. More broadly, equity is interrelated with diversity and inclusion. Equity is the ability to recognize the differences in the resources or knowledge needed to allow individuals to fully participate in society, including access to higher education, with the goal of overcoming obstacles to ensure fairness (Kranich, 2001). To have equitable systems all people should be treated fairly, unhampered by artificial barriers, stereotypes, or prejudices (Cooper, 2016). https://www.aacnnursing.org/Diversity-Inclusion/Publications-on-Diversity/Position-Statement

As the demographics of the population rapidly change in the 21st century there have been numerous strategies to recruit and retain minority nursing faculty, students, and practicing nurses in the profession to better reflect the population demographics. Just as contributions of diverse cultural groups are increasingly valued, the profession has begun to value the need for diversity in their students and faculty and to view this diversity as strength.

Strategies for Recruitment and Retention of Minorities in the Nursing Workforce

All national nursing organizations, the federal Division of Nursing, hospital associations, nursing philanthropies, and other stakeholders within the health care community agree that recruitment of underrepresented groups into nursing is a priority for the nursing profession in the United States. Nursing's leaders recognize a strong connection between a culturally diverse nursing workforce and the ability to provide quality, culturally competent patient care. Though nursing has made great strides in recruiting and graduating nurses that mirror the patient population, more must be done before adequate representation becomes a reality. The need to attract students from underrepresented groups in nursing—specifically men and individuals from African American, Hispanic, Asian, American Indian, and Alaskan native backgrounds—is a high priority for the nursing profession. For more information, visit AACN's web page on resources in enhancing workforce diversity (https://www.aacnnursing.org/news-data/fact-sheets/enhancing-diversity-in-the-nursing-workforce http://www.aacnnursing.org/News-Information/Fact-Sheets/Enhancing-Diversity).

Nursing shortage reports, including those produced by the American Hospital Association, the Robert Wood Johnson Foundation (RWJF), The Joint Commission, and the Association of Academic Health Centers, point to minority student recruitment as a necessary step to addressing the nursing shortage. For more information on these reports visit https://www.aacnnursing.org/news-data/fact-sheets/enhancing-.

Nursing Workforce. A lack of minority nurse educators may send a signal to potential students that nursing does not value diversity or offer career ladder opportunities to advance through the profession. Students looking for academic role models to encourage and enrich their learning may be frustrated in their attempts to find mentors and a community of support. Academic leaders are addressing this need by working to identify minority faculty recruitment strategies, encouraging minority leadership development, and advocating for programs that remove barriers to faculty careers.

There also is a need to increase the number of nurse educators and researchers from diverse, marginalized, and vulnerable populations. Raising consciousness involves increasing the level of awareness of nurses and other health care professionals about the issues surrounding diversity. This can be accomplished by encouraging participation in forums related to different aspects of various cultural phenomena, such as environmental control, communication, and health beliefs. Such forums might be offered by state and local professional nurses' organizations and health care facilities.

Another successful strategy for recruiting and retaining minorities in education and clinical practice is matched mentoring, which involves matching same-culture mentors in either the same institution or different institutions. A different mentoring strategy involves teaching and modeling by nurses who have been trained in cross-cultural care. Cross-cultural nursing consultants in the care of specific groups are available to agencies, professional groups, licensing bodies, and individual nurses. (Organizations should contact the Transcultural Nursing Society at http://www.tcns.org to obtain the names of consultants in the field of transcultural nursing.)

Audiovisual media should be used to teach the importance of human health conditions cross-culturally. Video conferencing can provide international links for students and faculty who cannot travel. Students from various cultures can share their clinical experiences. One of the greatest benefits is the discovery that thinking, values, and decision-making differ in various cultures. Collaborative arrangements should be encouraged between colleges and universities so that exchange programs can be offered to students. Such exchanges can give students firsthand in-depth experience with cultures that are different from their own. Interactive media can be used to gain a clearer perspective than can be obtained through the print medium on particular cultures.

Strategies such as mentoring by the same-culture professional are effective in recruiting and retaining minorities in nursing. In addition, the value of workshops, continuing education programs, and use of consultants to promote culturally competent care should not be overlooked.

CULTURAL COMPETENCE IN NURSING

Health professionals, educators, and health care systems must all respond to the consequences of increasing cultural diversity for the future well-being of all populations. The worldwide shortage of nurses and the global immigration of both nurses and populations have heightened the need to educate nurses to deliver culturally competent care for increasingly diverse populations, regardless of geographic location.

Cultural Competence in Nursing Practice

Cultural competency is a vital skill for delivering quality nursing care across culturally diverse groups The importance of cultural competence in nursing focuses on health equity through patient-centered care, which requires seeing each patient as a unique person Nurses must be able to understand and appreciate different cultural backgrounds to provide culturally competent person-centered care. Nurses must demonstrate willingness to understand and interact with people of different cultures, races, ethnicities, genders, and sexuality.

This approach allows nurses to successfully treat patients even when patients' beliefs, practices, and values directly conflict with their own or with conventional medical and nursing guidelines. Nurses can develop the ability to tailor and explain treatment plans according to patients' needs, which may be influenced by cultural practices that don't fall within the parameters of conventional medicine (Deering, 2023).

Culturally competent care as shows consists of four components: awareness of one's cultural worldview, attitudes toward cultural differences, knowledge of different cultural practices and worldviews, and cross-cultural skills. Together these components contribute to a high degree of cultural competency, and nurses can integrate them into the care of their patients.

Lenburg and colleagues (1995) suggest that it is essential that nurses take responsibility to:

- Be sensitive to and show respect for the differences in beliefs and values of others.
- Take responsibility to inquire, learn about, and integrate beliefs and values of others in professional encounters.
- Take responsibility to try to change negative and prejudicial behaviors in themselves and others.

In light of societal changes responsible persons at all levels in education and health care delivery systems acknowledge the need to reassess the influence of culture on achieving expected health outcomes. There is a significant need for nurse educators, administrators, students, and others to promote sensitivity to, acceptance of, and respect for the rights of all individuals within the context of their cultural orientation and society as a whole. Nurses must be culturally competent because:

- The nurse's culture often is different from the client's culture.
- Care that is not culturally competent may be costlier.
- Care that is not culturally competent may be ineffective.
- Specific objectives for persons in different cultures need to be met as outlined in the federal government's *Healthy People 2030* initiative.
- Racial and minority groups experience profound disparities in health and health care.
- Nursing is committed to social justice, diversity, and inclusion, providing safe quality care to all.
- Nurses are expected to respond to global infectious disease epidemics.

Achieving cultural competence should be our goal, although it may take most of us a lifetime to attain. However, we can all aspire to achieve cultural humility, which incorporates a lifelong commitment to self-evaluation and self-critique, to redressing the power imbalances in the patient–clinician dynamic, and to developing mutually beneficial and advocacy partnerships with communities on behalf of individuals and defined populations (Tervalon & Murray-Garcia, 1998). If we acquire cultural humility, we should also demonstrate cultural sensitivity, which shows appreciation of the diversity of others. Health care providers who have cultural humility and sensitivity will provide culturally congruent care.

Cultural Competence in Nursing Education

Since the 1960s there has been a united effort to include concepts sensitive to cultural diversity in nursing education. The National League for Nursing (NLN) and the AACN have made this effort mandatory for accreditation of nursing programs. In 2008 the AACN developed five end-of-program competencies for graduates of baccalaureate nursing programs, as well as a faculty toolkit for integrating these competencies into undergraduate education (AACN, 2008a). *The Essentials of Baccalaureate Education for Professional Nursing Practice* (2008) mandates the inclusion of culturally diverse nursing care concepts in the curriculum with attention to cultural, spiritual, ethnic, gender, and sexual orientation diversity. The AACN (2008b) developed the following five competencies to serve as a framework for integrating cultural content into existing curricula:

1. Apply knowledge of social and cultural factors that affect nursing and health care across multiple contexts.

2. Use relevant data sources and best evidence in providing culturally competent care.
3. Promote achievement of safe and quality outcomes of care for diverse populations.
4. Advocate for social justice, including commitment to the health of vulnerable populations and the elimination of health disparities.
5. Participate in continuous cultural competence development.

The AACN endorsed the New Essentials in 2021 to guide professional nursing education. This document does not list culture as a domain, but uses the terminology *person-centered care*. Foundational to person-centered care is respect for diversity, differences, preferences, values, needs, and determinants of care unique to the individual.

The Essentials: Core Competencies for Professional Nursing Education (AACN, 2021) Domain 2, Person-Centered Care, focuses on the individual within multiple complicated contexts, including family and/or important others. Person-centered care is holistic, individualized, just, respectful, compassionate, coordinated, evidence-based, and developmentally appropriate. Person-centered care builds on a scientific body of knowledge that guides nursing practice regardless of specialty or functional area.

Contextual Statement: Person-centered care is the core purpose of nursing as a discipline.

This purpose intertwines with any functional area of nursing practice, from the point of care where the hands of those that give and receive care meet, to the point of systems-level nursing leadership. Foundational to person-centered care is respect for diversity, differences, preferences, values, needs, resources, and the determinants of health unique to the individual.

The person is a full partner and the source of control in team-based care. Person-centered care requires the intentional presence of the nurse seeking to know the totality of the individual's lived experiences and connections to others (family, important others, community).

As a scientific and practice discipline, nurses employ a relational lens that fosters mutuality, active participation, and individual empowerment. This focus is foundational to educational preparation from entry to advanced levels irrespective of practice areas.

With an emphasis on diversity, equity, and inclusion, person-centered care is based on best evidence and clinical judgment in the planning and delivery of care

across time, spheres of care, and developmental levels. Contributing to or making diagnoses is one essential aspect of nursing practice and critical to an informed plan of care and improving outcomes of care (Olson et al., 2019). Diagnoses at the system-level are equally as relevant, affecting operations that impact care for individuals. Person-centered care results in shared meaning with the healthcare team, recipient of care, and the healthcare system, thus creating humanization of wellness and healing from birth to death. —Direct quote from *The Essentials: Core Competencies for Professional Nursing Education* (AACN, 2021).

Also, in collaboration with leading foundations and stakeholders, the AACN took the following steps to enhance diversity in nursing education:

New Careers in Nursing (NCIN) was a national scholarship program of the Robert Wood Johnson Foundation (RWJF) and the American Association of Colleges of Nursing (AACN). Founded in 2008 to help alleviate the nursing shortage and increase the diversity of nursing professionals, NCIN awarded its final grants in 2015 to schools with accelerated baccalaureate and master's degree nursing programs. In total grants have provided scholarships to 3517 students at 130 unique schools of nursing (http://www.newcareersinnursing.org/).

The Future of Nursing Scholars program, another effort supported by RWJF, created "a diverse cadre of PhD prepared nurses who are committed to a long-term leadership career; advancing science and discovery through research; strengthening nursing education; and furthering transformational change in nursing and health care" (Future of Nursing Scholars, 2018). In December 2017 the RWJF "announced the 31 schools of nursing selected to receive grants to support up to 58 nurses as they pursue their PhDs. These 31 schools comprise the fifth and final cohort of grantees of the *Future of Nursing Scholars* program" (Future of Nursing Scholars, 2018).

In 2013 AACN and the RWJF initiated the Doctoral Advancement in Nursing (DAN) Project to enhance the number of minority nurses completing PhD and Doctor of Nursing Practice (DNP) degrees. DAN's expert committee has developed a white paper featuring student recruitment and retention strategies that can be used by schools of nursing; comprehensive approaches to leadership and scholarship development for students; suggestions for model doctoral curriculum; and more. For more information, see DAN's web page (http://www.newcareersinnursing.org/doctoral-advancement-nursing.html).

In April 2008 the RWJF joined with the AACN to launch funding for Nursing Workforce Development Programs, including funding for Nursing Workforce Diversity Grants. This program provides funding for projects to increase nursing education opportunities for individuals from disadvantaged backgrounds, including racial and ethnic minorities underrepresented among RNs.

CULTURAL BELIEF SYSTEMS

A value is a standard that people use to assess themselves and others. It is a belief about what is worthwhile or important for well-being. There is a tendency for people to be "culture bound" (i.e., to assume that their own values are superior to, more sensible than, or more correct than that of others). Cross-cultural health promotion requires the nurse to work with clients without making judgments as to the superiority of one set of values over another.

Each culture has a value system that dictates behavior directly or indirectly by setting norms and teaching that those norms are right. Health beliefs and practices tend to reflect a culture's value system. Nurses must understand each patient's value system to foster health promotion.

CULTURAL PHENOMENA

Giger & Haddad (2021) have identified six cultural phenomena that vary among cultural groups and affect health care. These phenomena are environmental control, biological variations, social organization, communication, space, and time orientation.

Environmental Control

Environmental control is the ability of members of a particular culture to control nature or other environmental factors. Some groups perceive humans as having mastery over nature; others perceive humans to be dominated by nature; and still other groups see humans as having a harmonious relationship with nature (Giger & Haddad, 2021).

People who perceive that they have mastery over nature believe that they can overcome the natural forces of nature. Such individuals would expect positive results from medications, surgery, and other treatment modalities. Persons who believe that they are subject to the forces of nature or that they have little control over what happens to them may not be compliant with treatments because they believe that whatever happens to them is part of their destiny. Included in this concept are the traditional health and illness beliefs, the practice of folk medicine, and the use of traditional and nontraditional healers. Environmental control plays an important role in the way clients respond to health-related experiences and use health resources (Giger & Haddad, 2021).

Biological Variations

Biologic variations, such as body build and structure, genetic variations, skin characteristics, susceptibility to disease, and nutritional variations, exist among different cultures. For example, babies who are born in Western culture weigh more than non-Western babies. Other common variations include skin color, eye shape, hair texture, adipose tissue deposits, shape of earlobes, and body configuration (Giger & Haddad, 2021).

Social Organization

Social organization refers to the family unit (nuclear, single-parent, or extended family) and the religious or ethnic groups with which families identify. *Family* is defined differently among cultures. Families depend on the extended family for emotional and financial support in times of crisis.

Communication

Communication differences include language differences, verbal and nonverbal behaviors, and silence. Language can be the greatest obstacle to providing multicultural care. If the client does not speak the same language as the nurse a skilled interpreter is mandatory (Giger & Haddad, 2021).

Comfort with direct eye contact during communication is an area that varies among cultures. Although some cultures value direct eye contact as a sign of attention, other cultures may view direct eye contact as rude behavior.

Health professionals should not assume that a first-name basis is appropriate for client relationships. With any client terms of endearment such as "honey" and "dear" are unacceptable and can be interpreted as disrespectful, derogatory, or condescending. The best solution to the challenge of different communication styles and preferences is always to ask the client how they prefer to be addressed.

If the nurse and the client do not speak the same language an interpreter should be consulted. An interpreter can help the nurse establish rapport with the client and explain concepts to the patient that are foreign to the patient. When interpreters are needed they should be selected carefully. Friends are possible choices, as are bilingual staff and community volunteers. Nurses should be aware that some ethnic groups consider it a breach of confidentiality to have a stranger interpret, whereas certain individuals may not want other family members or friends to know the specifics of their medical condition.

The nurse also should be careful to consider the different dialects spoken in the same country and the culture's view of women and children. Children should not be used as interpreters because of the subject matter and because of certain cultural views of authority. Many cultures view adults as having more authority than children. In many cultures women would not be acceptable interpreters because of the cultural view of women.

Nurses should be aware of the possibilities for interpreter services. A language line can be accessed 24 hours a day, 7 days a week by calling 1-800-528-5888 and asking for the language wanted. A live translator comes on the line to serve in any of 77 languages. The nurse can conference call, use two phones on the same line, or simply pass the phone back and forth to the person with whom they wish to converse. For more information visit http://www.languageline.com.

Health care facilities may get a reasonable subscription rate that is less costly than the individual rate for these services.

Space

Space refers to people's attitudes and comfort level regarding the personal space around them. There are vast cultural differences in the comfort level associated with the distance between persons. Most nurses tend to feel comfortable with an intimate zone of 0 to 18 inches. This usually is the distance between the nurse and the patient when the nurse performs certain parts of a physical assessment, such as an eye or ear examination. Entering this zone could be uncomfortable for clients and nurses who have not had time to establish a trusting relationship. This discomfort would be greater for persons whose culture is not comfortable at all with such a limited space (Giger & Haddad, 2021).

Time

Time orientation is the view of time in the present, past, or future. Present-oriented persons enjoy what they are experiencing at the moment and move on to the next event or activity only "when the time is right." Punctuality and "watching the clock" are definitely part of Western culture, but many cultural groups do not view time in the same way. This difference in time orientation can have implications for the present-oriented professional in the work setting, who may always be late for work without thinking it is an important issue. In addition, there are implications for health teaching. For example, when teaching medication schedules to a patient it would be important to consider how that individual views time.

Clients who view the past as more important than the present or the future may focus on memories of the past. For instance, some ethnic groups may take actions that they believe are consistent with the views of their ancestors and look to them for guidance (Giger & Haddad, 2021).

In some cultures, time is viewed as being more flexible than in Western culture, and being on time for appointments is not a priority (Giger & Haddad, 2021).

People who are future-oriented are concerned with long-range goals and health care measures that can be taken in the present to prevent illness in the future. These persons plan ahead in scheduling appointments and organizing activities. They may be seen as having "distant" or "cold" personalities because they are not always engaged in communication at the moment, commonly because they may be thinking about their plans for the future. Persons who are oriented more to the present may be late for appointments because they are less concerned with planning ahead.

PRACTICE ISSUES RELATED TO CULTURAL COMPETENCE

Health Information and Education

According to the Task Force on Black and Minority Health of the US Department of Health and Human Services (DHHS), some minority populations are less knowledgeable about specific health problems than are White people. Successful programs to increase public awareness about health problems are being offered to minority groups but efforts must be continued to reach more of the population. Families, churches, employers, and community organizations need to be involved in facilitating behavior changes that will result in healthier lifestyles. Education programs have the greatest effect on diseases that are affected by lifestyle, such as hypertension, obesity, and diabetes. For example, if patients with diabetes could improve their self-management skills, complications could be prevented, saving human suffering and health care dollars (Nies & McEwen, 2022).

Education and Certification

Increasingly more universities and colleges offer graduate programs in transcultural, cross-cultural, and international nursing. Many nurses have not been exposed to transcultural nursing in their basic education program. Therefore the availability of graduate study in this area often is an unrecognized possibility.

Transcultural nursing is the study of differences and similarities of various cultural health values and beliefs among different ethnic and minority groups. The Transcultural Nursing Society has been certifying nurses in transcultural nursing since 1988. Certification as a transcultural nurse is based on oral and written examinations and evaluation of the nurse's educational and experiential background. Certification has increased recognition of transcultural nursing as a legitimate nursing specialty. Transcultural nurses are interested in finding universal care for clients that will improve, maintain, and restore health and improve client satisfaction.

International Marketplace

Nurses trained in the United States work, teach, and consult in hundreds of foreign countries on every continent. They often are recognized as international pacesetters and are viewed as "commodities for import" by both the more developed countries and the less developed third- or fourth-world nations. Nurses can make a difference in the health outcomes of people all over the world. Technology has enhanced global communication and facilitated travel. As nurses help solve emerging health problems in countries throughout the world, they are the most valuable assets of the health care system. They will be called on to design, implement, and evaluate international projects, educational endeavors, and research with an intercultural focus. Therefore it is important that nurses understand the intercultural issues related to our global society (Nies & McEwen, 2022).

Nursing Literature

The number of journal articles about culturally diverse clients, transcultural nursing research, international nursing, and the inclusion of transcultural concepts in nursing curricula has increased considerably since the 1950s. The *Journal of Transcultural Nursing* is a refereed journal that was first published in 1989. This journal was created to advance transcultural nursing knowledge and practices. It focuses on theory, research, and practice dimensions of transcultural nursing and provides a forum for researchers. Other journals that address cultural issues include the *Western Journal of Medicine: Cross Cultural Issues*, the *Journal of Cultural Diversity*, the *Journal of Multicultural Nursing*, the *International Journal of Nursing Studies*, the *International Nursing Review*, and the *Journal of Holistic Nursing*. Nurse writers also need to be encouraged to publish articles related to clients' cultural views and health care needs in nursing specialty and practice journals that are more widely read by nurses who actually are providing care on a daily basis to clients from diverse cultures.

Although research articles on transcultural issues are becoming a common feature in health care journals, there is a need for additional research that examines individual behavioral responses to normal life processes, such as pregnancy, birth, death, and human growth and development. There also is a need for well-designed studies that explore the biologic, psychologic, sociologic, and spiritual differences within, between, and among cultural groups. Dr. Madeline Leininger created the theory of culture care diversity and universality to guide transcultural research. Even though numerous research studies have been conducted on cultural diversity issues, a significant time gap often exists between the identification of findings and the publication of results. The limited dissemination of research findings inhibits widespread acceptance of new interventions that could improve health care practices of culturally diverse populations. Computer information technology and online networks help narrow this gap and distribute research findings in a timely manner.

Responsibility of Health Care Facilities for Cultural Care

Nursing policies should reflect openness to including extended family members and folk healers in the nursing care plan, provided that their presence is not harmful to the client's well-being. Most hospital chaplaincy programs have access to religious representatives available for patients of various religions.

Clients may need to consult with their support persons and folk healers before making medical decisions. Nurses must respect the client's right to privacy and allow time for the client to interact with their spiritual or cultural healers. Nurses must respect unconventional beliefs and health practices, and they must work with clients to develop a plan of care that builds on the client's beliefs and incorporates nontraditional health practices that are not harmful. These nontraditional healers should be received with respect and provided privacy to enable the healers to interact with their patients (Nies & McEwen, 2022).

Health care facilities should provide resources for nurses and other health care professionals to assist with the culture-specific needs of clients. Health care facilities should have a list of interpreters fluent in the major languages spoken by persons typically using the organization. Translators who have knowledge of health-related terminology are more effective than those who do not. Gender, birth origin, and socioeconomic class need to be considered in the selection of a translator. Gender is an important consideration because many cultures prohibit discussion of intimate matters between women and men. Birth origin of the client and translator should be determined because often many dialects are spoken within the same country, depending on the particular region (Stanhope & Lancaster, 2024). Differences in socioeconomic class between client and interpreter can lead to problems of interpretation.

Clinical nurse specialists (CNSs) in transcultural nursing should be added to the staff of institutions serving large numbers of culturally diverse individuals. The transcultural CNS could be a role model to the staff in delivery of culturally sensitive and competent care, provide in-service education to staff related to cultural differences, and conduct research related to cultural and social issues. In addition, consultants should be used to deal with specific cultural issues.

Continuing education programs for nurses should be offered by health care institutions. Programs should focus on promoting awareness of the nurses' own culturally based values, beliefs, and attitudes; cultural assessment; biologic variations of cultural groups; cross-cultural communication; and culture-specific beliefs and practices related to childbearing and childrearing, death and dying, issues of mental health, and cultural aspects of aging.

Recommended Standards for Culturally and Linguistically Appropriate Services (CLAS)

Culture and language have a considerable effect on how patients access and respond to health care services. To ensure equal access to quality health care by diverse populations, the Office of Minority Health in the DHHS developed guidelines for health care organizations. In its report *Assuring Cultural Competence in Health Care: Recommendations for National Standards and an Outcomes Focused Research Agenda*, the following standards are recommended (Fortier et al., 1999):

- Promote and support the attitudes, behaviors, knowledge, and skills necessary for staff to work respectfully and effectively with patients and each other in a culturally diverse work environment.
- Have a comprehensive management strategy to address culturally and linguistically appropriate services, including strategic goals, plans, policies, procedures, and designated staff responsible for implementation.
- Utilize formal mechanisms for community and consumer involvement in the design and execution of service delivery, including planning, policymaking, operations, evaluation, training, and, as appropriate, treatment planning.
- Develop and implement a strategy to recruit, retain, and promote qualified, diverse, and culturally competent administrative, clinical, and support staff members that are trained and qualified to address the needs of the racial and ethnic communities being served.
- Require and arrange for ongoing education and training for administrative, clinical, and support staff in culturally and linguistically competent service delivery.
- Provide all clients with limited English proficiency (LEP) access to bilingual staff or interpretation services.
- Provide oral and written notices, including translated signage at key points of contact, to clients in their primary language informing them of their right to receive interpreter services free of charge.
- Translate and make available signage and commonly used written patient educational material and other materials for members of the dominant language groups in service areas.

- Ensure that interpreters and bilingual staff can demonstrate bilingual proficiency and receive training that includes the skills and ethics of interpreting as well as knowledge in both languages of the terms and concepts relevant to clinical or nonclinical encounters. Family or friends are not considered adequate substitutes because they usually lack these abilities.
- Ensure that the clients' primary spoken language and self-identified race or ethnicity are included in the health care organization's management information system, as well as any patient records used by provider staff.
- Utilize a variety of methods to collect and use accurate demographic, cultural, epidemiologic, and clinical outcome data for racial and ethnic groups in the service area. Become informed about the ethnic and cultural needs, resources, and assets of the surrounding community.
- Undertake ongoing organizational self-assessments of cultural and linguistic competence; integrate measures of access, satisfaction, quality, and outcomes for CLAS into other organizational internal audits and performance-improvement programs.
- Develop structures and procedures to address cross-cultural ethical and legal conflicts in health care delivery and complaints or grievances by patients and staff about unfair, culturally insensitive, or discriminatory treatment; difficulty in accessing services; or denial of services.
- Prepare an annual progress report documenting the organizations' progress with implementing CLAS standards, including information on programs, staffing, and resources.

CULTURAL ASSESSMENT

Cultural Self-Assessment

The first step to becoming a culturally sensitive and competent health care provider is to conduct a cultural self-assessment. The nurse should engage in a cultural self-assessment to identify individual culturally based attitudes about clients who are from a different culture. Cultural self-assessment requires self-honesty and sincerity, as well as reflection on attitudes of parents, grandparents, and close friends toward different cultures. Through identification of health-related attitudes, values, beliefs, and practices, the nurse can better

understand the cultural aspects of health care from the client's perspective. Everyone has ethnocentric tendencies that must be brought to a level of consciousness so that efforts can be made to temper the feeling that one's own culture is best.

Cultural Client Assessment

After the nurse performs a cultural self-assessment they should obtain a cultural assessment of the client. Nursing assessments in institutional and community settings should include the gathering of data pertinent to cultural beliefs and practices. Cultural assessments lead to culturally relevant nursing diagnoses and give direction to effective nursing intervention. Basic cultural data include ethnic affiliation, religious preference, family patterns, food patterns, and ethnic health care practices. Cultural assessments should be used as an adjunct to other patient assessments. These data will give the nurse sufficient information to determine whether a more in-depth assessment of cultural factors is needed. A major reason that cultural assessments are performed is to identify patterns that may assist or interfere with a nursing intervention or treatment regimen (Giger & Haddad, 2021). The nurse needs to find out whether the client's beliefs, customs, values, and self-care practices are adaptive (beneficial), neutral, or maladaptive (harmful) in relation to nursing interventions. For example, if a client who is diagnosed with hypertension insists on taking garlic instead of an antihypertensive, this practice could be harmful. If the client agrees to take the garlic in addition to the antihypertensive, this practice would be neutral. An adaptive or beneficial practice would include daily exercise in addition to the garlic and antihypertensive.

In some cultures dermal methods are perceived as ways to relieve headaches, muscle pains, sinusitis, colds, sore throats, diarrhea, or fever. Cupping involves placing a heated cup on the skin; as it cools it contracts, drawing what is believed to be toxicity into the cup. A circular ecchymosis is left on the skin. Pinching may be done at the base of the nose or between the eyes. Bruises or welts are left at the site of treatment. Rubbing or "coining" involves rubbing lubricated skin with a spoon or a coin to bring toxic "wind" to the body surface. A similar practice is burning, which involves touching a burning cigarette or piece of cotton to the skin, usually the abdomen, to compensate for "heat" lost through diarrhea (Nies & McEwen, 2011). These practices nurture the client's sense of well-being and security in being able to do something to correct disturbing symptoms. In most cases the practice would be considered adaptive (beneficial) or neutral. However, if the client had a clotting disorder the practices would pose a threat to physical integrity and therefore would be considered maladaptive (harmful) (Nies & McEwen, 2011).

Cultural Client Nutrition Assessment

A cultural nutrition assessment should be obtained for clients who are minorities. It is necessary to assess the client's cultural definition of food. For example, certain cultures do not consider greens to be food. Therefore when asked to keep a food diary individuals would not list greens, which are an important source of vitamins and iron. Frequency and number of meals, amount and types of food eaten, and regularity of food consumption are other important factors to consider.

In cultures in which obesity is a problem it is helpful for the nurse to have an idea of food preferences to help the client select low-calorie, low-fat foods. Asians tend to prefer spicy foods, which may lead to their high incidence of stomach cancer, ulcers, and gastrointestinal bleeding (Giger & Haddad, 2021).

Nurses should avoid cultural stereotyping as it relates to food because not all Italians necessarily like spaghetti, nor do all Chinese like rice. However, knowing the clients' food preferences makes it possible to develop therapeutic interventions that do not conflict with their cultural food practices (Stanhope & Lancaster, 2024).

Cultural Beliefs about Sickness and Cures

It also is important for the nurse to consider the nontraditional beliefs of sickness and cure of various cultures. For example, there are diseases that are not classified as Western culture diseases. For different cultural groups they are real diseases for which the group has medicines and treatments. Examples of such diseases are mal ojo, susto, bilis, and empacho.

It is important to determine how culturally diverse clients define health and illness and whether their health beliefs and practices differ from the norm in the Western health care delivery system (Spector, 2016).

Health represents a balance within the body, mind, and spirit. It is strongly affected by the family and the community (Box 10.1). Spector (2016) has developed a guide that can be used to assess clients' personal methods for maintaining, protecting (preventing illness), and restoring health (Table 10.2).

BOX 10.1	**Health Traditions Assessment Model**
Maintaining Health	
Physical	Are there special clothes one must wear; foods one must eat or not eat, or combinations to avoid; exercises one must do?
Mental	Are there special sources of entertainment; games or other ways of concentrating; traditional "rules of behavior?"
Spiritual	Are there special religious customs; prayers; meditations?
Protecting Health and Preventing Illness	
Physical	Are there special foods that must be eaten after certain life events, such as childbirth; dietary taboos that must be adhered to; symbolic clothes that must be worn?
Mental	Are there special sources of entertainment, games, or other ways of concentrating; traditional "rules of behavior?"
Spiritual	Are there special religious customs, superstitions, amulets, oils, or waters?
Restoring Health	
Physical	Are there special folk remedies; liniments; procedures, such as cupping, acupuncture, and moxibustion?
Mental	Are there special healers, such as curanderos, rituals, folk medicines?
Spiritual	Are there special rituals and prayers, meditations, healers?

From Spector, R. (2016). *Cultural diversity in health and illness* (9th ed.) Prentice-Hall.

TABLE 10.2 Assessment Guide for Personal Methods to Maintain, Protect (Prevent Illness), and Restore Health

	Physical	Mental	Spiritual
Maintain health	Are there special clothes you must wear at certain times of the day, week, or year? Are there special foods you must eat at certain times? Do you have any dietary restrictions? Are there any foods that you cannot eat?	What do you do for activities, such as reading, sports, or games? Do you have hobbies? Do you visit family often? Do you visit friends often?	Do you practice your religion and attend church or other communal activities? Do you pray or meditate? Do you observe religious customs? Do you belong to fraternal organizations?
Protect health or prevent illness	Are there foods that you cannot eat together? Are there special foods that you must eat? Are there any types of clothing that you are not allowed to wear?	Are there people or situations that you have been taught to avoid? Do you take extraordinary precautions under certain circumstances? Do you take time for yourself?	Do you observe religious customs? Do you wear any amulets or hang them in your house? Do you have any practices, such as always opening the window when you sleep? Do you have any other practices to protect yourself from "harm?"
Restore health	What kinds of medicines do you take before you see a doctor or nurse? Are there herbs that you take? Are there special treatments that you use?	Do you know of any specific practices your mother or grandmother may use to relax? Do you know how big problems can be cared for in your community? Do you drink special teas to help you unwind or relax?	Do you know any healers? Do you know of any religious rituals that help to restore health? Do you meditate? Do you ever go to a healing service? Do you know about exorcism?

From Spector, R. (2016). *Cultural diversity in health and illness* (9th ed.) Prentice-Hall.

▮ SUMMARY

To summarize the chapter let's review the questions posed at the beginning of the chapter and see what you have learned.

1. What strategies can you implement to overcome prejudice? Assess and challenge your own biases and remove stereotypes,

    Nurses must keep themselves accountable. A prejudice is a handicap to your perspective as it prevents you from thinking beyond your assumptions. Your own implicit and explicit attitudes toward individuals of a different race, for example, strongly predict how interactive you will be toward them (both verbally and nonverbally). When dealing with internalized stereotypes ask yourself questions such as "Why do I feel this way?" and "Where does this belief come from?" Acknowledge your own biases and prejudices and actively replace them with more reasonable alternatives. For example, if you think something stereotypical about a certain gender, religion, culture, or race (i.e., older adults are crabby), remind yourself that this is a bias against that group and that you are over-generalizing. To reduce prejudice or bias in yourself it may be helpful to identify and understand the negative effects that your biases can have on others.

2. How can nurses provide effective care to different cultural groups who each have a unique set of beliefs about illness?

    The first step to becoming a culturally sensitive and competent health care provider is to conduct a cultural self-assessment. The nurse should engage in a cultural self-assessment to identify individual culturally based attitudes about clients who are from a different culture. Cultural self-assessment requires self-honesty and sincerity, as well as re-flection on attitudes of parents, grandparents, and close friends toward different cultures. Through identification of health-related attitudes, values, beliefs, and practices the nurse can better under-stand the cultural aspects of health care from the client's perspective. Everyone has ethnocentric tendencies that must be brought to a level of con-sciousness so that efforts can be made to temper the feeling that one's own culture is best.

After the nurse performs a cultural self-assessment, they should obtain a cultural assessment of the client. Nursing assessments in institutional and community settings should include the gathering of data pertinent to cultural beliefs and practices.

Cultural assessments lead to culturally relevant nursing diagnoses and give direction to effective nursing intervention.

3. How can nursing research affect the attitudes and beliefs of health professionals in regard to minority populations?

Research that examines individual behavioral re-sponses to normal life processes, such as pregnancy, birth, death, and human growth and development is needed. Research findings from well-designed studies that explore the biologic, psychologic, socio-logic, and spiritual differences within, between, and among cultural groups can guide nursing practice to achieve optimal outcomes for patients.

REFERENCES

American Academy of Nursing (AAN). (1995). *Diversity, marginalization, and culturally competent health care issues in knowledge development.* American Academy of Nursing.

American Nurses Association. (2021). *Nursing: Scope and standards for practice* (4th ed., p. 31). Nursebooks.org

American Association of Colleges of Nursing (AACN). (2008a). *The essentials of baccalaureate education for professional nurs-ing practice.* American Association of Colleges of Nursing.

American Association of Colleges of Nursing (AACN). (2008b). *Cultural competency in baccalaureate nursing education.* http://www.aacnnursing.org/Portals/42/AcademicNursing/CurriculumGuidelines/Cultural-Competency-Bacc-Edu.pdf?ver=2017-05-18-143551-883

American Association of Colleges of Nursing (AACN). (2021). *The Essentials: Core competencies for professional nursing education of baccalaureate education for professional nursing practice.* American Association of Colleges of Nursing.

American Association of Colleges of Nursing. (2023). *Position statement: Enhancing Diversity in the Nursing Workforce.* https://www.aacnnursing.org/news-data/fact-sheets/enhancing-diversity-in-the-nursing-workforce

American Academy of Nursing Expert Panel on Cultural Competence. (2007). *American Academy of Nursing standards of cultural competence.* American Academy of Nursing Expert Panel on Cultural Competence.

Bessent, H. (1997). *Strategies for recruitment, retention and graduation of minority nurses in colleges of nursing.* American Nurses Foundation.

Cooper, C.L. (2016). *The Blackwell encyclopedia of manage-ment.* Blackwell Publishing, Blackwell Reference Online, http://www.blackwellreference.com/public/book.html?id=g9780631233176_9780631233176.

Coulter-Thompson, E.I. (2023). Bias and discrimination against lesbian, gay, bisexual, transgender, and queer parents access-ing care for their children: A literature review. *Health Educa-tion & Behavior. 50*(2):181–192. doi: 10.1177/10901981221148959. Epub 2023 Feb 1. PMID: 36722720

Deering, M. (2022). Cultural competence in nursing. *Nurse Journal, November 29, 2022.* https://nursejournal.org/resources/cultural-competence-in-nursing/

Deering, T.F., Reiffel, J.A., Solomon, A.J., & Tamirisa, K.P. (2023). Chapter 6: AAD use in different patient popula-tions, and a patient-centric approach to optimal patient management. *The American Journal of Cardiology. 205*(Suppl. 1), S19–S21. doi:10.1016/j.amjcard.2023.08.018

Fang, D., et al. (2023a). *2022–2023 Enrollment and gradua-tions in baccalaureate and graduate programs in nursing.* American Association of Colleges of Nursing.

Fang, D., et al. (2023b). *2022–2023 Salaries of instructional and administrative nursing faculty in baccalaureate and graduate programs in nursing.* American Association of Colleges of Nursing.

Fortier, J.P., et al. (1999). *Assuring cultural competence in health care: Recommendations for national standards and an outcomes-focused research agenda.* US Department of Health and Human Services. Office of Minority Health.

Future of Nursing Scholars. (2018). *About the program.* https://infocus.ibxfoundation.org/future-of-nursing-scholars-program/

Giger, J., & Haddad, L. (2021). *Transcultural nursing: assessment and intervention* (8th ed.) Elsevier.

Harrison, L.E., White, B.A., Hawrylak, K., & McIntosh, D. (2019). Explicit bias among fourth-year medical students. *Baylor University Medical Center Proceedings, 32*(1):50–53

Lenburg, C.B., et al. (1995). *Promoting cultural competence in and through nursing education: A critical review and comprehensive plan for action.* American Academy of Nursing.

Kranich, N. (2001). *Libraries and democracy.* American Library Association.

Minority Nurse. (Oct 13, 2020). Common barriers for nursing students & how to overcome them. *Minority Nurse.*

National Council of State Boards of Nursing and The Forum of State Nursing Workforce Centers. (2022). Results from the 2022 National Workforce Survey.

Nies, M., & McEwen, M. (2011). *Community/Public health nursing: Promoting the health of populations* (5th ed.) Elsevier.

Nies, M., & McEwen, M. (2022). *Community/Public health nursing: Promoting the health of populations* (8th ed.) Elsevier Saunders.

Olson, A., Rencic, J., Cosby, K., Rusz, D., Papa, F., Croskerry, P., Zierler, B., Harkless, G., Giuliano, M.A., Schoenbaum, S., Colford, C., Cahill, M., Gerstner, L., Grice, G.R., & Graber, M.L. (2019). Competencies for improving diagnosis: An interprofessional framework for education and training in health care. *Diagnosis.* 6(4):335–341. doi:10.1515/dx-2018-0107

Promotion. (2021). *Healthy people 2030.* https://health.gov/healthypeople/objectives-and-data/browse-objectives/lgbt

Smiley, R., Allgeyer, R., Shobo, Y., Lyons, K., Letourneau, R., Zhong, E., Kaminski-Ozturk, N., & Alexander, M. (2023). *The 2022 National Nursing Workforce Survey.* 14(1): Supplement 2, SI–S90, p. 85.

Spector, R. (2016). *Cultural diversity in health and illness/culture care: Guide to heritage assessment health.* In R. Spector (Eds.), *Cultural diversity in health and illness* (9th ed.) Prentice-Hall.

Stanhope, M., & Lancaster, J. (2024). *Public health nursing: Population-centered health care in the community* (11th ed.) Mosby.

Tervalon, M., & Murray-Garcia, J. (1998). Cultural humility versus cultural competence: A critical distinction in defining physician training outcomes in multicultural education. *Journal of Health Care for the Poor and Underserved.* 9(2), 117.

Todt, K. (July 2023). Strategies to combat implicit bias in nursing. *American Nurse Journal.18*(7):18–23.

US Census Bureau. (2020). Census Bureau releases new American community survey 5-year estimates. https://www.census.gov/newsroom/press-releases/2020/acs-5-year.html

US Depratment of Health and Human Services. (2010). Healthy People 2020.

US Department of Health and Human Services. (2018). *Distribution of RNs, by race/ethnicity, relative to the working-age population.* US Department of Health and Human Services.

US Department of Health and Human Services. (2020). *Public health service: Healthy people 2030.* US Government Printing Office.

US Department of Health and Human Services, Office of Disease Prevention and Health

Vespa, J., et al. (2020). Demographic turning points for the United States: Population projections for 2020 to 2060. *Current Population Reports.* P25–1144. US Census Bureau.

Wilson, T.D., Lindsey, S., & Schooler, T.Y. (2000). A model of dual attitudes. *Psychological Review 107*(1):101–126

The 2020 National Nursing Workforce Survey Journal of Nursing Regulation Volume 12/Supplement April 2021: pp 84–86 https://www.ncsbn.org/public-files/2020_NNW_Executive_Summary.pdf

World Health Organization Health Innovation Group. (2021). Promoting health through the life course. Retrieved from https://www.who.int/life-course/ablut/who-health-innovation-group/en/

11

Complementary and Alternative Healing

Charlotte Eliopoulos, PhD, MPH, ND, RN

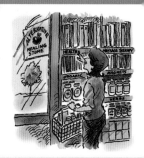

Consumers are increasingly seeking natu[ral] remedies for health promotion and dise[ase] management; nurses have a responsib[ility] to be aware of the potential effects.

e Additional resources are available online at: http://evolve.elsevier.com/Cherry/

LEARNING OUTCOMES

After studying this chapter, the reader will be able to:
1. Describe various complementary and alternative healing practices.
2. Identify how to incorporate effective complementary and alternative therapies into care.
3. Provide patient education regarding uses, limitations, and precautions associated with selected complementary and alternative healing practices and products.

KEY TERMS

Complementary and alternative medicine (CAM) Healing philosophies, practices, and products that are outside of what Western society considers mainstream medicine and are not typically taught in the educational programs of physicians, nurses, and other health professionals.

Conventional medicine Western style of medicine practiced in the United States; also called allopathic medicine.

Energy therapies Qi gong, Reiki, therapeutic touch, healing touch, magnet therapy.

Integrative medicine Care that combines the use of complementary and alternative medicine with conventional (Western) medicine.

Manipulative and body-based methods Chiropractic, massage, and related techniques (e.g., manual lymph drainage, Alexander technique, Feldenkrais method, pressure point therapies, Trager psychophysical integration), osteopathy.

Mind–body interventions Acupuncture, aromatherapy, art therapy, biofeedback, dance therapy, hypnosis, imagery, meditation, music therapy, prayer, qi gong, progressive relaxation, self-help support groups, tai chi, yoga.

Movement therapies Alexander technique, Feldenkrais method, Rolfing, Trager psychophysical integration.

Natural products Herbal therapies, individual and orthomolecular biologic therapies, special diets.

PROFESSIONAL/ETHICAL ISSUE

Mr. Jensen is a 50-year-old man who has been diagnosed with a rare liver cancer that is typically fatal within 1 year. His oncologist has recommended a form of chemotherapy that cannot offer a cure but could possibly slow the cancer's spread and offer a few added months of life to Mr. Jensen.

Mr. Jensen, accompanied by his wife, is meeting with the oncologist, who is your employer and whom you are assisting. Mr. Jensen informs the oncologist that, after giving it thought, he has decided against the chemotherapy. "I saw what my brother went through with his chemo for lung cancer and I don't want to do the same," Mr. Jensen states. "My wife found this natural health practitioner who offers some kind of touch therapy and uses herbal blends. I've seen him a couple of times now and have to tell you, I feel great so I'm going that route," he adds.

The oncologist is noticeably annoyed and responds, "You are wasting your time and money on that foolishness. If anything is going to help you it is what medicine has to offer, so I'd think about scheduling your next chemotherapy. The nurse will help you with that." He then exits the room.

Mr. and Mrs. Jensen appear upset and somewhat confused. You heard what the oncologist recommended and understand that there is no evidence supporting the effectiveness of the natural healing methods, yet you also know that the chemotherapy offers no cure and does carry risks and side effects. What do you do?

VIGNETTE

Ruth Jeffers is a registered nurse (RN) who works in a rehabilitation unit in which many clients suffer from chronic musculoskeletal pain. Ms. Jeffers has noted that a growing number of clients have a history of independently using acupuncture, nutritional supplements, and other alternative and complementary healing therapies to improve their symptoms. Although they report beneficial results, most do not tell their physicians that they are using these therapies.

Last year, Ms. Jeffers completed a course in the use of therapeutic touch and has used this therapy to promote relaxation and pain control with friends and family with considerable success. She is aware of many positive reports on the benefits of these unconventional approaches.

She believes therapeutic touch and some other complementary healing therapies could benefit clients on the rehabilitation unit, and informally introduces the topic to the team with whom she works. With the exception of one nurse who states that she believes these therapies are associated with the occult and wants no part of them, the nursing staff is enthusiastic and eager to implement complementary therapies. The physical and occupational therapists believe that complementary therapies could prove helpful to clients but that only therapists within their departments, not nurses, should provide them. The physician on the team opposes the use of all alternative and complementary therapies, stating, "I'm not about to put my license on the line for these unproven ideas."

Questions to Consider While Reading This Chapter:

1. What is the best course of action for Ruth Jeffers, RN, if she really believes that complementary and alternative therapies could benefit clients on the unit?
2. What would a hospital need to do to prepare for the inclusion of complementary and alternative therapies in its existing services?
3. What are some of the potential obstacles to introducing complementary and alternative therapies into a conventional setting?
4. What discipline(s) should be responsible for providing and/or coordinating or supervising the practitioners who provide complementary and alternative therapies in the hospital?

CHAPTER OVERVIEW

This chapter presents an overview of complementary and alternative medicine (CAM) therapies and products, which have gained popularity in Western society and are being integrated into health care. As increasing numbers of consumers and clinical settings become interested in and actually use CAM therapies, nurses must become knowledgeable about the uses, limitations, and precautions associated with these new practices and products. Professional nurses have an obligation to understand such practices and products so as to advise patients and effectively incorporate pertinent therapies into patients' care. Nurses who have knowledge and skills in this area are in key positions to empower patients for self-care that complements conventional medicine.

USE OF COMPLEMENTARY AND ALTERNATIVE HEALING METHODS

Complementary and alternative healing methods include healing philosophies, practices, and products that fall outside what Western society considers mainstream (conventional) medicine and that are not typically taught in the educational programs of physicians, nurses, pharmacists, and other health professionals.

The past few decades have seen CAM progress from a fringe movement to highly popular, widely used therapies that are being integrated into conventional care. According to a nationwide government survey, more than 38% of US adults 18 years and older and approximately 12% of children use some form of CAM, spending between $27 and $34 billion for these services out of their own pockets (Nahin et al., 2016; National Center for Complementary and Integrative Health, 2021).

Rather than emerging from the leadership of health care professionals, the growing popularity of CAM has been consumer driven. Several factors contribute to consumers' desire for CAM:

- *Dissatisfaction with the conventional health care system:* The impersonal nature of health care has grown with costs. Shorter hospital stays, several months' waiting periods to see a physician, hurried staff that barely have time to provide basic care, and horror stories of the adverse effects of medications are causing consumers to look for alternative approaches that are safer, less costly, and more responsive and personalized than conventional health care.
- *Increased empowerment of consumers in the health care system:* The Internet and growing assertiveness of consumers in all areas has affected health care. Consumers expect to have a voice in their care planning activities and to be able to utilize all available options for health promotion and disease management, including therapies outside mainstream medicine.
- *Unwillingness to "grin and bear" the effects of diseases:* Today's consumers are less willing than previous generations to live with symptoms that alter their lifestyles, or to passively accept terminal diagnoses and wait to die. They want to have options and to be empowered to do everything conceivable to promote the best possible quality and quantity of their lives, and they are willing to look to alternative healing measures to do so.

- *Shrinking world:* The rapid pace and ease of information sharing have enabled individuals to learn about diverse practices of cultures throughout the world.
- *Growing evidence of effectiveness:* The body of research supporting the effectiveness of alternative therapies increases almost daily. People hear testimonials from friends and family about the way they have been helped by acupuncture, herbs, and other forms of CAM. In addition, the media regularly report these findings, contributing to consumers' awareness of the body of evidence.

People who use CAM practices and products have been shown to hold values, beliefs, and philosophic orientation to engage in positive health behavioral changes and have greater motivation to do so when they use CAM (Bishop et al., 2019). With rare exceptions, consumers prefer natural approaches that afford them an active role in their care over high-tech interventions that relegate them to a passive, obedient role. They want to connect with their health care providers, have their individuality recognized, and gain education and skills to effectively make decisions and direct their care. Increasingly, consumers are seeking measures to enhance not just their bodies but also their minds and spirits. The quality of their lives is equally if not more important in comparison with the quantity of years they live. Consumers often discover that CAM promotes many principles of holistic care that they value, such as individual empowerment, self-care, attention to all facets of one's being, and a high quality of life. Fortunately CAM is becoming increasingly accepted by conventional practitioners (Phutrakool & Pongpirul, 2022).

PRINCIPLES UNDERLYING ALTERNATIVE HEALING

A wide range of healing therapies are encompassed in CAM, yet most are based on some common principles:

- *The body has the ability to heal itself.* Most conventional medicine works from the premise that the elimination of sickness requires an intervention "done to" the body (e.g., giving medications, surgery). In CAM, there is the assumption that the body has the potential to heal itself. Complementary and alternative healing therapies enhance the body's ability to self-heal.
- *Health and healing are related to a harmony of mind, body, and spirit.* The mind, body, and spirit are

inseparable—what affects one affects all. Healing and the improvement of health demand that all facets of a person be addressed, not merely a single symptom or system.

- *Basic, positive health practices build the foundation for healing.* Good nutrition, exercise, rest, stress management, and avoidance of harmful habits (e.g., smoking) are essential ingredients in health maintenance and the improvement of health conditions. Practitioners of healing therapies are more likely than conventional practitioners to look at total lifestyle practices rather than the diseased body part.
- *Approaches to healing are individualized.* The unique composition and dynamics of each person are recognized in CAM. Practitioners of healing therapies explore the underlying cause of a problem and customize approaches accordingly. It is rare in CAM to find a standing protocol that treats everyone with similar conditions alike.
- *Individuals are responsible for their own healing.* People can use a wide range of therapies, from conventional prescription drugs to herbal remedies, to treat illness. However, it is the responsibility of competent adults to seek health advice, make informed choices, gain necessary knowledge and skills for self-care, engage in practices that promote health and healing, and seek help when needed. Clients are responsible for getting their minds, bodies, and spirits in optimal condition to heal rather than looking externally for a physician or nurse to heal them.

A holistic philosophy, promotion of positive health habits, and the client's responsibility for facilitating their own health and healing are common threads among healing therapies.

OVERVIEW OF POPULAR CAM HEALING THERAPIES

Hundreds of healing therapies are practiced throughout the world, with varying degrees of evidence to support their effectiveness. As the use of these therapies grew in the United States the National Institutes of Health (NIH) established the Office of Alternative Medicine in 1992 to evaluate these complementary and alternative practices and products. In 1998 the Office of Alternative Medicine became a freestanding center within the NIH and was named the National Center for Complementary and Alternative Medicine. The name

---

> ### BOX 11.1   Categories and Examples of Complementary Health Approaches
>
> **Natural Products**
> Herbs (botanicals), vitamins, minerals, probiotics
>
> **Psychological and Physical Approaches**
> Acupuncture, chiropractic and osteopathic manipulation, healing touch, hypnotherapy, massage therapy, meditation, movement therapies (Alexander technique, Feldenkrais method, Pilates, Rolfing Structural Integration, Trager psychophysical integration), relaxation techniques (breathing exercises, guided imagery, progressive relaxation), tai chi
>
> **Other Approaches**
> Ayurvedic medicine, homeopathy, naturopathy, traditional Chinese medicine

---

was changed to the National Center for Complementary and Integrative Health (NCCIH) to reflect the wider acceptance and use of CAM in mainstream health care. NCCIH has categorized CAM into several major fields of practice (Box 11.1); the Center supports research and serves as a clearinghouse for information on alternative practices and products.

Consumers' growing use of CAM therapies, as well as the increased integration of such therapies into conventional care, places a demand on nurses to become familiar with these therapies. Some of the frequently used CAM therapies are discussed in the following sections.

Acupuncture

Practiced in China for more than 2000 years, acupuncture is a major therapy within traditional Chinese medicine. It is based on the belief that there are invisible channels throughout the body, called *meridians*, through which energy flows. This energy, called qi (pronounced "chee"), is considered the vital life force. It is believed that illness and symptoms develop when the flow of energy becomes blocked or imbalanced. Health is restored when the energy becomes unblocked; unblocking is achieved by stimulating acupuncture points on the meridian(s) affected (Fig. 11.1).

The acupuncturist typically begins the treatment by taking a history, examining the tongue, and evaluating pulses. On the basis of where the acupuncturist assesses the energy imbalance to be, they place needles at specific points. The placement of the needles may have no

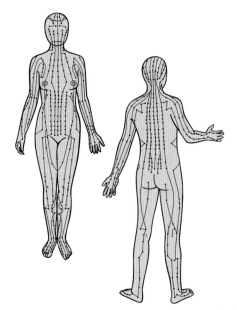

Fig. 11.1 Acupuncture meridians. (From Eliopoulos, C. [1999]. *Integrating alternative and conventional therapies.* Mosby.)

obvious relationship to the area of the body that is symptomatic. Sometimes the acupuncturist applies heat to the acupoints by burning a dried herb on the top of the needle or skin; this procedure is known as *moxibustion*. Electroacupuncture, a process in which a small current of electricity is applied to the tip of the needle, is another means of stimulating acupoints.

Pain relief is the most common reason people seek acupuncture treatment, and research supports its effectiveness for this problem (Huang et al., 2023; Lee et al., 2020; Montgomery & Ottenbacher, 2020). The use of acupuncture for dental pain and chemotherapy-induced nausea and vomiting has also been supported by research. There is some evidence that acupuncture can be of help for nicotine withdrawal, asthma, stroke rehabilitation, carpal tunnel syndrome, and a growing list of other conditions.

Insurance companies vary in their coverage of acupuncture, so it is best for clients to call their individual insurer for determination of benefits. State health departments can be consulted for licensing requirements for acupuncturists in a given state.

Ayurveda

Although it has gained popularity because of the writings and lectures of Deepak Chopra, Ayurveda has existed in India for more than 5000 years and is considered an accepted form of medical care in that country. Ayurveda, which means "the science of life," is a system of care that promotes spiritual, mental, and physical balance. Noninvasive approaches are used to achieve balance; they include yoga, massage, diet, purification regimens, breathing exercises, meditation, and herbs.

Individuals are believed to have distinct metabolic body types called *doshas*, which are *vata, pitta,* and *kapha* (Table 11.1). Signs of illness occur when the delicate balance of the doshas is disturbed.

The treatment to restore balance is influenced by the body type a client possesses and could include:

- Cleansing and detoxification
- Palliation
- Rejuvenation through special herbs and minerals
- Mental hygiene and spiritual healing

There is no process for licensing or certifying Ayurvedic practitioners. Because some of the treatments have the potential to cause complications (e.g., dehydration from cleansing enemas, herb–drug interactions, toxicity from preparations containing high levels of lead and mercury), finding a reputable trained practitioner is important. There is a need for continued research because scientific evidence supporting the effectiveness

TABLE 11.1	**Ayurvedic Metabolic Body Types**
Type	**Characteristics**
Vata	Unpredictable; moody; vivacious; hyperactive; imaginative; intuitive; impulsive; fluctuating energy levels; slender; prominent features and joints; eats and sleeps at varying times throughout day; prone to insomnia, premenstrual syndrome (PMS), muscular cramps, and constipation
Pitta	Predictable; orderly; efficient; perfectionist; intense; passionate; short-tempered; medium build; follows routine schedule; warm skin; prone to heavy perspiration, thirst, acne, ulcers, hemorrhoids, and stomach problems
Kapha	Relaxed; graceful; tendency toward procrastination; affectionate; forgiving; compassionate; sleeps long and deeply; cool, pale, and oily skin; eats slowly; prone to high cholesterol, obesity, allergies, and sinusitis

of Ayurvedic practices is minimal, and more rigorous research is needed to determine which practices are safe and effective.

Biofeedback

A popular mind–body intervention, biofeedback is a technique in which the client is taught to alter specific bodily functions (e.g., heart rate, blood pressure, muscle tension) by using various relaxation and imagery exercises. Machinery, such as electroencephalograms, electromyelograms, and thermistors, is used to measure and offer feedback about the function that the client is trying to alter. As the client becomes familiar with ways to successfully alter bodily responses, the equipment may no longer be necessary.

There are many conditions for which biofeedback can offer benefit, including urinary incontinence, anxiety, stress, irritable bowel syndrome, and neck and back pain. People with cardiac or dermatological problems should consult with their medical provider before using biofeedback to treat their conditions.

Chiropractic Medicine

Chiropractic medicine, a manipulative and body-based method, is a popular and widely accepted CAM therapy in the United States, perhaps because it was developed there and has been practiced for more than a century. Chiropractors must hold a Doctor of Chiropractic degree and become licensed in their state by passing the National Board of Chiropractic Examiners' exam. Most insurance companies pay for chiropractic treatments.

Chiropractic medicine is based on the belief that misalignments of the spine, called *subluxations,* put pressure on the nerves, leading to pain and disruptions in normal bodily function. The misalignment is treated by manipulation and adjustment of the spine. Typically, the chiropractor's hands do the alignment, although chiropractors increasingly are using heat, electrical stimulation, and other treatments. Chiropractors often incorporate other methods of treatment, such as nutritional counseling and exercise.

Dietary Supplements

The past advice that vitamin and mineral supplements are unnecessary if one is eating well has been replaced with the recommendation that everyone should take a daily vitamin and mineral supplement. This shift in

thinking has resulted from the realization that many people do not consume the proper nutrients through their diets. Pollutants, stress, and other factors that are more common today than in previous generations heighten the body's need for added protection. Unlike our ancestors who consumed produce that was picked the same day, we tend to eat more processed foods and produce that may have been in transit for several days before reaching us; therefore the foods we consume contain fewer vitamins and minerals. Given these factors, the National Research Council of the National Academy of Sciences is reevaluating the need to increase the recommended dietary allowances (RDAs).

Specific dietary supplements are thought to be beneficial for specific health conditions. However, too much of a good thing could prove harmful, and high doses of vitamins and minerals can lead to serious complications (National Center for Complementary and Integrative Health, 2019b). For example, high doses of folic acid can mask a vitamin B12 deficiency (a cause of dementia), calcium in excess of 2500 mg/day can cause kidney stones and impair the body's ability to absorb other minerals, and antioxidants can impair the effects of chemotherapy. In addition, because new research may disprove earlier claims about supplements, nurses need to keep abreast of new findings so that they can use supplements wisely and educate consumers to do the same.

Herbs

Herbs are a major entity under the category of natural products. Plants have been used for medicinal purposes for nearly as long as humans have inhabited the earth. There are thousands of plant species that have been used by various cultures throughout the world for medicinal purposes. Botanical medicine was a mainstream practice in the United States until the early 19th century, when medicine's shift toward a more scientific approach caused drugs to be viewed more favorably than herbs. But in the 1960s, when the movement toward natural health began to grow, interest in herbal products increased. The use and sales of herbal remedies have grown significantly since.

In reality, herbs are not that foreign to conventional medicine. Many modern drugs are derived from plants, including:
- Atropine from *Atropa belladonna*
- Digoxin from *Digitalis purpurea*
- Ipecac from *Cephaelis ipecacuanha*
- Reserpine from *Rauwolfia serpentina*

With more than 20,000 herbs and related products on the market, staying current of uses, dosage, interactions, and adverse effects is a near impossibility. However, nurses would be wise to become familiar with some of the most commonly used herbs (Box 11.2) and to know where to obtain information on other herbs when needed. Because of consumers' widespread use of herbs, questions regarding use of all supplements and education to ensure their safe use are significant nursing responsibilities.

BOX 11.2   Facts about Commonly Used Herbs

Cannabis (Marijuana)

Uses: Appetite stimulant, antianxiety, anorexic, antiemetic, and treatment of chronic pain, Crohn's disease, severe muscle spasms, and seizures.

Caution: Can cause dizziness, fatigue, tachycardia, hypotension, slower reaction times, impaired short-term memory, impaired judgment, anxiety, hallucinations, paranoia, acute psychosis (in large doses). Use during pregnancy can cause lower birth weight of infant. Further study is needed to determine short- and long-term risks. States vary in their laws concerning medicinal marijuana use; individuals should check with their own state laws regarding legality and conditions of use.

Chamomile

Uses: Antianxiety; calming an upset digestive tract, healing mouth ulcers caused by chemotherapy or radiation although these effects resulted when used in combination with other herbs.

Caution: There have been reports of interactions between chamomile and warfarin and cyclosporine; persons using anticoagulants or who have had organ transplants should consult with their medical provider before using this herb. Limited information exists as to the use of chamomile during pregnancy and when breastfeeding. People are more likely to experience allergic reactions to chamomile if they are allergic to related plants in the daisy family, which includes ragweed, chrysanthemums, marigolds, and daisies.

Echinacea

Uses: Stimulates the immune system to treat or prevent colds, flu, and other infections.

Caution: Although immunosuppressive effects with long-term use are inconclusive at present, it's best to limit to short-term use. It should not be used in people with autoimmune diseases. People are more likely to experience allergic reactions to echinacea if they have asthma or are allergic to related plants in the daisy family, which includes ragweed, chrysanthemums, marigolds, and daisies. Gastrointestinal side effects are common.

Feverfew

Use: Relief of migraines (although more evidence is needed).

Caution: Contraindicated for clients with allergies to ragweed and other members of the Compositae family. People who have used feverfew for an extended period may have headaches, difficulty sleeping, nervousness, and joint and muscle stiffness when they stop taking it. Women who are pregnant should not use feverfew because it may cause the uterus to contract, increasing the risk of miscarriage or premature delivery.

Garlic

Uses: Can lower total cholesterol and low-density lipoprotein (LDL) cholesterol; believed to aid in lowering blood pressure but evidence is limited.

Caution: Close monitoring necessary if taken by person using an anticoagulant because it can prolong bleeding time. Can reduce the effectiveness of saquinavir and some other drugs. Should not be used by women who are breastfeeding.

Ginger

Uses: Antiemetic, particularly helpful for pregnancy-related nausea and vomiting and nausea resulting from chemotherapy. Insufficient evidence regarding ginger's benefit for rheumatoid arthritis, osteoarthritis, or joint and muscle pain.

Caution: Few side effects are linked to ginger when it is taken in small doses. Powdered form can cause gas, bloating, heartburn, and diarrhea.

Ginkgo

Use: Was believed to increase circulation to the brain and improve cognitive performance in persons with dementia; however, research has not shown ginkgo to be effective in improving memory or cognitive function.

Caution: Close monitoring necessary if taken by person using an anticoagulant because ginkgo can prolong bleeding time; can reduce effectiveness of anticonvulsants. Should not be used by people who have fragile blood

BOX 11.2   Facts about Commonly Used Herbs—cont'd

vessels and a tendency to easily bleed. Side effects of ginkgo may include headache, nausea, gastrointestinal upset, diarrhea, dizziness, and allergic skin reactions. More severe allergic reactions have occasionally been reported. Fresh (raw) and roasted ginkgo seeds should be avoided; they can cause serious adverse effects because they contain high amounts of ginkgotoxin (which is present only in small amounts in standardized ginkgo leaf extracts, which do not pose the same risk).

Ginseng

Uses: Used to improve resistance to stress, boost energy, and as an immune stimulant; however, current research supporting its benefits are inconclusive.

Cautions: Can cause breast tenderness in some menstruating women. Asian ginseng may lower blood glucose levels; this effect may be seen more in people with diabetes. Therefore, people with diabetes should use extra caution with Asian ginseng, especially if they are using medicines to lower blood glucose or taking other herbs thought to have the same effect, such as bitter melon and fenugreek. Most common side effects are headaches, insomnia, increased heart rate, and gastrointestinal problems. Should be avoided in women who are pregnant or breastfeeding.

Green Tea

Uses: Laboratory studies suggest that green tea may help protect against or may slow the growth of certain cancers, but studies in people have shown mixed results. Some evidence suggests that the use of green tea preparations improves mental alertness, most likely because of its caffeine content. Green tea has been promoted to aid in weight loss; however, this has not been supported by research. Although there have not been many studies supporting its effectiveness, there is some limited evidence that green tea can have a beneficial effect on the heart and lower blood pressure and blood cholesterol levels.

Caution: There have been some case reports of liver problems in people taking concentrated green tea extracts, but this problem does not seem to be connected with green tea infusions or beverages. Although these cases are very rare and the evidence is not definitive, experts suggest that concentrated green tea extracts be taken with food and that people should discontinue use and consult a heath care practitioner if they have a liver disorder or experience symptoms of liver trouble, such as abdominal pain, dark urine, and jaundice. Green tea and green tea extracts contain substantial amounts of caffeine, which can cause insomnia, anxiety, irritability, upset stomach, nausea, diarrhea, or frequent urination in some people.

Lavender

Uses: Used for treatment of anxiety, restlessness, and insomnia. Inhaled at low concentrations lavender has been shown to reduce colic symptoms in infants resulting in reduced parental stress (Sahebkaram et al, 2022). Some early results from research show that scalp massage with lavender oil when combined with other herbal oils can aid in preventing hair loss in persons with alopecia areata.

Caution: Topical use of diluted lavender oil or use of lavender as aromatherapy is generally considered safe for most adults. However, lavender oil can be poisonous if taken orally, and applying lavender oil to the skin can cause irritation.

Saw Palmetto

Uses: Has been promoted for urinary tract symptoms associated with prostatic enlargement; however, major studies funded by the National Institutes of Health showed it to be no more effective than a placebo.

Caution: Saw palmetto appears to be well tolerated by most users. It may have mild side effects, including stomach discomfort and headache.

Soy

Uses: May slightly lower levels of low-density lipoprotein (LDL; "bad") cholesterol when taken daily. Some studies suggest that soy isoflavone supplements may reduce hot flashes in women after menopause; however, the effects are minimal.

Caution: Minor stomach discomfort and diarrhea are the most common side effects. Individuals deficient in iodine could experience changes in thyroid function with the use of soy. The safety of the long-term use of soy isoflavones has not been established.

St. John's Wort

Uses: Short-term treatment of mild to moderate depression. Although some studies have reported benefits for more severe depression, others have not; for example, a large study sponsored by NCCIH found that the herb was no more effective than placebo in treating minor, moderate, or major depression. Results are inconclusive of its benefits for menopausal symptoms, PMS, obsessive–compulsive disorder, or other conditions.

Continued

BOX 11.2   Facts about Commonly Used Herbs—cont'd

Caution: Can cause photosensitivity, particularly in fair-skinned individuals; contraindicated when other antidepressants are used. Other side effects include anxiety, dry mouth, dizziness, gastrointestinal symptoms, fatigue, headache, and sexual dysfunction. Can interact with antidepressants, birth control pills, cyclosporine, digoxin, indinavir (and possibly other drugs used to control human immunodeficiency virus [HIV] infection), irinotecan (and possibly other drugs used to treat cancer), seizure-control drugs (e.g., dilantin and phenobarbital), and warfarin and related anticoagulants.

Valerian

Use: Although there is not enough conclusive evidence from well-designed studies to confirm its effectiveness, it is used for insomnia, anxiety, depression, and menopausal symptoms. Safe to use in adults for short periods (4 to 6 weeks).

Caution: Can have mild side effects, such as headaches, dizziness, upset stomach, and tiredness the morning after its use. Should not be taken with alcohol or sedatives. The American Academy of Sleep Medicine recommended against using it for chronic insomnia in adults.

Cannabis sativa (marijuana) is a psychoactive herb produced by the cannabis plant. In recent years there has been growing popularity in the use of medical cannabis for nausea, vomiting, anorexia, muscle spasms, and chronic pain. Although the medical use of cannabis has existed for centuries in other cultures, it had been an illegal substance in the United States, where it had been primarily used for recreational purposes. California became the first state to legalize the medical use of marijuana in 1996, and since then a majority of states have made medical marijuana legal. Advocates of its use claim it is safe, and although its effectiveness for the intended uses has been supported, research is needed as to its long-term safety.

Medical cannabis can be administered by inhalation through a vaporizer, orally (solution or pill), sublingually, or by topical application. The quickest action is obtained by administration via vaporizer. Side effects include dizziness, slower reaction time, hypotension, tachycardia, depression, hallucinations, poor coordination, and impaired judgment. It can interact with other medications, causing other side effects. Although research is limited it is recommended that medical cannabis not be used by people with a history of serious mental illness (e.g., psychosis, schizophrenia, bipolar disorder, depression); women who are pregnant or breastfeeding; minors; individuals with a history of alcohol or drug abuse; and those with serious heart, liver, kidney, or lung disease.

Persons using medical cannabis will test positive on drug tests. This could prove to be an issue with drug testing done on employees or preemployment screening. Although a growing number of states are prohibiting employers from firing or not hiring someone using medical cannabis for having a positive drug screening result, there still are states that support employers' right to do so. Human resources department personnel can advise as to the law in their states. Every state prohibits people from operating or driving vehicles when they have cannabis is their systems, so using medical cannabis could affect employment in jobs involving this. Individuals using medical cannabis need to be aware that although they may not have used this drug on a workday, there still could be sufficient amounts remaining in their systems from the use on previous days, which could result in a positive drug test at work.

The American Nurses Association is among the professional organizations that have supported the use of medical cannabis, and because most nurses have not learned about cannabis in nursing school they urge nurses to independently seek information about its use (Theisen & Konieczny, 2019; Worster et al, 2021). The American Cannabis Nurses Association was formed to promote education, research, and policy development related to the use of medical cannabis (information on their activities can be obtained on their website https://cannabisnurses.org/). Laws related to conditions for which medical cannabis can be used, dispensing, and other issues vary by state; the National Conference of State Legislatures offers a description of state medical marijuana laws at https://www.ncsl.org/health/state-cannabis-policy-enactment-database.

Homeopathy

Homeopathy is a branch of medicine developed in the late 18th century by Samuel Hahnemann. It was widely practiced in the United States until the early 1900s, when modern (i.e., conventional) medicine discredited it as being unscientific and ineffective. Homeopathy remained popular in other parts of the world, however, and has regained popularity in the United States.

The origin of the word *homeopathy* helps in understanding this therapy. In Greek the word *homos* means "similar" and *pathos* means "suffering." At the foundation of homeopathy are the laws of *similars,* the *minimum dose,* and *cure* (Box 11.3).

Although the reason for their effectiveness is not fully understood, homeopathic remedies have been used for wellness promotion, disease prevention, and a

variety of conditions such as allergies, asthma, chronic fatigue syndrome, depression, digestive disorders, ear infections, headaches, and rashes.

It should be noted that although there have been positive experiences with the use of homeopathic remedies, research supporting its use has been minimal (Nelson et al., 2019). The Homeopathic Research Institute is supporting efforts to increase evidence supporting homeopathy's effectiveness (Roberts et al, 2023).

Hypnotherapy

Although the use of trance states for healing purposes dates back to primitive cultures, hypnotherapy was not approved as a valid medical treatment until the 1950s. This mind–body therapy is now widely and successfully used for a broad range of conditions, including chronic pain, menopausal symptoms, migraines, asthma, smoking cessation, and irritable bowel syndrome.

In the process of hypnosis the therapist first guides the client into a relaxed state and then creates an image that focuses attention to the specific symptom or problem that needs to be improved. The client must be in a state of deep relaxation to be receptive to a posthypnotic suggestion. Most people are capable of being hypnotized if they are willing.

Imagery

Imagery, another mind–body intervention, is the process of creating a "picture" (image) in the mind that can cause a specific bodily response. Hypnosis also uses imagery, but in hypnosis an image and suggestion are presented to the person, whereas in imagery the person creates an image on their own. The process of imagery begins with the client establishing a desired outcome (e.g., to relieve stress, enhance circulation, reduce blood pressure). The nurse or other practitioner assists the client in creating an image that helps achieve the outcome (e.g., the nurse may describe how the blood circulates through the body, help the client develop an image of how cancer cells can be eliminated, or suggest that the client think of a peaceful place where cares can "melt away") and guides the client in reaching a relaxed state. As an alternative to having someone guide them through an imagery exercise a client can learn the process from books or use commercially prepared audiotapes.

Imagery is not a difficult mind–body healing therapy to master and can be easily implemented in virtually every practice setting.

BOX 11.3 Principles Underlying Homeopathy

Law of Similars

This law builds on the idea of prescribing remedies that produce symptoms similar to those of the illness being treated, the same principle on which vaccines are based. In homeopathy, a dilute preparation is made from a plant or other biologic material; the more dilute the preparation, the higher its potency. The solution is typically added to a sugar tablet or powder for oral use or to a lotion or ointment for external use.

Law of Minimum Dose

This law, also known as the *principle of dilutions,* states that the lower the dosage of the substance, the greater its effectiveness. In the preparation of homeopathic remedies, substances are diluted and shaken vigorously; a portion of that substance is then diluted and shaken. This procedure is repeated to the point that the final substance is so dilute that no molecules of the original plant or substance remain. This process, known as *potentiation,* is believed to transmit some form of information or energy from the original substance to the final diluted remedy. It is believed that the substance has left its imprint or "essence," which stimulates the body to heal itself (this theory is called the "memory of water").

Law of Cure

This is the principle used to evaluate the effectiveness of a remedy. If the treatment is successful, symptoms should travel from vital to less-vital organs of the body, move from within the body outward, and disappear in reverse order of appearance. If symptoms do not follow this sequence, a new or additional treatment is used. In homeopathic medicine a worsening of symptoms after a remedy is given is considered a positive sign that healing is taking place.

Magnet Therapy

Although a mainstream therapy in Germany and Japan, the use of magnets has only lately become popular in the United States. The most common uses of magnet therapy are for pain and wound healing.

The mechanism by which magnets work is not completely understood and is being investigated. It is believed that magnets relieve pain by creating a slight electrical current that stimulates the nervous system and consequently blocks nerve sensations. Magnets are hypothesized to speed wound healing by dilating vessels and increasing circulation to an area. Distributors of magnet products make additional claims about the health benefits of magnets, ranging from improving attention deficit disorder to boosting the immune system, although these benefits are yet to be proven.

There are two major types of magnets: static or permanent magnets and eletromagnets. Static magnets are metal or alloy forms that produce a consistent magnetic field. They come in a variety of forms, strengths, and prices: magnet disks that can be strapped to limbs, magnet mattresses that one can sleep on, and magnet jewelry. To be effective for therapeutic purposes, the magnet needs to have a strength of at least 500 gauss (which is about eight times stronger than the magnets used for attaching things to a refrigerator door). There is no research supporting the effectiveness of static magnets for pain management. Eletromagnets are created by an electric current passing through an electric coil that contains magnetic material.

Preliminary scientific studies of magnets for pain have produced mixed results (NCCIH, 2023a; Fan et al., 2021). Overall, there is no convincing scientific evidence to support claims that static magnets can relieve pain of any type. Although inconclusive at this time, there is some evidence that electromagnets relieve musculoskeletal and osteoarthritic pain. More research on magnets for pain is needed before any firm conclusion can be reached.

Persons with pacemakers and insulin pumps should not use magnets, and because the effects of magnets on fetal growth are not fully understood they should not be applied to the abdomen of a pregnant woman.

Massage, Bodywork, and Energy Therapies

Massage for healing purposes has been used for thousands of years to maintain health. Many people today receive regular massages as an important component of their self-care to aid in stress management. In addition to promoting relaxation massage can be beneficial for reducing edema, promoting circulation and respirations, and relieving pain, anxiety, and depression.

A form of manipulative and body-based method, massage is the manipulation of soft tissue through rubbing, kneading, rolling, pressing, slapping, and tapping movements. The term *bodywork* is applied to the combination of massage with deep-tissue manipulation, movement awareness, and energy balancing. Touch therapies include techniques in which the hands of the nurse or therapist are near the body, in the client's energy field. Examples of various types of massage, bodywork, and touch therapies are described in Box 11.4.

Because therapeutic touch (TT) is a popular alternative healing therapy among nurses, it deserves some discussion. TT, a form of energy therapy, became popular in nursing in the 1970s with the work and research of Delores Krieger (Krieger, 1979; Therapeutic Touch International Association, 2023). Krieger advanced the theory that people are energy fields and that obstructed energy could be responsible for unhealthy states. She proposed that the nurse could draw on the universal field of energy and transfer this energy to the client. This incoming energy could help the client mobilize their own inner resources for healing and help unblock the client's obstructed energy.

In TT there is little direct physical contact between the practitioner and the individual being treated. Rather, TT is an energy-based therapy; the nurse enters the client's energy field to assess and treat energy imbalances.

In the first step of TT the nurse centers themself and focuses on the intent to heal (this is sometimes referred to as *healing meditation*). During this phase the nurse quiets their mind and prepares physically and psychologically to connect with the client. This is considered a crucial step in the process, to enable the nurse to be fully present in the moment with the client. Then the nurse passes their hands over the client's body to assess the energy field and mobilize areas in which energy is blocked or sluggish by directing energies to that area. TT is used to reduce anxiety, relieve pain, and enhance immune function. The Therapeutic Touch International Association website (https://therapeutictouch.org) offers information about the therapy and credentialing.

Healing touch (HT) is an energy therapy that is an offshoot of TT. It combines additional healing approaches to the basic ones of TT to open energy blockages, seal

BOX 11.4 Types of Massage, Bodywork, and Touch Therapies

Alexander Technique
Teaches improved balance, posture, and coordination by using gentle hands-on guidance and verbal instruction

Feldenkrais Method
Teaches movement re-education by using gentle manipulations to heighten awareness of the body; based on belief that each person has an individualized optimal style of movement

Healing Touch
A multilevel energy healing program that incorporates aspects of therapeutic touch with other healing measures

Reflexology
Application of pressure to pressure points on the hands and feet that correspond to various parts of the body

Reiki
A therapy that uses techniques to direct universal life energy to specific sites

Rolfing (Structural Integration)
Use of manual manipulation and stretching of body's fascial tissues to establish balance and symmetry

Swedish Massage
Most prevalent form of massage; uses long strokes, friction, and kneading of muscles

Therapeutic Touch
Energy therapy in which the practitioner detects and manipulates a person's energy field

Trager Approach
Use of gentle, rhythmic rocking and touch to promote relaxation and energy flow

energy leaks, and rebalance the energy field. There is a six-level educational program for HT. The Healing Beyond Borders (formally Healing Touch International) website offers a full description of their program in addition to a bibliography of recent research related to this therapy (http://www.healingbeyondborders.org).

Reiki is a practice in which the Reiki practitioner (of which there are several levels) channels energy to others using a series of hand positions. It is believed that healing energy flows through the hands without the need for any special skills. Like other forms of energy work Reiki is believed to be useful for pain management, wound healing, stroke rehabilitation, and general relaxation; however, research is insufficient to suggest that Reiki is an effective treatment for any condition. Despite the limited research supporting the existence of the energy field thought to affect healing or its effectiveness, the low risk of side effects, affordability, and desire of a person to utilize this therapy make an ethical case for its use (NCCIH, 2023b).

With the use of healing energy therapies, nurses need to be aware that some individuals may feel spiritual distress if they receive healing energy because they may be concerned about what and who the source of the energy is. For example, a Christian who believes that healing comes directly from Jesus Christ may react negatively to receiving healing energy that is drawn from a vague universal force. Assessing the client's spiritual beliefs, explaining the therapy clearly, and obtaining consent before offering the treatment are useful.

Meditation and Progressive Relaxation

Meditation, a mind–body intervention that involves the act of focusing on the present moment, has been used for centuries throughout the world. This practice gained considerable attention in the United States in the 1970s when Harvard Medical School cardiologist Herbert Benson published research on the relaxation response (Benson et al., 1974). Benson and his associates reported that after 20 minutes of meditation, participants' heart rates, respirations, blood pressure, oxygen consumption, carbon dioxide production, and serum lactic acid levels decreased. This discovery led to the use of meditation for a variety of conditions, including stress, anxiety, pain, and high blood pressure.

Progressive relaxation is another exercise that shares some of the benefits of meditation. Typically, a person learns to guide themself through a series of exercises that relax the body, such as tightening and relaxing various muscle groups. Many CDs are available in bookstores and health food stores that offer scripts to guide meditation and progressive relaxation exercises.

Naturopathy

An intense interest in natural cures in Europe during the 19th century led to the development of spas that offered natural treatments to promote health and healing.

Soon the movement spread to the United States, and in 1896 the American School of Naturopathy was founded. Naturopathic physicians and treatment facilities using natural cures became popular in the early part of the 20th century. For example, John Kellogg ran such a facility in Battle Creek in which he subsequently became famous for the natural breakfast cereals that he used. As time progressed medications and high-tech interventions caused naturopathy to pale by comparison; however, as consumers seek more natural approaches this form of alternative medicine is making a comeback.

Naturopathy is based on the principle that the body has inherent healing abilities that can be stimulated to treat disease. Naturopathic physicians assess and treat the cause of the disease rather than merely alleviate symptoms. They help clients identify unhealthy practices, encourage healthy lifestyle habits, counsel them, and guide them in managing health problems using natural approaches such as herbs, homeopathic remedies, diet modifications, dietary supplements, and exercise.

There are a limited number of accredited schools of naturopathic medicine (e.g., Bastyr University, Southwest College of Naturopathic Medicine and Health Sciences, National University of Natural Medicine, and National University of Health Sciences). A handful of states license naturopaths and require that they graduate from an accredited program. However, there are many individuals practicing as naturopaths who have obtained their education and experience through other means or who practice in states that do not require licensure; thus learning about the credentials of a naturopath before receiving services is beneficial for clients.

Prayer and Faith

Many people consider their faith to be an integral part of their total being rather than a therapy, but now there is scientific evidence supporting the therapeutic benefits of faith and prayer in health and healing. Hundreds of well-conducted studies have revealed that people who profess a faith, pray, and attend religious services are generally healthier, live longer, have lower rates of disability, recover faster, have lower rates of emotional disorders, and otherwise enjoy better health states than those who do not (Kaye, 2020; O'Brien, 2017; Victor & Treschuk, 2019; Singh et al, 2023). Not only do the faith and religious practices of individuals themselves affect health and healing, but research also supports the benefit of intercessory prayer.

Nurses need to appreciate that many people believe in the healing power of prayer and may expect their health care providers to join them in prayer if requested. This fact does not suggest that nurses or other health professionals should be forced into prayer if it is contrary to their beliefs; rather, if there is no objection from either party prayer by the client and health care provider can be used as a valuable healing measure.

Tai Chi

Tai chi is another practice from traditional Chinese medicine used to stimulate the flow of qi, the life energy. It is a combination of exercise and energy work that looks like a slow, graceful dance using continuous, slow, controlled movements of the arms and legs. There is a specific sequence of steps to follow in doing tai chi, but fortunately there are many inexpensive videos that can be used in addition to classes that are offered to aid people in learning this practice.

Tai chi has some demonstrated benefits, including reduced falls, improved coordination in older adults, and better function in persons with arthritis (NCCIH, 2023c; Purdie, 2019). Many people find that tai chi helps reduce stress and promotes a general sense of well-being.

Yoga

Yoga has changed from a mystical form of Hindu worship practiced more than 5000 years ago to what is now known as a system of exercises involving various postures, meditation, and deep breathing. The word *yoga* means "union;" the union of body, mind, and spirit is achieved through yoga. Research suggests that yoga has many beneficial effects, such as reducing stress, improving mood and sense of well-being, decreasing heart rate and blood pressure, increasing lung capacity, improving flexibility, and promoting relaxation and healthy sleep (NCCIH, 2023d). Yoga can be adapted to any level and capability so that it can be easily used. While the risk of injury is lower than for higher impact physical activities, sprains and strains can occur; more older adults than younger adults experience injuries doing yoga.

Conclusion

There are many other alternative healing modalities, and new ones are appearing regularly. Some may be safe and effective but lack sufficient experience or clinical research to support their claims; others may be worthless and merely an attempt to sell a product or service.

Discretion is crucial. Assistance in gaining objective information regarding CAM therapies can be obtained from the National Center for Complementary and Integrative Health website (http://www.nccih.nih.gov) or by calling 1-888-644-6226.

NURSING AND COMPLEMENTARY AND ALTERNATIVE MEDICINE THERAPIES

A Holistic Approach

The use of natural or "alternative" healing measures is hardly new to nursing. From Florence Nightingale (1860), who wrote about the importance of creating an environment in which natural healing could occur, through contemporary nurse theorists who discussed human and environmental energy fields (Hover-Kramer, 2012; Meleis, 2017; Rogers, 1975), nurses have long realized that healing quite effectively occurs in ways not encompassed within the conventional biomedical system. Nursing also has promoted many of the same principles evident in CAM, particularly care of the body, mind, and spirit. In fact, this is the essence of holistic nursing (Box 11.5). Nurses must ensure that the integration of CAM into their practice is done within a holistic paradigm to truly make them healing therapies and not merely disconnected procedures within an already fragmented health care system.

Facilitating Use of Complementary and Alternative Medicine

Nurses need to integrate CAM into their nursing practice. This integration begins during the assessment process when the nurse explores clients' use of CAM practices and products. Because it is not unusual for clients to use them without the knowledge of their physicians, nurses may be the first health professional with whom clients have discussed this issue. Factors to assess include:

- CAM practices and products being used and their sources
- Appropriateness of use of CAM practices and products
- Side effects and risks associated with use of CAM
- Conditions for which CAM currently is not used that could benefit by its use

Through the assessment process, nurses may identify the need to educate clients about the appropriateness of the CAM products and practices they are using.

> ## BOX 11.5   Beliefs Guiding Holistic Nursing Practice
>
> - The uniqueness of each individual is honored.
> - Health is a harmonious balance of body, mind, and spirit.
> - The needs of individuals' bodies, minds, and spirits are assessed and addressed in the caregiving process.
> - Health and disease are natural parts of the human experience.
> - Disease is an opportunity for increased awareness of the interconnectedness of body, mind, and spirit.
> - Individuals have the capacity for self-healing; the nurse facilitates this process.
> - Nurses empower individuals for self-care.
> - Individuals' cultural values, beliefs, and practices are honored and incorporated into the caregiving process.
> - Individuals have a dynamic relationship with their environment; the environment is part of the healing process.
> - Nurses, through their presence and being, are tools of the healing process.
> - Nurses engage in self-care and an ongoing process of unfolding inner wisdom.

Nurses can learn about holistic nursing and network with holistic nurses through the American Holistic Nurses Association (AHNA) website (https://www.ahna.org).

For example, a client with a pacemaker who uses magnets needs to be advised against continuing this practice; likewise, a client who drinks ginseng tea at bedtime requires an explanation that his insomnia may be the result of the stimulant effects of the herb. There may be situations in which nurses identify that specific conditions could benefit from the use of CAM therapies. As client advocates nurses could bring this possibility to the attention of the physician and other members of the health care team and make recommendations accordingly.

Nurses traditionally have been responsible for the coordination of client care. As CAM therapies are integrated into conventional care, nurses are the logical professionals to oversee the various parts and ensure that they are working in harmony for the client's benefit.

Nurses can learn to use many alternative healing measures to enhance nursing care. Among these are acupressure, aromatherapy, biofeedback, imagery, massage, and TT. Nurses should seek whatever additional education and training are required to gain competency in these therapies and ensure compliance with state licensing laws.

Integrating Complementary and Alternative Medicine Into Conventional Settings

Nurses can demonstrate leadership in helping conventional clinical settings integrate CAM therapies. In fact

nursing's holistic orientation and traditional coordination responsibilities make nurses logical for this role. Case Study 11.1 describes how one nurse accomplished this task.

Using Complementary and Alternative Medicine Competently

As increasing numbers of consumers and clinical settings are interested in or actually using CAM therapies,

---

CASE STUDY 11.1

Becky Blake, RN, recently joined the nursing staff in a combined coronary care and step-down unit. It did not take her long to note the expert technical skill of her colleagues, who could read monitors in a flash and respond to emergencies without missing a beat. The skill, efficiency, and organization of the nursing staff were evidenced by the lack of medication errors, infections, and pressure ulcers, coupled with the shortest length of stays of comparable hospital units in the area.

Yet there seemed to be something missing. Clients and their families often showed signs of anxiety and fear that were not addressed. Familiar faces reappeared as some clients were readmitted because they failed to alter lifestyle habits that contributed to their conditions. The same nursing staff who cared for people with hearts damaged by the effects of smoking, poor diet, and stress were guilty of the same unhealthy practices themselves.

It came to a head for Ms. Blake one morning when she was at a bedside changing an intravenous bag and checking equipment. The client, a man in his fifties, pulled at her arm, looked Ms. Blake in the eyes, and tearfully said, "How do you think I'm going to do? I've been awake all night wondering if I'll be able to do my job, take care of my wife, see my grandkids grow up, do the things I like to do." For the first time, Ms. Blake saw beyond the body in the bed to a human being experiencing considerable emotional distress—distress that was hardly beneficial to his condition. "We have managed to get this man's heart repaired," she thought, "but we have not begun to help him heal the emotional and spiritual pain that this illness created." This began a journey for Ms. Blake of discovering measures to help clients that went beyond the conventional treatments that were regularly prescribed.

Ms. Blake found a local network of holistic nurses and began attending their meetings. Through this group she learned of the difference between healing and curing and the importance of addressing the needs of body, mind, and spirit. She also heard nurses discussing their own

need to be nurtured and committed to positive self-care practices. She met nurses who shared how they were using alternative healing practices and who led her to resources from which she could learn more.

In the months that followed Ms. Blake attended several workshops and learned how progressive relaxation, meditation, TT, and aromatherapy could be used to benefit the clients on her unit. As her understanding of holism grew Ms. Blake recognized that stress reduction and improved health habits for her coworkers were sorely needed.

After planting seeds through informal discussions and sharing of articles Ms. Blake requested a formal meeting with the interdisciplinary team on the unit. In this meeting she described her areas of concern, which included the need to:

- Address clients' emotional and spiritual needs more effectively.
- Promote improved health habits of the staff.
- Develop practices that would reduce stress for clients, their families, and staff.

The staff concurred with these needs and expressed a desire to take actions to address them. Ms. Blake offered some suggestions:

- Coordinate with the staff development instructor to have classes offered on progressive relaxation, imagery, meditation, TT, and stress reduction.
- Form an ad hoc committee to develop guidelines, policies, and procedures on how these healing therapies could be safely and legally implemented.
- Begin to include healing therapies into care plans.
- Arrange for the nutritionist to offer classes to staff on healthy eating.
- Add healthy snacks to the break room.
- Coordinate with the housekeeping and maintenance departments to introduce aromatherapy diffusers, plants, and piped-in music in the unit.
- Develop a system to remind staff to use stress reduction measures throughout their shift.

CASE STUDY 11.1—cont'd

- Collaborate with the nutritionist, social worker, spiritual care counselor, and nursing clinical resources to provide group sessions for clients and their families on topics such as coping with illness, stress management, and promoting healthy lifestyle habits.
- Request that the quality improvement coordinator monitor and evaluate the effect of these interventions.

It did not take long for the effects of these new approaches to be realized. Clients requested fewer sedatives and analgesics. Surveys of clients and families revealed higher levels of satisfaction. Staff sick days were reduced, and there seemed to be a greater sense of team spirit and cooperation. Soon staff in other parts of the hospital began requesting that similar interventions be implemented in their units.

---

nurses are challenged to become knowledgeable about the uses, limitations, and precautions associated with these new practices and products. Maintaining a resource library and becoming familiar with websites to stay current are beneficial measures.

Nurses must become familiar with cultural factors that can influence acceptance and use of alternative healing practices. For instance, some individuals may object to energy therapies (e.g., TT, HT) on the grounds that they associate them with occult practices, or they may have anxiety about meditation because they believe evil spirits could invade their minds. As comforting as a massage can be some people who come from cultures that believe it is inappropriate to touch a person of the opposite sex could become distressed by this measure. Knowledge and sensitivity to personal and cultural preferences are essential.

Legal Considerations

The use of CAM could present some legal issues for which nurses need to be concerned. As growing numbers of practitioners of healing therapies advocate for recognition and separate licensure, some of the healing therapies once considered part of nursing care may require separate licensure. Such is the case with massage. In some states nurses may not provide a massage unless they are licensed as massage therapists. Acupressure and biofeedback are among the other areas in which the nurse could be challenged if using them without a license. Nurses need to clarify the therapies that fall within the realm of nursing practice and take a proactive role in ensuring that other disciplines do not attempt to limit them.

Another legal concern for nurses in the growing arena of CAM is the question of to whom the nurse is responsible when practicing CAM therapies. New, nonconventional practice settings are developing. For example, a nurse may be employed in a setting in which there is an acupuncturist, hypnotherapist, and homeopath. Some questions that could arise include: Who supervises the nurse? Can these therapists delegate responsibilities to the nurse? How does the nurse ensure that in such a practice setting diagnoses are not being made or treatments being prescribed that are beyond the scope of the CAM practitioners? Nurses need to begin to consider the implications of new practice models and to develop clear practice guidelines that ensure a legally sound practice.

▮ SUMMARY

To summarize the chapter let's review the questions posed at the beginning of the chapter and see what you have learned.

1. What changes are occurring in our health care system to help reduce overall health care costs?

   Changes in the US health care system bring new challenges for professional nurses. Health care has moved from an emphasis on illness to an emphasis on wellness and prevention and is shifting from acute care services to preventive and community-based services such as ambulatory care and home care, which are less expensive sites for care than the acute-care setting. Financing of health care services has gone from retrospective, fee-for-service payment systems to prospective payment and managed care and continues to evolve through implementation of the ACA to expand insurance coverage and new models of financial rewards and incentives (e.g., never events, value-based purchasing, readmission reduction programs) to improve quality and reduce costs. US leaders and legislators agree that health care costs are too high, but they differ in the best ways to stop the increased costs. Most agree that when citizens practice healthy lifestyles they require less health care and enjoy a better quality of life.

2. What do health care economics and finance have to do with me as I provide patient care?

Nursing practice in a cost- and quality-conscious environment is here to stay. Nurses must constantly challenge current practice for quality improvement and cost-effectiveness. Accurate data must be collected to show cost containment and positive patient outcomes. Roles on clinical teams, in administration, with insurance companies, and with the government hold promise for empowered change. Nurses can take the lead by being healthy role models, educating consumers, and encouraging personal responsibility for improved health practices. Managing care brings nurses back to the basics as society recognizes that healthy people are good business.

3. Why do I need to understand health care reimbursement and its implications for individuals who do not have health insurance?

As visualized in the opening Vignette, Callie's understanding of the reimbursement mechanism for home health allows her to advocate for her patients to ensure they are receiving care that is paid for by Medicare while also helping her to educate her patients about actions to better manage their chronic illnesses or prevent readmissions. Nurses should also understand that uninsured patients may lack preventive care, poorly manage their chronic conditions, and/or not seek care until the later stages of a disease. Finding innovative strategies to help the uninsured patients achieve better health is an important role for the nurse in conjunction with the interprofessional team. Regardless of the nurse's practice setting, they must understand how health care services are being paid so they can contribute to leading and implementing nursing practices that promote health and reduce costs.

An opportunity exists for nurses to demonstrate leadership in the integration of CAM with conventional care. Representing the largest number of health care professionals, nurses can have a significant effect on implementing CAM throughout the health care system. Nurses' historical holistic orientation to care enables them to ensure that the integration of CAM and conventional services is done in a manner that addresses the client's body, mind, and spirit. Without such coordinated efforts there is the risk that these new therapies will merely be additional ingredients in an already fragmented system of care. Nurses have shown that they can coordinate and promote comprehensive care like practitioners of no other discipline. Therefore nursing is the logical discipline to be the hub of the wheel of integrative services.

REFERENCES

Benson, H., Beary, J.F., & Carol, M.P. (1974). The relaxation response. *Psychiatry, 37*(1), 37–46. https://doi.org/10.1080/00332747.1974.11023785

Bishop, F.L., (2019). Health behavior change and complementary medicine use. *Medicina (Kaunas), 55*(10), 632. https://doi.org/10.3390/medicina55100632

Fan, Y., Ji, X., Zhang, L., & Zhang X. (2021). The analgesic effects of static magnetic fields. *Bioelectromagnetics, 42(2):115-127.*

Hover-Kramer, D. (2012). *Healing touch: Essential energy medicine for yourself and others.* Sounds True.

Huang, L., Xu, G., Sun, M., Yang, C., Luo, Q., et al. (2023). Recent trends in acupuncture for chronic pain: A bibliometric analysis and review of the literature. *Complementary Therapies in Medicine, 72*:102915. https://www.sciencedirect.com/science/article/pii/S096522992300002X

Kaye, E.C. (2020). Finding faith. *Journal of the American Medical Association, 323*(7), 609–610. https://doi.org/10.1001/jama.2020.0580

Krieger, D. (1979). *The therapeutic touch.* Prentice Hall.

Lee, I.S. (2020). Bibliometric analysis of research assessing the use of acupuncture for pain treatment over the past 20 years. *Journal of Pain Research, 13,* 367–376. https://doi.org/10.2147/JPR.S235047

Meleis, A.I. (2017). *Theoretical nursing: Development and progress* (6th ed.) Lippincott.

Montgomery, A.D., & Ottenbacher, R. (2020). Battlefield acupuncture for chronic pain management in patients on long-term opioid therapy. *Medical Acupuncture, 32*(1), 38–44. https://doi.org/10.1089/acu.2019.1382

Nahin, R.L., (2016). Expenditures on complementary health approaches: United States. *National Health Statistics Reports, No. 95*, National Center for Health Statistics.

National Center for Complementary and Integrative Health. (2023a). *Magnets for pain: What you need to know.* https://nccih.nih.gov/Health/magnets-for-pain-what-you-need-to-know

National Center for Complementary and Integrative Health. (2023b). *Reiki.* https://nccih.nih.gov/health/reiki-info

National Center for Complementary and Integrative Health. (2023c). *Tai chi: What you need to know.* https://www.nccih.nih.gov/health/tai-chi-what-you-need-to-know

National Center for Complementary and Integrative Health. (2023d). *Yoga: What you need to know.* https://nccih.nih.gov/health/yoga-what-you-need-to-know

National Center for Complementary and Integrative Health. (2019b). *Using dietary supplements wisely.* https://nccih.nih.gov/health/supplements/wiseuse.htm

National Center for Complementary and Integrative Health (2021). *Complementary, alternative, or integrative: What's in a name?* https://www.nccih.nih.gov/health/complementary-alternative-or-integrative-health-whats-in-a-name

Nelson, D.H., Perchaluk, J.M., Logan, A.C., & Katzman, M.A. (2019). The bell tolls for homeopathy: Time for change in the training and practice of North American naturopathic physicians. *Journal of Evidence-Based Integrative Medicine, 24*, 1–11. https://doi.org/10.1177/2515690X18823696

Nightingale, F. (1860). *Notes on nursing.* Harrison.

O'Brien, M.E. (2017). *Spirituality in nursing: Standing on holy ground* (6th ed.) Jones & Bartlett.

Phutrakool, P., & Pongpirul, K. (2022). Acceptance and use of complementary and alternative medicine among medical specialist: A 15-year systematic review and data synthesis. *Systematic Reviews*, 11, 10. https://doi.org/10.1186/s13643-021-01882-4

Purdie, N. (2019). Tai chi to prevent falls in older adults. *British Journal of Community Nursing, 24*(11), 550–552. https://doi.org/10.12968/bjcn.2019.24.11.550

Roberts, E.R., Eizayaga, J.E., van der Werf, E.T., & Tournier, A.L. (2023). HRI Online 2022: Leading experts illustrate the positive impact of increased collaboration in homeopathy research. *Homeopathy,* Feb;112(1):65–69.

Rogers, M. (1975). *An introduction to the theoretical basis for nursing* (3rd ed.) FA Davis.

Sahebkaram, Z., Bahrami, R., Azima, . & Akbarzadeh, M. (2022). Efficacy of aromatherapy for night crying in infants with infantile colic: A double-blind randomized controlled study. *International Journal of Preventive Medicine,* 13:159.

Singh, S., Kshtriya, S. & Valk, R. (2023). Health, hope, and harmony: A systematic review of the determinants of happiness across cultures and countries. *International Journal of Environmental Research and Health, 20*(4):3306. https://doi.org/10.3390/ijerph20043306, 13 February 2023.

Theisen, E., & Konieczy, E. (2019). *Medical cannabis: What nurses need to know.* https://www.myamericannurse.com/medical-cannabis-what-nurses-need-to-know/

Therapeutic Touch International Association. (2023). *A brief overview of TTIA.* https://therapeutictouch.org/about-us/

Victor, C.G.P., & Treschuk, J.V. (2019). *Critical literature review on the definition clarity of the concept of faith, religion, and spirituality.* https://doi.org/10.1177/0898010119895368

Worster, B., Ashare, R.L., Hajjar, E., Smith, K. & Kelly, E.L. (2021). Clinician attitudes, training, and beliefs about cannabis: An interprofessional assessment. *Cannabis Cannabinoid Research,* Dec 31, published online: http://doi.org/10.1089/can.2021.0022

ADDITIONAL RESOURCES

Barr, T.L., & Nathenson, S.L. (2022). A holistic transcendental leadership model for enhancing innovation, creativity, and well-being in health care. *Journal of Holistic Nursing, 40*(2):157–168.

Black, T. (2020). *Hospice and palliative care acupuncture.* Singing Dragon.

Braza, J. (2020). *Practicing mindfulness: Finding calm and focus in your everyday life.* Tuttle Publishing.

Carrere, E., & Lambert, J. (2023). *Yoga.* Picador.

Chevalier, A. (2023). *Encyclopedia of herbal medicine: 560 herbs and remedies for common ailments.* (4th ed.) DK Publishing.

Cohen, M.R. (2020). *The Chinese medicine companion: A modern guide to ancient healing.* Fair Winds Press.

Cooper, K.L. (2022). Spirituality and standards for practice: A critical discourse analysis. *Journal of Holistic Nursing, 40*(1):16–24.

Corasaniti, M.T., Bagetta, G., Morrone, L.A., et al. (2023). Efficacy of essentials oils in relieving cancer pain: A systematic review and meta-analysis. *International Journal of Molecular Science, 24*(8):7085.

Crawford, C., Brown, L.L., Costello, R.B., & Deuster, P.A. (2023). Immune supplements under the magnifying glass: An expert panel develops priorities and evidence-based recommendations for future research regarding dietary supplements. *Journal of Integrative and Complementary Medicine, 29*(4):261–267.

Danell, J.A.B. (2019). "I could feel it!": A qualitative study on how users of complementary medicine experience and form knowledge about treatments. *Journal of Holistic Nursing, 37*(4), 338–353. https://doi.org/10.1177/0898010119837427

Deleemans, J., MacLeod, J., Fuentes, E., et al. (2023). Exploring the roles of patient advocates in integrative oncology. *Journal of Integrative and Complementary Medicine, 29*(3): 134-138.

Deutsch, J.K. (2020). Complementary and alternative medicine for functional gastrointestinal disorders. *American Journal of Gastroenterology, 115*(3), 350–364. https://doi.org/10.14309/ajg.0000000000000539

Eliopoulos, C. (2018). *Invitation to holistic health: A guide to living a balanced life* (4th ed.) Jones & Bartlett.

Fontaine, K.L. (2018). *Complementary & alternative therapies for nursing practice* (5th ed.) Prentice Hall.

Frisch, N.C., & Rabinowitsch, D. (2019). What's in a definition? Holistic nursing, integrative health care, and integrative nursing: Report of an integrated literature review. *Journal of Holistic Nursing, 37*(3), 260–272. https://doi.org/10.1177/0898010119860685

Golden, J., Kenyon-Pesce, L., & Guerra, M.P. (2023). Disclosure of complementary and alternative medicine use among older adults: A cross sectional study. *Gerontology and Geriatric Medicine,* Published online June 6, 2023, https://journals.sagepub.com/doi/10.1177/23337214231179839

Hamwee, J. (2020). *Experiencing acupuncture.* Singing Dragon Press.

Harris, B. (2022). *A comprehensive approach to complementary and alternative medicine.* Murphy & Moore Publishing.

LaForge, K., Gray, M., Livingston, C.J., et al. Clinician perspectives on referring Medicaid back pain patients to integrative and complementary medicine: A qualitative study. *Journal of Integrative and Complementary Medicine, 29*(1):55–60.

Lara-Cinisomo, S. (2019). Feasibility of a mindfulness-based intervention for caregivers of veterans: A pilot study. *Journal of Holistic Nursing, 37*(4):322–337. https://doi.org/10.1177/0898010119831580

Maddocks, W. (2023). Aromatherapy in nursing and midwifery practice: A scoping review of published studies since 2005. *Journal of Holistic Nursing, 21*(1):62–89.

Micozzi, M.S. (2019). *Fundamentals of complementary and alternative medicine* (6th ed.) Saunders.

Murley, B. (2019). Influence of Tai Chi on self-efficacy, quality of life, and fatigue among patients with cancer receiving chemotherapy: A pilot study brief. *Journal of Holistic Nursing, 37*(4), 354–363. https://doi.org/10.1177/0898010119890389

National Center for Complementary and Integrative Health. (2023.). Cannabis (marijuana) and cannabinoids: What you need to know. https://www.nccih.gov/health/cannabis-marijuana-and-cannabinoids-what-you-need-to-know

National Center for Complementary and Integrative Health. (2023). *Herbs at a glance.* https://www.nccih.nih.gov/health/herbsataglance

National Agriculture Library. (2023). *Dietary reference intakes (DRIs).* https://www.nal.usda.gov/fnic/dietary-reference-intakes.

Newcombe, R. (2023). *Natural remedies guide.* Thunder Bay Press.

O'Brien, M.E. (2021). *Spirituality in nursing: Standing on holy ground* (7th ed.) Jones & Bartlett Learning.

Paquette, L., Haring, E., Jones, M. et al. (2023). *Radiant spirits: Holistic coaches share how radiant life can be.* Radiant Publishing.

Pizzorno, J.E., & Murray, M.T. (2020). *Textbook of natural medicine* (5th ed.) Churchill Livingstone.

Rediger, J. (2020). *Cured: The life-changing science of spontaneous healing.* Flatiron Books.

Rosenberg, K. (2020). Mind-body therapies can improve pain and opioid-related outcomes. *American Journal of Nursing, 120*(3):68. https://doi.org/10.1097/01.NAJ.0000656376.74649.a1

Rustica, S. (2020). *Advanced herbal pharmacy: The practitioner's guide to preparation, formulation and compounding.* Lincoln Town Press.

Sanogo, F., Xu, K., Cortessis, V.K., et al. (2023). Mind- and body-based interventions improve glycemic control in patients with type 2 diabetes: A systematic review and meta-analysis. *Journal of Integrative and Complementary Medicine, 29*(2):69–79.

Sherman, K.J. (2020). T'ai C'hi for chronic low back pain in older adults: A feasibility trial. *Journal of Alternative and Complementary Medicine, 26*(3), 176–189. https://doi.org/10.1089/acm.2019.0438

Simkin, D.R., Swick, S., Taneja, K.S., & Ranjbar, N. (2023). Complementary and integrative medicine for anxiety in children, adolescents, and young adults. *Child and Adolescent Clinics of North America, 32*(2):193–216.

Stefanon, L. (2023). The science and art of holistic wound care. *Journal of Wound Care, 32*(5):262–263.

Sulak, D. (2020). *Handbook of cannabis for clinicians. Principles and practices.* W.W. Norton & Co.

Swanberg, S. (2019). *A patient's guide to acupuncture: Everything you need to know.* Althea Press.

Swanberg, S. (2020). *Aromatherapy for self-care: Your complete guide to relax, rebalance, and restore with essential oils.* Rockridge Press.

Tselios, K. (2023). *The essential book of Ayurveda: Secrets of ancient healing wisdom.* Sirius.

Wexler, T.M. & Schellinger, J. (2023). Mindfulness-based stress reduction for nurses: An integrative review. *Journal of Holistic Nursing, 41*(1):40–59.

Yifang, Z. (2020). *A comprehensive handbook of traditional Chinese medicine: Prevention & healing.* Shanghai Press.

12

Palliative Care

Patricia R. Keene, DNP, ACNP-BC, ACHPN

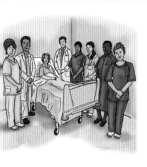

Palliative care: A team concept.

ⓔ Additional resources are available online at: http://evolve.elsevier.com/Cherry/

LEARNING OUTCOMES

After studying this chapter, the reader will be able to:

1. Describe the palliative care model and its effectiveness today.
2. Summarize the key elements and issues of palliative care.
3. Integrate palliative care knowledge and skills into the professional nursing role.

KEY TERMS

Advance care plan This is a *process* of examining one's thoughts and feelings about what gives one's life value. By determining what gives value to one's life, one is then able to determine the goals for their health care. For example, watching and understanding a 6-year-old grandchild's baseball game could be a strong value for an elderly grandfather. This requires that the man have ears that can hear and a brain that can understand. Should this same patient have a catastrophic stroke and in light of his cited value, he would choose to not have his life artificially prolonged but rather to die in the comfort of his home with hospice care. This is an example of the *process* that a patient might go through to determine health care goals. Further, the advance care plan consists of two parts: the advance directive documenting decisions made for the future, and listing the decision-makers who will decide for the patient if the patient is unable to do so.

Advance directive A *document* in which a person with decision-making capacity gives permission about future medical care and/or designates the person to make decisions for them if decision-making capacity is impaired or lost.

Decision-making capacity The ability of one to make decisions about their health care. They must be able to understand the facts, to appreciate the alternatives that may exist, and to communicate these decisions to the health care team.

Disease trajectory The decline that is seen as a particular disease progresses.

Double effect In the care of seriously ill and dying patients, the intent of any treatment is to relieve pain and suffering—not to hasten the patient's death; however, the patient's death is a foreseeable potential effect of the treatment. An example would be escalating doses of morphine to relieve a patient's pain with the double effect of depressing respirations, resulting in death.

End-of-Life Nursing Education Consortium (ELNEC) A national project funded by the Robert Wood Johnson Foundation.

Hospice care This is not only a type of care but also a philosophy of care that focuses on comfort for the patient and family at the end of life.

Informed consent Permission given by a patient or caregiver to treat a medical condition with understanding of the risks/benefits of a medical procedure, costs that may accrue, and alternative therapies.

Interprofessional team A group of professionals that works together to provide comprehensive care to the patient/family.

Palliative care Care that seeks to improve the quality of life of patients who are facing serious illness.

Patient Self-Determination Act (PSDA) A federal law that requires health care institutions to give patients

a copy of their decision-making rights, determine whether patients have advance directives, and assist them in completing them. The PSDA promotes patients making their own decisions about the health care they want to receive or refuse.

Prognostication A physician's prediction about the course and outcome of a disease, often made with consideration of survival, symptoms, function, and quality of life with or without treatment.

PROFESSIONAL/ETHICAL ISSUE

Mrs. P. is an 85-year-old widowed female admitted to the hospital with end-stage Parkinson's disease, which was diagnosed 5 years ago. Her family reports that she has had three falls in the past 2 weeks and during the past 6 months has lost 20 pounds. The weight loss is more than 10% of her body weight. She scores 40% on the Palliative Performance Scale and was recently diagnosed with right lower lobe pneumonia. The family states that she is having difficulty communicating her needs and is having dysphagia. It was thought that her recent pneumonia was secondary to aspiration. Two of her daughters want to start enteral feedings via a percutaneous endoscopic gastrostomy tube. When asked about advance directives, the family reports that Mrs. P. does not have any. A third daughter indicates that she would not want artificial nutrition and that they had talked about it. The first two daughters are concerned that she would starve to death.

As the RN on the palliative care team, what steps will you take to help the family come to consensus about whether to provide artificial nutrition?

Schwarz and Tarzian (2010) demonstrate a method of analyzing situations that are ethically challenging (Table 12.1).

VIGNETTE

Christine Glover is a 32-year-old divorced female who has been undergoing aggressive cancer chemotherapy for 4 years. Her physician has informed her that her disease continues to spread in spite of these therapies. He tells her that there are two primary options: a Phase I clinical trial and hospice care. She longs to see her young

children settled in with her parents before she dies, but she suffers with constant pain and intermittent nausea, and gravitates between anxiety and deep periods of depression, which she hides as best as she can from her family. She struggles between the two options of care, but doesn't know what questions to ask related to treatment. How does she tell her children? How does she prepare her parents for the role of parenting their grandchildren? How can she prepare herself for what lies ahead? She feels the depression enveloping her again.

Questions to Consider While Reading this Chapter:

1. What patient experiences have you had related to serious illness?
2. What do you think is important to include in serious illness/end-of-life discussions?
3. Have you considered how you would like to live during serious illness?
4. Have you completed your advance directive?
5. How can nursing research affect end-of-life care?

CHAPTER OVERVIEW

Someone should tell us, right at the start of our lives, that we are dying. Then we might live life to the limit, every minute of every day. Do it! I say. Whatever you want to do, do it now! There are only so many tomorrows.

Pope Paul VI, 1897–1978

Palliative care is one of the newest subspecialties. The focus of palliative care is to give comfort to patients

TABLE 12.1 Steps to Analyze Situations Seen as Ethically Challenging and to Explore the Context in Which These Situations Have Arisen	
Steps to Analyze Ethically Challenging Situations	**Context of the Situation**

1. Review the overall situation—identify what is going on in the case.
2. Identify the ethical dilemma(s).
3. Gather all relevant facts:
  • Significant medical and social history
  • Involved family
  • Decision-making capacity
  • Existence of advance directives—written, appointed, or verbal—and any pertinent institutional policies
  • Surrogate or health care agent if decision-making capacity is absent
4. Identify the parties or stakeholders involved in the situation, including those who will be affected by the decision(s) made.
5. Identify relevant legal data, including state and federal laws.
6. Identify religious or cultural issues.
7. Identify specific conflicts of ethical principles or values. Identify and consider nursing guidelines and the profession's code and position statements.
8. Identify possible options, their purpose, and their probable consequences to the welfare of the patient. Identify and make use of interdisciplinary and institutional resources, including ethics committee, social workers, chaplains, and other experienced colleagues.
9. Identify practical constraints, including institutional, legal, organizational, and economic.
10. Review and evaluate the situation after action has been taken—debrief and support the staff.
	1. Mrs. P. has a disease that is end stage (Parkinson's disease).
	2. Mrs. P. no longer has capacity and is nonverbal. There are no advance directives. Daughters are in disagreement regarding mother's wishes for health care.
	3. The patient has a history of decline starting 4 years earlier, culminating to her present state. She does not have decision-making capacity. She did tell one daughter that she did not want a feeding tube.
	4. Stakeholders include the patient and three daughters.
	5. There is no relevant legal data.
	6. No religious or cultural beliefs identified.
	7. Ethical principles involved are: autonomy, beneficence, maleficence, and double effect.
	8. Options include feeding tube placement, artificial hydration. Risks of providing artificial nutrition and hydration (ANH) include aspiration, third spacing of fluids, diarrhea/constipation.
	9. The team recognizes patient is unable to participate in the decision-making process. The daughters report that they want what is best for their mother.
	10. The decision is made not to start fluids or place a feeding tube. The patient is offered food and fluids orally until she is unable to swallow. She is allowed to die a natural death.

From Schwarz, J.K., & Tarzian, A.J. (2010). Ethical aspects of palliative care. In Matzo, M., & Sherman, D.W. (Eds.). *Palliative care nursing: Quality care to the end of life* (pp. 119–141). Springer.

with serious illness. It can begin with the diagnosis of a serious illness and continue to the death of the patient, followed by continued support of the family. The purpose of this chapter is to describe the benefits, barriers, and challenges of palliative care as well as to discuss the role of the palliative care nurse.

INTRODUCTION

The world of health care is constantly changing; yet for Western health care, the growth and advancement of new and innovative treatments are mind-boggling.

With these new therapies come an increasing emphasis on care and rehabilitation of those with serious illness. Today, we live longer; by 2030 20% of the American population will be more than 65 years of age (Meier et al., 2010).

Palliative care was coined by Dr. Balfour Mount in 1974. It comes from the Latin root word *pallium*, which referred to an outer garment that cloaked a person. This derivation suggests that palliative care "covers" or "cloaks" the symptoms of serious illness, providing comfort and relief. Palliative care recognizes the same needs, stressors, symptoms, and suffering that a hospice patient might endure, but supports and enhances the best quality of life during the time of diagnosis, treatment, and life with serious illness.

The World Health Organization defined palliative care in 1990:

> *Palliative care is an approach that improves the quality of life of patients and their families facing the problem associated with life-threatening illness, through the prevention and relief of suffering by means of early identification and impeccable assessment and treatment of pain and other problems, physical, psychosocial, and spiritual (Sepúlveda et al., 2002).*

The Hospice and Palliative Nurses Association (HPNA) developed standards of practice for registered nurses. HPNA defines a palliative nurse as one who:

- Provides age-appropriate culturally, ethically, and spiritually sensitive care and support.
- Maintains a safe environment.
- Educates patients/families to identify appropriate settings and treatment options.
- Ensures continuity of care and safe transitions to the next appropriate setting.
- Coordinates care across settings and among caregivers.
- Manages information and protects confidentiality.
- Communicates promptly and effectively.

However, nurses must recognize the need for palliative care in all settings and in all specialties. In 2007 Stjernswärd and colleagues recognized that palliative care should be seen as a public health issue and as such all health care clinicians would do well to become palliative care generalists. As stated in the American Nurses Association (ANA) *Code of Ethics for Nurses,* "Nursing care is directed toward meeting the comprehensive needs of patients and their families across the continuum of care. This is particularly vital in the care of patients and their families at the end of life to prevent and relieve the cascade of symptoms of suffering that are commonly associated with dying" (ANA, 2015).

THE NATURAL COURSE OF SERIOUS ILLNESS

As a patient's health declines, decisions about care must be made. With the initial diagnosis, palliative care can help guide therapy. With disease progression to an end-stage condition, hospice is an option of care. Prior to palliative care, the care model showed disease progression and then death. The palliative care continuum model of care (Fig. 12.1) begins comfort care at the time of diagnosis: Early in the disease process therapies are aggressive, but as the disease progresses comfort care increases. Included in this model is the introduction of hospice care and bereavement services.

As patient decline occurs, palliative care or hospice care becomes the focus. Frequently the terms are used synonymously, which is incorrect because they differ. Both offer comfort care to the patient with serious illness, but in hospice care the disease is considered end stage with progression to death. Hospice care provides support to not only the patient but also the family.

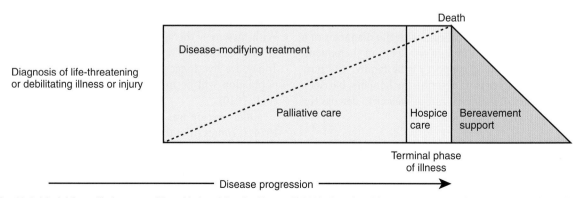

Fig. 12.1 Model for palliative care. (From National Quality Forum. [2006]. *A national framework and preferred practices for palliative and hospice care quality: A consensus report.* http://www.qualityforum.org/Publications/2006/12/A_National_Framework_and_Preferred_Practices_for_Palliative_and_Hospice_Care_Quality.aspx.)

Support includes physical assistance but also emotional, psychologic, and spiritual support. Hospice is underutilized by much of the population, and this lack of use can be due to cultural beliefs, lack of understanding, fear, or decreased availability. Table 12.2 compares hospice and palliative care services.

Prognostication

Patients with serious illness question the time they have until death. Predicting a patient's death is not a simple task. Research shows that when physicians prognosticate, they are optimistic in predicting survival by up to as much as 300% (von Gunten, 2014). Physicians are faced with the task of telling a patient that their time to live is limited. This is difficult not only because of medical complexity but also because emotions come into play when there has been a patient–physician relationship. The disease process is distinguished by its severity and ability to be cured. Laboratory and diagnostic findings help to track the progress of the disease—is it improving or progressing? Current functional status of the patient, including a history of falls, can be helpful for predicting as well. When functional status is examined, cognitive ability and the ability to perform activities of daily living are reviewed (Singh et al., 2019).

A number of tools are used to help with prognostication. The Palliative Performance Scale (PPS) (Table 12.3) and the Karnofsky Scale (Table 12.4) are two such tools. The PPS is a more general tool that identifies functional decline and scores it. Scores are an indication about disease progression to death. The Karnofsky Scale is more appropriate for the patient with a cancer diagnosis.

TABLE 12.2 Comparison of Hospice and Palliative Care Services

Component	Palliative Care	Hospice
Focus of care	To address the specific needs of patients and families experiencing serious illness	To address the specific needs of the dying patient and their family, including bereavement services
Onset of care	Begins at the time of diagnosis of a serious illness	Begins with a prognosis of 6 months or less
Medicare benefit	Physicians (MDs) and nurse practitioners may bill	Yes
Beneficiary entitled to levels of care	No specific levels of care	Yes. Routine home care, respite care, general inpatient care, continuous care
Settings where care delivered	All inpatient settings, outpatient, private practice, home care	Home, nursing home, residential, hospice, inpatient (on designated unit or designated beds)
Interprofessional team approach	Yes	Yes
Supplies and symptom management medications covered	No	Yes
Therapies limited	No. Palliative care is delivered with aggressive treatment and therapies	Yes. Therapies with significant burden but that may prolong life are restricted
Quality components include safety, timeliness, patient-centered care, beneficial/effective care, equity, and efficiency	Yes	Yes
Expertise on pain and symptom management	Yes	Yes
Appropriate at any age	Yes	Yes
Effective initiation of life planning	Most effective	Effective if discussions occur prior to hospice or if earlier referrals to hospice

TABLE 12.3 Palliative Performance Scale

%	Ambulation	Evidence of Disease	Self-Care	Intake	Level of Consciousness
100	Full	Normal No disease	Full	Normal	Full
90	Full	Normal Some disease	Full	Normal	Full
80	Full	Normal with effort Some disease	Full	Normal or reduced	Full
70	Reduced	Can't do normal job or work Some disease	Full	As above	Full
60	Reduced	Can't do hobbies or housework Significant disease	Occasional assistance needed	As above	Full or confusion
50	Mainly sit/lie	Can't do any work Extensive disease	Considerable assistance needed	As above	Full or confusion
40	Mainly in bed	As above	Mainly assistance	As above	Full or drowsy or confusion
30	Bedbound	As above	Total care	Reduced	As above
20	Bedbound	As above	As above	Minimal	As above
10	Bedbound	As above	As above	Mouth care only	Drowsy or coma
0	Death	—	—	—	—

From Anderson, F., Downing, G.M., Hill, J., et al. (1996). Palliative performance scale (PPS): A new tool. *Journal of Palliative Care, 12*(1):6. Copyright: Institut universitaire de gériatrie de Montréal.

TABLE 12.4 Karnofsky Performance Status Scale

Score	Criteria	Definitions
100	Normal, no complaints, no evidence of disease	Able to carry on normal activity and to work, no special care needed
90	Able to carry on normal activity, minor symptoms	
80	Normal activity with some symptoms	
70	Cares for self, unable to carry on normal activities	Unable to work; able to live at home and care for most personal needs; various degrees of assistance needed
60	Requires occasional assistance, cares for most needs	
50	Requires considerable assistance and frequent care	
40	Disabled, requires special care and assistance	Unable to care for self; requires equivalent of institutional or hospital care; disease may be progressing rapidly
30	Severely disabled; hospitalized but death not imminent	
20	Very sick; active supportive care needed	
10	Moribund; fatal processes are progressing rapidly	
0	Death	

From Callin, S.E., & Bennett, M.I. (2009). Assessment of mobility. In Walsh, T.D., Caraceni, A., Fainsinger, R., et al (Eds.). *Palliative medicine*. Saunders.

It is helpful to compare the patient's status at 12 months, 6 months, and 1 month previously as well as the current status. The patient's ability to perform activities of daily living, a change in appetite, weight loss, anorexia/cachexia, and/or dysphagia all help paint the picture of serious illness with decline. Laboratory findings and diagnostic test results can also help validate the presence of serious illness. For example, by examination of laboratory data one is able to assess the extent of organ decline.

After the nurse has gathered the objective and subjective data, a meeting with the patient and family is imperative. With *family* being defined by the patient, a family conference is invaluable. A group meeting allows everyone to hear the same thing at the same time from the health care provider. There is less room for misinterpretation as information is presented at a level understood by the patient and family. There must be time for questions. Information given must be realistic but should not take away hope.

There are different types of hope: hope for a cure; hope for more time; hope for no pain; hope for a good death. Often physicians shy away from specific time frames because the disease course can vary from patient to patient and it may take away hope. What is helpful is if the patient/family can understand the "usual course of the illness." Some disease states follow a more predictable pattern—for example, metastatic cancer. Deaths due to heart failure, emphysema, or dementia, however, are not as easily predicted. With these disease states, it is helpful to review with the patient and family the decline that has already occurred. Plotting it on paper shows the decline and makes it more real. This discussion of prognostication does not end with one meeting but is ongoing as the disease progresses toward the end of life. Additionally, education is ongoing throughout the disease process for the patient and family.

Two Roads to Death. Ferris and colleagues (2003) describe two roads to death: the usual road and the difficult road. The usual road is what most would describe as a peaceful death, in which the patient begins sleeping more and being less and less responsive. They progress to a comatose state and dies. Caregivers describe the death as peaceful and comfortable. The difficult road, on the other hand, is one of restlessness with increased confusion and frequently with hallucinations. To avoid the difficult death, health care providers must view not only the physical aspects of patient care but also the emotional, spiritual, and psychosocial aspects. Physical pain can be medicated; however, emotional/spiritual pain is complicated and medications cannot always erase it. Health care providers must be open to listening and encouraging the patient to deal with difficult issues while able to do so.

When death occurs, it can be verified by the absence of heartbeat and respirations, fixed and dilated pupils, and absence of the corneal reflex. Other signs that are seen include a change in skin color and temperature. Frequently, eyes do not close completely and the jaw may remain open. Urine and stool may also be expelled. Depending on the setting, the patient is pronounced deceased by a nurse or physician.

Criteria for Palliative Care

For most institutions, a physician's order is required for hospice/palliative care services. Patients can be referred on admission as well as during their hospital stays. On admission patients who have had multiple hospitalizations over a relatively short time for the same condition (e.g., heart failure, urinary tract infection, sepsis) should be considered. Things that may trigger a palliative care consult include (Weissman & Meier, 2011):

- Receiving a positive response when asking oneself the "surprise" question: "Would I be surprised if this patient died within 6 months to a year?"
- Patients who are receiving multifaceted care such as ventilator support, parenteral feedings, and assistance with functional needs
- A patient's place of residence in a long-term care facility (e.g., nursing home)
- The age of the patient
- Cognitive impairment
- Metastatic cancer
- Current or past enrollment in hospice care
- A patient who has not participated in advance care planning

Throughout a hospital stay, other triggers can indicate the need for a palliative care consult. These triggers may include the patient's desire to change health care providers, patient or family request for palliative care, and dissension about therapy/treatments being offered. Other triggers are a prolonged stay in the intensive care unit and symptoms that have not been controlled. Palliative care can assist with decisions about long-term use of feeding tubes, need for tracheostomy, dialysis, placement of a left ventricular assist device or automatic implanted cardioverter-defibrillator (AICD), and other life-prolonging therapies.

Palliative care can assist patients and their families with decision-making regarding goals of care. For example, the initial intent of therapy may have been cure, but the disease was found to be widespread. The focus could then change to comfort. The patient may hear "There is nothing more we can do," but there is always care to be provided. It is the focus of the care that changes: the quality of time may now be the focus rather than the quantity.

Hospice Services

The term *hospice*, derived from the word *hospitality,* can be traced back to medieval times when it referred to a place of shelter and rest for weary or ill travelers on a long journey. The name was first applied to specialized care for dying patients by physician Dame Cicely Saunders, who began her work with the terminally ill in 1948 and eventually went on to create the first modern hospice—St. Christopher's Hospice—in London. She was also responsible for coining the term *total pain* to describe the full experience of physical, emotional, spiritual, and social distress and suffering of many hospice patients.

Saunders introduced the idea of specialized care for the dying to the United States in a lecture at Yale University. Her lecture on holistic hospice care launched a chain of events that resulted in the development of hospice care in the United States. This chain of events was spearheaded by Florence Wald, MS, RN, a former dean of Yale University School of Nursing.

Definition and Criteria for Hospice Care

Considered the model for quality, compassionate care at the end of life, hospice care involves a team-oriented approach of expert medical care focused on symptom management and is expressly tailored to the patient's wishes. Support is also extended to the family and loved ones. Generally, this care is provided in a number of settings. Medicare, private health insurance, and Medicaid in most states cover hospice care for patients. A patient is deemed an appropriate candidate for hospice care if they have a terminal diagnosis—that is, the patient has been assessed according to disease factors defined by Medicare that determine a person's eligibility for hospice care. Examples of these factors include a patient's ability to breathe or patient's refusal of dialysis.

Hospice recognizes that the dying process is a part of the normal process of living and focuses on enhancing the quality of remaining life. Hospice affirms life and neither hastens nor works to postpone death. The hospice team is interdisciplinary and develops a care plan that meets each patient's individual needs for pain management and symptom control. Team members include the same disciplines as those for palliative care. Included in hospice responsibilities are managing the patient's pain and symptoms; assisting the patient with the emotional, psychosocial, and spiritual aspects of dying; providing needed drugs, medical supplies, and equipment; and coaching the family on caring for the patient as well as addressing family distress and suffering.

KEY ELEMENTS OF PALLIATIVE CARE

Eight Elements of End-of-Life Nursing Education Consortium

The End-of-Life Nursing Education Consortium (ELNEC) is a project started in February 2002 by Bettye Ferrell at City of Hope with a grant from the Robert Wood Johnson Foundation. The ELNEC core curriculum identifies eight modules: nursing care at the end of life, pain management, symptom management, ethical/legal issues, cultural considerations, communication, loss/grief/bereavement, and final hours. The goal of this project was to improve palliative care. Now there are ELNEC curricula for pediatrics, critical care, oncology, veterans, geriatrics, and advanced practice nursing. The newest model is integrating palliative oncology care into the Doctor of Nursing Practice. The ELNEC program went international in May 2008, again with the goal of educating nurses (http://www.aacnnursing.org/ELNEC).

The Eight Domains of the National Consensus Project

The National Consensus Project (NCP) for Quality Palliative Care, which began in 2001, is a task force of organizations that strives to improve palliative care. The organizations involved are: American Academy of Hospice and Palliative Medicine (AAHPM), Center to Advance Palliative Care (CAPC), Hospice and Palliative Care Nurses Association, and National Hospice and Palliative Care Organization (NHPCO). NCP identifies eight practice domains for palliative care to follow:

- *Domain 1: Structure and Processes of Care.* This domain describes the use of the interprofessional team to work together assessing and planning care with patients and families.

- *Domain 2: Physical Aspects of Care.* This domain emphasizes the use of validated tools for assessment and the treatment of physical symptoms.
- *Domain 3: Psychological and Psychiatric Aspects of Care.* This domain stresses the need to address assessment and treatment of psychiatric concerns and diagnoses. Included also in this domain are the requirements of a bereavement program.
- *Domain 4: Social Aspects of Care.* This domain's focus emphasizes engaging patients and families in the patient's care and taking advantage of their strengths. The team social worker begins this process.
- *Domain 5: Spiritual, Religious, and Existential Aspects of Care.* This domain focuses on involving the chaplain in the plan of care throughout the disease trajectory. Spiritual and religious practices are encouraged as a means to obtain comfort.
- *Domain 6: Cultural Aspects of Care.* This domain focuses on the inclusion of cultural aspects when providing care and holds that the interprofessional team should be culturally competent.
- *Domain 7: Care of the Patient at the End of Life.* This domain emphasizes communication and physical signs and symptoms of the dying process. Again the patient/families/interprofessional team should be involved with scrupulous assessment and management of pain and other symptoms. Ongoing education about the dying process is of utmost importance for families.
- *Domain 8: Ethical and Legal Aspects of Care.* This domain addresses advance care planning and ethical/legal aspects. Advance care planning is seen as something that is ongoing and may change throughout the disease course. This domain reaffirms that ethical issues are common and must be addressed. The identification of complex legal and regulatory issues of palliative care is also addressed in this domain. (For more information, see https://www.nationalcoalitionhpc.org/ncp/.)

BENEFITS OF PALLIATIVE CARE

Palliative care can be viewed as both a model of care and a philosophy of serving our patients. It is built of multiple components as expressed in the ELNEC's curriculum (ELNEC, 2020).

- The family is the unit of care and the patient defines family.

- The role of the nurse as an advocate is vital to the care of patients and their families.
- Culture is honored as an important aspect of the patient/family.
- Palliative care further carries an important focus to special populations such as the vulnerable, the prisoner, and the substance abuser.
- Serious illness affects all systems of care. Put another way: Where there are patients, there are patients who are suffering needlessly.
- Sensitivity to the reality of financial issues that affect quality of life is critical.
- Palliative care is not confined to just those with cancer and acquired immunodeficiency syndrome (AIDS), but to those with all life-threatening illnesses.
- The interprofessional care of the patient/family is integral to high-quality palliative care.

To understand the benefits of palliative care, one must grasp the depth and breadth of symptoms, stress, and suffering of serious illness. This section examines a broad overview of these concepts; however, the reader is encouraged to continue to pursue more in-depth knowledge.

The numbers speak for themselves. We live in a time of unprecedented numbers of older Americans who are living with chronic illnesses. In 2010 there were 403 million people 65 years or older, 12 times the number in 1900 (US Census Bureau, 2016). Additionally, a baby born in the United States today can expect to live to 78 years old (US Census Bureau, 2016). With this longer lifespan comes an expectation that all illnesses can be treated, as many successes in public health and medical care have shown (Meier et al., 2010). However, "the sheer numbers of the elderly with chronic disability means an unprecedented number will experience prolonged functional dependency and frailty" (Meier et al., 2010). Approximately 57% of Americans 80 years and older report a severe disability (Meier et al., 2010). Individuals with five or more chronic illnesses account for 66% of Medicare spending and are the largest consumers of health care (Meier et al., 2010).

Technology offers the ability to prolong life but does not consistently restore life to its former level of quality. Many Americans live with one or more chronic illnesses. Although these persons are living longer, many suffer from illnesses that limit their lives (Meier et al., 2010). Furthermore, degenerative diseases have replaced communicable disease as the leading causes of death in the United States. Today 54% of Americans die in acute care facilities surrounded by strangers and suffer from prolonged chronic illnesses and, in many cases, receiving futile treatment that may result in financial burden for the family (Grant & Dy, 2012).

The stress, symptoms, and suffering experienced in chronic illness by both the patient and the family also exact a tremendous burden. In 1995 the SUPPORT (Study to Understand Prognoses and Preferences for Outcomes and Risks of Treatment) "demonstrated a lack of communication between patients, families, and health care providers about goals of care, a significant pain burden in seriously ill patients, and discrepancies between patient preferences for care and the aggressive care received" (SUPPORT Principal Investigators, 1995). This study became the impetus for increasing research and education in palliative care at the end of life.

Pain and Symptom Management

Pain and symptom management and communication are commonly recognized aspects of quality care for persons with serious illness. Dr. Nathan Cherny (2015) best delineates the impact of unrelieved pain in his description related to cancer:

> Unrelieved pain is incapacitating and precludes a satisfying quality of life; it interferes with functioning and social interaction, and is strongly associated with heightened psychological distress. It can provoke or exacerbate existential distress, disturb normal processes of coping and adjustment, and augment a sense of vulnerability contributing to a preoccupation with the potential for catastrophic outcomes. Persistent pain interferes with the ability to eat, sleep, think, interact with others, and is correlated with fatigue in cancer patients.

In palliative care, the prevalence of pain varies by diagnoses and demographics. Moreover, the fear of unrelieved pain expressed by patients and families is often reflective of what they have experienced (American Geriatrics Society, 2009). The experience of pain for the individual patient has multiple dimensions and includes such factors as the meaning of pain, knowledge of pain and pain management, expectation and goals of pain management, cultural beliefs, and the support received from family and others.

Pain is further complicated by the presence of other symptoms that can occur during serious illness: dyspnea, insomnia, constipation, nausea and vomiting, anxiety, depression, delirium, and fatigue. These symptoms seriously affect quality of life and may limit functional activity to the detriment of the patient's overall well-being. Through comprehensive assessment and management of patient and family, palliative care is able to improve quality of life as evidenced by these benefits:

- Relief of suffering
- Optimization of function
- Promotion of healing and comfort
- Fostering of appropriate hope
- Genuine coordination of care at times of transitions between health care providers
- Providing opportunity and assistance in exploring and preparing for hospice care as appropriate.

Suffering

In 1982, Dr. Eric Cassel published one of the earliest articles on suffering to enter the medical literature, and it opened discussions about suffering for professionals. In this article, he defines suffering as "a state of severe distress associated with events that threaten the intactness of a person" (Cassel, 1982). Suffering is the experience of a person, whereas pain and other symptoms are the result of physical body or organ changes. Suffering and pain can coexist together, although one can be present without the other. However, "the transition from pain to suffering can occur when pain is unrelieved and out of control or when the source of pain is unknown. The persistence of pain and uncertainty therefore can increase suffering" (Matzo & Sherman, 2019).

Relieving a patient's and family's suffering is central to the work of palliative care. Spiritual and existential distress is prevalent but also goes under-recognized in the hospice and palliative care populations (Puchalski et al., 2009). Excellent pain and symptom management becomes the foundation for relief of suffering because active symptomatology can dominate a patient's life. However, once physical symptoms are resolved or controlled, spiritual assessment can reveal areas of loss, such as loss of hope, loss of meaning, loss of value, or loss of relationships (Quill et al., 2010). Once this suffering is discovered, practical strategies including counseling are methods to relieve it.

Family Caregiving

Family caregivers also benefit from palliative care services. The National Alliance for Caregiving defines a family caregiver as "someone who is responsible for attending to the daily needs of another person. They are responsible for the physical, emotional, and often financial support of another person who is unable to care for himself or herself due to illness, injury or disability" (National Alliance for Caregiving, 2020). The average period of caregiving is 4.6 years, with 31% of caregivers involved in caregiving for longer than 5 years. The average time of caregiving is 20.4 hours weekly, with females providing more caregiving time than males (National Alliance for Caregiving in Collaboration with AARP, 2020). The stresses of caregiving are multifactorial, including compassion fatigue with neglect of their own needs and health (Family Caregiver Alliance, 2020), role changes with stress (Dumont et al., 2008; Herbert et al., 2009), and the development of depression and other emotional complications (Family Caregiver Alliance, 2020). Matzo and Sherman (2019) define four general areas where strategies can successfully affect caregiving:

1. Setting realistic goals
2. Having difficult discussions
3. Finding help
4. Negotiating expectations

These strategies begin with a comprehensive family assessment, including an assessment of family strengths and weaknesses.

BARRIERS TO PALLIATIVE CARE

Four significant barriers form the basis for the growth and progress of palliative care for the future. First is the lack of a general understanding on the part of health care professionals as well as the consumers of the role and nature of palliative care. With that strong linkage, patients and families, and often health care providers, believe "It's just not time yet"; that is, "I'm not dying yet." The lack of recognition of the true nature of palliative care prevents patients and families from obtaining the care they need to address needs of the whole person. Further, the lack of recognition of the negative impact of a disease condition on the whole person results in distress—physical, social, psychologic, and spiritual. The denial of death in our American culture also affects the lack of acceptance of palliative care. Woody Allen has been quoted as saying, "I don't want to achieve immortality through my work. I want to achieve it by not dying." The combination of this "stigma of death with widely held beliefs that modern medicine and hospitals can perform miracles in the battle against death" has meant that "hospitals and nursing homes have become the dominant site for gravely ill, dying people" (Meier, et al., 2010), with more than 70% of deaths in the United States occurring in an institution (Meier et al., 2010).

The second barrier to the growth and progress of palliative care is the limited numbers of palliative care–trained professionals. Although there has been remarkable growth of palliative care programs, which has continued to the present, "These numbers have not matched the number of trained clinicians to lead and staff these programs" (Meier et al., 2010). As Meier and colleagues (2010) further report, "A number of strategies have been employed to improve medical and nursing education in palliative care, including the pursuit of subspecialty status for palliative medicine and nursing advocacy for changes in undergraduate and graduate accreditation standards; and numerous philanthropically funded efforts to train mid-career physicians and nurses."

The third barrier to palliative care growth and progress is the question, "How is palliative care paid for?" Although palliative care providers do bill Medicare and other payers for the care they deliver, the reimbursement is for time-intensive care and not procedural services. This reimbursement fails to cover the salaries of the professionals, much less the overhead expenses for running a business. As a result, the growth in hospital palliative care services has been financed "not by fee-for-service reimbursement to hospitals and providers but rather by hospitals' operating budgets" (Meier et al., 2010). But first these hospitals and their administrators must be persuaded of the value during economic times of decreased reimbursement. R. Sean Morrison and colleagues analyzed administrative data from eight hospitals with established palliative care teams from 2002 to 2004, and they matched their patients with patients receiving usual care. "The palliative care patients who were discharged alive had an adjusted net savings of $1696 in direct costs per admission and patients who died had a cost savings of almost $5000" (Hannon, 2018).

Communication is the fourth barrier, and it is a vital part of patient care; however, at the end of life it can be detrimental if poorly done. Patients and their families deserve appropriate information to help them make difficult decisions. As patients and families face serious illness, conversations must be kept simple. Trying to tell everything is overwhelming. Unfortunately, health care providers have not been educated in the delivery of difficult news.

COMMON CHALLENGES

Providing quality palliative care is not perfect and there are struggles. Giving up their independence can be devastating for patients as they decline. In a qualitative study Smucker and colleagues (2014) described safety concerns from 17 hospices in 13 states. Hospice workers described harm from falls and uncontrolled symptoms, especially pain. Some of the factors identified as contributing to the safety issues included patients who were living alone and/or cognitively impaired, caregivers who were cognitively impaired, and caregivers with their own physical limitations. These barriers related to patient safety and independence need to be addressed.

Another common challenge is treating the patient for the family's sake. Families may want intravenous fluids, antibiotics, and other therapies. It is not easy helping them understand that these can be more of a burden than help and may hasten death. Frequently, the family/caregiver is not considering the best interest of the patient during decision-making.

Families/caregivers frequently struggle with the care that is given as well as the care that is not given. They also struggle with whether the right decisions have been made. They want the best care for their loved one, but emotions may cloud judgment as to what is the best care. If the diagnosis is new, patients/caregivers find it more difficult to change the focus of therapies. There is often a fear that death will be hastened if therapies are stopped or changed. Caregivers providing the care may fear they will hasten death. When asked about pain and suffering, families do not want the patient to suffer yet they do not want the patient sedated. There is often a fine line of acceptable level of symptoms and a decreased level of consciousness. If the patient is alert enough to participate in the level of acceptance, they should be included. Education of caregivers/patients should be continuous throughout the process of disease management. For example, once families understand

the burden of numerous medications they often agree to simplify the list. Helping caregivers to understand the pros and cons of therapies can help. Support and encouragement for caregivers is essential. It helps them to understand they are providing the best care possible. The goal for all is a peaceful death. The family will be left to review the care given. If they are educated, they will understand that the care the patient received was appropriate and provided comfort.

Withholding or withdrawing food and fluids or treatments is a challenge for palliative care providers. Withholding and withdrawing have both ethical and legal components. The principle of autonomy comes into play, and the individual ultimately has the right to refuse or accept a therapy. Ideally, the patients should speak for themselves but unfortunately they may not be able to. Advance directives, if present, can speak for patients and their wishes. When therapies are considered, a time frame should also be discussed and the question asked, "Will the therapy be time sustaining or life prolonging?"

Families view food and fluids as essential. Food and fluids are very important in our society. Many things revolve around food—for example, birthdays, holidays, and even funerals! We talk about comfort foods. Caregivers fear the patient will starve to death when food or fluids are withheld or not started. In truth, patients frequently stop eating gradually as they age or their disease progresses. Patients say, "I'm not hungry" or "Food just doesn't taste good anymore." Families fear that the health care provider is starving their loved one. It is the progression of the disease that has caused decreased intake of food and fluids. Health care providers do not withhold nutrition from those patients who still want to eat. The introduction of artificial nutrition is just that: artificial! It is helpful to discuss the benefits and burdens of intravenous fluids and feeding tubes and the purpose of these therapies. Although both serve a useful purpose in the acute care setting for individuals whose prognosis is good, they are a burden for an individual who has a terminal illness. Historically, prior to the advent of intravenous therapy or tube feedings, patients ate and drank as long as they were able. When feeding became a burden, families continued to care for them, offering food and fluids, but not forcing them. The patient was allowed to die naturally. Further, it has not been found that artificial feedings show improved survival (Adile, 2018).

PROFESSIONAL ISSUES IN PALLIATIVE CARE

The HPNA's *Scope and Standards of Practice* identifies the following specific areas of expertise for hospice and palliative care nurses (Dahlin & Glass, 2007):
1. Clinical judgment
2. Advocacy and ethics
3. Professionalism
4. Collaboration
5. Systems thinking
6. Cultural competence
7. Facilitator of learning
8. Communication

Certification

Currently, there are three levels of certification for the palliative care nurse. At the generalist level is the CHPN designation—certified hospice palliative nurse; for the palliative nurse administrator is the CHPA—certified hospice palliative administrator. The hospice palliative advanced practice nurse usually has specialty training or certification in palliative care. The advanced-level certification is the ACHPN (advanced certified hospice palliative nurse).

At the institutional level, palliative care programs can now achieve recognition for high-quality palliative care through The Joint Commission. This voluntary certification is based on the National Consensus Project for Quality Care and the National Quality Forum's National Framework and Preferred Practices for Hospice and Palliative Care.

Quality Assessment and Improvement

The National Hospice and Palliative Care Organization is a hospice and palliative care national organization committed to social change for the care of patients at the end of life. As part of their mission, they are committed to the improvement of multiple areas of quality, including patient-centered measures related to management of pain within 48 hours of admission, avoiding unwanted hospitalizations, avoiding unwanted cardiopulmonary resuscitation (CPR), and patient safety. In the area of bereavement, a survey has been designed to evaluate bereavement service and is completed by family members or primary caregivers. A postdeath survey is completed by family members of hospice patients regarding their perceptions about the quality of the care given to their loved ones at end of life. Lastly, a staff job satisfaction survey has been designed specifically for hospice field staff.

The CAPC is the nation's leading resource for palliative care program development. It provides multiple learning opportunities to assist health care institutions in building hospital programs, from strategic planning, to funding, to operations, and sustainability. CAPC is a national organization dedicated to increasing the availability of quality palliative care service for people facing serious, complex illness. They have numerous references and resources available, including information on quality assessment and improvement.

Research

Research in palliative care is lacking, in part because it is a relatively new subspecialty but also because palliative researchers are faced with numerous ethical quandaries (Chen et al., 2014). Palliative care research must meet the same rigor as other disciplines, and barriers can include lack of funding, lack of staff, and lack of trained researchers. Obtaining subjects can also be a barrier, especially when patients/families as well as health care providers have poor understanding of palliative care. Because patients have life-limiting diseases, they may die before a study can be completed.

Ethical Concerns

Ethical challenges arise when the ethically appropriate course of action or range of choices is unclear, or when there are competing ethical claims that may not be reconcilable (Berlinger et al., 2013). For purposes of this chapter, the following four areas will be briefly examined: advance care planning, double effect, palliative sedation, and medically futile care.

Advance Care Planning. In December 1991 all hospitals, nursing facilities, hospice programs, and health maintenance organizations that serve Medicare or Medicaid patients were mandated to provide new patients with written information describing their rights under state law to make decisions about medical care, including their right to execute a living will or durable power of attorney for health care (Berlinger et al., 2013). This was the Patient Self-Determination Act (PSDA) of 1991. The living will or advance directive outlines one's decisions for health care for when one is unable to speak or decide. These documents were intended to foster communication between the doctor and the patient, and at the same time, respect the patient's right to autonomy. Ethical dilemmas can arise because an advance directive "requires a person to predict accurately the final illness and what medical interventions might be available to postpone death and living wills require physicians to make decisions on the basis of their interpretation of the document, rather than a discussion of treatment options with a person acting on behalf of the patient" (Meier et al., 2010). The suggested solution now in practice is for the patient to appoint a health care agent or decision-maker who can speak on the patient's behalf with detailed knowledge of their health care wishes.

Double Effect. Day to day, nurses face issues related to beneficence and nonmaleficence, or doing no harm. This principle becomes particularly important with seriously ill or dying patients who are often in a weakened condition, frail, frightened, and vulnerable. Nurses often become distressed when being requested to give opioid therapy to an actively dying patient. Although these medications are intended to relieve pain and symptoms such as dyspnea, they also have a foreseeable risk of hastening death by respiratory depression.

Nash and Nelson (2012) have explained that according to the rule of double effect, an action with two possible effects—one good and one bad—is ethically acceptable if these four conditions are satisfied:

- The good effect has to be intended and therefore is not morally wrong.
- The bad effect is not intended but can be foreseen; that is, causing respiratory depression can result in death.
- The bad effect cannot be the means to the good effect. In this example, pain relief is not achieved by ending a patient's life.
- The symptom must be severe enough to warrant taking risks; that is, administering this dose at this time is needed to relieve the pain.

Palliative Sedation. At times in palliative care and particularly in patients receiving hospice care, patients present with intolerable symptoms that cannot be controlled by standard methods of pain management. Examples of symptoms that become intolerable are dyspnea, pain, and delirium with agitation.

To appropriately manage these symptoms, palliative sedation can be considered. *Palliative sedation* is the use of sedating medications to relieve refractory or intolerable symptoms when other pharmacologic measures have failed. The education and informed consent discussion with the patient and/or the patient's decision-maker includes the purpose of therapy, the expected outcomes, and how the patient and symptoms will be monitored. In consideration of the stress that family members are under during episodes of palliative sedation, continuing education and explanation of the patient's condition and status are important. Further, nursing and the interdisciplinary team require around-the-clock monitoring to ensure that symptoms are controlled, that limited numbers of breakthrough episodes are occurring, and that the need for increased medications are identified promptly.

Medically Futile Care. A medically futile treatment is a treatment option that offers no possibility of physiologic benefit related to diagnosis, prognosis, or the current medical condition. Ethically, a physician is not obligated to provide such a treatment; however, the physician should be aware of any state laws relevant to these decisions.

When decisions of medical futility are being made, a patient/family meeting is a critical strategy to ensure that all pertinent parties are involved in the decision-making process. These relevant parties include the physician, the patient and/or decision-maker, the family, and members of the interdisciplinary team. Often, members of the hospital-based ethics committee are also involved.

The first step is to establish common ground of mutual understanding of the patient's condition. In this process the members of the interdisciplinary team ask open-ended questions of the patient/family to clarify that information is indeed understood. Once common ground is established, the next step is to determine and verbalize the patient's/family's goals and expectations of treatment. Then the physician explains the treatment options and, in the case of futile treatments, explains why a treatment cannot provide benefit. Lastly, the team clarifies the questions and misconceptions; and once these are clarified to the satisfaction of the patient/family, an explicit statement of the medical plan of action is made for everyone present to hear.

LEGAL CONCERN: RIGHT TO REFUSE TREATMENT

"The right to refuse is the belief that medical care is optional for adults with appropriate capacity" (Berlinger et al., 2013). The landmark cases of Quinlan and Cruzan and others have established that patients have a legal right to refuse life-sustaining medical treatment.

In April 1975 21-year-old Karen Ann Quinlan suffered an anoxic brain injury. Her medical care included a tracheostomy, artificial ventilation, and a feeding tube with artificial nutrition and hydration (ANH). Her condition was later diagnosed as persistent vegetative state, at which time her father sought to be appointed by the courts as her legal guardian so that he could discontinue the respirator that assisted her breathing. Karen's physician refused to do so because this choice was not in accordance with medical standards of the day. After years and multiple court battles, the ventilator was removed, and she died several years later of an infection. The outcome of this woman's experience was the endorsement by the legal system of the use of hospital ethics committees to review decisions to withdraw life-sustaining treatments.

The second young woman to affect decisions to refuse medical treatment was Nancy Cruzan. She was 25 years old in January of 1983 when she was seriously injured in a motor vehicle accident. She was treated to restore her breathing and heartbeat both at the accident site and en route to the hospital, and she was admitted in a coma. A gastrostomy tube was inserted with her husband's permission. She was diagnosed as being in a persistent vegetative state.

Over time, her parents requested that the ANH be discontinued but the hospital refused to do so without a court order. Once more, a series of court interventions were sought, including involvement of the US Supreme Court. The legal outcome of this series of legal events was that the Court stated that "incompetent patients need certain protections given when they cannot exercise their right of refusal"; therefore, it was appropriate at the state level "to impose additional safeguards in the form of the clear and convincing evidence standard in light of its interest in preserving life" (Nash & Nelson, 2012).

After this decision the Cruzan family petitioned the state court in Missouri to grant the request to discontinue the ANH. The discontinuation was approved, and Nancy Cruzan died shortly thereafter. This case affects us today through the increased interest in advance care planning and health care decision-makers and also "generated support for the Patient Self-Determination Act" of 1991 (Nash & Nelson, 2012).

SUMMARY

To summarize the chapter let's review the questions posed at the beginning of the chapter and see what you have learned.

1. What patient experiences have you had related to serious illness?

   Each nurse will have had individual experiences. The novice nurse will not have had many unless they themselves have had serious illness or had a family member with serious illness. A novice nurse can benefit from a mentor who can help them through this less-familiar territory. As one considers experiences of serious illness, they should think about how it made them feel. Frequently if the patient is near the same age as the nurse, it becomes more real for that nurse. The seasoned nurse can have many experiences, identifying what went well and what could have been different to help the patient.

2. What do you think is important to include in serious illness/end-of-life discussions?

   Serious illness discussions should include the patient's understanding of the disease process and expected therapies and outcomes. Also, the patient should be asked what their treatment–cure goals are. Prolongation of life? Comfort care? Are their goals realistic? Included in these discussions is the desire for resuscitation and intubation and their likelihood to help the patient. The desire for antibiotic, fluids, enteral and parenteral feedings, and other therapies should be reviewed. In this discussion the risks and benefits of therapies should be integrated into the discussion. For example, will the therapy prolong suffering or will it increase suffering? Oftentimes the patient and/or caregivers believe that death will be hastened with the omission of certain therapies. Helping the patient/caregiver understand the dying process can be helpful in managing the patient's/caregiver's understanding that therapies at the end of life may increase suffering. For the terminally ill patient, the focus should be on comfort including physical, psychological, and spiritual comfort. Comfort care can be explained as care that relieves physical symptoms such as pain, dyspnea, nausea/vomiting, and constipation/diarrhea. These are most often treated with some type of drug therapy. Psychological distress may also be treated with drug therapy but may also include conversations with health care providers, family members, or volunteers. Spiritual distress can be addressed by any team member but frequently the chaplain is an important part of guiding the patient to spiritual distress. An important part of serious illness/end-of-life conversations is the emphasis that the patient and caregivers will be supported in their journey as individuals.

3. Have you considered how you would like to live during serious illness?

   Frequently the young nurse has not given a lot of considerations to serious illness unless they have had a family member with a serious illness or work in an area that cares for patients with serious or terminal illness. The older nurse may be experiencing health issues themselves and must consider what they want.

4. Have you completed your advance directives?

   Just as each nurse reviews advanced care plans with patients, they should either complete an advanced care plan or five wishes form for themselves. The reflection on their own wishes can help them understand what the patient is experiencing.

5. How can nursing research affect end-of-life care?

   Nursing research can help nurses provide care that leads to a good death. Research can also help families understand what is happening and why certain therapies are given while others are withheld or withdrawn. When research is used to guide the care, patients and caregivers benefit from the gold standard of care. They are receiving care that has been found to help rather than care that is guesswork.

You matter because you are you, and you matter to the end of your life. We will do all we can not only to help you die peacefully, but also to live until you die.

Dame Cicely Saunders, 1918–2005; nurse, social worker, physician, founder of modern-day hospice

REFERENCES

Adile, C. (2018). *Feeding tube and survival among patients with severe cognitive impairment.* In D. Hui, A. Reddy, E. Bruera (Eds.). *50 studies every palliative doctor should know.* Oxford University Press.

American Geriatrics Society. (2009). American Geriatric Society clinical practice guidelines: Pharmacological management of persistent pain in older persons. *Journal of the American Geriatric Society, 57*(8), 1331–1346. https://doi.org/10.1111/j.1532-5415.2009.02376.x

American Nurses Association. (2015). *Code of ethics for nurses with interpretive statements.* http://www.nursingworld.org/MainMenuCategories/EthicsStandards/CodeofEthicsforNurses/Code-of-Ethics-For-Nurses.html

Anderson, F., Downing, G.M., & Hill, J., (1996). Palliative performance scale (PPS): A new tool. *Journal of Palliative Care, 12*(1):6.

Berlinger, N., Jennings, B., & Wolf, S.M. (2013). *The hasting center guidelines for decisions on life-sustaining treatment and care near end of life* (2nd ed.) Oxford University Press.

Callin, S.E., & Bennett, M.I. (2009). Assessment of mobility. In T.D. Walsh, A. Caraceni, R. Fainsinger (Eds.). *Palliative medicine.* Saunders.

Cassel, E.J. (1982). The nature of suffering and the goals of medicine. *New England Journal of Medicine, 306*(11), 639–645. https://doi.org/10.1056/NEJM198203183061104

Chen, E.K., Riffin, C., Reid, M.C., Adelman, R., Warmington, M., Mehta, S.S., & Pillemer, K. (2014). Why is high-quality research on palliative care so hard to do? Barrier to improved research from a survey of palliative care researchers. *Journal of Palliative Medicine, 17*(7), 782–787. https://doi.org/10.1089/jpm.2013.0589

Cherny, N.I. (2015). *Pain assessment and cancer pain syndromes.* In G. Hanks, N.I. Cherny, N.A. Christakis (Eds.), *Oxford textbook of palliative medicine.* Oxford University Press.

Dahlin, C., & Glass, E. (2007). *Hospice and palliative nursing: Scope and standards of practice.* Hospice and Palliative Nurses Association and American Nurses Association.

Dumont, I., Dumont, S., & Mongeau, S. (2008). End-of-life care and the grieving process: Family caregivers who have experienced the loss of a terminal phase cancer patient. *Qualitative Health Research, 18*(8), 1049–1061. https://doi.org/10.1177/1049732308320110

End-of-Life Nursing Education Consortium. (2020). *Core curriculum.* http://www.aacnnursing.org/ELNEC

Family Caregiver Alliance (2020). *Caregiver assessment: Principles, guidelines, and strategies for change, Report from a Consensus Development Conference,* Vol. I: Family Caregiver Alliance.

Ferris, F.D., von Gunten, C.F., & Emanuel, L.L. (2003). Competency in end-of-life care: Last hours of life. *Journal of Palliative Medicine, 6*(4), 605–613. https://doi.org/10.1089/109662103768253713

Grant, M., & Dy, S.L. (2012). *UNIPAC #1: The hospice and palliative care approach to serious illness* (4th ed.) American Academy of Hospice Palliative Medicine.

Hannon, B. (2018). *Cost savings associated with palliative care.* In D. Hui, A. Reddy, E. Bruera (Eds.), *50 Studies every palliative care doctor should know.* Oxford University Press.

Herbert, R. S., Schulz, R., Copeland, V. C., & Arnold, R. M. (2009). Preparing family caregivers for death and bereavement: Insights from caregivers of terminally ill patients. *Journal of Pain and Symptom Management, 37*(1), 3–12. https://doi.org/10.1016/j.jpainsymman.2007.12.010

Matzo, M., & Sherman, D.W. (Eds.). (2019). *Palliative care nursing: Quality care at the end of life* (5th ed.) Springer Publishing Company.

Meier, D.E., Isaacs, S.L., & Hughes, R.G. (2010). *Palliative care: Transforming the care of serious illness* (3rd ed.) Jossey-Bass.

Nash, R.R., & Nelson, L.J. (2012). *Ethical and legal issues.* American Academy of Hospice and Palliative Medicine.

National Alliance for Caregiving in Collaboration with AARP. (2020). *Caregiving in the US.*

National Alliance for Caregiving. (2020). *Care for the family caregiver: A place to start.* http://www.caregiving.org/data/emblem_cfC10_Final12.pdf

Puchalski, C., Ferrell, B., Virani, R., Otis-Green, S., Baird, P., Bull, J., Chochinov, H., Handzo, G., Nelson-Becker, H., Prince-Paul, M., Pugliese, K., & Sulmasy, D. (2009).

Improving the quality of spiritual care as a dimension of palliative care: The report of a consensus conference. *Journal of Palliative Medicine, 12,* 885–904. https://doi.org/10.1089/jpm.2009.0142

Quill, T.E., Holloway, R.G., Shah, M.S., et al. (2010). *Primer of palliative medicine* (5th ed.) American Academy of Hospice and Palliative Medicine.

Schwarz, J.K., & Tarzian, A.J. (2010). *Ethical aspects of palliative care.* In M. Matzo, D.W. Sherman (Eds.). *Palliative care nursing: Quality care to the end of life.* Springer.

Sepúlveda, C., Marlin, A., Yoshida, T., & Ullrich, A. (2002). Palliative care: The world health organization's global perspective. *Journal of Pain and Symptom Management, 24*(2), 91–96. https://doi.org/10.1016/s0885-3924(02)00440-2

Singh, S., Graham, Z., Rodriguez, A., Lee, D., Wenger, B., Min, S., & Fescher, S. (2019). Accuracy of the surprise question on an inpatient oncology service: A multidisciplinary perspective. *Journal of Hospice and Palliative Nursing, 21*(4), 300–304. https://doi.org/10.1097/NJH.0000000000000558

Stjernswärd, J., Foley, K.M., & Ferris, F.D. (2007). The public health strategy for palliative care. *Journal of Pain and Symptom Management, 33*(5), 486–493. https://doi.org/10.1016/j.jpainsymman.2007.02.016

Smucker, D.R., Regan, S., Elder, N.C., & Gerrety, E. (2014). Patient safety incidents in home hospice care: The experiences of hospice interdisciplinary team members. *Journal of Palliative Medicine, 17*(5), 540–544. https://doi.org/10.1089/jpm.2013.0111

SUPPORT Principal Investigators(1995). A controlled trial to improve care for the seriously ill hospitalized patients: The study to understand prognoses and preferences for outcomes and risks of treatment. *Journal of the American Medical Association, 274*(20), 1591–1598

US Census Bureau(2016). *65+ in the United States: 2010.* US Government Printing Office.

von Gunten, C.F. (2014). Prognosis: How long do we wait for the doctor? *Journal of Palliative Medicine, 7*(6), 634–635.

Weissman, D.E., & Meier, D.E. (2011). Identifying patients in need of a palliative care assessment in the hospital setting: A consensus report from the center to advance palliative care. *Journal of Palliative Medicine, 14*(1), 17–23. https://doi.org/10.1089/jpm.2010.0347

13

Workplace Advocacy for a Professional Nursing Practice Environment

Katie Boston-Leary, PhD, MBA, MHA, RN, NEA-BC

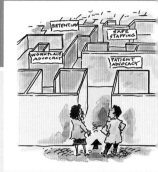

A dynamic, ever-changing workplace requ[...]
nurses to embrace workforce advoca[...]
ensure quality care and a healthy work [...]
ronment.

ⓔ Additional resources are available online at: http://evolve.elsevier.com/Cherry/

LEARNING OUTCOMES

After studying this chapter, the reader will be able to:

1. Identify issues that affect the practice of professional nursing in the workplace.
2. Identify available resources to assist in improving the workplace environment.
3. Define the role of nurses in advocating for safe and effective workplace environments.
4. Describe workforce strategies that support efficient and effective quality patient care and promote improved work environments for nurses.

KEY TERMS

Patient advocacy The nurse and the nursing profession's powerful voice at local, state, and national levels in advancing policies that protect health-care consumers and support the nursing workforce along with enforcing accountability for quality by promoting safer health care systems. Patient advocacy is foundational to the nursing profession, and patients depend on the nurse to ensure that they receive quality care.

Workplace advocacy Nurses taking actionable steps to promote a healthy work environment, quality patient care, safety, and policies to support nurses and patients.

Workplace issues An array of complex issues nurses face in the workplace on a regular basis. These issues affect the nurse, the patient, the organization, and the profession. Examples include the nursing shortage, adequate staffing levels, errors in care delivery, and violence in the workplace.

PROFESSIONAL/ETHICAL ISSUE

Elizabeth Gordon, registered nurse (RN), is a medical-surgical nurse at an acute care hospital in a rural town—a position she has held for the past 5 years. She considers herself experienced and routinely volunteers to precept new staff. When news broke of a new respiratory virus, Elizabeth and her team followed the news closely. As the situation rapidly evolved they sought to prepare and learn about this novel virus as quickly as possible, recognizing the need to be knowledgeable to properly care for infected patients. Within a few weeks' time Elizabeth's facility reached capacity treating both confirmed and suspected positive cases. At the same time

Elizabeth began to learn of nursing staff shortages in her organization due to staff who were mandated to undergo quarantine following exposure to the virus. Upon arriving for her shift today Elizabeth was informed that the ICU is understaffed and she will need to be reassigned to work the ICU during her shift. The ICU is at capacity and she knows she will be caring for patients requiring various life support measures, including mechanical ventilation. The assignment makes Elizabeth uneasy. She has never cared for a patient on a ventilator and has never actively cared for patients within the ICU. She is concerned about patient safety and her own risk of providing care in an unfamiliar unit. What options, if any, does Elizabeth have regarding this assignment that she believes to be unsafe? After reading the chapter, discuss how Elizabeth should approach the situation with her supervisor and what questions she should ask to advocate for herself and for patient safety.

VIGNETTE

As a new graduate 26-year-old Elena Gonzalez is searching for her first position as an RN in a large metropolitan city. As part of her education she learns about the importance of a nurse's role in advocating for a workplace conducive to delivering safe and effective quality care. She also understands that a workplace is filled with numerous challenges including but not limited to chronic staff shortages, incivility, occupational hazards and exposures, and supply shortages, which affect nurses, patients, the organization, and the profession overall. Elena constantly receives attention from various organizations interested in hiring her. However, she wisely chooses not to accept any new role at "face value" and investigates her opportunities more thoroughly. She searches the websites of hospitals in her target area. She is looking for the answers to questions such as:

- What are the organization's mission and values, and do they align with her own?
- Does the organization have a formal plan to advance diversity, equity, inclusion, and belonging?
- Are organizations within her area designated as centers of excellence (Magnet, Pathway to Excellence, Baldridge, Leapfrog, etc.)?
- Which organizations have shared governance models and structures that elevate nurses' voices?

- How is nursing and departmental orientation structured for successful onboarding?
- Does the organization embrace a just culture framework, safety principles, and safe staffing principles?
- What is the current state of the organization's staffing and how are challenges being managed?
- Does the organization have meaningful growth and development and reward and recognition programs?
- What models are in place for continuous quality improvement?

Answers to some of these questions are typically found on health care organizations' websites, from nurse recruiters or nurse educators, and during the interview process when meeting with unit or department nurse managers. It is also good practice to request meeting or shadowing prospective team members as part of the interview process. After getting most of her questions answered, Elena decides to accept a position with a large tertiary care center that she believes has an environment most supportive of nurses and ensures the delivery of quality patient care. Elena also recognizes that she still has a role to improve and advance policies and practices to improve the work environment and patient care.

Questions to Consider While Reading This Chapter:

1. What strategies can Elena use to promote quality patient care and a safe work environment?
2. What is the importance of shared governance to Elena's individual nursing practice?
3. What resources are available to help Elena learn more about important workplace issues and workforce advocacy?

CHAPTER OVERVIEW

In today's modern health care system, nurses are faced with many workplace issues. The objective of this chapter is to identify select critical issues facing nurses and the nursing profession and provide strategies for nurses to assess and improve care delivery and the work environment. Workplace advocacy is defined above, and its specific strategies are highlighted. Success, sustainability, and accountability require nurses to be aware of current issues within their work settings and externally and know their support systems and resources for effective workplace advocacy.

As we revisit Elena Gonzalez's story 6 months after she assumed her new position it is evident that she has become involved in advocating for a safe work environment. Elena and other nurses working on the medical unit are concerned because there is limited availability of safe patient handling equipment. Their patients often have mobility issues, and the nurses are worried about suffering musculoskeletal injuries when transferring and repositioning patients. Where will they find information about ergonomic safety and other workplace safety issues? What legal rights do nurses have to demand safe patient handling equipment? Is there an avenue to work with hospital leaders to decrease liabilities associated with unsafe practices and to move toward a user-friendly work environment? Seeking answers to these questions is workplace advocacy.

PROMOTING WORKPLACE ADVOCACY AND A PROFESSIONAL PRACTICE ENVIRONMENT

Historically, nurses have advocated for the profession and for the safety of their patients and surrounding communities. Key research has validated the contribution and value of registered nurses in:

- Preventing hospital readmissions (Azevedo et al., 2022; Ma, et al. 2015)
- Decreasing length of stay (Lasater et al., 2021)
- Decreasing patient mortality (Lasater et al., 2021, Olds et al., 2017)

Within this context of the important contributions that nurses make to patients, hospitals, and health care in general, nurses are challenged to deliver quality care while facing barriers and headwinds and high acuity with limited resources. Nurses' strong commitment to patient care and their role as patient advocates at times place them in direct conflict with those who have more power and influence. How nurses respond to such conflicts within the workplace but remain steadfast to advocate to improve patient care is workplace advocacy.

Think about workplace advocacy as you consider the situation Elizabeth Gordon (from the Professional/ Ethical scenario) is in with being reassigned to an unfamiliar unit. The reassignment of nurses to address shortages and surges during times of crisis and the principles of safety and quality of care remain applicable, as does the need to match the level of staff competence with clinical interventions and the overall complexity of patient needs. However, during public health emergencies redeployment of staff is not unreasonable. The American Nurses Association (ANA)'s *Crisis Standard of Care: COVID-19 Pandemic* (2020) maintains that professional nurses have a duty to care for patients in crises such as pandemics, and their employers have a duty to reduce the physical and emotional risks they face while supporting work–life balance to the greatest degree possible. Furthermore, institutions have a responsibility to safeguard employees through evidence-based policies and practices that are "transparently decided and have clear accountabilities" (ANA, 2020, p. 2).

It is stated within Provision 4 of ANA's *Code of Ethics for Nurses with Interpretive Statements* (2015, p. 16) that "Nurses in management or administration should facilitate open communication with health care personnel allowing them, without fear of reprisal, to express concerns or even to refuse an assignment for which they do not possess the requisite skill." When discussing this assignment with her manager, Elizabeth should ask what policies are in place for implementation during public health emergencies. It is also reasonable to inquire about the organization's overall plan for surge capacity, staffing, and allocation of scarce resources. Quality and safety continue to underpin care during a crisis. Knowing and understanding her own clinical capabilities, it is appropriate for Elizabeth to request orientation to the unfamiliar unit and just-in-time training for any unfamiliar clinical procedures and medical equipment. It is also appropriate to suggest consideration of alternate staffing models, such as a team-based care approach to balance patient care needs and optimize each unique skill set offered by the members of the interprofessional team.

For more than a century, the ANA and its state affiliates have advocated for the professional nurse and quality patient care. Through research, continuing education, and knowledge sharing among today's nursing community, ANA offers powerful resources to nurses seeking to overcome workforce challenges and realize opportunities. ANA's commitment to workplace advocacy was advanced with the creation of the *Nurses Bill of Rights* (ANA, 2022a), which sets forth basic principles concerning workplace expectations and environments that every nurse has a fundamental right to see fulfilled (Box 13.1).

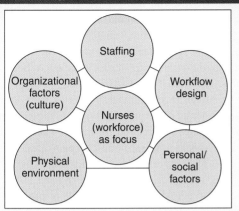

1. Nurses have the right to practice in a manner that fulfills their obligations to society and to those who receive nursing care.
2. Nurses have the right to practice in environments that allow them to act in accordance with professional standards and legally authorized scopes of practice.
3. Nurses have the right to a work environment that supports and facilitates ethical practice, in accordance with the *Code of Ethics for Nurses with Interpretive Statements.*
4. Nurses have the right to freely and openly advocate for themselves and their patients, without fear of retribution.
5. Nurses have the right to fair compensation for their work, consistent with their knowledge, experience, and professional responsibilities.
6. Nurses have the right to a work environment that is safe for themselves and for their patients.
7. Nurses have the right to negotiate the conditions of their employment either as individuals or collectively, in all practice settings.

For the full Nurses Bill of Rights, visit the ANA website at https://www.nursingworld.org/practice-policy/work-environment.

NURSING SHORTAGES AND WORKPLACE CHALLENGES

The nursing profession has a long history of cyclic shortages, which have been documented since World War II, but the shortage following the Covid-19 pandemic may be the most serious in history. The *2022 National Nursing Workforce Survey*, the first comprehensive analysis of the nursing workforce since the pandemic, confirms that an estimated 200,000 experienced RNs left the workforce from 2020 to 2022 due to the pandemic (Smiley et al., 2023). According to the survey the active RN and LPN/LVN licenses in the United States were 5,239,499 and 973,788, respectively (Smiley et al., 2023), with approximately 89% of licensed RNs employed in nursing and approximately 70% working full time. Of concern for the continued nursing shortage is that 28% of nurses who responded to the survey plan to retire in the next 5 years, which is an increase from the 21% who reported plans to retire in 2020 (Smiley et al., 2023). Nurses also report higher workloads since the pandemic and increased feelings of stress, exhaustion, and burnout (American Nurses Foundation [ANF], 2023; Smiley et al., 2023).

This concerning data should compel employers to develop plans to retain experienced nurses while recruiting and mentoring new nurses in their roles. Additionally, as we continue to understand the long-term impact of the COVID-19 pandemic on the nursing workforce it is essential for employers to develop the necessary sustained support systems to address burnout and the need for psychologic support for the overall well-being and long-term retention of the nursing workforce. New nurses entering the workforce need to be prepared to work with their nursing leaders to promote key nurse retention strategies, which include a focus on work–life balance, appropriate compensation for their work, a safe work environment, and caring and trusted teammates (ANF, 2023). The following sections take a closer look at the challenges to ensuring an appropriate supply of nurses to meet the nation's health care needs.

Current and Future RN Employment Opportunities

The good news for nurses is that future employment opportunities are very bright! Professional nursing is the largest US health care occupation with employment of RNs expected to grow by 6% from 2022 to 2032, much faster than the average for all occupations, with 193,100 openings for RNs projected each year through 2032 (US Bureau of Labor Statistics, 2023). RN employment will be affected by:

- The need to replace experienced nurses who leave the occupation.
- An increased emphasis on population health, preventive care, and wellness.

- The rapid growth in the older population, who are much more likely than younger people to need nursing care.
- Increased rates of chronic conditions and co-morbidities.
- An increased emphasis on employment opportunities for nurses in case management, care coordination, public health, and Advanced Practice Registered Nurses (APRNs) roles, which include Family Nurse Practitioners, Pediatric Nurse Practitioners, and Adult-Gerontology Acute Care Nurse Practitioners.

The RN vacancy rate for hospitals remains critical and is 15.7% nationally with more than 75% of hospitals reporting an RN vacancy rate greater than 10% (NSI Nursing Solutions, 2023). Hospital leaders report that it takes more than 3 months to recruit an experienced RN, with medical/surgical nurses presenting the greatest challenge (NSI Nursing Solutions, 2023). Planning for an adequate workforce will remain one of the most critical challenges of the new century but also represents great opportunities for new nurses.

Nursing School Challenges: Recruitment, Enrollment, Education, and Preparation

Numerous efforts have been undertaken over the past decade to recruit more students into nursing—efforts that have been largely successful. Unfortunately, even with successful attempts most schools and universities increasingly find themselves unable to expand their nursing programs to accept the qualified applicants because they are faced with a serious shortage of nursing faculty. The American Association of Colleges of Nursing (AACN) reports a national faculty vacancy rate of 8.8%, which is just the tip of the iceberg (AACN, 2022). A wave of faculty retirements across the United States is expected over the next decade, which could be one-third of the nursing faculty workforce in baccalaureate and graduate programs (AACN, 2022). In addition to recruiting more nurses into faculty positions nursing education leaders must take intentional actions to increase the recruitment and retention of faculty from racial and ethnic minority groups (Thompson, 2021). This increasing faculty shortage, compounded by a lack of diversity among its members, is contributing to the current nursing shortage by limiting the number of students admitted to nursing programs. The impact is significant. More than 91,000 qualified applicants were turned away from baccalaureate and graduate nursing programs in 2021 due to an insufficient number of faculty (AACN, 2022).

Concurrently, the complexity of care continues to intensify, leading to a demand for more RNs with critical thinking, leadership, quality improvement, case management, and health promotion skills who are capable of delivering care across a variety of health care settings. Demand has also increased for experienced RNs; for nurses in key clinical specialties, such as critical care, emergency department (ED), operating room, and neonatal intensive care; and for master's and doctorally prepared RNs in advanced clinical specialties, teaching, and research. Fortunately, the nursing workforce is becoming more educated with more than 70% of the RN workforce holding a baccalaureate or higher degree (Smiley et al., 2023).

Nurse Retention

Retaining nurses in the workforce became THE challenge in 2023 and beyond for health care leaders. A meta-analysis of 106 primary studies found the strongest predictors of nurse turnover were job strain, role tension, work–family conflict, job control, job complexity, rewards and recognition, and team cohesion (Nei et al., 2015). Research conducted by McKinsey & Company in collaboration with the ANA Enterprise found that 45% of nurses who work in hospitals reported they are likely to leave their role in the next 6 months (Berlin et al., 2023). Among those who reported an intent to leave, the top two reasons cited were not feeling valued by their organization and not having a manageable workload (Berlin et al., 2023). In other surveys, more than 80% of nurses reported the following factors would help reduce stress and keep them in the workforce (AMN Healthcare, 2023; ANF, 2023):

- Better work–life balance
- Additional nurse input into decision-making
- Safer work environments
- Increased salaries
- Reduced patients per nurse
- Added support staff

Our health care system cannot exist without nurses. Thus health care leaders must work to improve work environments to keep nurses in the workplace by addressing those issues identified as most important to them. And nurses must advocate as leaders to create healthy work environments using their expertise and innovative spirits to keep nurses in the workforce.

Transition to Nursing Practice

Transition to practice for nurses can be extremely stressful. Without the appropriate support, turnover rates for newly licensed registered nurses can run as high as 60% at the end of the first year of employment (Eckerson, 2018). While traditional new graduate nursing orientation programs are still offered in health care organizations, formal nurse residency programs are gaining popularity in both community-based and academic medical centers as they have demonstrated better outcomes, such as improved satisfaction and decreased turnover rates (Eckerson, 2018). In addition, formal, standardized residency programs such as those developed by the American Nurses Credentialing Center (ANCC), University Health Consortium or Versant had significantly better outcomes compared to organization-based residency programs (Asber, 2019). Chapter 25 provides information about strategies to ease the transition from novice to professional nurse.

Diversity, Equity, Inclusion, Belonging, and Justice

Diversity, equity, inclusion, belonging, and justice are drivers of nurse retention and improved patient outcomes. In the most recent data available the RN workforce is comprised of 20% racial and ethnic minorities while 80% are white/Caucasian, a slight decrease from 2020; RNs who reported being of Hispanic or Latino ethnicity increased to 7% of the workforce in 2022 compared to 4% of the RN workforce in 2015 (Smiley et al., 2023). Direct correlations exist between workplace diversity and job satisfaction within an organization. In a 2019 survey of nurses who report their organization supports diversity extremely well, 59% of them reported being extremely likely to remain in their current job 1 year from now compared to 18% of those who say their organizations do not support diversity well (AMN Healthcare, 2019).

In 2021 leading nursing organizations launched *The National Commission to Address Racism in Nursing* (the *Commission*) to lead a national discussion for the nursing profession to exemplify inclusion, diversity, and equity and to create antiracist practice and work environments that are safe and liberating for all nurses (ANA, 2022b). In 2022 the *Commission* released the results of a survey, which revealed that 63% of nurses surveyed say that they have personally experienced an act of racism in the workplace with the transgressors

being either a peer (66%), patients (63%), or a manager or supervisor (60%) (ANA, 2022b). To support culturally congruent care, it is essential that health care leaders, workforce advocates, and nurse educators promote actions to ensure a nursing workforce representative of the diverse population seeking care. The *Commission* "urges all nurses across every health care setting and environment to join us in boldly confronting individual and systemic racism. Nurses need to take the time to educate themselves on this issue to gain a deeper knowledge of racism's impact on the profession, patients, and colleagues" (ANA, 2022b). For more information about *The National Commission to Address Racism in Nursing*, visit their website at www.nursingworld.org and go to the "Practice and Advocacy" link.

Aging Workforce and Retention

As the nation works to increase the supply of professional nurses through education, strategies must be developed to retain tenured expert professional nurses. The following statistics detail the extent of the aging workforce issues:

- In 2022, the median age of RNs was 46 years, which reflects a decrease of 6 years from the 2020 data; this decline in the median age was associated with the large numbers of nurses who left the profession as a result of the Covid-19 pandemic (Smiley et al., 2023).
- In 2022 nearly 43% of the RN workforce was 50 years old or older (Smiley et al., 2023).
- The average ages of doctorally prepared nurse faculty holding the ranks of professor, associate professor, and assistant professor were 62.5, 56.7, and 50.6 years, respectively (AACN, 2022).
- For master's-prepared nurse faculty, the average ages for professors, associate professors, and assistant professors were 55.0, 54.7, and 48.6 years (AACN, 2022).

To complicate the aging of the nursing workforce, up to 28% of nurses surveyed report they may retire in the next 5 years (Smiley et al., 2023). As one can see, the aging of the nursing workforce and potential retirements are serious, complex issues that must be addressed by nursing leaders. Although nursing literature is replete with the many positive aspects of continuing in nursing, suggestions on ways to keep older nurses practicing include flexible scheduling, preceptor positions, fostering positive relationships between older and younger nurses, and better ergonomics and health care facility design to decrease the time nurses spend walking and reduce the physical demands of their work, including aids such as mechanical lifts, decentralized supply storage, and better lighting at the bedside (Parsons et al., 2018; Stichler, 2013).

Emerging Workforce Recruitment and Retention

In addition to planning for retention of an aging workforce, health care is challenged to become the employer of choice for the younger workforce. Several studies have focused on the work and management expectations of today's young workers, who want work–life balance and emotional support in the workplace. Nurses with fewer than 10 years' work experience reported feeling less valued, less supported, and less hopeful, with 61% of nurses under 35 indicating that they felt anxious in the past 14 days compared to only 33% of nurses 55 or older (ANF, 2023). Additionally, younger and more inexperienced nurses are struggling more with their emotional health than their more-experienced colleagues, with nearly one-third of nurses with fewer than 10 years of experience citing being "not" or "not at all" emotionally healthy (ANF, 2023).

The good news is that there are ample opportunities and strategies to support new nurses in the workplace and help them become successful as professional nurses. Such opportunities to support emerging nurses include offering advanced training, education, and certification as they seek to be more marketable in professional nursing roles and providing feedback on performance to help refine skills and build confidence. Younger nurses identified other needs to feel supported such as stability, flexible work schedules, recognition, opportunities for professional development, and nursing leadership support (Christensen et al., 2018; Dols et al., 2019). Nurse leaders need to take a personal interest in the professional development and career aspirations of younger nurses and support their career. New nurses also need to take responsibility for communicating their needs to their colleagues and nurse leaders.

Nursing Salaries

RN salaries show a consistent pattern in alignment with nursing shortages. The hospital RN shortages through the early 1990s were transitory until wage increases brought the demand and supply of RNs into equilibrium. Unfortunately, during the 1990s nursing salaries remained flat—low salaries definitely contributed to the nursing shortage. Another concern with nursing salaries in the past is the small opportunity for significant salary increases as nurses gain more experience.

In today's climate of severe nursing shortages following the COVID-19 pandemic, nurses have made significant improvements related to salaries. The average RN salary for a hospital staff nurse reported in 2023 (includes 25.9% for benefits) was $51.66 hourly or $107,445 annually (NSI, 2023). In addition to higher salaries nurses may expect other benefits that include (Nurse.com, 2022):

- More flexible work schedules
- Sign-on bonuses and relocation packages
- Loan forgiveness and tuition assistance
- Child-care discounts
- Better retirement plans
- Incentives for pursuing certifications and other career development opportunities

The top three benefits that nurses prefer but did not have were bonuses, malpractice insurance, and profit sharing (Nurse.com, 2022). Because of the nursing shortage nurses are in a strong position to negotiate their employment benefits and salary and are encouraged to consider the entire benefits package when looking at employment opportunities—if there is something they want they should ask for it!

Work Environment

A healthy work environment is vital to creating workplaces where nurses can thrive and provide the best care possible. Research has shown the positive impact of a healthy work environment on staff satisfaction, retention, improved patient outcomes, and organizational performance (Aiken et al., 2009; McHugh et al., 2016; Ulrich et al., 2019). The importance of the work environment is clear—increasing the overall supply of nurses and improving patient care are unlikely to be successful if nurses' work environments are not addressed. In recent surveys issues identified by nurses to support healthy work environments were more qualified nurses in leadership positions, reduced patients per nurse, increase in support staff, caring and trusting teammates, safer work environments, more input into decision-making, and more support from employers for work–life balance and mental health resources (ANF, 2023; AMN Healthcare, 2023; AMN Healthcare, 2019).

Two national initiatives have been undertaken to promote healthy work environments for nurses. The Nursing

Organizations Alliance, a coalition of more than 65 national nursing organizations, developed the *Elements of a Healthy Practice Environment*, which provides a framework for organizations to improve nurses' work environments (Nursing Organizations Alliance, 2019). The American Association of Critical Care Nurses (AACN) promotes a healthy work environment as one of their three major advocacy issues and has developed standards along with measurement tools (AACN, n.d.). AACN's six standards for promoting healthy work environments are (1) skilled communication; (2) true collaboration; (3) effective decision-making; (4) appropriate staffing; (5) meaningful recognition; and (6) authentic leadership (AACN, n.d.). New nurses are encouraged to learn more about these two national initiatives as they advance in their professional nursing role and help to create healthy work environments.

SAFE STAFFING

Many nurses across the country are concerned about the inadequacies of staffing to meet patient care needs (AMN Healthcare, 2023). A landmark study by Aiken and colleagues (2002) found that in hospitals with fewer nurses per patient, surgical patients were more likely to experience higher death rates from failure to rescue (insufficient nursing care) and death from complications. The same study also found that nurses working in institutions plagued by insufficient staffing and workforce shortages were more likely to experience emotional exhaustion and greater job dissatisfaction. Subsequent research has reinforced the importance of appropriate nurse staffing for positive patient and nurse outcomes (Aiken & Sloane, 2020; Shin et al., 2018). Safe staffing definitely must be a priority for health care organizations!

Given concerns about resources and cost reductions in health care, challenges continue about determining optimal staffing and how to appropriately delegate to other personnel to care for patient populations who are more acutely ill, those who require high-tech care, and those with relatively long lengths of stay. Federal regulations require hospitals to staff patient care areas with the appropriate numbers of nurses and other health care personnel needed to provide adequate care to patients. With such nebulous language, it has been left to the states to ensure that staffing is appropriate to meet patients' needs safely. Three general approaches to ensure

sufficient nurse staffing have been utilized at the state level include:

1. Require hospitals to have a nurse-driven staffing committee to create staffing plans that reflect the needs of the patient population and match the skills and experience of the staff. ANA endorses this approach and recommends staffing committees be composed of a minimum of 55% staff RNs (ANA, n.d.a). Such an approach provides for flexible staffing levels that can account for the intensity of patient needs, number of admissions, discharges and transfers during a shift, level of experience of nursing staff, layout of the unit, and availability of resources (e.g., ancillary staff, technology). As of 2023 nine states require hospitals to have staffing committees responsible for staffing plans and policy (Davidson, 2023).

2. Require facilities to disclose staffing levels to the public and/or a regulatory body. As of 2023 five states, whether voluntarily or mandated by legislation, have some form of disclosure/public reporting (Davidson, 2023).

3. Enact legislation to mandate specific nurse-to-patient ratios. As of 2023 California is the only state with a legislative mandate for specified nurse-to-patient ratios in all areas of hospital care. Massachusetts enacted legislation mandating staffing ratios only for intensive care units (ICUs) (Davidson, 2023).

As nurses consider their positions on staffing, they will be faced with many decisions, including prospective employers' approaches, methodologies and philosophies, how to advocate and implement safe staffing, nurses' involvement in staffing decisions, and real-time decision-making. When considering future employers, nurses should ask the questions regarding safe staffing that are listed in Box 13.2. Resources to help nurses' decision-making relative to adequate staffing are shown in Box 13.3. Box 13.4 identifies questions to help the staff nurse decide whether to accept an assignment. These questions are designed to help nurses think critically about assignments and provide guidance on discussions with leaders if there are concerns about safety.

Floating and Mandatory Overtime

As nurse staffing issues persist, floating and mandatory overtime continue to be utilized as strategies for addressing immediate nurse staffing issues. When the

---

BOX 13.2   Questions to Ask About Safe Staffing Before Accepting Employment

1. Who is the chief nursing officer, to whom do they report, and do they have full authority over staffing decisions?
2. Are nurses empowered to make real-time staffing decisions?
3. Are there nurse-led staffing committees to review decisions on staffing?
4. Does the organization have an effective shared governance model?
5. How is input obtained from staff nurses about staffing concerns?
6. Is there a regular review of patient outcomes in relation to staffing?
7. How is nursing orientation managed for newly hired nurses?
8. How are nurses' concerns about unsafe staffing managed without retribution?
9. What is the frequency of floating to other nursing units?
10. What resources does the organization use to supplement staff during peak census?
11. What ancillary and nonnurse staffing are available to support nurses' work?
12. How are overtime, on-call time, and cancellation of regularly scheduled shifts handled?
13. Does the organization mandate overtime? If so, can the staff nurse refuse to participate without repercussions?
14. What is the turnover rate, and what is the average longevity of staff nurses?
15. What opportunities for advancement exist in the organization, such as clinical ladders or other systems of recognition?
16. Where does the organization expect discussions about staffing or practice issues to take place?
17. Is there a conflict resolution process in place?

From American Nurses Association. (n.d.). *Questions to ask about safe staffing before accepting employment.* https://www.nursingworld.org/practice-policy/workforce/questions-to-ask-about-safe-staffing-before-accepting-employment/.

BOX 13.3   Resources for Decision-Making Related to Safe Staffing and Mandatory Overtime

ANA's Nurse Staffing website: https://www.nursingworld.org/practice-policy/advocacy/state/nurse-staffing
ANA Principles for Nurse Staffing, 3rd Edition: Directs RNs on the major elements needed to achieve appropriate nurse staffing based upon today's complex health care system.
ANA's Principles for Delegation: Provides the principles and guidelines for delegation of tasks to others. Its purpose is to define relevant principles and provide RNs with practice strategies when delegating patient care to nursing assistive personnel.
Principles for Nursing Documentation: Focuses on managing the increasingly complex requirements of documenting patient care activities in both paper and electronic formats.
- These three documents are available as a *Principles for Practice* set at http://www.nursesbooks.org.

---

availability of nursing staff is limited, leaders may (1) require that professional nurses float to other patient care units for which they have little or no orientation, experience, or support and (2) implement mandatory overtime and/or mandatory on-call requirements. Particularly regarding mandatory overtime, such strategies can be challenging given research findings that inadequate rest among nurses is associated with nurse perceptions of lower quality and safety relative to patient care (Stimpfel et al., 2020). In addition, findings related to nurse fatigue and sleep deprivation showed that nurses are more likely to report clinical decision regret, which occurs when their behaviors do not align with professional nursing practice standards or expectations (Caruso et al., 2019).

Although the growing research and enactment of state-level laws on mandatory overtime and medical errors have caused many organizations to end or limit use of mandatory overtime, it continues to be a concern. Excessive and recurring use of overtime, at times used as a staffing strategy, has made it necessary for continued state-level legislation. Nurses should learn about their scope of practice and delegation authority with the state Board of Nursing where they practice and also learn about the rules and regulations related to mandatory overtime in that state.

BOX 13.4 Questions to Ask in Making the Decision to Accept a Staffing Assignment

1. *What is the assignment?*

   Clarify the assignment. Do not assume. Be certain that what you believe is the assignment is indeed correct.

2. *What are the characteristics of the patients being assigned?*

   Do not just respond to the number of patients; make a critical assessment of the needs of each patient, their age, condition, other factors that contribute to special needs, and the resources available to meet those needs. Who else is on the unit or within the facility that might be a resource for the assignment? How stable are the patients, and how long have they been stable? Do any patients have communication and/or physical limitations that will require accommodation and extra supervision during the shift? Will there be discharges to offset the load? If there are discharges, will there be admissions, which require extra time and energy?

3. *Do I have the expertise to care for the patients?*

   Am I familiar with caring for the types of patients assigned? If this is a float assignment, am I cross-trained to care for these patients? Is there a buddy system in place with staff who are familiar with the unit? If there is no cross-training or buddy system, has the patient load been modified accordingly?

4. *Do I have the experience and knowledge to manage the patients for whom I am being assigned care?*

   If the answer to this question is no, you have an obligation to articulate limitations. Limitations in experience and knowledge may not require refusal of the assignment but rather an agreement regarding supervision or a modification of the assignment to ensure patient safety. If no accommodation for limitations is considered, the nurse has an obligation to refuse an assignment for which they lack education or experience.

5. *What is the geography of the assignment?*

   Am I being asked to care for patients who are in proximity for efficient management, or are the patients at opposite ends of the hall or on different units? If there are geographic difficulties, what resources are available to manage the situation? If my patients are on more than one unit and I must go to another unit to provide care, who will monitor patients out of my immediate attention?

6. *Is this a temporary assignment?*

   When other staff are located to assist, will I be relieved? If the assignment is temporary, it may be possible to accept a difficult assignment, knowing that there will soon be reinforcements. Is there a pattern of short staffing, or is this truly an emergency?

7. *Is this a crisis or an ongoing staffing pattern?*

   If the assignment is being made because of an immediate need on the unit, a crisis, the decision to accept the assignment may be based on that immediate need. However, if the staffing pattern is an ongoing problem, the nurse has the obligation to identify unmet standards of care that are occurring as a result of ongoing staffing inadequacies. This may result in a request for "safe harbor" and/or peer review.

8. *Can I take the assignment in good faith? (If not, you will need to get the assignment modified or refuse the assignment.)*

   Consult your individual state's nurse practice act regarding clarification of accepting an assignment in good faith. In understanding good faith it is sometimes easier to identify what would constitute bad faith. For example, if you had not taken care of pediatric patients since nursing school and you were asked to take charge of a pediatric unit, unless this were an extreme emergency, such as a disaster (in which case you would need to let people know your limitations, but you might still be the best person, given all factors for the assignment), it would be bad faith to take the assignment. It is always your responsibility to articulate your limitations and to get an adjustment to the assignment that acknowledges the limitations you have articulated. Good faith acceptance of the assignment means that you are concerned about the situation and believe that a different pattern of care or policy should be considered. However, you acknowledge the difference of opinion on the subject between you and your supervisor and are willing to take the assignment and await the judgment of other peers and supervisors.

From American Nurses Association. (n.d.). *Questions to ask in making the decision to accept a staffing assignment.* https://www.nursingworld.org/practice-policy/workforce/questions-to-ask-in-making-the-decision-to-accept-a-staffing-assignment-for-nurses.

PATIENT ADVOCACY

Patient advocacy is a fundamental element of being a nurse, and patients depend on nurses to ensure that they receive quality care. Today's health care systems have created an environment in which errors and adverse events are attributed to complex systems and complicated uses of technology. This complex environment demands that the nursing profession assert its powerful voice in the role of patient advocate by supporting public policies that protect consumers and enhance accountability for quality by ensuring and advancing safer systems of health care delivery. (See Chapter 23 about how to advocate for public health policy.)

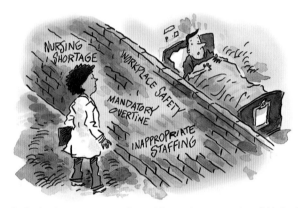

Professional nurses are struggling to deliver patient care against all kinds of barriers and with dwindling resources.

Patient Safety

A landmark report on patient safety by the Institute of Medicine (IOM) (now known as the National Academy of Medicine), *To Err Is Human,* focused heavy empirical data and awareness on the importance of patient safety when it reported that between 44,000 and 98,000 patients die in US hospitals each year from preventable medical errors (Kohn et al., 2000). Subsequently, the IOM released its report, *Keeping Patients Safe: Transforming the Work Environment of Nurses,* which examined patient safety from the perspective of the work environment in which nurses provide patient care (Page, 2004). This second landmark report provided evidence of the critical role nurses have in the health care system and found that the typical work environment of nurses is characterized by many serious threats to patient safety. These two reports have spurred the development of nursing-focused quality and safety programs, which are discussed in the following sections.

The National Database for Nursing Quality Indicators. The National Database for Nursing Quality Indicators (NDNQI) is a national nursing quality measurement program that enables hospitals to compare measures of nursing quality against national, regional, and state norms for similar units and hospitals. It was instituted by the ANA in 1998 and is maintained by Press Ganey as a tool for nursing quality measurement through data collection at the nursing unit level that allows for empirical linkages between nursing care and patient outcomes. Indicators such as patient falls, physical restraints, nosocomial infections, nursing care hours provided per patient day, and RN satisfaction surveys are used for quality improvement, reporting requirements (e.g., TJC, Magnet® Recognition Program), staff retention efforts, budget allocation, and research.

Quality and Safety Education for Nurses. Recognizing the need to strengthen nurses' competencies in the science of patient safety and quality, *The Essentials: Core Competencies for Professional Nursing Education* (AACN, 2021) has been updated to require entry-level nurses to understand principles of safety and improvement science and achieve such competencies as "recognize nursing's essential role in improving health care quality and safety; establish and incorporate data-driven benchmarks to monitor system performance; identify sources and applications of national safety and quality standards to guide nursing practice; use national safety resources to lead team-based change initiatives; and implement standardized, evidence-based processes for care delivery" (AACN, 2021). For the full description of the AACN Essentials and the quality and safety competencies, go to the following link: www.aacnnursing.org/essentials.

High Reliability Organizations. An increased focus on patient safety has led to interest from health care leaders in adapting the principles of high reliability to health care organizations. High reliability organizations (HROs) are those in which there is a potential for failures and errors that could result in catastrophic outcomes, thus individuals in HROs have an excessive preoccupation to prevent failure and errors. The airline industry is an example of an industry that functions as an HRO. A positive impact on patient outcomes has been demonstrated when high-reliability principles have been successfully applied to care bundles designed to improve nursing sensitive measures such as falls and catheter-acquired urinary tract infections (Oster & Deakins, 2018). Many organizations are adopting methods used in high-reliability science to create safer work and practice environments and reduce the likelihood that patients will come to harm through error or defects in the provision of care.

Whistle-Blower Protection

Nurses want the assurance that they will be able to speak up for their patients through appropriate channels without fear of retaliation. State and federal whistle-blower protection legislation seeks to prohibit health care organizations from retaliating against the professional nurse who in good faith discloses information or participates in agency investigations. Specifically, whistle-blower protection protects nurses who speak out about unsafe situations from being fired or subjected to other disciplinary actions by their employers.

As a real-world example of the value of whistle-blower protection, two nurses in Texas filed a complaint against a physician, citing unsafe medical practice. The case made national headlines when both nurses were charged with harassment and ultimately fired from their hospital jobs. Charges against one of the nurses were dropped. The second nurse endured a 4-day trial and was found not guilty. The nurses filed a federal civil suit against their accusers and won a $750,000 settlement. ANA and the Texas Nurses Association strongly supported the nurses, advocating for the importance of protecting whistle-blowers from prosecution. Ultimately, the county sheriff, county attorney, and hospital administrator were charged and received jail sentences for their roles in trying to silence the two nurses, and the physician was fined, received 60 days in jail and 5 years of probation, and surrendered his medical license. These actions sent a powerful message in support of whistle-blower protection.

Box 13.5 provides an overview of things to know about whistle-blowing. Nurses should check with their state nurses' association to assess the status of whistle-blower protection in their state.

BOX 13.5 Things to Know About Whistle-Blowing

- If you identify an illegal or unethical practice, reserve judgment until you have adequate documentation to establish wrongdoing.
- Do not expect those that are engaged in unethical, illegal, and questionable conduct to welcome your questions or concerns about this practice.
- Seek the counsel of someone you trust outside of the situation to provide you with an objective perspective, keeping specific patient and organizational information private.
- Consult with your state nurses' association or legal counsel if possible before taking action to determine how best to document your concerns.
- Remember that you are not protected in a whistle-blower situation from retaliation by your employer until you blow the whistle.
- Blowing the whistle means that you report your concern to the national and/or state agency responsible for

regulation of the organization for which you work or, in the case of criminal activity, to law enforcement agencies as well.
- Private groups, such as The Joint Commission (TJC) or the National Committee for Quality Assurance, do not confer protection. You must report to a state or national regulator.
- Although it is not required by every regulatory agency, it is a good rule of thumb to put your complaint in writing.
- Document all interactions related to the whistle-blowing situation, and keep copies for your personal file.
- Keep documentation and interactions objective.
- Remain calm and do not lose your temper, even if those who learn of your actions attempt to provoke you.
- Remember that blowing the whistle is a very serious matter. Do not blow the whistle frivolously. Make sure you have the facts straight before taking action.

From American Nurses Association. (n.d.). *Things to know about whistle-blowing*. https://www.nursingworld.org/practice-policy/workforce/things-to-know-about-whistle-blowing/.

WORKPLACE SAFETY

Nurses strive to provide safe, quality care for patients in an environment that is inherently hazardous to their health and well-being. The occupational safety and health of nurses is an ongoing concern for individual nurses, as well as professional nursing associations, because of numerous hazards that exist in the health care workplace. See the Centers for Disease Control and Prevention (CDC), National Institute for Occupational Safety and Health (NIOSH) web page for detailed information about current health hazards that exist in the health care workplace (http://www.cdc.gov/niosh/topics/healthcare). The following sections focus on four key hazards of concern to nurses: bloodborne pathogens, ergonomic injuries, workplace violence, and fatigue.

Exposure to Bloodborne Pathogens

Nurses and other health care professionals are at major risk for exposure to bloodborne diseases, including hepatitis B, hepatitis C, and human immunodeficiency virus–acquired immunodeficiency syndrome (HIV-AIDS), primarily due to accidental exposure from the use of sharps (needles). In 1991 the Occupational Safety and Health Administration (OSHA) issued the bloodborne pathogens standard to protect health care workers from this risk; the standard was revised by the Needlestick Safety and Prevention Act of 2000 (CDC, 2000). This law requires the use of safer needle devices to protect employees from sharps injuries, input of employees responsible for direct patient care who are at-risk for sharps injuries in the selection of effective work-practice controls, and that employers maintain a sharps injury log. See the ANA website for more information and resources about needlestick safety: https://www.nursingworld.org/practice-policy/work-environment/health-safety/safe-needles/.

Ergonomic Injuries

Nurses and other members of the health care team are at risk for ergonomic injuries. Recent data from the US Department of Labor indicates that individuals working in health care experienced the highest rate of musculoskeletal disorders (MSDs). Nurse assistants, orderlies, and attendants reported the highest incidence of illness and injuries and days away from work (US Department of Labor, 2022). Two decades of research have demonstrated that use of a single approach (e.g., engineering controls, administrative changes, or worker training) to reduce the incidence of MSDs has been ineffective. Rather than one approach health care organizations need a comprehensive program to prevent injuries that include no-lift policies, appropriate safe patient handling and mobility technology, training programs for staff, and a comprehensive tracking system of MSD injuries that includes ongoing evaluation of the program.

Additionally, every organization should have specific policies concerning reporting of workplace injuries, and employees should be encouraged to report workplace injuries. Workplace injuries may be highly underreported with nurses citing various reasons for not reporting workplace injuries such as thinking the injury was insignificant or they were too busy to report. OSHA's recordkeeping standard requires employers to keep a log of workplace injuries and to keep the OSHA 300 Log available to employees (OSHA, 2019). The OSHA standard also prevents discrimination against employees who report a work-related injury, illness, or fatality.

To support and protect nurses the ANA has led major initiatives aimed at reducing workplace injuries, including the *Safe Patient Handling Interprofessional Standards and Implementation Guide* (ANA, 2021). These standards outline the role of employers and health care workers in safe patient handling and mobility. For more information about these standards, see the Handle with Care resources on the ANA website at https://www.nursingworld.org/practice-policy/work-environment/health-safety/handle-with-care/.

Incivility, Bullying, and Violence in the Workplace

Unfortunately, incivility, bullying, and violence continue to be problems in the health care workplace. Data from the *Healthy Nurse, Healthy Nation* survey revealed that almost 14% of nurses agree or strongly agree that they have been assaulted by a patient or family member; almost 25% agree or strongly agree that they had experienced verbal and nonverbal aggression from a person of authority; and more than 30% agree or strongly agree that they have experienced verbal and nonverbal aggression from a peer (Healthy Nurse Healthy Nation, 2023). Another survey found that one in four nurses have been assaulted, only 20% to 60% of incidents are reported, and 13% of days missed at work are due to workplace violence (ANA, n.d.b). It is important to recognize that the spectrum of workplace violence also includes peer-to-peer "lateral violence," defined as acts of incivility or bullying behavior between colleagues. Complicating the situation is that many of these acts of aggression go unreported. These behaviors, which include covert or overt acts of verbal and nonverbal aggression, have been reported to affect the nurse's ability to provide quality care and may have a negative impact on the RN's level of job satisfaction, organizational commitment, and even their physical and mental health (ANA, n.d.b).

To address this very serious problem in nursing, the ANA developed an *Issue Brief: Reporting Incidents of Workplace Violence* that outlines the responsibilities and actions that both individuals and organizations must undertake to create and maintain a violence-free workplace (ANA, 2019). Nurses in all settings must proactively advocate for interventions that ensure personal safety and a safe work environment, including a strong Workplace Violence Prevention Program that (ANA, 2019):

- Has a zero-tolerance policy for workplace violence, verbal and nonverbal threats, and actions;
- Ensures that no employee who reports or experiences workplace violence faces reprisals;
- Maintains detailed recordkeeping to assess risk and measure progress;
- Contains a comprehensive plan for maintaining security in the workplace;
- Demonstrates management commitment from leadership; and
- Provides periodic employee education about violence prevention in the workplace.

Another great resource for nurses to help stop workplace incivility, bullying, and violence is the *#EndNurseAbuse Resource Guide* available on the ANA website. Also see Chapter 17 for more information on strategies to prevent violence, bullying, and incivility in the workplace.

Fortunately, there is increasing awareness of the gravity of this issue at the federal level. *The Workplace Violence Prevention for Health Care and Social Service Workers Act*, officially introduced in the US House of Representatives, would mandate that OSHA create a federal standard requiring health care and social service employers to develop and implement comprehensive workplace violence prevention plans. As of 2023 this bill had passed in the US House of Representatives and

moved to the Senate. To track this legislation, visit the ANA website at www.nursingworld.org.

Nurse Fatigue

Nurses may work long and variable hours, owing to the nature of round-the-clock care delivery, forgoing adequate rest and sleep, which may result in chronic fatigue. Restorative sleep is critical to the health of the nurse and to ensure that the nurse can provide the highest quality patient care possible (Caruso et al., 2019). Yet almost 40% of nurses reported experiencing excessive fatigue while almost 30% believe they are at significant risk for excessive fatigue (Healthy Nurse Healthy Nation, 2023). Research studies have found that short duration of sleep (less than 7 hours) was statistically significantly correlated to lower ratings of patient care quality (Bae & Fabry, 2014; Stimpfel et al. 2020). In addition to the increased risk for work-related errors, the effects of fatigue on the health and well-being of the nurse are well documented. Shift work and long hours have been linked to a multitude of health-related disorders, including diabetes, cardiovascular disease, depression, sleep disturbances, and physical injuries (Bae & Fabry, 2014; Bannai & Tamakoshi, 2014). The data is clear—nurse fatigue is a major problem for nurses.

Both individual nurses and health care organizations have responsibilities to address this very serious issue of nurse fatigue. Working with a panel that included nurses from all areas of the professional nursing community, ANA released a position statement to address the safety and health issues related to nurse fatigue and outlined responsibilities of both nurses and employers (ANA, 2014). The position statement available on the ANA website—*Joint Responsibilities of Registered Nurses and Employers to Reduce Risks*—contains a substantive list of recommendations ranging from limitation of hours worked to no more than 40 hours in one week and 12 hours in one shift, to elimination of mandatory overtime, to redesign of work schedules to minimize the occurrence of fatigue in the workplace (ANA, 2014). Both the nurse and the employer have ethical responsibilities to ensure the safety and well-being of those who work in health care settings and the patients they care for. The nurse must take the steps necessary to ensure that they have adequate rest prior to the start of a work shift, and their employer must develop and maintain policies and procedures that support a healthy work environment and adequate rest.

Advocating for a Safer Workplace

ANA has emerged as a leader in health care worker health and safety, working in collaboration with other nursing organizations, including the American Association of Occupational Health Nurses, the Association of periOperative Registered Nurses, the Emergency Nurses Association, and labor unions representing health care workers. These organizations advocate for administrative controls, such as adequate staffing and health and safety committees; engineering controls, such as ventilation and safer needlestick devices; and personal protective equipment, such as respirators and synthetic gloves that prevent exposure to hazardous substances and/or prevent illness or injury from unavoidable exposure. Although the health care industry can be a hazardous place to work, many of the risks are avoidable and dangerous exposures preventable.

STRATEGIES TO PROMOTE NURSING EXCELLENCE AND HEALTHY WORK ENVIROMENTS

For the past 50 years, the nursing profession has focused on promoting excellence and healthy work environments to ensure quality patient care and to attract and keep nurses in the profession. The following discussion details some important programs and strategies to promote excellent work environments for nurses.

Magnet® Recognition Program

During the nursing shortage of the 1970s and 1980s the American Academy of Nurses, an ANA affiliate, undertook a national study of 163 acute care hospitals to identify the factors associated with retaining qualified nurses during a nursing shortage (McClure et al., 1983). The ANA's credentialing arm, the ANCC, used the study findings to create the Magnet® Recognition Program, which includes best practice standards to improve nurse satisfaction and the work environment of nurses, as well as to reduce turnover rates.

The Magnet® program has five domains that must be demonstrated with a strong emphasis on outcomes: Transformational Leadership, Structural Empowerment, Exemplary Professional Practice, New Knowledge and Innovation, and Empirical Outcomes (ANCC, n.d.a). Research has consistently shown that Magnet® hospital nurses have higher levels of autonomy, more control over the practice setting, and better relationships with physicians as well as improvements in patient satisfaction, failure to rescue rates, and mortality rates (Connor et al., 2023; Hamadi et al. 2020; Kutney-Lee et al., 2015). Nurses advocating for a strong workplace should advocate for their hospital to achieve Magnet® status. For more information about the *Magnet® Recognition Program,* go to https://www.nursingworld.org/organizational-programs/magnet/.

Some organizations may choose to pursue Pathway to Excellence designation. Based on the Texas Nurse-Friendly Program originally developed for small/rural hospitals, the standards were revised by the ANCC to meet national criteria and were renamed the Pathway to Excellence program. Pathway practice standards were developed according to evidence-based practices and expert nurse input that promote and support a positive practice environment (ANCC, n.d.b). For more information about the Pathway to Excellence Program, go to https://www.nursingworld.org/organizational-programs/pathway/.

Shared Governance

Introduced in the 1970s, *shared governance* has been identified by RNs as a cornerstone of excellence in nursing practice (Kutney-Lee et al., 2016). Shared governance provides an organizational framework for nurses in direct care to engage in creating and sustaining an optimal nursing practice and work environment, ensuring that nurses are active participants in decision-making and have shared accountability for the outcomes of those decisions. Magnet® Recognition Program standards support the formation of formal shared governance or decision-making models as foundational to professional practice. In organizations that do not have shared governance, it is important that nurses have access to and input into decisions that affect nursing practice and patient outcomes. Box 13.6 identifies questions that should be asked about shared governance or participatory management models when nurses are trying to identify the organization that would be most conducive to the delivery of quality nursing care.

Conflict Resolution

All organizations should provide nurses with conflict resolution policies and procedures that illustrate processes they should follow if they are in disagreement with the organization's policies and/or leadership. Examples

---

BOX 13.6   Questions to Ask About Shared Governance Models

- Are nurses encouraged to participate in shared governance?
- How do nurses become involved in the shared governance process?
- What is the ratio of staff nurses to managers involved in shared governance within the organization?
- Is adequate work time allowed to participate in governance councils?
- How does the organization communicate shared governance decisions with all staff nurses?

- How does shared governance improve nursing care delivery in the organization?
- Do nurses feel shared governance within their organization is beneficial to their practice?
- Does the organization have outcomes data related to shared governance?
- If so, how have those data helped to drive changes in nursing practice?

From American Nurses Association. (n.d.). *Questions to ask about shared governance models.* https://www.nursingworld.org/practice-policy/workforce/questions-to-ask-about-shared-governance-models-in-nursing/.

---

include open-door policies, ombudsman programs, and dispute–resolution processes. When seeking dispute resolution, the nurse may use a third party or resources internal to the organization to assist in the resolution. Some states have processes such as peer review, safe harbor, and mandatory reporting to help resolve patient care or professional issues. All nurses should be aware of the requirements as set forth by their state's Board of Nursing for these processes—safe harbor, peer review, and mandatory reporting.

SUMMARY

As we summarize this chapter let's revisit Elena and the questions posed at the beginning of the chapter following the opening Vignette.

1. What strategies can Elena use to promote quality patient care and a safe work environment?

   Fortunately, Elena and her nursing team have multiple resources available to them such as needlestick safety laws; comprehensive programs to prevent workplace injuries; programs to protect nurses from workplace violence, bullying, and incivility; and an increased focus on addressing nurse fatigue and providing mental health support for nurses. Most health care organizations have realized the impact of safe staffing on patient outcomes and nurse satisfaction and are undertaking initiatives to address staffing from multiple approaches including nurse recruitment and retention programs; staffing committees or other legislative mandates; and using data from the NDNQI to quantify the value of safe staffing to nursing sensitive outcomes. This chapter provides key information about each of these areas to help all nurses promote quality patient care and a safe work environment.

2. What is the importance of shared governance to Elena's individual nursing practice?

   Shared governance has long been recognized as a key strategy to promote excellence in nursing practice. Shared governance provides Elena and her team with an organizational framework to engage direct-care nurses in decision-making to create and sustain optimal nursing practice and work environments. New nurses are encouraged to learn about the shared governance structures in their practice settings and get involved!

3. What resources are available to help Elena learn more about important workplace issues and workforce advocacy?

   Working together with the resources of organizations such as ANA, specialty professional nursing organizations, state Boards of Nursing, and the health care organization's shared governance structures, Elena and all nurses can learn more about critical workplace issues and help to create a workplace that promotes career satisfaction and quality patient care.

   This chapter has covered a variety of significant workplace issues and has identified workforce advocacy strategies and resources for a nurse to use to improve their work environment and quality of patient care. A rapidly changing health care environment, significantly affected by a serious nursing shortage, creates a challenge for all nurses.

Nurses must be aware of the issues facing the profession and know where to seek assistance, information, and resources to address workplace issues.

CLINICAL JUDGMENT AND NEXT-GENERATION NCLEX® EXAMINATION-STYLE QUESTIONS

Cindy Scoggins, RN, BSN, a seasoned nurse with 11 years of experience, is working in a medical step-down unit. A male patient under her care makes inappropriate remarks about her physical appearance, including a small tattoo on her arm. Later in the shift his demeanor becomes more aggressive and at one point he threatens to strangle her. Cindy is very upset by the encounter with the patient. She notifies her manager, who reassigns the patient to another nurse and recommends that Cindy file a report with hospital security and the local police department, which Cindy does. In the interview that follows, the Director of Security and the police officer downplay the incident, telling her that she should "expect this sort of thing" from men of a certain age. What should Cindy do next? She has several options to protect herself from the threat of violence now and in the future.

Multiple Response: Select All That Apply:

A. Plan time to fully debrief with her supervisor and possibly other colleagues about the incident and how to minimize the risk of similar events occurring in the future.

B. Accept the advice from the Director of Security and forget about the incident.

C. Accept violence from patients as a normal part of the job and, if it occurs again, do not report it.

D. Engage the support of the Shared Governance Council or the Unit Council to promote actions to prevent and address violence in the workplace and ensure an appropriate Workplace Violence Program is implemented.

E. Ask for training in violence de-escalation strategies to use with patients and/or others who become violent or may be potentially violent.

F. Understand that violent acts may be a symptom of the patient's illness and should be accepted by nurses as a normal part of their job that must be tolerated.

G. Request a worksite analysis to identify trends and risk factors for violence specific to the workplace and the patient population being cared for.

REFERENCES

Aiken, L.H., Clarke, S.P., Sloane, D.M., Sochalski, J., & Silber, J.H. (2002). Hospital nurse staffing and patient mortality, nurse burnout, and job dissatisfaction. *JAMA, 288*(16), 1987–1993. https://doi.org/10.1001/jama.288.16.1987

Aiken, L.H., Clarke, S.P., Sloane, D.M., Lake, E.T., & Cheney, T. (2009). Effects of hospital care environment on patient mortality and nurse outcomes. *The Journal of Nursing Administration, 39*(Suppl 7–8), S45–S51. https://doi.org/10.1097/NNA.0b013e3181aeb4cf

Aiken, L.H., & Sloane, D.M. (2020). Nurses matter: More evidence. *BMJ Quality & Safety* (29), 1. https://qualitysafety.bmj.com/content/29/1/1.full

American Association of Colleges of Nursing. (2021). *The essentials: Core competencies for professional nursing education.* Essentials-2021.pdf (aacnnursing.org).

American Association of Colleges of Nursing. (2022). *Fact sheet: Nursing faculty shortage.* https://www.aacnnursing.org/Portals/0/PDFs/Fact-Sheets/Faculty-Shortage-Factsheet.pdf

American Association of Critical Care Nurses. (n.d.). *Healthy Work Environments.* https://www.aacn.org/nursing-excellence/healthy-work-environments

American Nurses Association (n.d.a). *Principles for nurse staffing.* https://www.nursingworld.org/practice-policy/nurse-staffing/staffing-principles

American Nurses Association. (n.d.b). *Workplace violence/# EndNurseAbuse.* https://www.nursingworld.org/practice-policy/work-environment/end-nurse-abuse/

American Nurses Association. (2014). *Addressing nurse fatigue to promote safety and health.* https://www.nursingworld.org/practice-policy/nursing-excellence/official-position-statements/id/addressing-nurse-fatigue-to-promote-safety-and-health/

American Nurses Association. (2015). *Code of ethics for nurses with interpretive statements.* https://www.nursingworld.org/practice-policy/nursing-excellence/ethics/code-of-ethics-for-nurses/coe-view-only

American Nurses Association. (2019). *Issue brief: Reporting incidents of workplace violence.* https://www.nursingworld.org/,4a4076/globalassets/practiceandpolicy/work-environment/endnurseabuse/endabuse-issue-brief-final.pdf

American Nurses Association. (2020). *Crisis standard of care COVID-19 pandemic.* https://www.nursingworld.org/,496044/globalassets/practiceandpolicy/work-environment/health—safety/coronavirus/crisis-standards-of-care.pdf

American Nurses Association. (2021). *Safe Patient Handling Interprofessional Standards and Implementation Guide.* https://www.nursingworld.org/,4a011a/globalassets/practiceandpolicy/work-environment/health—safety/ana-1650-sphm-infographic-updates_final.pdf

American Nurses Association (2022a). Nurses Bill of Rights. https://www.nursingworld.org/,498d25/globalassets/practiceandpolicy/work-environment/health—safety/nurses-bill-of-rights.pdf.

American Nurses Association (2022b). National commission to address racism in nursing. https://www.nursingworld.org/practice-policy/workforce/racism-in-nursing/national-commission-to-address-racism-in-nursing

American Nurses Credentialing Center. (n.d.a). *ANCC Magnet® Recognition Program.* https://www.nursingworld.org/organizational-programs/magnet/

American Nurses Credentialing Center. (n.d.b). *ANCC American Nurses Credentialing Pathway to Excellence®.* https://www.nursingworld.org/organizational-programs/pathway/

AMN Healthcare. (2023). *2023 AMN Survey of registered nurses: The pandemics consequences.* https://www.amnhealthcare.com/amn-insights/nursing/surveys/2023

AMN Healthcare. (2019). *2019 AMN Survey of registered nurses: A challenging decade ahead.* https://www.amnhealthcare.com/amn-insights/nursing/surveys/2019-survey-of-registered-nurses-a-challenging-decade-ahead

American Nurses Foundation (2023). *Three-year annual assessment survey: Nurses need increased support from their employer.* https://www.nursingworld.org/,48fb88/contentassets/23d4f79cea6b4f67ae24714de11783e9/anf-impact-assessment-third-year_v5.pdf

Asber, S.R. (2019). Retention outcomes of new graduate nurse residency programs: An integrative review. *JONA: The Journal of Nursing Administration, 49*(9), 430–435. https://doi.org/10.1097/nna.0000000000000780

Azevedo, A.V., Tonietto, T.A., & Boniatti, M.M. (2022). Nursing workload on the day of discharge from the intensive care unit is associated with readmission. *Intensive and Critical Care Nursing, 69*(10), 31–62.

Bae, S.H., & Fabry, D. (2014). Assessing the relationships between nurse work hours/overtime and nurse and patient outcomes: Systematic literature review. *Nursing Outlook, 62*(2), 138–156. https://doi.org/10.1016/j.outlook.2013.10.009

Bannai, A., & Tamakoshi, A. (2014). The association between long working hours and health: A systematic review of epidemiological evidence. *Scandinavian Journal of Work, Environment & Health, 40*(1), 5–18. https://doi.org/10.5271/sjweh.3388

Berlin, G., Bilazarian, A., Chang, J. & Hammer, S. (2023). *Reimagining the nursing workload: Finding time to close the workforce gap.* https://www.mckinsey.com/industries/healthcare/our-insights/reimagining-the-nursing-workload-finding-time-to-close-the-workforce-gap

Caruso, C.C., Baldwin, C.M., Berger, A., Chasens, E.R., Edmonson, J.C., Gobel, B.H., Landis, C.A., Patrician, P.A., Redeker, N.S., Scott, L.D., Todero, C., Trinkoff, A., & Todero, C. (2019). Policy brief: Nurse fatigue, sleep, and health, and ensuring patient and public safety. *Nursing Outlook, 67*(5), 615–619. https://doi.org/10.1016/j.outlook.2019.08.004

Centers for Disease Control. (2000). *Needlestick Safety and Prevention Act 2000.* http://www.cdc.gov/sharpssafety/pdf/Neelestick%20Saftety%20and%20Prevention%20Act.pdf

Christensen, S.S., Wilson, B.L., & Edelman, L. S. (2018). Can I relate? A review and guide for nurse managers in leading generations. *Journal of Nursing Management, 26*(6), 689–695. https://doi.org/10.1111/jonm.12601

Connor, L., Beckett, C., Zadvinskis, I., Melnyk, B.M., Brown, R., Messinger, J., & Gallagher-Ford, L. (2023). The association between Magnet® Recognition and patient outcomes. *The Journal of Nursing Administration, 53*(10), 500–507.

Davidson, A. (2023). Nurse-to-patient staffing ratio laws and regulations by state. *Nurse Journal.* https://nursejournal.org/articles/nurse-to-patient-staffing-ratio-laws-by-state/#:,:text=California%20is%20the%20only%20state,ratio%20in%20every%20hospital%20unit

Dols, J.D., Chargualaf, K.A., & Martinez, K.S. (2019). Cultural and generational considerations in RN retention. *JONA: The Journal of Nursing Administration, 49*(4), 201–207. https://doi.org/10.1097/nna.0000000000000738

Eckerson, C.M. (2018). The impact of nurse residency programs in the United States on improving retention and satisfaction of new nurse hires: An evidence-based literature review. *Nurse Education Today, 71*, 84–90. https://doi.org/10.1016/j.nedt.2018.09.003

Hamadi, H.Y., Martinez, D., Palenzuela, J., & Spaulding, A.C. (2020). Magnet hospitals and 30-day readmission and mortality rates for Medicare beneficiaries. *Medical Care, 59*(1), 6–12. https://doi.org/10.1097/mlr.0000000000001427

Healthy Nurse Healthy Nation. (2023). Celebrating five years. *American Nurse Journal, 18*(4), 1–12. https://www.healthynursehealthynation.org/,497fe5/globalassets/hnhn-assets/all-images-view-with-media/about/2023-hnhn_5-years_final.pdf

Kohn, L., Corrigan, J., & Donaldson, M. (2000). *To err is human: Building a safer health system.* National Academies Press.

Kutney-Lee, A., Stimpfel, A.W., Sloane, D.M., Cimiotti, J.P., Quinn, L.W., & Aiken, L. (2015). Changes in patient and nurse outcomes associated with Magnet hospital recognition. *Medical Care,* 53(6), 550–557. doi: 10.1097/MLR.0000000000000355

Kutney-Lee, A., Germack, H., Hatfield, L., Kelly, M.S., Maguire, M.P., Dierkes, A., Guidice, M.D., & Aiken, L.H. (2016). Nurse engagement in shared governance and patient and nurse outcomes. *The Journal of Nursing Administration,* 46(11), 605. https://doi.org/10.1097/nna.0000000000000412

Lasater, K.B., Aiken, L.H., Sloane, D., French, R., Martin, B., Alexander, M., & McHugh, M.D. (2021). Patient outcomes and cost savings associated with hospital safe nurse staffing legislation: An observational study. *BMJ Open, 11*(12): doi: 10.1136/bmjopen-2021-052899

Ma, C., McHugh, M.D., & Aiken, L H. (2015). Organization of hospital nursing and 30-day readmissions in Medicare patients undergoing surgery. *Medical Care, 53*(1), 65. https://doi.org/10.1097/mlr.0000000000000258

McClure, M., Poulin, M., Sovie, M.D., & Wandelt, M.A. (1983). Magnet® hospitals: Attraction and retention of professional nurses: Task Force on Nursing Practice in Hospitals, American Academy of Nursing. *American Nurses Association Publications (G–160),* 1–135 i–xiv. 382. https://doi.org/10.1097/01.nna.0000435145.39337.d5

McHugh, M.D., Rochman, M.F., Sloane, D.M., Berg, R. A., Mancini, M.E., Nadkarni, V.M., Merchant, R.M., Aiken, L.H., & American Heart Association's Get with The Guidelines-Resuscitation Investigators. (2016). Better nurse staffing and nurse work environments associated with increased survival of in-hospital cardiac arrest patients. *Medical Care, 54*(1), 74. https://doi.org/10.1097/mlr.0000000000000456

Nei, D., Snyder, L.A., & Litwiller, B.J. (2015). Promoting retention of nurses: A meta-analytic examination of causes of nurse turnover. *Health Care Management Review, 40*(3), 237–253. https://doi.org/10.1097/hmr.0000000000000025

NSI Nursing Solutions (2023). *2023 NSI National Health Care Retention & RN Staffing Report.* https://www.nsinursingsolutions.com/Documents/Library/NSI_National_Health_Care_Retention_Report.pdf

Nurse.com. (2022). *2022 Nurse Salary Research Report.* https://advertise.nurse.com/wp-content/uploads/2022/05/B2B_NurseSalaryReport_2022.pdf

Nursing Organizations Alliance. (2019). *Elements of a healthy practice environment.* https://www.aonl.org/system/files/media/file/2020/02/elements-healthy-practice-environment_1.pdf

Occupational Safety and Health Administration. (2019). *OSHA injury and illness recordkeeping and reporting requirements.* https://www.govinfo.gov/content/pkg/FR-2019-01-25/pdf/2019-00101.pdf

Olds, D.M., Aiken, L.H., Cimiotti, J.P., & Lake, E.T. (2017). Association of nurse work environment and safety climate on patient mortality: A cross-sectional study. *International Journal of Nursing Studies, 74*, 155–161.

Oster, C.A., & Deakins, S. (2018). Practical application of high-reliability principles in healthcare to optimize quality and safety outcomes. *JONA: The Journal of Nursing Administration, 48*(1), 50–55. https://doi.org/10.1097/nna.0000000000000570

Page, A. (2004). *Keeping patients safe: Transforming the work environment of nurses. Institute of Medicine.* National Academies Press.

Parsons, K., Gaudine, A., & Swab, M. (2018). Older nurses' experiences of providing direct care in hospital nursing units: A qualitative systematic review. *JBI Database of Systematic Reviews and Implementation Reports, 16*, 669–700. https://doi.org/10.11124/JBISRIR-2017-003372

Shin, S., Park, J.H., & Bae, S.H. (2018). Nurse staffing and nurse outcomes: A systematic review and meta-analysis. *Nursing Outlook, 66*(3), 273–282. https://doi.org/10.1016/j.outlook.2017.12.002

Smiley, R.A., Allgeyer, R.L., Shobo, Y., Lyons, K.C., Letourneau, R. Zhong, E., & Alexander, M. (2023). The 2022 national workforce survey. *Journal of Nursing Regulation, 14*(1), S1–S90.

Stichler, J.F. (2013). Healthy work environments for the ageing nursing workforce. *Journal of Nursing Management, 21*, 956–963. https://doi.org/10.1111/jonm.12174

Stimpfel, A.W., Fatehi, F., & Kovner, C. (2020). Nurses' sleep, work hours, and patient care quality, and safety. *Sleep Health, 6*(3), 314–320. https://doi.org/10.1016/j.sleh.2019.11.001

Thompson, R. (2021). Increasing racial/ethnic diversification of nursing faculty in higher ed is needed now. *Journal of Professional Nursing, 37*(4), A1–A3.

Ulrich, B., Barden, C., Cassidy, L., & Varn-Davis, N. (2019). Critical care nurse work environments 2018: Findings and implications. *Critical Care Nurse, 39*(2), 67–84. https://doi.org/10.4037/ccn2019605

US Department of Labor, Bureau of Labor Statistics. (2022). *Employer reported workplace injuries and illnesses – 2021.* https://www.bls.gov/news.release/pdf/osh.pdf

US Bureau of Labor Statistics. (2023). *Occupational outlook handbook, registered nurses.* https://www.bls.gov/ooh/healthcare/registered-nurses.htm#tab-6

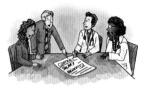

14

Collective Bargaining and Unions in Today's Workplace

Barbara Cherry, DNSc, MBA, RN, NEA-BC

*llective bargaining is a method to achieve
wer sharing in the workplace.*

(e) Additional resources are available online at: http://evolve.elsevier.com/Cherry/

LEARNING OUTCOMES

After studying this chapter, the reader will be able to:
1. Use terms associated with collective bargaining and unions correctly in written and oral communications.
2. List key events in the historical development of collective bargaining and unions.
3. Recognize questionable labor or management practices in the workplace.
4. Analyze collective bargaining as a method to achieve power sharing in the workplace.
5. Evaluate current controversies associated with collective bargaining by professional nurses.

KEY TERMS

Arbitration The process of negotiation sanctioned in the United States by the National Labor Relations Board. It is the method used for formal talks between management and labor within modern business, industry, and service organizations. "Binding arbitration" means that all parties must obey the arbitrator's recommendations.

Collective bargaining The process whereby workers organize under the representation of a union to share a degree of power with management to determine selected aspects of the conditions of employment.

Grievance A term associated with a negative workplace event that results in an allegation by an employee that they have not been treated fairly and equitably. Grievances can occur in union and nonunion settings. In a union setting, a grievance generally arises when two parties, such as an employee and a manager, interpret contract provisions differently. Grievances often involve job security or safety, which is a union priority, or job performance or discipline, which is a management priority.

Industrial unionism A type of union in which there is a single union for all workers in a corporation. For example, all people who work in an automobile manufacturing company may be grouped together under the United Auto Workers (UAW). It is possible that the industrial union, with its massive numbers of union members, is the strongest possible collective group.

Labor A group composed of those who work for others to receive a salary.

Management The group of people within a business or company that plans, organizes, leads, or controls the activities of employees who have agreed to work to receive a salary.

Occupational unionism A type of union in which each occupation within a given company has a separate union. White collar workers coming from a background of higher education and some measure of job security tend to prefer occupational unionism and organizing with like-minded professionals. In general, nurses prefer occupational unionism.

Picketing A form of protest in which people (called picketers) congregate outside a place of work or location where an event is taking place. Often this is done in an attempt to dissuade others from going in ("crossing the picket line"), but it can also be done to draw public attention to a cause.

Right-to-work laws Statutes enforced in just over half of US states, mostly in the southern and western United States, allowed under provisions of the Taft–Hartley Act, which prohibit the requirement for employees to be union members or pay union dues as a condition of employment.

Secret ballot elections To establish a union in a workplace, a majority of employees must express support for the union. The employees prove majority through a secret ballot election conducted by the National Labor Relations Board.

Strike A work stoppage caused by the refusal of a large portion of employees to perform work; usually takes place to enforce demands relating to employment conditions or to protest unfair labor practices. A sympathy strike occurs when one union stops work to support the strike of another union.

Unfair labor practices Actions that interfere with the rights of employees or employers as identified under the National Labor Relations Act. An unfair labor practice can be something as simple as suspicion by an employee that they were assigned to an unpopular task unfairly, or it can be as complex as the identification of a pattern of many employees receiving discriminatory treatment in the workplace because of being union supporters. Unfair labor practices are a frequent source of either strikes or the initiation of union activity within a setting.

Union A group of workers who band together to accomplish goals related to conditions of employment.

PROFESSIONAL/ETHICAL ISSUE

Samuel Lennon is a registered nurse (RN) in the cardiovascular lab at University Hospital. He is experiencing stress and internal conflict because the nurses are going through a union organizing effort. What he thought would be a fairly easy process to vote in a union to represent the nurses with a strong voice to improve their nurse-to-patient ratios has turned into a tension-filled, adversarial situation. Before the union efforts started, Samuel had a good relationship with his nurse manager; now they are pitted against each other because they have very different perspectives about unions. Samuel is also feeling tension and distrust with the same nurses he had supportive working relationships with only a few weeks ago. They are now against one another because of opposing views about unions. His once-collegial relationships with the pharmacists and physical therapists on his unit have also become strained. Samuel is having a great deal of self-doubt about the unionizing efforts and especially what some of his colleagues perceive to be the potential for patient abandonment in the event of a strike. Samuel's greatest concern is how this very difficult situation is affecting patient care.

How can Samuel resolve his feelings and ethical concerns about the unionizing effort yet remain true to the original goals of unionization?

VIGNETTE

Addison Mitchell graduated in June from nursing school. She passed the National Council Licensure Examination (NCLEX) and can now call herself an RN. As she drives to the hospital on the first day of her new job she is feeling a sense of pride and joy—mixed with sheer fright—as she realizes that this is the world-class place she has chosen for her first job. She had always dreamed of working at this hospital, and she will now have a chance to become a seasoned nurse at one of the finest hospitals in the country.

Addison is realistic enough to know that her feelings of joy may not last because her new job is likely to be very stressful, but she is unaware that she is on the verge of walking into a challenging situation. As she enters the drive leading to the hospital parking area, picketers are there with signs about unfair working conditions. Addison quickly learns that nurses are involved in organizing to be represented by a union.

As Addison walks to the building with her new name tag, which reads "Registered Nurse," she is approached by someone asking her to sign a card. Addison replies, "I'm sorry. I'm new here. I need to get my feet on the ground, and then I will be happy to talk to you about the card." Addison feels very anxious because she does not have a good understanding of union organizing efforts or the issues the nurses are facing.

Addison does not yet know that she will be approached many times in the coming days by coworkers who will tell her how she should feel and what she should do. She has much to consider before making a decision between two alternatives that she does not fully understand—supporting unionization or voting against it.

Questions to Consider While Reading This Chapter

1. What questions should the nurse ask about collective bargaining and labor relations?
2. What does signing a card mean, and what questions should Addison ask before signing?
3. How can Addison establish good relationships with both nurse managers and staff nurses in an atmosphere in which collective bargaining has put these two groups in adversarial positions?
4. What provisions in a union contract are in both the nurse's and patient's best interest?

CHAPTER OVERVIEW

Collective bargaining is a very complex and often emotionally charged issue. Because the future of nursing may be influenced by our collective and individual efforts to be fairly represented and to have a voice in the conditions of our work, it is important to understand the positives and negatives related to unionization and collective bargaining as well as the motives of those who would represent nursing. This chapter attempts to present a balanced view of collective bargaining and unionization in the hope that students, staff nurses, and nurses in managerial positions will use the information to make effective decisions when confronted with collective bargaining issues.

DEVELOPMENT OF COLLECTIVE BARGAINING IN AMERICA

Early Activities

During the late 19th century, when the Industrial Revolution was a force throughout North America, a cadre of thinkers arose who believed that workers needed to join together to protect themselves from circumstances such as long work hours, child labor, and unhealthy and unsafe factory conditions. These early groups sought such basic conditions as safety in work situations, adequate pay for hours worked, and the right not to be arbitrarily dismissed. This banding together of workers to accomplish goals was termed *trade unionism*. The technique was successful in many instances and remains with us today.

Federal Legislation

As a result of these early efforts at unionization, Congress passed the National Labor Relations Act (NLRA) in 1935. Under the terms of the NLRA, employees were given the right to self-organize, to form labor unions, and to bargain collectively. The National Labor Relations Board (NLRB) was established to implement provisions of the NLRA. The NLRB is an independent federal agency that continues to play a vital role in labor-management relations and, working through 26 regional offices in major US cities, the agency conducts union elections and prosecutes unfair labor practices.

With employees' rights protected by federal legislation, collective bargaining now occurs in companies across the country. Employees can legally organize themselves into units recognized under terms of the NLRA without fear of being fired for belonging to a union or for participating in union activities such as collective bargaining. Typical goals in collective bargaining activities are to establish reasonable working conditions and to make formal agreements between employees and management for wages and for health and retirement benefits. Unions can vary by the group or groups of employees represented. Industrial unionism is a single union representing all workers in a company, whereas occupational unionism is a separate union representing a distinct occupation within a given company.

However, exemptions to the 1935 NLRA were established for nonprofit companies. This provision meant that employees of nonprofit hospitals, such as nurses, were not protected under the NLRA and therefore were not legally protected for participation in collective bargaining activities. Hospitals' employees may have been excluded from protection by the NLRA because it was believed that services provided were so essential that organizing activities would be contrary to the public's interest. In 1974 legislation allowed for the inclusion of nonprofit hospitals in coverage under provisions of the NLRA. Nurses could form collective bargaining units. The 1974 amendments also included the requirement for a 10-day written notice of the intent to picket or to strike. This notice would give the health care facility time to prepare and would protect the relative health and safety of the public.

Development of Collective Bargaining in Nursing

Formal unionization in nursing began in 1946 when the American Nurses Association (ANA) endorsed collective bargaining as a way to gain economic security and influence employment issues for nurses. While the ANA worked to pave the way for collective bargaining, it also struggled with its role in representing nurses who were part of unions as well as nurses who did not support unionization. To help resolve ANA's role in representing different interests of nurses, a national nurses union—United American Nurses (UAN)—was established as an ANA affiliate to create an independent voice for union nurses. In 2009 the UAN dropped its affiliation with the ANA and merged with the California Nurses Association/National Nurses Organizing Committee and the Massachusetts Nurses Association to form National Nurses United (NNU).

Of the approximately 3.1 million employed RNs in the United States (US Bureau of Labor Statistics, 2023) 17.9% are represented by a collective bargaining unit (Hirsch, Macpherson, & Even, 2023). National Nurses United is the largest nursing union in the United States, representing almost 225,000 RNs in 2023 (NNU, 2023). Other unions that represent nurses include some state nurses associations, Service Employees International Union, and the American Federation of State, County and Municipal Employees.

THE COLLECTIVE BARGAINING PROCESS

Collective bargaining is a method of equalizing power between the employer and the employees. As such it involves negotiation and administrative agreements between employees and employers. Because the individual employee, or even a small group of employees, has limited power to bargain with the employer, banding together in a union gives the employees a stronger voice to negotiate with management. The goals of collective bargaining are achieved by imposing rules regarding how employers must treat employees represented by a union.

Nurses and nurse managers need to understand the steps involved in the union organizing and election process, as well as what are considered appropriate or inappropriate management responses and labor responses. Because union organizing involves power sharing and sometimes a temporary sense of distrust between direct-care nurses and management, it can become an anxious and emotional process. Knowing the allowable patterns for the process of union organizing can help alleviate some stress.

The following discussion is an overview of the general steps in the union organizing process based on information taken from the *Basic Guide to the National Labor Relations Act* (NLRB, 1997). The reader will see that careful attention is given to ensuring fairness for employer, employees, and the unions that may be involved in an election to determine whether employees agree to unionize.

Although this discussion provides a general overview of the union election process, readers are encouraged to visit the NLRB website (http://www.nlrb.gov) for more detailed information about the union election process.

The Preformal Period in Union Organizing

The goal of collective bargaining is the equalization of power between labor (e.g., direct-care nurses) and management. To initiate collective bargaining activities an organizing drive is instituted by union forces, who attempt to create an official NLRB-sanctioned bargaining unit in a particular institution. A union organizing drive may be initiated when nurses in a health care facility contact a union because they feel a need for help in negotiating with their employer. The stimulus for this initial contact is usually not frivolous. There is typically a pervasive feeling among the nurses on a particular unit, or in the health care facility as a whole, that working conditions are unsatisfactory and that there is no possibility of making improvements under the existing management circumstances.

It is helpful at this point to examine what is to be gained by those petitioning the NLRB for an election for union representation. For a group of nurses, a newly formed union will:

- Have the power to make certain demands of the employer, especially regarding salary, benefits, and nurse-to-patient ratios.
- Provide some degree of political power on a local level.
- Require nurses to pay dues to the union.

For the union organization, a newly formed union will:

- Give the union additional power by adding more members and more bargaining units, especially if the union is part of a larger national union.
- Increase monetary support for the union organization through dues paid by nurses. The additional money can be used to pay union officials' salaries, organize other bargaining units, or contribute to political causes or candidates.

Signing Cards.

Once a union has been contacted by nurses and told that there is some interest in establishing a collective bargaining unit, union forces try to determine whether efforts to organize the majority of nurses in the facility will be successful. This determination is made through a process of "signing cards." Union authorization cards help the union organizer, a person who works for the union, to decide whether there is enough interest in unionization on the part of nurses employed in the facility. Once signed by the nurse, the union authorization card designates the union as their bargaining agent. The signed authorization card is legally binding on the employee, despite any claims the union may make to the contrary. ***It is very important for the nurse to understand that their signature on a union authorization card is automatically authorizing the union to serve as their legal representative.***

If 30% of employed nurses sign cards, signaling an interest in representation by the union, the employer and the NLRB are officially notified, and the employer must refrain from antilabor action such as firing those who favor the union (NLRB, 1997). If 50% plus 1 of the nurses who are eligible to vote (nonmanagement nurses) respond in the affirmative to accept union representation, then nurses in the facility become represented by the union and are unionized.

Right-to-Work Laws.

An important exception to note here is that there are 27 states with right-to-work laws that allow employees to work without being compelled to join a union. A nurse in a right-to-work state can choose not to become a union member yet will receive the benefits resulting from the union contract. Thus in right-to-work states union member nurses may work alongside nonunion member nurses, possibly creating tension between the two groups. As of 2023, the 27 right-to-work states are Alabama, Arizona, Arkansas, Florida, Georgia, Idaho, Indiana, Iowa, Kansas, Kentucky, Louisiana, Michigan, Mississippi, Nebraska, Nevada, North Carolina, North Dakota, Oklahoma, South Carolina, South Dakota, Tennessee, Texas, Utah, Virginia, West Virginia, Wisconsin, and Wyoming.

Allowable Actions During the Union Organizing Effort.

To follow the process effectively, a nurse should be aware of details of what is and is not allowed and what is and is not likely to occur during union organizing efforts. When a specific union, such as NNU, initiates organizing activities in a particular facility an organizer goes to the facility. The organizer, who may be called a *business agent* or *field representative*, is responsible for developing and implementing plans to ensure success of the unionizing effort.

To form a core support group in the facility the organizer locates respected leaders in the workplace. Meetings are then held in nonwork settings such as homes or restaurants to gain initial information about grievances and workplace inequities. This information is used as a basis for campaign literature. To gain additional supporters, discussion and card signing take place in areas in the actual facility: locker rooms, bathrooms, lunch areas, lounges, and less-visible work areas. E-mail and social media such as Facebook and X are also used as means for union organizers to communicate with employees.

As the union drive surfaces to gain management's attention organizers begin to distribute cards more openly. At this point the union organizer sends a registered letter to the employer with the names of employees on the organizing committee. Management will probably have become aware of organizing activities through clues such as employee behavior changes during this period. There will be times when individuals seem distracted or when there is an increase in the number or aggressive quality of complaints about workplace conditions. Conversely, there may be a feeling of distancing between labor and management and an air of unnatural silence among employees.

Although peaceful strikes and picketing may occur for publicity or recognition, the NLRB prohibits certain behaviors during the preelection period. The union may not:

- Inflame racial prejudices.
- Lie about loss of jobs if the union loses the election.
- Forge documents or signatures.

- Meet or distribute literature in work areas during work times.
- Hold meetings within 24 hours of an election.
  During the preelection period, management may not:
- Solicit spying.
- Photograph employees engaged in union activities.
- Visit employees in their homes.
- Lie about what will happen if the union is the victor in an election.
- Question employees about their preferences regarding union activity.

The Election Process

The bargaining unit is either accepted or rejected through an election process in which nonmanagement employees (direct-care nurses) vote. If accepted the bargaining unit will be made up of union members who are workers at the unionized facility and will be protected against arbitrary treatment and unfair labor practices.

There are several steps in the election process. Either the union or the employer must petition the NLRB for an election. Once this petition is made the request is passed along to the regional NLRB director. Within 48 hours the union must submit proof of its claim that 30% of eligible nurses are interested in forming a collective bargaining unit. Eligible nurses are generally considered to be nurses who are engaged in patient care and are not in management positions. Normally, for a 10-day period, literature will be distributed to eligible employees. The union and the employer may circulate literature; however, both sides must cease such activities 24 hours before the election.

On the day designated for the election, the three parties (the NLRB, union representatives, and employer representatives) meet to review the list of those eligible to vote. A secret ballot election is then conducted by the NLRB. The three parties then count ballots, and in case of a true tie a victory for the employer is declared. However, any votes in dispute will be set aside for a later recount. Objections must be made within 5 working days after the election and may be made on the grounds of problems with the conduct of the election or unfair labor practices.

Postelection

After the election in the case of a union victory, federal law guarantees workers the right to collectively bargain and strike. Nurses may subsequently change a bargaining agent or remove the union representation by having 30% of nurses sign cards. An election would follow, requiring a vote of 50% plus 1 in favor of the change (NLRB, 1997).

The NLRA mandates that under the rules of collective bargaining meetings between management and labor be held at reasonable times for the purpose of conferring in good faith. Mandatory topics for arbitration include wages; the establishment of rules about the use of labor, such as hours of work and nurse-to-patient ratios; individual workers' rights; resolution of grievances; and methods of enforcement, interpretation, and administration of the union agreement. Negotiations between union and management occur in cycles following the initial year of collective bargaining. Negotiations are held before a contract is ratified (approved) by both union and management and again just before the contract expires.

Principles to Guide Fairness During Union Organizing

In an unprecedented collaboration between a major US health care employer and unions a set of guiding principles was established to ensure a fair process for union organizing efforts. The principles, which were adopted in 2009 and reaffirmed in 2019, can serve as a guide for employers and unions across the country, and they help ensure that health care employees are able to make informed decisions regarding unionization without undue influence or pressure from either side. On the basis of these seven principles employers as well as unions should agree in writing how they will act (Catholic Healthcare Association of America, 2009):

1. Demonstrate respect for each other's organization and mission.
2. Provide workers with equal access to information from both sides.
3. Adhere to standards for truthfulness and balance in their communications.
4. Create a pressure-free environment.
5. Allow workers to vote through a fair and expeditious process.
6. Honor employees' decision regardless of the outcome.
7. Create a system for enforcing these principles during the course of an organizing drive.

UNIONS AND PROFESSIONAL NURSING

Professionalism Vs Unionization

Nurses in the workplace are buffeted by cost cutting, nursing shortages, shuffled duties, and concerns about patient safety and quality care. Despite these challenges in the workplace, it is often problematic for nurses to come to grips with their feelings related to unionization. Nurses know that unions may present the possibility of having a stronger voice to improve their working conditions, but they also know that unions bring the requirements to pay monthly dues and participate in strikes against the hospital, among other things. See Table 14.1 for a summary of the positives and negatives related to unionization.

The process of joining a union can also be fraught with conflict between and among direct care nurses, their nurse managers, and even members of the interprofessional team as Samuel was experiencing in the opening Professional/Ethical Issue (at the beginning of the chapter). It is often difficult for nurses to reconcile feelings of professionalism and service with the perceived connotations of strife and discord sometimes associated with unions. The following four questions address important issues for nurses to contemplate as they approach any decisions about unionization and collective bargaining.

Questions to Answer

Four major questions need to be answered as nurses consider unionization.

1. Are there relevant gains to be made for the nursing profession and for improved patient care through collective bargaining?

2. Should nurses, who frequently are called on to supervise the work of others, be classified for collective bargaining purposes as management or labor?

3. Will nurses be too reluctant to strike? This is one of the most powerful tools that a union has at its disposal. There is concern that strikes by nurses could negatively affect patient care and destroy the public's image of nursing. More importantly, the strike is contrary to nursing ethics and licensure to do no harm and avoid patient abandonment.

4. How will nursing unions affect other members of the interprofessional team (e.g., physical therapy, dietary, pharmacy) who are essential for quality patient care? Will the nurses' collective bargaining contract create inequities for other professionals?

These questions are addressed in more detail in the following sections.

Gains for the Nursing Profession and Patient Care?

When considering unionization, nurses need to seriously reflect on issues that affect the practice of professional nursing and the patient care environment beyond the aspects that unions typically address during negotiations (wages and benefits, work hours, worker safety, and resolution of grievances). The primary triggers that spark interest in being represented by a union often are forgotten in the challenges confronted by nurses during the union organization process. Consider the following issues that may prompt a group of nurses to seek union representation:

- Staffing issues that lead to unsafe nurse-to-patient ratios

TABLE 14.1 Positive and Negative Points Related to Unionization	
Positive Points for Unions	**Negative Points for Unions**
• Improve wages and benefits	• Nurse is required to pay monthly union fees
• Ensure safe working conditions including appropriate breaks and safety equipment	• Nurse may be required to participate in strikes even if they do not personally support the cause behind the strike; nurses on strike are not paid
• Support to investigate grievances and ensure due process	• Seniority is rewarded above performance, making it difficult to address poor or inadequate work performance for nurses with seniority
• Ensure consistent standards for hiring, promotion, and termination	• Unions are designed to protect nurses and are not focused on improving patient care outcomes

Data from Feeney, A. (2024). What are the pros and cons of joining a nursing union? *Nursing Journal.* https://nursejournal.org/resources/nursing-union-pros-cons

- Lack of administrative support for collegial, professional relationships among nurses, physicians, and other interprofessional team members
- Deficient patient handoff procedures that cause errors, frustration, interdepartmental conflicts, and delay in care
- Inadequate time and resources for continuing education and training in unit-specific competencies

Nurses are cautioned that gains in wages and benefits have been associated with unionization (Catlin, 2020) but improvements in the nursing practice environment may or may not occur. The literature is scant and ambiguous about the effect of unionization on patient outcomes and nurse satisfaction but there are some relevant studies to consider:

- A study looking at job satisfaction and nurse turnover found that nurses who were union members were more likely to experience job dissatisfaction but less likely to report turnover when compared to nonunion nurses (Lee, Halleck, & Lee, 2023).
- A second study looking at the impact of unions on nurse job satisfaction found that union representation was negatively associated with job satisfaction (Seago et al., 2011); researchers in this study point out that a cause for this finding may be that union nurses could be more vocal about expressing their concerns or the dissatisfaction may have led to the unionization.
- A study with results favorable to unionization found 12 of 13 potentially nurse-sensitive patient outcomes improved among a group of California hospitals after nurses voted to be represented by a union (Dube et al., 2016).
- A study of nurse leaders' perception of union activities found a negative effect on the work environment as a result of union activities (Stichler et al., 2019).
- A study comparing 84 union and 84 nonunion hospitals in the United States found that hospitals with unions had significantly lower patient satisfaction (Koys et al., 2015).

As one can see we still have much to learn about the impact of unions on the professional practice environment!

Another professional practice issue to consider is that open dialog between nurses and their managers regarding patient care issues and concerns may be limited in a unionized facility. For example, the manager cannot discuss performance issues or concerns with a nurse directly; the union representative must serve as the intermediary between the nurse and the manager. This added layer to address the nurse's performance increases costs to the facility for both management time and legal expense. However, these communication issues in a union facility may be mitigated with proactive strategies allowing nurse leaders to meet with frontline nurses without union negotiators present; topics for discussion might include staffing, scheduling, floating, technology, education, career ladder, and the charge nurse role but would not include complementation and benefits (Stichler et al., 2019).

When faced with union organizing efforts, nurses need to carefully consider all factors, including the professional practice environment. Box 14.1 presents a list of questions the nurse should ask when considering a union organizing effort.

Promoting a Positive Work Environment. Regardless of whether the nurse works in a union environment, there are several strategies they can use to develop and encourage sound relationships between management and labor to promote a positive work environment:

- Assess your knowledge of the labor laws and practices in your area; seek to understand the unique

---

BOX 14.1   Questions to Ask When Confronted by a Union Organizer

- What measures has the union successfully used to improve quality of care and nurse-sensitive patient outcomes and to promote national patient safety goals?
- Will the union guarantee in writing that it will be getting employees a specified wage increase and better benefits or be liable to employees if it doesn't?
- How much are union dues? What portion of union dues goes to paying union salaries?
- Are there special union assessments? If so, how much are they and how often are they imposed?
- What are the consequences if employees violate the union constitution and/or bylaws?
- Will the union guarantee in writing that employees will not be permanently replaced during an economic strike?
- Will the union pay wages to employees if they are called on to strike?
- Will union members be expected to picket at other unionized facilities in the event of a strike or an informational picket?

culture of the facility; and seek transparent communication with nursing leaders before union activity begins or grievances are filed.

- Understand what protections are already in place through laws and regulations to protect your rights as a nurse (e.g., whistle-blower protection, staffing regulations, safe patient handling laws).
- Identify and be proactive in situations in which nurses or managers disrespect others, ignore serious staff and patient care concerns, or neglect appropriate communication and follow-up.
- Participate in education and training that will improve relationships with both staff and managers in union and nonunion environments.
- Be proactive in solving issues that compromise patient care; embrace your role in achieving timely outcomes that truly improve care.
- Develop an understanding of and respect for the health care facility's financial challenges and become part of the solution for more cost-effective care.

Management or Staff?

One of the difficult issues for nursing in relation to collective bargaining is that in the eyes of the NLRB certain nurses are singled out as management or supervisory personnel and are not allowed NLRA protection, which applies only to nonmanagement employees. Charge nurses and shift supervisors have traditionally been considered part of management rather than labor. But what about frontline nurses who routinely supervise others such as nursing assistants? Are these nurses acting exclusively on behalf of the company that employs them or are they routinely carrying out their responsibilities as professional nurses?

The definition of *manager* or *supervisor* is problematic even in nonhealth care settings. In nursing, things become even more complicated. Most experienced RNs are involved in some type of supervisory or management work. For example, most staff nurses who ordinarily provide bedside care have been called on to be in charge of a particular unit for a particular working shift. Does this mean that the nurse should no longer be considered nonmanagement?

Another trend that affects decisions about supervisory status is the increasing use of unlicensed personnel in health care workplaces and how these workers are supervised. More nurses could now be classified as supervisory because they direct the activities of unlicensed

workers. However, this issue about nurses as supervisors was addressed and clarified through the judicial system. In 1997 the decision of the US Court of Appeals for the Ninth Circuit ruled that RNs who performed charge nurse duties were not management and therefore were eligible for collective bargaining protection. In another case the court ruled that the judgment used by RNs in assigning patients and coordinating patient care was part of their professional role rather than part of any statutory supervision as defined by the NLRA.

Beyond the issue of recognizing who is management and who is staff is the uncomfortable prospect of pitting nurse managers against their colleagues in the workplace. A definite schism occurs when managers and staff are placed on opposite sides of the table. Bad feelings arise. For example, a nurse manager represents management but is not insulated in an executive office. In addition, the nurse manager must often assume duties routinely performed by staff nurses in the event of a strike. This situation can lead to lingering negative feelings even after the strike is resolved.

Techniques frequently used by nurse managers to maintain smooth and efficient job performance in their work settings may be relatively ineffective when unionization or collective bargaining initiatives occur. For example, the nurse manager who believes that open communication in both upward and downward directions is useful for problem solving may become frustrated during unionization initiatives. Union tactics may involve coaching nurses at staff levels to use the "silent treatment" and not cooperate with nurse managers' attempts to communicate.

To Strike or Not?

A nursing strike is defined as "a last resort effort, after significant bargaining on specific issues between nurses and management, which has not allowed for agreement, in which a work stoppage occurs, and nurses leave the bedside" (Catlin, 2020). Strikes can have very powerful effects. One can best understand the economic effect of a strike by noting that hospitals become concerned over lost revenues when the average daily census drops only a few percentage points. A hospital could possibly have to turn away patients because of a strike and could lose that market share permanently, resulting in long-term losses to the hospital. Thus a strike or the threat of a strike can be effective in gaining concessions (e.g., salary increases, better benefits) from management in an effort to avoid the strike completely or to end it as soon as possible. However, the nurse will not be paid while on strike, which can have a significant personal financial impact for the nurse. It is important to note that in some states collective bargaining contracts may contain "no strike" clauses, prohibiting the collective bargaining unit from having the power of the strike.

Nursing is a trusted profession, and for many nurses the strike is a symbol of negative behavior and the decision to strike can be very difficult for a nurse, especially because nurses have a strong sense of duty to their patients. To safeguard nursing's image and allow hospitals to react effectively in safeguarding patient care, a 10-day notice of intent to strike is required. On receipt of such notice, the NLRB attempts to mediate, and the hospital in question is encouraged to decrease census and halt elective admissions. Schedules are developed for covering the emergency department, operating room, and intensive care areas.

As nurses are confronted with making decisions about unionization it is important to consider the many issues that would affect their personal economic welfare, their practice environment, and the quality of patient care they are able to provide. There are no easy answers because the issues and challenges vary depending on each organization's unique set of circumstances. To successfully negotiate unionization initiatives and make good decisions nurses are encouraged to learn more about collective bargaining and unions.

Nursing Unions and Interprofessional Teamwork?

Nursing may be the only professional occupation in a health care setting to be represented by a union (i.e., occupational unionism). Unfortunately, having unionized nurses working alongside employees such as pharmacists and therapists, who are not represented by unions, may create ill will between the two groups. The benefit package for nurses represented by a union can be different from—and likely better than—the benefit package for other employees. As employment and practice issues arise, nurses have union representation as their go-between to work with management, whereas other disciplines work directly with management to resolve issues. The union contract for nurses' benefits will increase the overall costs to the organization, forcing the organization to cut in other areas not controlled by the union, such as benefits for nonunionized health professionals. Imagine how the relationship between two professionals might be strained if the nurse represented by the union has more paid time off and more frequent salary increases than a colleague they work with on a daily basis; plus the nonnursing professional knows that the cost of the union contract may be the reason they are not able to get a salary increase. Relationships between interprofessional team members is a very important issue as nurses consider unionization.

◼ SUMMARY

To summarize this chapter, let's revisit Addison from the opening Vignette as she is experiencing conflict related to the union organizing effort in the hospital where she just started working. First, the chapter provides Addison with a history and overview of the collective bargaining process, which can help her better understand what is happening in her workplace. As Addison has asked many questions of her new manager and fellow nurses, she has learned important issues that need to be considered including (1) what it means to sign a union authorization card, which automatically authorizes the union to serve as her legal representative; (2) the positive and negative points of unionization (Table 14.1); (3) how unionization may or may not improve the professional practice environment and quality care; (4) questions surrounding management versus labor in unionization; (5) the controversy of the strike as a strategy to gain concessions from the employer; and (6) the impact of nursing unions on the interprofessional team. Addison has also learned important questions to ask during the union organizing process (Box 14.1) and now understands strategies to promote a positive work environment regardless of working in a union or nonunion workplace. Nurses live in a new era in health care and will need to continue to grow in their knowledge of unions and collective bargaining.

REFERENCES

American Nurses Association. (2023). ANA membership. https://www.nursingworld.org/ana

Catlin, A. (2020). Nursing strike, America, 2019: Concept analysis to guide practice. *Nursing Outlook, 68*(4), 468–475. https://doi.org/10.1016/j.outlook.2020.03.002

Catholic Healthcare Association of America. (2009). *Respecting the just rights of workers: Guidance and options for Catholic health care and unions.* http://www.usccb.org/issues-and-action/human-life-and-dignity/labor-employment/upload/respecting_the_just_rights_of_workers.pdf

Dube, A., Kaplan, E., & Thompson, O. (2016). Nurse unions and patient outcomes. *ILR Review, 69*(4), 803–833. https://doi.org/10.1177/0019793916644251

Hirsch, B.T., Macpherson, D.A., & Even, W.E. (2023). *Union membership and coverage databases.* www.unionstats.com

Koys, D.J., Martin, W.M., Lavan, H., & Katz, M. (2015). Union density and hospital outcomes. *Hospital Topics, 93*(3), 69–76. https://doi.org/10.1080/00185868.2015.1108142

Lee, D., Halleck, J., & Lee, H. (2023). The impact of union membership on nursing turnover and job satisfaction. *The Journal of Nursing Administration, 51*(6), 353–360.

The National Labor Relations Board (1997). *Basic guide to the national labor relations act.* US Government Printing Office. https://www.nlrb.gov/sites/default/files/attachments/basic-page/node-3024/basicguide.pdf

National Nurses United. (2023). *About us.* https://www.nationalnursesunited.org/about

Seago, J.A., Spetz, J., Ash, M., Herrera, C.N., & Keane, D. (2011). Hospital RN job satisfaction and nurse unions. *The Journal of Nursing Administration, 41*(3), 109–114. https://doi.org/10.1097/nna.0b013e31820c726f

Stichler, J.F., Pelletier, L.R., & Thomason, T. (2019). An exploratory, descriptive study of nurse leaders' personal and work experiences during union negotiations and strike events. *Journal of Nursing Administration, 49*(1), 42–47. https://doi.org/10.1097/nna.0000000000000706

US Bureau of Labor Statistics. (2023). *Occupational employment and wage statistics.* https://www.bls.gov/oes/current/oes291141.htm#ind

15

Information Technology in the Clinical Setting

Stephanie H. Hoelscher, DNP, RN-BC, CPHIMS, CHISP, FHIMSS

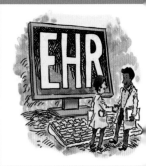

Electronic health records offer nurses other team members information w■ where, and how they need it.

ⓔ Additional resources are available online at: http://evolve.elsevier.com/Cherry/

LEARNING OUTCOMES

After studying this chapter, the reader will be able to:

1. Describe key attributes of electronic health record systems and their influence on patient safety and quality care.
2. Explain "meaningful use" and promoting interoperability program criteria as applicable to electronic health records.
3. Critique various types of point-of-care technology and their use in the clinical setting.
4. Assess how future trends in digital health technology will affect health care delivery.

KEY TERMS

Decision support tools Software programs that process data to produce or recommend decisions by linking with an electronic knowledge base controlled by established rules for combining data elements; the knowledge base and rules mimic the knowledge and reasoning an expert health professional would apply to data and information to solve a problem.

Digital Health Various health information technology falls under the "digital health" umbrella, including sensors, wearable devices, telehealth, mobile devices and applications, artificial intelligence, and machine learning (US Food & Drug Administration, 2020a).

Electronic health record (EHR) A digital version of a patient's chart with real-time patient records that make information available instantly and securely to authorized users; in addition to patient data, the EHR may allow for access to evidence-based tools to help providers make decisions about a patient's care and sharing of information with other health care providers and organizations (The Office of the National Coordinator for Health Information Technology [ONC], 2019a). The longitudinal electronic record of patient health information generated by one or more encounters in any care delivery setting has the ability to support other care-related activities such as evidence-based decision support, quality management, and outcomes reporting.

EHR interoperability EHR systems that have the ability to share and transfer patient data seamlessly across health care systems and settings in a standardized manner that protects the reliability, confidentiality, privacy, and security of the information.

EHR "meaningful use" (MU) A defined set of EHR capabilities and standards that EHR systems must meet to ensure that their full capacity is realized and for the users (hospitals and physician/provider practices) to qualify for financial incentives from Medicare (now known as the "Promoting Interoperability Program").

Health information technology (HIT) The use of various forms of technology to improve the quality of health services to individuals and communities.

Information technology The hardware and software that enable information to be stored, retrieved, communicated, and managed.

Point-of-care technology Technologies that allow real-time data retrieval, documentation, and decision support at the bedside or wherever direct care is provided.

Promoting Interoperability Program The Centers for Medicaid and Medicare Services (CMS) renamed "meaningful use" in 2018 to refocus efforts to increase interoperability and improve patients' access to their health care data.

PROFESSIONAL/ETHICAL ISSUE

Katherine is a recent registered nurse–bachelor of science in nursing (RN-BSN) graduate working in the intensive care unit of a small, community-based hospital. She receives a new patient and begins reviewing the patient's history. This patient, a 68-year-old male with multiple comorbidities, has transferred due to a deteriorating condition and has a developing coccyx bedsore. During her assessment, Katherine notes the bedsore and takes out her sanctioned facility phone for photographic documentation and upload into the EHR. Katherine notes that the facility phone battery has no charge and places it on the charger. She wishes to finish the assessment as she is busy, so she takes a picture with her personal cell phone for later use.

Knowing the legal and security risks with using personal cell phones for patient information, discuss how Katherine might have handled the situation differently and how a breach of inpatient health information can be a detriment to the patient as well as the nurse and the health care facility.

VIGNETTE

Victoria Ellis is finally living her dream. After 4 hard years in school, Victoria is working at a university medical center. Although she graduated from a well-respected nursing program, she is apprehensive about her new role, especially documenting care and accessing pertinent information. In nursing school, all of her clinical experiences were in facilities that used electronic health records (EHRs), but as a student, Victoria's access to the EHRs was limited. She could not log onto the system herself, she could not chart, and she could access only limited screens such as lab values, assessment information, and vital signs. Victoria learned in school that EHRs are a vital information technology tool in health care today, but according to her limited experience an EHR seems like it is nothing more than a paper chart on a computer. So what is all the hype about EHRs, information technology, and health care?

Questions to Consider While Reading This Chapter:

1. What are the potential benefits of EHRs to nurses, other health care providers, and patients?
2. What are the barriers to a universal US health information technology infrastructure?
3. What is meant by "meaningful use" of EHRs? What is meant by "promoting interoperability" for EHRs?
4. How might digital health technology and advanced point-of-care technology influence health care at the bedside?
5. What are your roles and responsibilities in protecting health data at your health organization and beyond?

CHAPTER OVERVIEW

Today's clinical setting is filled with a multitude of technological tools and equipment that are used by all health care providers. Nurses are likely to encounter voice communication systems, handheld mobile devices, robotic pharmacy dispensaries, wearable technologies, and complex computers and EHRs. These records present data in dashboards, graphs, tables, and charts that may reveal a different story from that told by words and numbers alone. Transforming patient data into meaningful bits of information is merely one advantage of health information technology (HIT). These data can also be shared with other health care settings, creating a comprehensive patient record, thereby reducing duplicate services and tests (potentially saving patients pain and financial burden) and creating continuity in care. In this chapter, we explore the important role of HIT in today's clinical environment, barriers to and opportunities with advanced HIT, and ways to educate consumers about health information on the Internet.

HEALTH INFORMATION TECHNOLOGY ACROSS THE GLOBE

Health information technology, or technology used to promote the health and well-being of patients and the community, is ever-increasing as technology rapidly advances. Consumer-driven demands for greater knowledge and access to care options have driven many of the technology integrations within health care settings, including nursing academia and practice. Additionally, regulatory and accrediting bodies require or strongly recommend integrating technology into all aspects of nursing academia and practice. Expansion of the Internet, through search engines and mobile device applications, is also responsible for promoting access to health resources and information. The need for EHR interoperability is changing the functionality of patient portals, mobile device applications, and EHRs. Global integration of technology has advanced the possibilities for networking, education, provider consultation, and disaster response without regard to geographic limitations.

Health Information Technology in the United States

Health information technology has been a hot topic for more than two decades, specifically in relation to the need for improved quality and safety of patient care. Since 2011 meaningful use (MU) has challenged health care leaders to implement certified EHR technology (CEHRT) across all settings, from hospitals to ambulatory care to home health agencies and nursing homes. Per The Office of The National Coordinator for Health Information Technology (ONC), in 2017 more than 99% of the nation's larger hospitals and 80% of office-based physicians had met MU criteria with CEHRT (ONC, 2019b). For EHR systems to have the greatest impact on cost and quality, they must be interoperable, with the ability to exchange information across systems and settings in a standardized manner that protects the

information's reliability, confidentiality, privacy, and security.

Within the United States there are two major influences on the adoption of EHRs: the federal government and America's health insurance plans. Both entities can set certain requirements regarding EHRs as a condition of payment for services. In the past measuring adoption rates of EHRs in the United States was a challenge because it depended on self-reporting. However, in 2011 the Centers for Medicare & Medicaid Services (CMS) offered payment incentives to providers—hospitals and physician/provider practices—that qualify and adopt certified EHRs that meet MU criteria. This was renamed in 2018 to the Promoting Interoperability Program (PIP) (CMS, 2020a).

ELECTRONIC HEALTH RECORDS

An EHR is a system that captures, processes, communicates, secures, and presents data about the patient. In addition to capturing patient data, other components of an EHR include clinical rules, patient education materials, evidence-based practice guidelines, and payer rules related to reimbursement. A certified electronic health record is an EHR meeting specific standards by CMS and the ONC (CMS, 2021). These standards must be met to qualify for PIP. Examples of these required standards include technological capability and functionality for reporting and data sharing, as well as data security and the ability to maintain patient confidentiality (CMS, 2020b). When these elements work together in an integrated fashion the EHR becomes much more than a patient record—it becomes a knowledge tool. The system is able to integrate information from multiple sources and provide decision support; thus the EHR serves as the primary source of information for patient care and quality improvements in the health care system.

Key Functions of the EHR

The Institute of Medicine (IOM) was an early leader in providing definitions for EHR components. In 2003 IOM published a letter report recommending that EHR systems offer the following eight functionalities: (1) health information and data capture; (2) results/data management; (3) provider order entry management; (4) clinical decision support; (5) electronic communication and connectivity among providers, the health care

TABLE 15.1	Core Functionalities for Electronic Health Record Systems as Recommended by the Institute of Medicine
Health information and data	Information to make sound clinical decisions, such as past medical history, laboratory tests, allergies, current medications, and consent forms
Results management	Electronic reports of laboratory results and radiology procedures with automated display of previous results; electronic consultation reports
Order entry and order management	Computerized provider order entry with or without decision support to eliminate lost orders and illegible handwriting, generate related orders automatically, monitor for duplicate or contradictory orders, and reduce time to fill orders
Decision support	Enhance clinical performance by providing reminders about preventive practices, such as immunizations, drug alerts for dosing and interactions, and clinical decision-making
Electronic communication and connectivity	Electronic communication between health care team members and other care partners, such as radiology and laboratory personnel, and connectivity to the patient record across multiple care settings
Patient support	Computer-based patient education and home monitoring where applicable
Administrative processes	Scheduling systems, billing and claims management, insurance eligibility, and inventory management
Reporting and population health management	Meeting of public and private sector reporting requirements at the federal, state, and local levels; addressing of internal quality improvement initiatives

Data from Institute of Medicine of the National Academies (IOM). (2003). *Key capabilities of an electronic health record system: Letter report*. National Academies Press. https://www.ncbi.nlm.nih.gov/books/NBK221802/pdf/Bookshelf_NBK221802.pdf

team, and patients; (6) patient support; (7) administrative process support; and (8) reporting and population health management. Table 15.1 provides more detailed information about these core functionalities. Similar to these original IOM recommendations, the current PIP core functions should also be considered (CMS, 2020b, 2020c):

- Coordination of care through patient engagement;
- Health information exchange (HIE);
- Public health reporting; and
- Collection and reporting of quality care measures.

To view sample screens from an EHR, see Figs. 15.1 and 15.2.

Clinical Decision Support (CDS). CDS is of particular relevance to nursing practice because it contributes to safety and quality by providing automatic reminders about preventive practices, such as computerized, evidence-based alerts and reminders, severity indexes for specific illnesses, preventative care screenings (e.g., mammograms) identification, immunizations, drug alerts for drug allergies, drug dosing and interactions (including drug, environment, and food interactions), and electronic resources for data interpretation and clinical decision-making. The ONC defines CDS as providing "clinicians, staff, patients, or other individuals with knowledge and person-specific information, intelligently filtered or presented at appropriate times, to enhance health and health care. CDS encompasses a variety of tools to enhance decision-making in the clinical workflow" (2018a, para. 1).

Since its start CDS has proven itself to have many benefits including (1) increased quality of care and health outcomes; (2) avoidance of errors and adverse/never events; and (3) improved efficiency, cost, and clinician satisfaction (ONC, 2018a). Downsides to CDS that must be considered in its development and implementation are alert fatigue, clinical burnout, and over-reliance on technology to replace critical thinking skills. These are all expected outcomes surrounding poorly designed EHR CDS. It is always of benefit to include nurses, as well as other applicable clinicians, at the decision-making table when it comes to implementing CDS (Bellucci, 2022; Hoelscher & McBride, 2020).

Computerized Provider Order Entry (CPOE). Another component of the EHR relevant to safety and quality is CPOE, defined as the "the process of providers

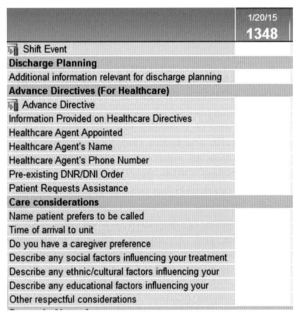

aspirin tablet 325 mg
325 mg, Oral, Once, Tomorrow at 0000, For 1 dose   Accept   Cancel

Dose: 325   mg   325 mg   650 mg

Administer Dose: **325 mg**
Administer Amount: **1 tablet**

Route: Oral   Oral

Frequency: Once   Once Daily Q4H PRN Q6H PRN

Starting: 1/21/2015   Today Tomorrow   At 0000
First Dose: **Tomorrow 0000**   Number of doses: **1**
Scheduled Times: Hide Schedule
1/21/15 0000

Admin. Inst.:   Click to add text
Comments (F6): Click to add text
(300 char max.)
Priority:

▶ Additional Order Details

⟳ Next Required   Link Order   Accept   Cancel

Fig. 15.1 Selected screen from a patient's EHR. (Courtesy of Epic.)

1/20/15
1348

⊠ Shift Event
Discharge Planning
Additional information relevant for discharge planning
Advance Directives (For Healthcare)
⊠ Advance Directive
Information Provided on Healthcare Directives
Healthcare Agent Appointed
Healthcare Agent's Name
Healthcare Agent's Phone Number
Pre-existing DNR/DNI Order
Patient Requests Assistance
Care considerations
Name patient prefers to be called
Time of arrival to unit
Do you have a caregiver preference
Describe any social factors influencing your treatment
Describe any ethnic/cultural factors influencing your
Describe any educational factors influencing your
Other respectful considerations

Fig. 15.2 Selected screen from a patient's EHR. (Courtesy of Epic.)

entering and sending treatment instructions—including medication, laboratory, and radiology orders—via a computer application rather than paper, fax, or telephone" (ONC, 2018b). CPOE contributes to safety and quality by eliminating lost orders and illegible handwriting; generating related orders automatically

(e.g., a laboratory test needed to monitor a specific medication); monitoring for duplicate or contradictory orders; and reducing time to fill orders (Bellucci, 2022; IOM, 2003; ONC, 2018b). Several of the proven benefits of CPOE integration include:

- Reduced error and improved patient safety (e.g., legible, complete orders);
- Improved efficiency; and
- Improved reimbursements.

Basically, CPOE has proven to be safer and more efficient for providers and patients (ONC, 2018b).

EHR Data Management

A fully functional EHR is a complex system. Consider a single data element (datum) such as a person's weight. The system must be able to capture, or record, the weight, then store it, process it, communicate it to others, and present it in a usable format such as a bar graph or chart. All of this must be done in a secure environment that protects the patient's confidentiality and privacy. The complexity of these issues and the development of the necessary systems help explain why adoption of fully functional, certified EHR systems has been slow.

Data Capture. *Data capture* refers to the collection and entry of data into an EHR. The origin of the data may be local or remote from patient-monitoring devices, direct from the individual recipient of health care, or even from others who have information about the recipient's health or environment, such as relatives, friends, and public health agencies. Data may be captured by multiple means, including key entry, pattern recognition (e.g., voice, handwriting, or biologic characteristics), and transmission from medical devices such as interoperable smart pumps used for medication and fluid delivery and vital sign machines.

Data Storage. *Storage* refers to the physical location of data. In EHR systems, data need to be distributed across multiple systems at different sites. For this reason, common access protocols, retention schedules, and universal identification are necessary. Access protocols permit only authorized users to obtain data for legitimate uses. The systems must have backup and recovery mechanisms in the event of failure. Retention schedules address the maintenance of data in active and inactive forms, as well as the permanence of the storage medium. A person's identity can be determined by many types of data in addition to common identifiers, such as name and number. Universal identifiers or other methods are required for integrating health data of an individual distributed across multiple systems at different sites.

Data Privacy and Security. A significant responsibility of the nurse leader is to have a working knowledge of essential data privacy and security best practices. Data privacy relates to properly handling personal or sensitive data; this includes data collection, storage, usage, and sharing. Data security centers more on protecting data from unauthorized access, such as cyberattacks and threats, through technical safeguards. These can include data encryption, access controls, and network security (Department of Health & Human Services [DHHS], n.d.-a).

Computer-based patient record systems provide better protection of confidential health information than paper-based systems because such systems incorporate controls designed to ensure that only authorized users with legitimate uses have access to health information. Security functions address the confidentiality of private health information and the integrity of the data. Security functions must be designed to ensure compliance with applicable laws, regulations, and standards. Security systems must ensure that access to data is provided only to those authorized and with a legitimate purpose

for its use. Security functions also must provide a means of auditing for inappropriate access. According to the Department of Health & Human Services (DHHS), with the implementation of the 1996 Health Insurance Portability and Accountability Act (HIPAA) there are safeguards to be addressed when keeping your EHR and patient data secure (DHHS, n.d.-b, p. 2):

- Access control, such as unique passwords and PINs to limit access to patient information to only authorized users;
  - This includes EHR access setup to control the "rights" each user has in the system
  - This includes not sharing passwords, securing monitors, etc.
- Encryption of stored patient information, meaning only a user with a "key" could read or understand your data;
- Audit trail feature that records keystrokes and who accessed patient information; and
- Federal law requiring clinicians, hospitals, and others to report data breaches to patients;
  - This also includes federal notification of large data breaches that impact more than 500 patients in a region.

Information Processing. EHR functions provide for effective retrieval and processing of data into useful information. These include decision support tools, such as "info buttons" and alerts and alarms for drug interactions, allergies, and abnormal laboratory results. Reminders can be provided for appointments, critical path actions, medication administration, and other activities. The systems also may provide access to consensus- and evidence-driven diagnostic and treatment guidelines and protocols. The nurse could integrate a standard guideline, protocol, or critical path into a specific individual's EHR, modify it to meet unique circumstances, and use it as a basis for managing and documenting care.

Outcome data communicated from various caregivers and health care recipients themselves also may be analyzed and used to continually improve guidelines and protocols. Data may also be downloaded into statistical software programs, such as IBM's SPSS Statistics®, Tableau, or Microsoft's Excel, for more sophisticated analysis for research purposes. Organizations are increasingly using EHRs for electronic surveillance to monitor trends and indications of potential critical incidents to prompt preventive and/or responsive actions in advance of an actual disease outbreak. An excellent example would be the use of EHR infectious disease CDS alerts for early detection and treatment of COVID-19 patients in 2020 (Hoelscher, 2020).

Information Communication. *Information communication* refers to the interoperability of systems and linkages for exchange of data across disparate systems. To integrate health data across multiple systems at different sites, identifier systems (unique numbers or other methodology) for health care recipients, caregivers, providers, payers, and sites are essential. Local, regional, and national health information infrastructures that tie all participants together using standard data communication protocols are essential. Hundreds of types of transactions or messages must be defined and agreed to by participating stakeholders. Vocabulary and code systems must permit the exchange and processing of data into meaningful information. EHR systems must provide access to point-of-care information databases and knowledge sources, such as pharmaceutical formularies, referral databases, and reference literature.

HEALTH INFORMATION TECHNOLOGY LAWS AND INITIATIVES

Since the early days of health information technology, there are been several landmark laws and initiatives put into place, specifically in the United States. The following addresses the most impactful to the nursing profession.

EHRs: "Meaningful Use" (MU) and Moving to Promoting Interoperability

The American Recovery and Reinvestment Act of 2009 directed the meaningful use of EHR systems for hospital and physician practice settings and provided for financial incentives from CMS to providers who adopt and use EHRs that meet the MU standards. "Meaningful use" refers to a complex set of capabilities and standards to be met by EHR use in a series of three stages over several years.

Stage 1 MU (2011–2012) criteria primarily addressed the capture of health information, access to comprehensive patient health data, exchange of clinical information among the health care team, and reports for quality improvement and public reporting requirements.

Stage 2 criteria, effective in 2014, focused on continuous quality improvement at the point of care and structured information exchange (for example, the electronic exchange of diagnostic test results). Stage 3, implemented in 2017, focuses on using CEHRT to improve health outcomes and also serves to introduce the final rule to ease reporting requirements and align with other quality reporting programs.

MU has been renamed to PIP. According to CMS (2020a) PIP historically has three stages:
1. **Stage 1** set the foundation for PIP; set requirements for EHI data, including providing patients with their EHI.
2. **Stage 2** focused on advancing clinical processes and ensuring that the MU of EHRs supported the National Quality Strategy; encouraged use of CEHRT for continuous quality improvement at the point of care.
3. **Stage 3** in 2017 to now, focuses on CEHRT to improve health outcomes.

Although great progress in EHR adoption and usage has been made, the full capacity has not yet been realized. This situation may be due in part to barriers that impede the universal adoption of EHRs in the United States, which is discussed in the following section.

Opportunities for and Barriers to Adoption of EHRs in the United States

Clearly the movement toward EHRs, along with financial incentives, was designed to promote universal adoption and interoperability of EHRs in the United States. This movement created not only opportunities but also some barriers for independent health care providers.

Meeting the guidelines for the original MU, as well as PIP, was and is strenuous and often costly for community-based ambulatory services and small rural inpatient centers. Nonetheless, federal dollars had been allocated for this endeavor, and incentive monies were available for facilities and providers meeting the criteria. Starting in 2011 Medicare providers had to have qualified for the maximum incentive payment. Medicaid providers came into the MU program in 2016 and their payments could be received through 2021. The MU system moved to penalties in 2015 for not adopting CEHRT for dual Medicare/Medicaid providers.

The power of sharing data across health care settings surpasses the benefits to an individual patient.

Obviously patients benefit when their different providers have access to the same comprehensive patient record. Shared records promote continuity of care across systems and potentially reduce costs by eliminating duplicate diagnostic testing and services. Moreover, much can be learned when data are shared across systems. Aggregate data from such systems can be evaluated and predict outcomes in a particular population, disease, complication, or extended hospital stay. The ability to predict outcomes from data entered across systems, termed *mining data* or *examining trends,* can be highly beneficial for examining population health outcomes.

Great strides have been made in using EHRs to increase patient and provider communication, decrease errors, and streamline the workflow process. However, despite the evidence for these positive results there is continued resistance to EHRs from providers and nurses (Gomes et al., 2016; ONC, 2019c). The integration of technology, including the use of EHRs, will continue to change the practice of nursing, prompting the need for more research to explore patient-centered care practices within this new paradigm.

EHRs and the Health Insurance Portability and Accountability Act (HIPAA)

Because of the increase in the number of EHRs in the 1990s and the anticipated penetration of EHRs in health care, experts advocated for standardized protocols and clinical practice guidelines to ensure privacy and security. HIPAA was signed into law in 1996. HIPAA regulations focus on the privacy and security of patient data, including standard formats for transmitting electronic patient information. By April 2005 health care institutions had to comply with federal HIPAA regulations.

HIPAA requires every organization or facility that gathers or collects personal health information (PHI) to name an individual as a privacy officer and to develop policies and procedures to ensure the privacy and security of PHI (or electronic/ePHI as the situation may dictate). The protection of PHI/ePHI extends to every employee, new hire, and patient. Those found in violation of HIPAA regulations may be subject to criminal penalties and civil monetary penalties. Related HIPAA rules of note include HIPAA Security Rule, HIPAA Breach Notification Rule, and HIPAA Omnibus Rule (DHHS, n.d.-c).

21st Century Cures Act

In the middle of the CMS MU/PIP initiatives came the 21st Century Cures Act. This act, signed into law in 2016, contains key provisions related to EHRs that will advance interoperability; promote access, exchange, and use of electronic health information (EHI); support patients' access to their EHI; and address information blocking (US Federal Register, 2020). Information blocking is defined as practices conducted by either a health IT developer or a health care provider that may prevent or interfere with access, exchange, or use of EHI (ONC, 2020). The 21st Century Cures Act legislated the final push for EHR certification requirements, full EHI interoperability, and easy access by patients.

Trusted Exchange Framework and Common Agreement (TEFCA)

Related to the ongoing efforts to improve interoperability, in 2022 ONC published Version 1 of TEFCA. The overall goal was to create a "universal floor" for interoperability across the United States via a Commons Agreement (ONC, 2023). This trusted exchange allows for different users in different networks to share clinical data securely. TEFCA was established formally through Section 4005(b) of the 21st Century Cures Act (ONC, 2022a, 2022b).

DIGITAL HEALTH TECHNOLOGIES

According to the US Food & Drug Administration (FDA), "Digital health includes categories such as mobile health (mHealth), health information technology (IT), wearable devices, telehealth and telemedicine, and personalized medicine" (FDA, 2020a, para. 1). The FDA created the Digital Health Center of Excellence to educate and empower digital health users and stakeholders. Services provided by the Center include (FDA, 2020b, para. 3):

- Digital Health Policy and Technology Support and Training
- Medical Device Cybersecurity
- Artificial Intelligence/Machine Learning
- Regulatory Science Advancement
- Regulatory Review Support and Coordination
- Advanced Manufacturing
- Real World Evidence and Advanced Clinical Studies
- Regulatory Innovation
- Strategic Partnerships

Their current timeline for education through sustaining capacity goes from Fall 2020 (Phase I–Raise Awareness and Engage Stakeholders) through Winter 2021 (Phase II–Build Partnerships) and beyond (Phase III–Build and Sustain Capacity). The Center has laid out the timeline for the FDA's goals related to digital health innovation, found at https://www.fda.gov/medical-devices/digital-health-center-excellence.

Point-of-Care Technology

With advancing technologies and the movement toward universal use of EHRs, there is a greater demand for HIT at the point of care. This means HIT directly at the bedside or within close proximity to the area where services are delivered. Point-of-care technology is no longer nonessential but is paramount to delivery of safe, efficient, high-quality patient care with access to patient data and evidence-based guidelines. The technology must provide access to past and current patient data, references, policies, procedures, and evidence-based literature to guide clinical decisions at the point of care. A variety of technology tools supports point-of-care decision-making and documentation such as handheld computers, tablets, and smartphones.

It is nearly impossible to visit a health care facility or office and not see providers using mobile technology. These small devices are as robust as laptops or desktop computers but are more convenient for on-the-go health care providers. These systems have wireless Internet capability so that patient information and other resources can be accessed anywhere, anytime, within the confines of the firewall-protected health care environment to maintain privacy, security, and confidentiality of the data. Small laptops also allow providers to access pertinent information at the point of care. These laptops are usually secured to a mobile cart, so they have names like *workstation on wheels (WOWs), mobile workstations (MWSs), mobile point-of-care (MPOC),* and *computer at bedside (CAB).*

Computer-based alerts and reminders provided by point-of-care technology are helpful in detecting and preventing potential adverse drug events related to drug–drug interactions and abnormal laboratory values. Point-of-care technology is an essential component of nursing as it shifts from a practice that relies on memory to one that emphasizes continuous use of as-needed resources. This means that nurses must transform from being technical experts to knowledge workers and must rely on the ever-increasing and reliable computer memory versus the overburdened and fallible human memory.

Wearables and Sensors

Wearable technologies and sensors are becoming more integrated into health care for continuous, remote patient monitoring. Digital health wearable devices have more than tripled from 2017 to 2020, and this number continues to grow as wearable technology becomes more accessible and standardized (Insider Intelligence, 2023; Sarkar, 2023). Wearables include technology such as smartwatches, fitness trackers, biosensors, and interoperable monitors. Fitness trackers have made many leaps recently, including the ability to track heart rates, sleep cycles, and daily steps. Fitness trackers have been around for some time but their more-powerful cousin, the smartwatch, is taking over in certain markets. No longer just tools to tell time and count your steps, they now have advanced functionality to contribute to health care in science in new and innovative ways.

The Apple Watch® is not only one of the first to incorporate an electrocardiogram (ECG) monitor (for rhythms such as atrial fibrillation) but also has "Movement Disorder API" that contributes to Parkinson's disease research (Insider Intelligence, 2023). There is new wearable technology for patients with Alzheimer's disease that tracks their progression by monitoring walking mechanics, or gait speed, symmetry, and stride length (Carfagno, 2019). Wearable technology has also progressed in the straight health care arena for tools such as wearable ECG monitors, oxygen saturation monitors, and blood pressure monitors. All are fully integrated and interoperable with either mobile applications, such as on a cell phone, or even the ordering provider's office. In December of 2019 Current Health produced the first FDA-approved artificial intelligence medical monitor wearable, called Current. It can monitor patients' vital signs from home or in an inpatient location (Carfagno, 2019).

Sensors and biosensors are also picking up speed in the realm of health care. Biosensors, such as a patch, are considered a type of wearable medical device but can function differently than the traditional smart watches. According to Zheng et al. (2023) sensor technology provides several health care benefits (para. 2):

1. The early diagnosis and prevention of human diseases by detecting critical biomarkers;

2. Health assessments by monitoring and analyzing human physiological signals in health care and biomedical applications; and
3. The efficient evaluation of human-health-relevant environmental factors by monitoring and measuring environmental determinants.

All wearables and sensors that are considered medical devices fall under the watchful eye of the FDA's regulation.

Mobile Devices and mHealth

Smartphones and tablets promote evidence-based clinical decision-making at the point of care. These palm-sized computers can store medical applications and access health care journals, calculators, databases, and more through their wireless capabilities. Nowadays, even EHR vendors have catered to the needs of clinicians using mobile devices (Sharma et al., 2022). This also includes vendors who design applications for direct patient interactions, such as patient portals or interoperable electronic signature devices used by patients to sign important documents.

One of the greatest advantages of smartphones and other mobile devices is the convenient and quick access to references and tools for patient education and care. For example, nurses can teach patients about tracking their health by using tools on smartphones or display pictures that show proper procedures. Some of the benefits of using smartphones for nursing include (Sharma et al., 2022; Zysk, 2018):

- Provides for enhanced coordination of care (two-way, instant support, team-building)
- Enables communication at the point of care
- Improves time management
- Helps lessen nursing burnout (fosters teamwork, lessens physical fatigue, lessens stress)
- Integrates communication streams and devices (less devices for a nurse to carry around)

Mobile health, or mHealth, devices such as tablets are being used in many organizations as standards of care to promote safety and quality via enhanced communications among team members. One example is the use of tablets for virtual handoffs. The virtual handoffs use video technology to include the patient and their family in the introductions and initial conversations about the transfer, reducing anxiety and promoting rapport. Nurses have found these virtual first encounters helpful in confirming patient information and

promotion of accountability (Santa & Roach, 2017). Another was the increased use of tablets for inpatient use in the communication efforts with COVID-19 patients who were isolated and alone, with limited clinician interaction as well as no family member visitations (Iyengar et al., 2020; Sharma et al., 2022).

Mobile health applications (apps) are increasingly being used in the clinical environment by providers and patients. One example is the use of mobile apps for home monitoring of infants recently discharged from the neonatal intensive care unit. Home monitoring has traditionally depended on the parents' ability to assess, record, and report significant data, which often results in delay and/or noncompliance in reporting of critical information that leads to complications, even deaths. With the use of mobile technology, data are collected via the app and securely transferred to the EHR, where nurses and caregivers can immediately review and revise the plans of care. Mobile apps have been found to greatly enhance the home monitoring of the elderly, infants, and those who may be homebound, to minimize delays in care and reduce at-home mortality (Sharma et al., 2022).

As today's health care environment focuses on safe, efficient, effective, and high-quality care, access to patient data, standardized protocols, and clinical practice guidelines through point-of-care technology has become the standard for patient care. Nurse scientists are increasingly focusing their research efforts on the benefits of using secured mobile devices that are HIPAA compliant. These research efforts are widely being translated into clinical environments to improve the quality and safety of patient care and contribute to the efficiency and satisfaction of nursing staff.

Telehealth

A discussion about digital health technology would be incomplete without mentioning *telehealth*—the use of telecommunications technology to assess, diagnose, and, in some cases, treat persons who are at a distance from the health care provider. Nurses, physicians, radiologists, psychiatrists, and others use this technology via telephone, computers, interactive videos, and teleconferencing. In many instances telehealth makes possible the delivery of health care services to underserved populations, such as rural communities, older adults, and prisoners, who may have difficulty accessing necessary services. Demonstrated benefits of telehealth include improved quality of care and continuity of care, improved decision-making, and higher-quality records related to the incorporation of digital information. During the COVID-19 pandemic telehealth also provided for improved limited physical contact to reduce exposure, reduced travel time and time off from work, tools to shorten wait time for appointments, and increased access to specialists and speciality care (Childs et al., 2020; Schulz et al., 2020).

Several telehealth modalities used by health care providers (HCPs) to deliver high-quality patient care have been identified, including (CDC, 2020, para. 3):

- **Synchronous:** This includes real-time telephone or live audio-video interaction typically with a patient using a smartphone, tablet, or computer. In some cases peripheral medical equipment (e.g., digital stethoscopes, otoscopes, ultrasounds) can be used by another HCP (e.g., nurse, medical assistant) physically with the patient while the consulting medical provider conducts a remote evaluation.
- **Asynchronous:** This includes "store and forward" technology where messages, images, or data are collected at one point in time and interpreted or responded to later. Patient portals can facilitate this type of communication between provider and patient through secure messaging.
- **Remote patient monitoring:** This allows direct transmission of a patient's clinical measurements to their HCP from a distance (may or may not be in real-time).
- **The virtual nurse:** A more recent addition to the telehealth/telemedicine toolkit, virtual nursing and virtual care can remotely support the primary health care team (American Nurses Association, 2023).

With the rapid surge of COVID-19 cases and the government relaxation of restrictions regarding the use of telehealth/telemedicine methods during the pandemic, interstate licensing, reimbursement, and data confidentiality, the use of telemetry as a primary source of patient care has increased very quickly (Bashshur et al., 2020).

These technological advances that enhance and improve health care delivery systems are only valuable for those who consume the technology: health care workers and patients, if they develop the skill set to use point-of-care technologies, EHRs, and telehealth (Sarkar, 2023). Further, patients must possess skills to evaluate and critique technologies and information that influence their health.

Artificial Intelligence and Machine Learning

The history of artificial intelligence (AI) in health care and academia can be traced back to the 1970s when researchers began exploring the use of computer programs to assist with medical diagnosis and treatment. Before that, with the birth of the Turing Test, Alan Turing started considering the concept of AI in the early 1950s. Over the years advances in technology and data science have led to the development of increasingly sophisticated AI applications for health care with several branches under the AI umbrella: machine learning, natural language processing, and large language models that fuel most "chatbots."

AI and machine learning are rapidly being adopted in health care for improved decision-making, diagnostic accuracy, digital dictation/voice-to-text, and predictive capabilities. As these technologies become more integrated into patient care, nurses need to have working knowledge of AI and how it can impact their role.

AI programs can analyze large datasets and identify trends undetectable to humans. AI can also power chatbots, personalized treatment plans, and early warning systems (such as sepsis advisors) for high-risk patients. All of these emerging technologies have the potential to improve patient outcomes and lower health care costs. AI technologies like automated documentation and virtual nursing assistants are changing workflows for nurses.

While AI cannot replace the skilled discernment of nurses, understanding how to maximize these technologies can augment nurses' abilities to deliver evidence-based, life-saving care. With solid foundations in nursing practice and AI capabilities nurses can genuinely transform patient care as health care evolves (Bellucci, 2022; Dell Technologies, 2023; Sarkar, 2023).

Virtual, Augmented, and Mixed Reality

Another fast-developing technology being incorporated into nursing and health care education is virtual reality (VR). This type of technology has three major aspects: virtual, augmented, and mixed reality.

VR provides a fully immersive, computer-generated experience that transports users into a different environment through a head-mounted display and controllers. VR aims to trick the senses into believing the simulated world is real by displaying imagery and playing sounds corresponding to the user's movements (Anthropic, 2023). VR can be used for immersive patient experiences to reduce pain and anxiety such as during physical therapy. VR simulation training allows nurses and other health care providers to practice skills and procedures repeatedly in a risk-free environment. This can include activities from taking vital signs to surgical procedures.

Augmented reality (AR) overlays digital information and virtual objects onto the real-world environment. AR uses mobile devices or headsets to blend digital elements with the physical surroundings, enhancing but not completely replacing reality. Well-known examples of AR include gaming, where game characters are mapped into real-world settings. AR is being used to overlay patient information and data directly into the nurse's field of vision during care, reducing the need to look away to monitors and charts. Another example is the use of AR to visualize patients' anatomy before and during surgery by overlaying CT scans and other imaging onto the patient (Anthropic, 2023).

Mixed reality (MR) seamlessly integrates physical and virtual worlds, allowing users to interact with and manipulate physical and digital objects. Using advanced sensing and imaging technologies such as MR headsets, users can map physical environments to anchor virtual objects, creating a hybrid environment in which real and virtual dynamically interact. MR headsets can provide three-dimensional holograms of anatomy and virtual demonstrations for nurse training programs. MR shows promise for overlaying patient vital signs and records for nurses, supporting clinical decision-making at the point of care (Anthropic, 2023).

These immersive technologies enhance nursing care, education, and training in a disruptive and innovative way. As adoption increases this method of learning will be seen more often.

CONSUMER HEALTH IT AND FUTURE TRENDS

Consumer Health Information Technology

Today individuals are more involved than ever in searching for information about their own health on "the Web," or the Internet. There are, historically, several versions of "the Web." Web 1.0 consisted of passive web page usage by individuals; typically not a lot of new content development was happening. This led us into

what we now refer to as Web 2.0, with tools such as social media, collaboration sites, interactive websites, and Internet bulletin boards or blogs, which encouraged individuals to be more involved and more knowledgeable about their own health.

Web 2.0 saw more individuals creating content, interacting with sites, and participating in the social media boom. The information that patients and families glean from such sites can be a challenge for providers because as patients are better informed, health care providers are required to answer more directed questions. Further, the health care provider must inform patients how to be good consumers of health information. Because providers are seen as the experts it is the provider's responsibility to ensure that patients are well informed about how to evaluate content. They also must protect the privacy of others while engaged in discussion via either the Internet or other forms of wireless connection.

Health consumers of all ages are increasingly turning to social media for information about health promotion such as healthy eating, exercise, and ways to reduce stress. Consumers often access YouTube, Facebook, Twitter, and LinkedIn to learn more about health, health prevention, and health promotion. Web 2.0 tools are designed to allow any Internet user to become an author of content. With the growing number of Internet users, content is expanding exponentially so that one can find information about virtually anything, including the most obscure illnesses, home remedies, procedures, and medications. For this reason, information accessible on the Internet may not necessarily be accurate or created by experts. Consumers of information on the Internet, especially health information, must be knowledgeable and must evaluate the credibility and accuracy of the source.

The current state is often referred to as Web 3.0, or 3D Web. Web 3.0 consists of five main features (Expert System, 2020): (1) Semantic Web (a virtual environment where data and information have an automated connection for processing and interpretation); (2) AI and machine learning; (3) 3D graphics/web; (4) expanded connectivity; and (5) ubiquity (something that's very common). Some of these concepts tie into a term called the Internet of Things (IoT), which simply refers to a networking of physical objects, or things, specifically to exchange data with other "things," such as other devices and systems (think smartwatches). It helps make data

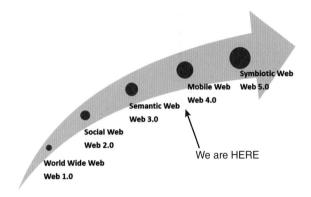

Fig. 15.3 Future of the Web. (Adapted from Spisak, K. [2019]). Eras of the Web - Web 0.0 through web 5.0. https://www.business 2community.com/tech-gadgets/eras-of-the-web-web-0-0-through-web-5-0-02239654; Expert System Team. [2020]. Web 3.0: Data growth and web 3.0.https://expertsystem.com/web-3-0/; Cook, A.V., Bechtel, M., & Anderson, S. (2020). The spatial web and web 3.0. Deloitte Insights. https://www2.deloitte.com/us/en/insights/topics/digital-transformation/web-3-0-technologies-in-business.html.)

collections simpler and much more dynamic (Rouse, 2019; Sarkar, 2023). For more information visit https://www.ibm.com/topics/internet-of-things.

How does this all relate to nursing and health care? Web 3.0 helps us move from reactive health care to proactive health care. The use of wearables, health care applications, AI, and machine learning all contribute to the vast transformative power of data creation and data needs. See Fig. 15.3 for the future of the Web.

Future Health IT Trends

With technology advancing at warp speed it is difficult to imagine the future, but some of our current technologies offer insight about the possibilities. To better understand how technology will shape health care, let us review some of the ways technology is currently shaping our lives.

- Social media will no longer be a source of informal content. With more than 3.5 billion users worldwide, it will be interesting to see the discussion around enforced regulation expand. Lack of regulation leads to "fake news," cyberbullying, and decreased trust in the sciences. Education to aid the public (and health care workers) to tell the difference between reputable and misleading resources will be paramount (Hint: Wikipedia is not considered a reliable source). To help improve overall health literacy nurses should consider educating themselves, as well as their patients, on safe, reputable social media and internet usage.
- Cloud computing (e.g., applications and data stored and accessed through the Internet) is making another surge in the computing world. A 2020 Cloud Computing Survey reported that 59% of respondents stated that most or all of their computing would be cloud-based within 18 months (Knorr, 2020; Sarkar, 2023).
- Personalized medicine and patient-centered care driven by rapid change and unlimited opportunity will include advancements in genomics, gene therapy, immunooncology, personalized medicine, artificial intelligence, and wearable digital devices (Collins, 2023).
- Gaming will continue to expand health technologies by promoting health maintenance, mental health, physical activity, and cognitive skills that may lead to improved health behavior. This includes developments for things such as patient physical therapy and virtual reality-based training tools for surgeons (Sarkar, 2023; Truong, 2019).
- The increased availability of biosensors, such as self-adhesive patches for vital sign data collection, will continue to advance. Preliminary data suggests that using such a device can provide up to an 89% reduction in cardiac or respiratory arrest (Insider Intelligence, 2023).

As previously discussed security is paramount for health data. Future health information technologies will integrate more biometric technology for authentication and security. Biometric technologies use human characteristics, such as fingerprints, retinas, irises, voices, and facial patterns, to authenticate or grant access to data or information. More and more health care information systems are including biometric options to provide an additional layer of security. It is almost incomprehensible to imagine health care in 2030 when one considers the evolution in technology and how technology has shaped health care since the invention of the stethoscope.

SUMMARY

Returning to Victoria in the opening Vignette, she certainly has great opportunities to advance her knowledge of EHRs and HIT. As a profession nurses must understand and manage information technology, promote interoperability of health technology and EHRs, and teach patients how to use health information wisely. As the largest group of organized health care professionals in the United States, nurses have a responsibility to patients and society to continually improve and refine their competencies and knowledge base related to HIT. Findings of multiple studies confirm that nurses in every role and at each level of education and practice exhibit large gaps in knowledge of and competencies in information technology. To overcome these gaps Victoria and all nurses need to be a lifelong learners. Take in-person or online classes. Arrange groups in your place of employment to learn more about HIT in the clinical setting. Review the resources that are available to you, and evaluate them to ensure they are valid,

current, and based on evidence. If the resources are not valid, take actions within your facility to replace outdated or inaccurate resources. If the sources are valid, integrate them into your everyday practice.

With health data and technology at the forefront of health care for the foreseeable future, the latest Future of Nursing Report, released in 2021, increased its reference to the importance of informatics, including nursing informatics (National Academies of Sciences, Engineering, and Medicine). The American Nurses Association defines nursing informatics as "the specialty that transforms data into needed information and leverages technologies to improve health and health care equity, safety, quality, and outcomes" (ANA, 2022, p. 3). Technology is an essential resource for nurses in their important role of tracking, interpreting, and improving quality of care, in addition to translating research into practice. Technology continues to change and evolve at an ever-increasing pace.

REFERENCES

American Nurses Association. (2022). *Nursing informatics: Scope and standards of practice* (3rd ed.) American Nurses Association.

American Nurses Association. (2023). *Virtual nursing, What is it?* https://www.nursingworld.org/practice-policy/innovation/blog/virtual-nursing-what-is-it/

Anthropic. (2023). *Claude* (September 23) [Larglanguage model]. https://claude.ai/chat/

Bashshur, R., Doarn, C.R., Frenk, J.M., Kvedar, J.C., & Woolliscroft, J.O. (2020). Telemedicine and the COVID-19 pandemic, lessons for the future. *Telemedicine and e-Health, 26*(5), 571–573. http://doi.org/10.1089/tmj.2020.29040.rb

Bellucci, N. (2022). Disruptive innovation and technological influences on healthcare. *Journal of Radiology Nursing, 41*(2022), 98–101. https://doi.org/10.1016/j.jradnu.2022.02.008

Carfagno, J. (2019). 5 new and emerging wearable medical devices. *Docwirenews.* https://www.docwirenews.com/docwire-pick/future-of-medicine-picks/top-5-wearable-medical-devices/

Centers for Disease Control and Prevention (CDC). (2020). *Using telehealth to expand access to essential health services during the COVID-19 pandemic.* https://www.cdc.gov/phlp/publications/topic/telehealth.html

Centers for Medicare & Medicaid Services (CMS). (2020a). *Promoting interoperability programs.* https://www.cms.gov/Regulations-and-Guidance/Legislation/EHRIncentivePrograms/index.html?redirect=/EHRIncentivePrograms/

Centers for Medicare & Medicaid Services (CMS). (2020b). *Certified EHR technology.* https://www.cms.gov/Regulations-and-Guidance/Legislation/EHRIncentivePrograms/Certification

Centers for Medicare & Medicaid Services (CMS). (2020c). *Medicare and Medicaid promoting interoperability program basics.* https://www.cms.gov/Regulations-and-Guidance/Legislation/EHRIncentivePrograms/Basics

Centers for Medicare & Medicaid Services (CMS). (2021). *2021 Medicare promoting interoperability program: Certified electronic health record technology fact sheet.* https://www.cms.gov/files/document/2021-cehrt-fact-sheet.pdf

Childs, A.W., Unger, A., & Li, L. (2020). Rapid design and deployment of intensive outpatient group-based psychiatric care using telehealth during COVID-19. *Journal of the American Medical Informatics Association, 27*(9), 1420–1424. https://doi.org/10.1093/jamia/ocaa138

Collins, J. (2023). 5 Leading healthcare trends for 2023. *Forbes.* https://www.forbes.com/sites/forbesagencycouncil/2023/02/16/5-leading-healthcare-trends-for-2023/?sh=156e6f8f6c7d

Dell Technologies. (2023). Leveraging AI and machine learning to protect and validate relevant patient data. *HealthcareITNews.* https://www.healthcareitnews.com/news/leveraging-ai-and-machine-learning-protect-and-validate-relevant-patient-data

Department of Health & Human Services (DHHS). (n.d.-a). Top 10 tips for cybersecurity in health care. https://www.healthit.gov/sites/default/files/Top_10_Tips_for_Cybersecurity.pdf

Department of Health & Human Services (DHHS). (n.d.-b). *Privacy, security, and electronic health records.* https://www.hhs.gov/sites/default/files/ocr/privacy/hipaa/understanding/consumers/privacy-security-electronic-records.pdf

Department of Health & Human Services (DHHS). (n.d.-c). HIPAA Privacy Rule. https://www.hhs.gov/hipaa/for-professionals/privacy/index.html

Expert System. (2020). *5 main features of Web 3.0.* https://expertsystem.com/web-3-0/

Gomes, M., Hash, P., Orsolini, L., Watkins, A., & Mazzoccoli, A. (2016). Nurses' beliefs about using an electronic health record and their ability to incorporate professional and patient-centered nursing activities in patient care. *Computers, Informatics, Nursing, 34*(12), 578–586. https://doi.org/10.1097/CIN.0000000000000280.

Hoelscher, S.H. (2020). *The future of health information technology: Digital health in the time of COVID-19,* September 22–25. Nursing Management Congress, Virtual [Conference session].

Hoelscher, S.H., & McBride, S. (2020). Digitizing infectious disease clinical guidelines for improved clinician satisfaction. *Computers, Informatics, Nursing, 38*(6), 303–311. https://doi:10.1097/CIN.0000000000000612

Insider Intelligence. (2023). Latest trends in medical monitoring devices and wearable health technology. *Insider Intelligence eMarketer.* https://www.insiderintelligence.com/insights/wearable-technology-healthcare-medical-devices/

Institute of Medicine of the National Academies (IOM). (2003). *Key capabilities of an electronic health record system: Letter report.* National Academies Press. https://www.ncbi.nlm.nih.gov/books/NBK221802/pdf/Bookshelf_NBK221802.pdf

Iyengar, K., Upadhyaya, G. K., Vaishya, R., & Jain, V. (2020). COVID-19 and applications of smartphone technology in the current pandemic. *Diabetes & Metabolic Syndrome: Clinical Research & Reviews, 14*(5), 733–737. https://doi.org/10.1016/j.dsx.2020.05.033

Knorr, E. (2020). *The state of cloud computing in 2020.* InfoWorld. https://www.infoworld.com/article/3561329/the-state-of-cloud-computing-in-2020.html

National Academies of Sciences, Engineering, and Medicine. (2021). *The Future of Nursing 2020-2030: Charting a Path to Achieve Health Equity.* The National Academies Press. https://doi.org/10.17226/25982

Rouse, M. (2019). *Definition: Web 3.0.* https://whatis.techtarget.com/definition/Web-30

Sarkar, S. (2023). Top healthcare technology trends for 2023. SelectHub. https://www.selecthub.com/medical-software/top-health-it-security-trends/

Santa, D., & Roach, D.E. (2017). Using mobile technology during patient handoffs. *American Nurse Today, 12*(9), 84–87.

Schulz, T., Long, K., Kanhutu, K., Bayrak, I., Johnson, D., & Fazio, T. (2020). Telehealth during the coronavirus disease 2019 pandemic: Rapid expansion of telehealth outpatient use during a pandemic is possible if the programme is previously established. *Journal of Telemedicine and Telecare,* 1–7. https://doi.org/10.1177/1357633X20942045

Sharma, S., Kumari, B., Ali, A., Yadav, R.K., Sharma, A.K., Sharma, K.K., Hajela, K., & Singh, G.K. (2022). Mobile technology: A tool for healthcare and a boon in pandemic. *Journal of Family Medicine and Primary Care, 11*(1), 37–43. https://doi.org/10.4103/jfmpc.jfmpc_1114_21

The Office of the National Coordinator for Health Information Technology (ONC). (2018a). *Clinical decision support: What is clinical decision support (CDS)?* https://www.healthit.gov/topic/safety/clinical-decision-support

The Office of the National Coordinator for Health Information Technology (ONC). (2018b). *What is computerized provider order entry?* https://www.healthit.gov/faq/what-computerized-provider-order-entry

The Office of the National Coordinator for Health Information Technology (ONC). (2019a). *What is an electronic health record?* https://www.healthit.gov/faq/what-electronic-health-record-ehr

The Office of the National Coordinator for Health Information Technology (ONC). (2019b). *Health IT Dashboard: Quick Stats.* https://dashboard.healthit.gov/quickstats/quickstats.php

The Office of the National Coordinator for Health Information Technology (ONC). (2019c). *How do I overcome resistance within my organization during electronic health record implementation?* https://www.healthit.gov/faq/how-do-i-overcome-resistance-within-my-organization-during-electronic-health-record

The Office of the National Coordinator for Health Information Technology (ONC). (2020). *$170.401 Information blocking.* https://www.healthit.gov/condition-ccg/information-blocking

The Office of the National Coordinator for Health Information Technology (ONC). (2022a). *Common agreement for nationwide health information interoperability*-Version 1. https://www.healthit.gov/sites/default/files/page/2022-01/Common_Agreement_for_Nationwide_Health_Information_Interoperability_Version_1.pdf

The Office of the National Coordinator for Health Information Technology (ONC). (2022b). *The Trusted Exchange Framework (TEF): Principles for trusted exchange.* https://www.healthit.gov/sites/default/files/page/2022-01/Trusted_Exchange_Framework_0122.pdf

The Office of the National Coordinator for Health Information Technology (ONC). (2023). *Trusted Exchange Framework and Common Agreement (TEFCA).* https://www.healthit.gov/topic/interoperability/policy/trusted-exchange-framework-and-common-agreement-tefca

Truong, K. (2019). Playing doctor: The evolution of videogames in healthcare. *MedCity News.* https://medcitynews.com/2019/05/from-joke-hour-to-digital-therapeutics-an-evolution-of-gaming-in-healthcare/

US Federal Register. (2020). *21st Century Cures Act: Interoperability, Information Blocking, and the ONC Health IT Certification Program.* https://www.federalregister.gov/documents/2020/05/01/2020-07419/21st-century-cures-act-interoperability-information-blocking-and-the-onc-health-it-certification

US Food & Drug Administration (FDA) (2020a). *What is digital health?* FDA, https://www.fda.gov/medical-devices/digital-health-center-excellence/what-digital-health

US Food & Drug Administration (FDA)(2020b). *About the Digital Health Center of Excellence.* FDA, https://www.fda.gov/medical-devices/digital-health-center-excellence/about-digital-health-center-excellence

Zheng, W., Liu, M., Liu, C., Wang, D., & Li, K. (2023). Recent advances in sensor technology for healthcare and biomedical applications (Volume II). *Sensors, 23*(10); 5949. https://doi.org/10.3390/s23135949

Zysk, T. (2018). Five benefits of using smartphones for nurse communication. *Healthcare innovation: People, process, technology transformation.* https://www.hcinnovationgroup.com/population-health-management/mobile-health-mhealth/article/13010711/five-benefits-of-using-smartphones-for-nurse-communication

16

Emergency Preparedness and Response for Today's World

Rebecca R. Keck, DNP, RN, NEA-BC and
Elizabeth E. Weiner, PhD, RN-BC, FACMI, FAAN

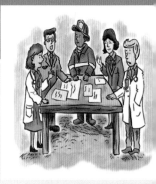

Partnering to respond to disaste

ⓔ Additional resources are available online at: http://evolve.elsevier.com/Cherry/

LEARNING OUTCOMES

After studying this chapter, the reader will be able to:

1. Describe the interaction between local, state, and federal emergency response systems.
2. Summarize the roles of public and private agencies in preparing for and responding to a mass casualty event.
3. Compare and contrast chemical, biologic, radiologic, nuclear, and explosive agents and treatment protocols.
4. Access resources related to disaster preparedness on the Internet.
5. Communicate effectively (using correct emergency preparedness terminology) in regard to a mass casualty incident.
6. Describe the need for personal preparedness for individuals and households.

KEY TERMS

Active shooter An individual actively engaged in killing or attempting to kill people in a confined and populated area; in most cases, active shooters use firearms and there is no pattern or method to their selection of victims.

All-hazards approach A process approach for all sectors to prepare for any emergency or disaster that may occur.

Biologic agents Microorganisms or toxins from living organisms with infectious or noninfectious properties that produce lethal or serious effects in plants and animals.

Chemical agents Solids, liquids, or gases with chemical properties that produce lethal or serious effects in plants and animals.

Cohorting Grouping residents or staff based on their risk of infection or whether they have tested positive for a disease during an outbreak; way to help prevent the spread of infection within a facility.

Crisis standard of care A substantial change in usual health care operations and the level of care it is possible to deliver, which is made necessary by a pervasive (e.g., COVID-19) pandemic or catastrophic (e.g., earthquake, hurricane) disaster. This change in the level of care delivered is justified by specific circumstances and is formally declared by a state government, in recognition that crisis operations will be in effect for a sustained period.

Disaster condition A significant natural disaster or human-caused event that overwhelms the affected state, necessitating both federal public health and medical care assistance.

Emergency As defined by federal legislation in the Stafford Act, any occasion or instance for which, in the determination of the president, federal assistance is needed to supplement state and local efforts and capabilities to save lives and protect property, public health, and safety; includes emergencies other than natural disasters.

Emergency Management Assistance Compact (EMAC) An organization authorized by the US Congress through which a state impacted by a disaster can request and receive assistance from other member states quickly and efficiently (EMAC, 2017).

Epidemic A sudden rapid disease outbreak that affects a large number of people in an identified region.

Global warming The long-term warming of the planet's overall temperature, which has significantly increased in the last hundred years due to the burning of fossil fuels.

Hospital incident command system (HICS) A multiagency operational structure that uses a model adopted by the fire and rescue community. The ICS can be used in any size or type of disaster to control response personnel, facilities, and equipment.

Lead agency As defined by the Federal Bureau of Investigation (FBI), the federal department or organization assigned primary responsibility to manage and coordinate a specific function—either crisis management or consequence management. Lead agencies are designated on the basis of their having the most authority, resources, capabilities, or expertise relative to accomplishment of the specific function.

Major disaster As defined under the Stafford Act, any natural catastrophe (including any hurricane, tornado, storm, high water, wind-driven water, tidal wave, tsunami, earthquake, volcanic eruption, landslide, mudslide, snowstorm, or drought) or, regardless of cause, any fire, flood, or explosion in any part of the United States that in the determination of the president causes damage of sufficient severity and magnitude to warrant major disaster assistance to supplement the efforts and available resources of states, local governments, and disaster relief organizations in alleviating the damage, loss, hardship, or suffering caused thereby.

Mass casualty incident (MCI) A disaster situation that results in a large number of victims who need the response of multiple organizations.

Mitigation Those activities designed to alleviate the effects of a major disaster or emergency or long-term activities to minimize the potentially adverse effects of future disasters in affected areas.

Pandemic Outbreak of disease that affects populations worldwide; for example, COVID-19 pandemic that causes serious illness and death worldwide.

Preparedness Activities that build capability and capacity to address potential needs identified by the threat and vulnerability study.

Recovery Activities designed to return responders and the facility to full normal operational status and to restore fully the capability to respond to future emergencies and disasters; activities traditionally associated with providing federal supplemental disaster relief assistance under a presidential major disaster declaration.

Response Activities to address the immediate and short-term effects of an emergency or disaster. Response includes immediate actions to save lives, protect property, and meet basic human needs.

Scene assessment The act of reviewing the location of an event to look for information that might help to determine treatment options.

Strategic National Stockpile A federal emergency response program that houses drugs and supplies that can be requested by local, regional, tribal, and state officials needed in an emergency situation.

Terrorist attack As defined by the FBI, a violent act or an act that is dangerous to human life, in violation of the criminal laws of the United States or of any state, and intended to intimidate or coerce a government, the civilian population, or any segment thereof in furtherance of political or social objectives.

Triage Process of prioritizing which patients are to be treated first; first action in any disaster response.

PROFESSIONAL/ETHICAL ISSUE

Jeannette Fraser, RN, worked in the emergency department (ED) of a major hospital system when, during her shift in the ED, an explosion occurred at a large factory near the city. As soon as the hospital determined that a disaster occurred with multiple injuries, the hospital's emergency operations plan (EOP) was activated. Fortunately, less than 1 month before the explosion, Jeannette had participated in a large-scale disaster drill conducted by the hospital in partnership with agencies from across the city, including the fire department, the police department, and the city's emergency operations center (EOC). Although extremely anxious, Jeannette knew exactly what to do and went to work in her assigned role to triage victims who were coming into the ED. Jeannette knew that the entire hospital staff was more successful in managing the disaster and helping victims because of the well-coordinated EOP that was in place.

Now Jeannette has moved to another state and accepted a nursing position in the outpatient clinic of a large academic medical center. As part of her orientation Jeannette asks her supervisor about the facility's EOP and the supervisor replies, "I am sure we have a written plan in the policy manual but I really don't know much about it. This is a very safe community so we don't need to worry about anything happening here. Besides, if something did happen the victims would go to the hospital, and it would not affect us." This response from her supervisor leaves Jeannette feeling very concerned and wondering whether she should get involved in helping the clinic understand the importance of having a good EOP that is coordinated with the hospital and other community agencies.

Think about Jeannette's situation as you consider the following questions:

- In the event of a major disaster, is it conceivable that victims might go to an outpatient or community-based clinic for treatment?
- What are some strategies Jeannette can use to persuade the clinic managers of the importance of having an up-to-date EOP in place?
- When might nurses in an ambulatory clinic be considered "first responders?"
- What local, state, and/or federal resources are available to help communities develop EOPs?

VIGNETTE

Tana Wolverton works as a staff nurse at the local Childrens' Hospital. It is the first day of school and she just learned that an elementary student was killed and 23 other students were injured after their school bus was hit by a minivan and overturned. The situation has caused her hospital to institute its incident command system to handle all the injuries.

Questions to Consider While Reading This Chapter:

1. How do we prepare for mass casualty events that will overwhelm the resources of our health facility?
2. How do we plan for a catastrophic event to ensure that the response offers the best care possible given

the resources at hand? How are response efforts coordinated so that the needs of the local area are met?

3. How do hospitals and other health care facilities organize themselves to manage disaster situations while continuing to communicate with other external agencies?
4. How does the response differ when the health care facility suffers damage and cannot function normally?
5. Where can I find current information about this ever-changing area?

CHAPTER OVERVIEW

The purpose of this chapter is to describe the various components of our nation's local, state, and federal National Response Framework and how these components interrelate in the event of a mass casualty incident (MCI). The problems associated with natural or terrorist disasters when the health care system is damaged or rendered ineffective because of the event are reviewed. The kinds of agents that may be used in a terrorist attack are described, along with the activities and response systems related to the preparedness, relief response, and recovery phases of a disaster. Readers will be particularly interested to note how standard triage and patient care priorities change when care is provided during an MCI. Additionally, readers are encouraged to closely review the list of key terms to understand and be able to use emergency preparedness terminology and explore the online resources about emergency preparedness and disaster management found throughout the chapter.

THE NATIONAL IMPERATIVE FOR EMERGENCY PREPAREDNESS

During the past three decades, we have seen many mass casualty events on US soil, some from natural disasters and some as a result of terrorist attacks. Examples of terrorist attacks include the bombing of the Alfred P. Murrah Federal Building in Oklahoma City in 1995; the attacks on the US embassies in Kenya and Tanzania in 1998; and the attack in 2000 on the *U.S.S. Cole*, an American warship refueling in Yemen. None of these events, however, had the same effect as the events of September 11, 2001, when the United States experienced devastating, well-coordinated attacks in New York City, Washington, D.C. and Shanksville, Pennsylvania, that led to the deaths of nearly 3000 people.

Later events have kept the threat of terrorism alive. The Boston Marathon bombings in 2013 killed 3 people and injured an estimated 264 others, who were treated in 27 local hospitals (Kotz, 2013). This event vividly demonstrated the need to have coordinated efforts among first responders: law enforcement/fire, medical and mental health services, emergency management, and related local and federal agencies. The brutal beheadings of journalists by Islamic extremists remind all of us that the ever-changing world is difficult to protect. Active shooter incidents such as the mass shooting occurrences at Sandy Hook Elementary School, Newtown (2012); Route 91 Harvest Music Festival, Las Vegas (2017); Pulse, Orlando (2016); Marjory Stoneman Douglas High School (2018); Walmart, El Paso (2019); and Uvalde (2022) continue throughout the United States with devastating personal and system-related impacts. Twenty-one people died in the Uvalde shooting with a delayed police response creating a public outcry for stricter gun controls. Investigations by officials found lapses in public safety communication and leadership that contributed to significant delays in law enforcement action and medical care.

The disasters unfolding in this century are frequently associated with global instability, economic decay, political upheaval and collapse of government structure, violence and civil conflicts, famine, and mass population displacements (Veenema, 2019a). The growing complexity and nature of disasters create considerable challenges for individuals responsible for disaster planning and related responses. The need for formalized plans for preparedness, mitigation, response, recovery, and evaluation is essential to minimizing the impact to individuals and society at large. Nurses serve in vital roles in planning development and overall response.

Although a great deal of attention has been focused on preparing for an MCI related to a terrorist attack, the United States has suffered major damage from natural disasters. Hurricane Katrina has become the classic example of massive system failure in emergency response. Most of the destruction was due to storm surge, and further flooding took place in New Orleans as the levee system catastrophically failed. Although the death toll from this event did not reach the level seen at the World Trade Center in New York City, the damage to the health care systems in the affected areas was substantial. It became evident very quickly that the response systems in place could not be effective in dealing with the destruction of the health care infrastructure and, in fact,

the health care agencies themselves were sites of mass casualties. The extensive need for immediate and long-term shelters for large numbers of victims also highlighted the need for nurses to have knowledge and skills in how to meet the needs of victims with psychologic and chronic diseases in a sheltered environment.

The year 2017 proved to be a devastating one for catastrophic hurricanes impacting numerous southern states (Florida, Texas, Louisiana), Puerto Rico, the Caribbean, Cuba, and Mexico. In particular, Hurricane Irma forced large-scale evacuations as it developed from a tropical storm to a category 5 hurricane. These natural disaster events caused infrastructure damage to power, water supply, gas, homes, industry, and health care facilities. Furthermore, there was an unprecedented number of hurricanes during the 2020 season, resulting in the naming of hurricanes using the Greek alphabet. Once again coordinated local, state, and federal responses were key in preparation for and response to these events. Post-event evaluations still indicate a need for further refinement in emergency operations planning and response.

Emergency management plans must address adequate response systems that can be used regardless of the cause of the MCI. A more reasonable approach has been the movement to plan and improve responses to a variety of hazards, called an all-hazards approach. Nurses have traditionally received disaster education as a part of community health content within nursing education programs; however, the education has been focused on responding to a disaster site of victims when the health care system is still intact. The same is true for other health care professional education programs. In addition, they have not routinely received education related to dangerous biologic agents or chemical agents or to nuclear, explosive, or radiologic hazards. It is imperative that all health care providers become knowledgeable about how to provide care for victims of all types of hazards and in situations in which the health care system itself either has been damaged or destroyed or has no contact with the other parts of the community.

It is recognized by all federal agencies that the most serious knowledge deficit for health care providers is in the area of bioterrorism attacks and pandemic events. Unlike the other hazards, these situations place the health care providers in a position of being first responders. Traditionally, first responders to emergencies have been the law enforcement, firefighters, and emergency medical technicians who respond with ambulances. In a biologic event (covert or natural transmission), however, victims first appear in EDs, physicians' offices, nurse-managed clinics, or even in school health settings. Health care professionals need to be able to identify symptoms, patterns of similar events, and other irregularities. If they fail to recognize or report significant events, a biologic event could go unrecognized until it is of epidemic proportions.

The same principles of responding to a bioterrorist event are pertinent for coping with a natural biologic outbreak such as a pandemic flu event, severe acute respiratory syndrome (SARS), or, most recently, the coronavirus (COVID-19). In these types of diseases and exposures education not only for the health care community but also for the general community at large is critical to foster cooperation to mitigate the spread of a disease as well as the subsequent morbidity and mortality that follows.

THE BASICS OF EMERGENCY PREPAREDNESS AND RESPONSE

Nurses have experience in dealing with natural disasters and are familiar with the work of the Red Cross in bringing disaster relief to affected areas. A disaster condition is defined as a significant natural disaster or human-caused event that overwhelms the affected state and necessitates both federal public health and medical care assistance (Federal Emergency Management Agency [FEMA], 2014). The disaster condition must be of significant impact to warrant federal resources. Understanding the responsibilities of the multiple agencies that respond to a disaster is imperative to be able to communicate with patients, families, and other health care providers.

In some situations the number of victims is so large that multiple organizations are called to respond. When casualties occur at this level, the event is termed an MCI. Although the situation may be unfamiliar for some nurses, it is important to remember that the nursing fundamentals practiced in other settings and during smaller crises are generally still applicable. Traditionally, triage that is practiced in most health care agencies categorizes patients into low risk, intermediate care, and critically ill (those who need immediate care to save their lives). With such large numbers, however, there is a paradigm shift to crisis standards of care in which priorities change into doing the greatest good for the greatest number of people. Care is given to those

patients who have the greatest chance of survival. This type of triage typically places nurses in ethical situations in which they experience discomfort, particularly if patients are triaged and tagged to receive only pain management rather than the typical extensive treatment that might be provided during normal health care conditions. Furthermore, the public responds to the visible tags placed on patients and can provide added stress when calling out to health care providers to provide further care.

Community disaster plans need to clearly define the care processes to be used when the needs shift from those of one patient to the needs of the populations. Nurses may also find themselves in positions in which there is a lack of necessary resources, and they will then have to come up with creative solutions.

Harmful Agents used by Terrorists

Terrorism has created the need for us to prepare against a variety of different agents. A standardized nomenclature has been developed for five categories using the acronym CBRNE, which stands for chemical, biologic, radiologic, nuclear, and explosive. Table 16.1 describes the similarities and differences related to the CBRNE agents and provides information about treatment protocols for each.

PHASES OF DISASTER

FEMA (2023) trains emergency managers to think of disasters as recurring events with four phases: mitigation, preparedness, response, and recovery. All communities are in at least one phase of this cycle at any time. The mitigation phase includes actions taken to prevent or reduce the cause, impact, and consequences of disasters. Preparedness includes planning, training, and educational activities for events that cannot be mitigated. The response phase occurs in the immediate aftermath of a disaster. During the recovery period, restoration efforts occur concurrently with regular operations and activities. This period can be prolonged.

Nursing as a profession has a long history of being creative and visionary in its continuous efforts to meet the needs of patients and their families. Nursing leadership, in tumultuous times such as during a disaster continuum or an MCI, will require significant amounts of the same creativity and vision (Veenema, 2019b). Thus it is important for nurses to understand the phases

TABLE 16.1   CBRNE Agents

Agents	Action	Advantages	Disadvantages	Treatment
Chemical	Agents injure or kill through variety of means: vesicant, nerve, blood, respiratory	Spread easily through air; cause immediate effects; require decontamination	Less toxic than biologic agents; need to be used in large quantities; subject to dispersion by wind; terrorists need to protect themselves; require trained HAZMAT teams	Dependent on agent used; in some cases, there are agent-specific medications; require decontamination; require use of personal protective equipment by personnel
Biologic	Disease-causing organisms (bacteria, viruses, toxins)	Available; small quantities can have large effect; spread through large areas; can remain in air or on surfaces; difficult to prepare against	Delayed effects; production hazardous to terrorists; difficult to develop	Dependent on agent used; most cause flu-like symptoms; plague and smallpox most contagious; timing of specific treatment critical; in some cases, there are vaccines
Radiologic	Ionizing radiation is able to strip electrons from atoms, causing chemical changes in molecules; expression may be delayed; radiation depends on time, distance, shielding, and quantity of radioactive material	Available; psychologic effect likely to be substantial; often used in conjunction with explosive devices ("dirty bombs")	Delayed effects of radiation materials; difficult to shield against	Dirty bomb causes immediate effects (radiation burns, acute poisoning) and long-term effects (cancer, contamination of drinking water); decontamination must occur before patient care can be safely provided by the health care worker
Nuclear	Depends on yield of nuclear weapon, but consists of blast range effects, thermal radiation, nuclear radiation, and radioactive fallout	Requires decontamination; contamination can remain for many years; psychologic effect likely to be substantial	Large, heavy, and dangerous weapons; hazardous to terrorists; making weapons of this type expensive and difficult to make	Symptomatic treatment of thermal burns, shrapnel injuries, and radioactive fallout; depends on distance from source and time of exposure
Explosive	Most common method for terrorists; capable of violent decomposition; pressure, temperature changes, and propellants cause injury and/or death	Available materials to construct explosive device; large devices can be placed in abandoned vehicles; smaller device can be placed on the body of a person willing to commit suicide by igniting the device	Volatile ingredients could cause premature explosion of device, thus creating danger for terrorists; government agencies have improved training and processes for identifying incendiary devices	Symptomatic; often requires treatment for burns

of a disaster, described in the following sections, to know which actions are necessary in each phase.

Preparedness Phase

The Joint Commission's (TJC) disaster preparedness standards require emergency management and community involvement in the management process. All accredited organizations must take an "all-hazards" approach to disaster planning—reviewing, analyzing, and addressing all hazards that are determined to be credible and serious threats to the community. Following the terrorist attacks on September 11, 2001, TJC added to its disaster preparedness a standard requiring organizations to communicate and coordinate with one another (TJC, 2023).

Local Planning. Every disaster, regardless of the cause, begins as a local event. Each locale has the responsibility for responding to the emergencies within its community first. Thus the heaviest burden falls on the local community when a mass casualty occurs. Assistance from state and federal levels is appropriated when the local system is unable to provide the necessary level of care. It is imperative, then, that communities plan for the services that will be needed in a time of disaster and train providers within each agency about responding to all hazard types of MCIs. Efforts must be directed toward the interrelationship of roles and responsibilities of agencies and services that will be needed at the time of a disaster. Key elements of a community preparedness program include:

- Assessing the community for risks and determining the types of events that may occur
- Planning the emergency activities to ensure a coordinated response effort
- Building the capabilities that are necessary to respond to the consequences of the events

There must be agreements between agencies within the community and between neighboring communities for entities such as emergency response units, hospitals, long-term care facilities, clinics, and health departments to be able to provide mutual aid and transfer of people and materials during a time of disaster. The Institute of Medicine (IOM) report *Crisis Standards of Care* (2012) emphasizes that integrated planning for coordinated response by state and local governments, emergency medical services, health care organizations, and health care providers in the community is critical to successfully

respond to disasters. It is key to include mental health professionals as a component of the response for the individuals impacted by the event, as well as the health care providers who may need additional support to debrief after a disaster/mass casualty situation.

Medical Reserve Corps. Agreements should be in place that address issues related to credentialing health care providers who may be shared among institutions. The Medical Reserve Corps (MRC) was initiated in 2002 to improve the health and safety of communities across the country by organizing and utilizing public health, nursing, medical, and other volunteers to serve their communities. There are 800 MRC units and 300,000 volunteers throughout the United States and its territories (Administration for Strategic Preparedness & Response, 2023). Part of the requirements for membership in the MRC is to complete an emergency response curriculum.

The MRC is the responsibility of the local area, with many states receiving funding to establish the network of volunteers. They function as a way to locally organize and utilize volunteers who want to donate their time and expertise to prepare for and respond to emergencies and promote healthy living throughout the year. MRC volunteers supplement existing emergency and public health resources. There are situations (such as Hurricane Katrina) for which local units deployed outside of their region respond to the additional needs that were not being met. Visit https://aspr.hhs.gov/MRC/Pages/Become-a-Volunteer.aspx for more information about how to volunteer to participate in the MRC system.

Local Emergency Operating Plans. Plans and contracts need to be developed with school systems, YMCA buildings, churches, and other large facilities to provide shelter for large numbers of victims. The interface with volunteer agencies such as the Red Cross also needs to be arranged. Each agency should have a well-developed emergency operating plan (EOP) that includes its responsibilities and capabilities for responding to an MCI, an identified chain of command, and a plan for interaction with other community agencies. Agency personnel should be knowledgeable about their role in the EOP and should receive education concerning the ways to respond to all types of hazards.

Several federal-level programs are designed to assist communities in planning their emergency response to

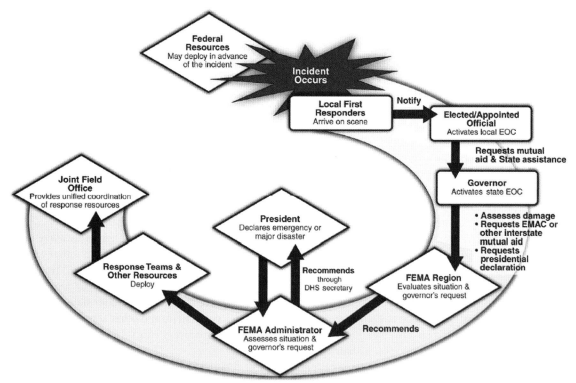

Fig. 16.1 Emergency response flows from the community to the state to the federal level. *DHS*, Department of Homeland Security; *EMAC*, Emergency Management Assistance Compact; *EOC*, emergency operations center; *FEMA*, Federal Emergency Management Agency. (Department of Homeland Security. [2008]. *National response framework.* https://www.fema.gov/pdf/emergency/nrf/nrf-overview.pdf)

an MCI and to provide assistance during a time of disaster. Agency and community EOPs should outline their relationship with the federal system. The National Response Framework is a guide to how the nation conducts an all-hazard response—from the smallest incident to the largest catastrophe—using a comprehensive, national, all-hazards approach to domestic incident response (FEMA, 2020). Fig. 16.1 illustrates the relationship among local, state, and federal response systems. The following is a description of the key components of the federal response system.

Metropolitan Medical Response System. The Metropolitan Medical Response System (MMRS) program builds a cadre of specialty trained responders and equipment in local or sub-state jurisdictions. The system is coordinated with area and state-wide planning systems and integrates the efforts of all of the emergency response teams. The MMRS includes plans for expanding

hospital-based care, enhancing emergency medical transport and emergency department capabilities, locating specialized pharmaceuticals to respond to an MCI, managing mass fatalities, and providing mental health care for the community, victims, and health care providers. Scenarios designed to test the effectiveness of the MMRS in the community in providing an integrated response to an MCI are conducted on a regular basis.

National Disaster Medical System. The National Disaster Medical System (NDMS) is a federally coordinated system that augments the nation's medical response capability during times of major peacetime disasters and provides support to the military and the Department of Veterans Affairs medical systems in caring for casualties evacuated back to the United States from armed conventional conflicts overseas (US Department of Health and Human Services [USDHHS], 2023). The National Response Framework utilizes the

NDMS under Emergency Support Function #8, Health and Medical Services, to support the federal medical response to major emergencies and federally declared disasters, including national disasters, major transportation accidents, technologic disasters, and acts of terrorism. For more information about becoming involved in NDMS visit the website https://aspr.hhs.gov/NDMS/Pages/join-ndms.aspx.

Disaster Medical Assistance Teams. Disaster Medical Assistance Teams (DMATs) are regionally organized teams of health care professionals and administrative staff designed to be the rapid-response component to support local medical care needs until federal resources can be deployed; DMATs can be sent into areas outside their own regions to assist in providing care for ill or injured victims at the location of a disaster or emergency. DMATs provide triage, medical or surgical stabilization, and continued monitoring and care of patients until they can be evacuated to locations to receive definitive medical care. Specialty DMATs can also be deployed to address, for example, mass burn injuries, pediatric care requirements, and chemical injury or contamination. For more information about DMATs, visit the website https://aspr.hhs.gov/SNS/Pages/Disaster-Medical-Assistance-Teams.aspx.

Commissioned Corps. The Commissioned Corps emergency response teams are managed by the Office of the Surgeon General and are part of the US Public Health Service. These teams are an additional asset capable of responding in times of extraordinary need when the public health needs exceed the capability of the local or state agencies. The Commissioned Corps comprises more than 6500 health care professionals who can be deployed to respond to a disaster, either as a large group or in small numbers, to support the DMAT's effort. For example, Commissioned Corps teams were deployed to support hospitals that were overwhelmed during the COVID-19 pandemic. For more information, visit the website https://www.surgeongeneral.gov/corps/index.html.

Strategic National Stockpile. The Centers for Disease Control and Prevention (CDC) host a Strategic National Stockpile (SNS) that has large quantities of medicine and medical supplies to protect the American public if there is a public health emergency severe enough to cause local supplies to be depleted. The SNS has a national repository of antibiotics, chemical antidotes, antitoxins, IV administrations, airway supplies, and other medical–surgical items. A 12-hour "push pack" of supplies can be deployed within 12 hours of the decision to activate the SNS. The community emergency plan should include procedures to receive the push pack. Follow-up pharmaceutical or medical supplies can be shipped within 24 to 36 hours if required. This supply can be tailored to the specific needs of the event if the needs are known at that time (CDC, 2023).

Emergency Management Assistance Compact. The Emergency Management Assistance Compact (EMAC) was authorized by the US Congress to allow states to request and receive assistance from other states impacted by a governor-declared disaster. This program allows states to quickly and efficiently request and receive assistance from other member states in the form of personnel, equipment, and other supplies for emergency response and recovery efforts (EMAC, 2017).

Using Response Resources. Community EOPs must include strategies for the community's interaction with these various state and federal response teams and systems to efficiently use the services and materials provided for mass casualty response. Hospital EOPs should include descriptions of the federal responses and how they will be incorporated into the emergency operations.

Individual Citizen Preparedness. Although not formally part of emergency operations, individuals and households play an important role in the overall emergency management strategy. Individuals can contribute by reducing hazards in and around their homes, preparing emergency supply kits and household emergency plans, and monitoring emergency communications carefully. The government website *Ready* provides additional disaster response information (http://www.ready.gov) including a FEMA Mobile App that has preparedness strategies and real-time weather and emergency alerts.

Relief Response Phase

Response Activities. Response activities are first initiated during the impact phase of disasters. These activities begin at the time of the event and are focused on providing the first emergency response to victims of the disaster, stabilizing the situation, and giving adequate treatment to victims. This phase requires the interaction of emergency responders from fire and police departments, emergency medical services, hazardous materials teams, health care agencies, and health departments and enables the group to triage, provide assistance, conduct a scene assessment, and stabilize the scene. Typically the first unit responding establishes an incident command post from which to coordinate the activities. However, as other units arrive and as the cause of the incident becomes known, one of the law enforcement agencies may assume control as the lead agency if there is suspicion of a crime before the establishment of a community-based emergency operations center (EOC).

National Incident Management System. Emergencies breed chaos, and it is essential that order be brought to the situation for an effective response. The National Incident Management System (NIMS) provides a systematic proactive approach to guide departments and agencies at all levels to work seamlessly during disaster situations (FEMA, 2023). The system is designed to expand from one person or agency performing all roles to having hundreds of people involved in the process. An efficient NIMS requires a hierarchical chain of command led by the incident manager or commander. Assigned personnel who refer to specific job action sheets consistently follow job assignments. A NIMS is established at the scene of the disaster and includes representatives of all agencies needed to provide the emergency services.

At the time of a mass casualty each hospital system initiates its emergency response plans. Structures may vary from hospital to hospital, but most are using the system called the hospital incident command system (HICS). The assumption is that in a time of crisis communication will be improved if all disaster responders begin from a common structure. The HICS defines responsibilities, reporting channels, and common terminology for hospitals, fire departments, local governments, and other agencies (California Emergency Medical Services Authority, 2017). The HICS can be customized for organizations of varying sizes. (The most current edition of the *HICS Guidebook* can be downloaded online at no charge at https://emsa.ca.gov/disaster-medical-services-division-hospital-incident-command-system).

Regardless of the structure of the NIMS, the ultimate aim is to coordinate the safe and effective response of emergency resources to an incident. In the HICS, there is only one incident commander, supported by

clearly identified levels in the command structure. The hierarchy of command is important so that there is no confusion as to who reports to whom or about who is managing the incident. The chain of command is established to allow for communication to flow from the top down or the bottom up.

Personal Protection and Safety. Personal protection and safety are important regardless of the situational factors causing an MCI. What is important to note, however, is that situational factors dictate how to be personally protected and safe. Protecting the lives of emergency responders takes precedence over other incident issues because if emergency responders are exposed or injured they will be unable to provide care to others.

Because of the varied routes of exposure from CBRNE agents personal protective equipment (PPE) must be designed to impede the most vulnerable route(s), thereby blocking the agent from entering the body. Specially designed PPE is available in a variety of levels, each designed to meet specific protection needs:
- *Level A* equipment consists of a totally encapsulated chemical-resistant suit, including supplied air. As a result, maximum respiratory and skin protection is provided. This level of equipment is used to protect against liquid splashes or in situations when agents are still unidentified.
- *Level B* equipment is a chemical splash-resistant suit with hood and self-contained breathing apparatus (SCBA). It provides maximum respiratory protection but less skin protection than level A equipment.
- *Level C* equipment is chemical-resistant clothing with a hood and an air-purifying respirator. The respirator can remove all anticipated contaminants and concentrations of chemical materials, thus providing adequate protection against airborne biologic agents and radiologic materials.
- *Level D* protection may consist of a uniform or scrubs and is appropriate when it has been determined that no respiratory or skin hazard is present.

Although each level provides some protection, it is important to understand the limitations of all PPE. Typically first responders to community emergencies are firefighters, police, and emergency medical technicians. These professionals have traditionally been trained in the effective use of PPE and can be a good community resource. In addition hospital infection control personnel can be an excellent resource for the use of PPE. As health care providers assume the care of patients who may have been contaminated it is important to note whether patients have been decontaminated and require no further protective equipment or what additional level of protection is required.

Communication Within the Health Care Facility. At the initial time of the event, when news stories are first breaking, staff, patients, and families may hear of the incident before the EOP and HICS have been initiated. In this case it is crucial for the facility information officer to take charge of communicating with the news media and for administrators to initiate a plan to communicate within the health care facility. Crisis intervention strategies to prevent group panic must be instituted immediately. Communication officers need to:

- Determine the effects the crisis will have on the audience.
- Speak clearly and simply about the facts.
- Be direct, honest, and to the point.
- Reassure and calm the audience.

Regular updates of information (every 30 minutes) need to be planned and distributed to all hospital units as quickly as possible. Patients and families need to be informed of measures that will be taken with the initiation of the EOP, such as early discharge or relocation of less ill patients to other areas of the hospital or to other facilities. Family members may not be able to leave the hospital to return home; if so, arrangements must be made to care for them, including providing medications that they take regularly.

Lessons Learned from Mass Casualty Incidents

Staff and Family Considerations. Although preparation for all types of causes of MCIs (natural or human-caused) is necessary, nurses must understand the actions needed when the health care agency is damaged and how health care providers must function during these times. Issues related to use of personnel, rotation and resting of personnel, use of family or volunteers, methods of evacuation, and care of hospital staff and families must be included in emergency preparedness preparations and education. Alterations in the standard of care during an MCI need to be understood. Hospitals are viewed by the community and employees as places of safe haven when a disaster strikes. Incoming staff will be limited, and decisions about how care will be provided must be made. Places to provide rest and measures to encourage staff to rest should be determined early in the MCI. Mechanisms for staff to contact their families or significant others

should be initiated as soon as possible. Arrangements need to be made for the care of children, other dependents, and pets for those staff members who will be staying at the hospital for extended periods.

In addition measures must be included to provide information to the staff for those who are not able to locate their family because of the disaster. The role of the information liaison office of the HICS is most important for this function. In addition to these considerations mass casualty incidents have the potential to create widespread civil unrest and violence, which may occur immediately following the event. Safety/security resources, if available, should be put in place as quickly as possible. Personal safety and the safety of others must remain at the forefront in response efforts. This principle is particularly true for vulnerable populations such as women, children, elderly, and those with disabilities.

Power Outages and Building Damage. Staff need to be prepared to cope with power outages and damage to the institution. All hospitals and most other health facilities are equipped with emergency generators, and most staff members assume that these will be operational. Emergency plans and drills must include scenarios of how to adapt care if the generators are not functioning. It is important that the staff delivering care have the skill set to know how they will function in these situations. Lessons learned from previous disasters emphasize the necessity to include the care delivery staff in this level of detail. Some examples of decisions that have had to be made were how to:

- Deliver medications when the usual pumps were not functioning.
- Decide which medications would be given when the medication supply was depleted.
- Provide ventilation and suctioning without electricity.

Nurses and staff on the nursing units need to be prepared for these situations. Composing unit-based scenarios for discussion can be helpful in preparing for an MCI.

BIOLOGIC CAUSES OF MASS CASUALTY

Pandemic Influenza and COVID-19

Nurses also need to be prepared to respond to MCIs that result from biologic agents. Although terrorist dissemination of biologic agents was initially the focus of emergency preparedness efforts following the World Trade Center attack, the natural dissemination of biologic agents such as influenza, respiratory syncytial virus (RSV), and COVID-19 has been the priority for disaster preparedness efforts for communities. A *pandemic* is a global outbreak that occurs when a new virus emerges in the human population, causing serious illness and death as it spreads worldwide.

During the memorable flu pandemic of 2018 21 million died worldwide (later estimated to be 50 million) and 675,000 died in the United States (Pan American Health Organization [PAHO], 2003). Many of the flu prevention strategies again surfaced during the recent COVID-19 pandemic, which left 6,957,216 dead worldwide with 770,563,467 confirmed cases (WHO, 2023). As 2023 drew to a close, COVID-19 was no longer considered to be a pandemic but cases of hospitalization were on the rise.

Tracking and predicting pandemic flu and coronavirus is an important component of the response to this potential serious threat to the nation's health. The most up-to-date information for flu and COVID-19 tracking and reporting is now found on the CDC (www.cdc.gov) and WHO (www.who.int) websites. The CDC has also developed competencies for response to a pandemic flu epidemic. Health care providers are directed to these websites to determine virus outbreaks in their own areas and those within the region, country, and world. Although most people believe that virus transmission is a local problem, it has become a global issue with the amounts of international travel and transmission that now occur.

It is important to note that when COVID-19 reached global proportions and was declared an international pandemic, academic and pharmaceutical communities united to develop and produce vaccine within months of the virus' initial detection. These vaccines were based on a copy of a molecule messenger RNA (mRNA) to produce an immune response. While this science had been years in the making, there were many who were hesitant to get the vaccines because they were developed so soon after the outbreak. Additional cultural and political reasons for not taking the vaccines arose, thus the outbreak continued, although with declining rates. In the meantime, RSV cases rose during 2022–23, creating higher risks for infants and the elderly. As a result vaccines are recommended according to CDC guidelines for those eligible for the flu, COVID, and RSV vaccines.

As with other MCIs, planning is aimed at saving the largest number of people. It is likely that flu varieties, RSV, and COVID-19 would strike nearly simultaneously in many different geographic regions and cause multiple waves of disease lasting several weeks to months in communities. Thus local communities need to make their plans self-sufficient because other areas would be dealing with the same

problem. Control methods include isolation, quarantine, and restrictions. Limitations include suspension of large public gatherings, school closures, and social distancing.

The term *social distancing* refers to keeping people as far apart as possible to limit the possibilities of spreading germs. For COVID-19 these guidelines include additional actions such as mask wearing, handwashing, crowd gathering limitations, and other mitigation efforts. Health care providers are advised to treat patients symptomatically without encouraging them to come to offices or emergency departments. Many health care facilities set up separate screening facilities for those who have flu-like symptoms, while telehealth visits have become a rapidly growing method of connecting patients with providers for assessment and treatment during the COVID-19 pandemic.

As a health care provider you need to take the time to become familiar with your institution's preparedness plan. Most have a plan specific to the threat of pandemic flu and now for COVID-19. Know what your role is, how you would be notified, and where and how you would report if an emergency is declared. The response of the entire health workforce will make the difference in morbidity and mortality, the degree of suffering, and the rate at which recovery occurs in the community. Being ready to adapt and provide essential care under crisis conditions is a professional responsibility (ANA, 2020).

Being prepared means that you and your family need to be prepared as well. Practice good health hygiene and follow the general principles of sound public health. Teach family members how to cover their mouths when coughing, how to appropriately dispose of used tissues, and how and when to wash their hands. Develop contingency plans to address school and business closures, unavailability of public transportation, and disruption in social activities. Grocery stores and gas stations may not be open during their typical hours. That means that personal stockpiling of food and medications would help you and your family get through the event with minimal contact with others. Ideally the goal is to keep the number of people infected within range of existing medical capabilities.

HUMAN CAUSES OF MASS CASUALTY: ACTIVE SHOOTER EVENTS

The federal government defines an active shooter as "an individual actively engaged in killing or attempting to kill people in a confined and populated area; in most cases, active shooters use firearm(s) and there is no method to their pattern or selection of victims." (DHS, 2008). The FBI

(2019) analyzed 333 active shooter incidents from 2000 through 2019 to look for common elements that might guide law enforcement officials in more effective prevention and response efforts. In the 333 events reviewed, 1062 individuals were killed and 1789 were wounded. Businesses open to pedestrian traffic had the highest number of incidents with 96, followed by open spaces with 50, and schools (PreK–12) with 44 (FBI, 2019).

Active shooter events can take place in various locations, including schools, health care facilities, and office settings. With the recognition of the increased active shooter threat and the swiftness with which active shooter incidents unfold there is greater emphasis on the importance of training and exercises for all employees. It is important, too, that training and exercises include not only an understanding of the threats faced but also the risks and options available in active shooter incidents. Recommendations for response to an active shooter are shown in Table 16.2.

Active shooter events in a health care setting present unique challenges: a potentially large vulnerable patient population, hazardous materials (including infectious disease), locked units, and other special challenges. During the 2010–2020 timeframe The Joint Commission received reports from its accredited organizations of 39 shootings that resulted in 39 deaths: 21 were staff members (10 shot by a patient, 5 shot by a visitor, 4 shot by a family member, and 2 shot by a current or former staff member); 18 were patients: 15 were shot by a family member; 2 were shot by a visitor; and 1 was shot by another patient (TJC, 2020).

Since every health care organization is different because of its patient population, location, size, and other variables, health care settings present a unique set of challenges when planning for active shooters. Planning should take into consideration what works best for each organization's particular circumstances. Prior planning will allow employees to choose the best option during an active shooter situation, with the goal of maximizing lives saved.

TABLE 16.2 Recommended Response to an Active Shooter

1. Evacuate (RUN)	2. Hide Out (HIDE)	3. Take Actions Against the Active Shooter (FIGHT)
If there is an accessible escape path, attempt to evacuate the premises. Be sure to: • Have an escape route and plan in mind • Evacuate regardless of whether others agree to follow • Leave your belongings behind • Help others escape, if possible • Prevent individuals from entering an area where the active shooter may be • Keep your hands visible • Follow the instructions of any police officers • Do not attempt to move wounded people • Call 911 when you are safe	If evacuation is not possible, find a place to hide where the active shooter is less likely to find you. Your hiding place should: • Be out of the active shooter's view • Provide protection if shots are fired in your direction (e.g., an office with a closed and locked door) • Try not to trap yourself or restrict your options for movement To prevent an active shooter from entering your hiding place: • Lock the door • Blockade the door with heavy furniture If the active shooter is nearby: • Lock the door • Silence your cell phone and/or pager • Turn off any source of noise (e.g., radios, televisions) • Hide behind large items (e.g., cabinets, desks) • Remain quiet If evacuation and hiding out are not possible: • Remain calm • Dial 911, if possible, to alert police to the active shooter's location • If you cannot speak, leave the line open and allow the dispatcher to listen	As a last resort, and only when your life is in imminent danger, attempt to disrupt and/or incapacitate the active shooter by: • Acting as aggressively as possible against them • Throwing items and improvising weapons • Yelling • Committing to your actions

From US Department of Homeland Security. (2008). *Active shooter: How to respond.* https://www.dhs.gov/xlibrary/assets/active_shooter_booklet.pdf

SUMMARY

Preparing for an MCI requires a complex set of activities. All nurses need to be aware of the emergency response system at the local, state, and federal levels and to know how to interface with the systems. They should be involved in developing and evaluating the emergency response plans for their health care agencies and communities. Consider Tana in the opening Vignette. Her understanding of the resources available in the community's emergency response system will help her better cope with the disaster at the hospital where she works. Just as in Tana's situation, disaster can strike any time, and preparation for an effective emergency response is absolutely critical to ensure the very best outcome for everyone involved. Nurses are well positioned to serve in leadership roles within health care agencies during the time of a disaster because of their excellent communication and collaboration skills.

REFERENCES

Administration for Strategic Preparedness & Response. (2023). *About the Medical Reserve Corps (MRC)*. https://aspr.hhs.gov/MRC/Pages/About-the-MRC.aspx.

American Nurses Association (ANA). (2020). *Crisis standard of care COVID-19 pandemic*. https://www.capc.org/documents/download/796/#:~:text=Definition%3A%20Crisis%20Standards%20of%20Care,e.g.%20earthquake%2C%20hurricane)%20disaster

California Emergency Medical Services Authority. (2017). *Disaster medical services: Hospital incident command system (HICS)*. https://emsa.ca.gov/disaster-medical-services-division-hospital-incident-command-system-resources

Centers for Disease Control and Prevention (CDC). (2023). *Strategic national stockpile*. https://aspr.hhs.gov/SNS/Pages/default.aspx

Department of Homeland Security (DHS). (2008). *Active shooter: How to respond*. https://www.dhs.gov/xlibrary/assets/active_shooter_booklet.pdf

Emergency Management Assistance Compact (EMAC). (2017). *EMAC*. https://www.emacweb.org

Federal Bureau of Investigation (FBI). (2019). *Active shooter incidents in the United States: 2000–2019*. https://www.fbi.gov/file-repository/active-shooter-incidents-20-year-review-2000-2019-060121.pdf/view

Federal Emergency Management Agency (FEMA). (2014). *A guide to the disaster declaration process and federal disaster assistance*. https://www.fema.gov/pdf/rrr/dec_proc.pdf

Federal Emergency Management Agency (FEMA). (2020). *National Response Framework*. https://www.fema.gov/emergency-managers/national-preparedness/frameworks/response

Federal Emergency Management Agency (FEMA). (2023). *National incident management system*. http://www.fema.gov/national-incident-management-system

Institute of Medicine. (2012). Crisis standards of care: A systems framework for catastrophic disaster response. https://nap.nationalacademies.org/catalog/13351/crisis-standards-of-care-a-systems-framework-for-catastrophic-disaster#:~:text=Crisis%20Standards%20of%20Care%20provides,a%20disaster%20response%20should%20address

Kotz, D. (2013). Injury toll from Marathon bombs reduced to 264. *The Boston Globe*, http://www.bostonglobe.com/lifestyle/health-wellness/2013/04/23/number-injured-marathon-bombing-revised-downward/NRpaz5mmvGquP7KMA6XsIK/story.html

Pan American Health Organization (2003). *Purple death: The great flu of 1918*. https://www.paho.org/en/who-we-are/history-paho/purple-death-great-flu-1918

The Joint Commission (TJC). (2020). *Quick safety 4: Preparing for active shooter situations (Updated June 2021)*. https://www.jointcommission.org/resources/news-and-multimedia/newsletters/newsletters/quick-safety/quick-safety—issue-4-preparing-for-active-shooter-situations/preparing-for-active-shooter-situations-addendum-february-2017/

The Joint Commission (TJC). (2023). *Emergency management: The Joint Commission's emergency management resources portal*. https://www.jointcommission.org/resources/patient-safety-topics/emergency-management/

US Department of Health and Human Services (USDHHS). (2023). *National disaster medical system*. https://www.phe.gov/Preparedness/responders/ndms/Pages/default.aspx

US Department of Homeland Security. (2008). *Active shooter: How to respond*. http://www.dhs.gov/xlibrary/assets/active_shooter_booklet.pdf

Veenema, T.G. (2019a). *Essentials of disaster planning*. In T.G. Veenema (ed.), *Disaster nursing and emergency preparedness for chemical, biological, and radiological terrorism and other hazards*. Springer, pp. 3–30.

Veenema, T.G. (2019b). *Leadership and coordination in disaster healthcare systems: The U.S. disaster response network*. In T.G. Veenema (ed.), *Disaster nursing and emergency preparedness for chemical, biological, and radiological terrorism and other hazards*. Springer, pp. 31–61.

World Health Organization (WHO). (2023). *WHO Coronavirus disease (COVID-19) dashboard*. https://covid19.who.int/

17

Nursing Leadership and Management: The Foundations

Barbara Cherry, DNSc, MBA, RN, NEA-BC

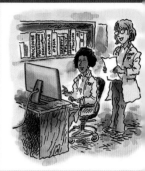

All nurses—regardless of their role setting—must step up as leaders to mote joy and engagement in the work ting for healthier patients and happier s.

(e) Additional resources are available online at: http://evolve.elsevier.com/Cherry/

LEARNING OUTCOMES

After studying this chapter, the reader will be able to:

1. Discuss the responsibility of being a leader in any role or setting where professional nursing is practiced.
2. Relate leadership and management theory to nursing leadership and management functions.
3. Integrate principles of patient-centered care in professional nursing practice.
4. Implement effective team-building skills as an essential component of nursing practice.
5. Implement the clinical judgment model as a method of problem-solving and decision-making.
6. Apply principles and strategies of change theory in nursing practice.
7. Employ strategies to create joy and engagement in the work setting.

KEY TERMS

Authority The legitimate right to direct others, given to a person by the employer through an official position, such as manager or director.

Health care organization Any business, company, institution, or facility (e.g., hospital, home health agency, ambulatory care clinic, health insurance company, nursing home) engaged in providing health care services or products.

Leadership The ability to guide or influence the beliefs, opinions, or actions of individuals, groups, or organizations.

Management Coordination of resources, such as time, people, and supplies, to achieve outcomes; involves problem-solving and decision-making processes.

Organizational chart A visual picture of the organization that identifies lines of communication and authority.

Productivity The amount of output or work produced (e.g., home visits made) by a specific amount of input or resources (e.g., nursing hours worked).

Resources Personnel, time, and supplies needed to accomplish the goals of the organization.

PROFESSIONAL/ETHICAL ISSUE

Marybeth Rodgers graduated from nursing school 5 years ago and worked at a renowned academic medical center in a busy medical-surgical unit since graduation. She recently took a job as a staff registered nurse (RN) in a small community hospital closer to her home to reduce her commute time and give her more time with her family. Marybeth was confident in her skills and knowledge to care for adult medical-surgical patients because of her experience over the past 5 years, but she knew she would have a lot to learn in this new setting. After a few weeks working on her new unit in the community hospital Marybeth began to sense that one of her nurse colleagues was resentful toward her. Initially the nurse was refusing to help Marybeth when she had questions, but she has now begun to openly criticize Marybeth with statements such as "I guess you think you are smarter than everyone else because you worked at that academic medical center downtown" and "I think you are just lazy and don't want to think for yourself; after all, you had all those medical students to think for you." Marybeth senses that she is being talked about by the other nurses and is being excluded from some conversations. She is coming to deeply regret her decision to move to the community hospital; she is having trouble sleeping and now dreads coming to work every day. Marybeth is deeply concerned about reporting the situation to the nurse manager because she knows that the nurse who is causing the problems has worked on the unit for many years and seems well-liked by the supervisor and other nurses. What are Marybeth's options for addressing this situation? What does the American Nurses Association (ANA) Code of Ethics tell us about a nurse's ethical obligation to support colleagues? What resources can Marybeth access to learn more about disruptive behaviors and how to handle them?

VIGNETTE

Nancy Caballero, a new RN, has accepted a position in a busy outpatient dialysis unit. During nursing school Nancy worked in the facility as a patient care technician, and she is confident in her clinical skills because of this experience. Amanda, the nursing director of the dialysis unit, has scheduled Nancy to attend the new-nurse orientation. Although Nancy thinks to herself, "I know what the RNs do around here; I'd like to jump right in

without attending orientation," she readily accepts the assignment.

The nursing director begins the orientation program with a discussion about the mission of the organization and the RN's responsibility to ensure that quality patient care is provided in a safe and cost-effective manner. As Nancy progresses through the orientation program her confidence quickly fades. She becomes overwhelmed as she listens to a description of her new responsibilities as an RN. The RN's duties involve much more than the expected physical assessment and developing and implementing care plans. Some of Nancy's many new responsibilities as a staff RN are to:

- Supervise patient care technicians and manage assignments and supply use for a group of patients.
- Meet with the interprofessional team, including the social worker, dietitian, nephrologist, nurse manager, and the patient and family, to develop the patient's care plan and then follow up to coordinate and implement the plan.
- Serve on a task force charged with developing and implementing a zero-tolerance policy for bullying and incivility in the workplace.
- Perform chart audits to review nursing documentation, identify problems, develop recommendations, and report to the quality improvement committee.

As Nancy is trying to assimilate the information being presented she almost fails to hear Amanda say that within 6 months of employment all staff RNs are expected to begin orientation for the charge nurse position to provide backup coverage. At the end of the orientation Nancy has a new perspective about professional nursing practice—it seems to be as much about managing the delivery of patient care as actually giving the care!

Questions to Consider While Reading This Chapter:

1. What skills will assist Nancy as she begins her new role as a staff RN with many leadership and management responsibilities?
2. Why is it important for the nursing staff to understand the mission and values of the organization to provide direct patient care?
3. What type of team-building skills will help Nancy as she learns to work with the interprofessional team and coordinate the patient's plan of care with a diverse group of health professionals?
4. What resources are available to help Nancy learn and enhance her management and leadership skills?

5. How can Nancy contribute to creating joy in the workplace and building a healthier work environment for all staff?

CHAPTER OVERVIEW

During nursing school students are often more concerned with developing clinical knowledge and skills and are less concerned with management and leadership skills. However, immediately after graduation the new nurse is placed in many situations that require leadership and management skills—managing a group of assigned patients, serving on a task force or committee, supervising assistive personnel and licensed vocational nurses (LVNs) or licensed practical nurses (LPNs), or addressing difficult situations such as incivility and bullying. In addition to providing safe, evidence-based, high-quality clinical care the challenges for RNs today are to manage nursing units that are constantly admitting and discharging higher-acuity patients, to motivate and coordinate a variety of diverse health professionals and assistive personnel, and to look for ways to improve the work environment to support healthier patients and happier staff.

Regardless of the position or area the nurse is employed in, the health care organization will expect the professional nurse to have leadership skills to:

- Use good clinical judgment to ensure all aspects of care are safe, high quality, cost-effective, ethical, and patient-centered.
- Promote evidence-based practice. (See Chapter 6.)
- Lead quality improvement initiatives in the work environment. (See Chapter 22.)
- Coordinate patient care activities for the interprofessional team.
- Promote team morale, patient satisfaction, and healthy work environments.
- Support compliance with governmental regulations and accreditation standards.

As the reader can easily visualize, leadership and management activities are a primary responsibility for the RN. In fact, professional nursing within a health care organization has as much to do with managing the delivery of care as it does with actually providing that care. This chapter presents key leadership and management concepts that will guide the nurse to grow and develop in this important aspect of the professional practice role.

Throughout this chapter, the term *organization* is used to refer to the hospital, home health agency, post–acute care facility, long-term care facility, ambulatory clinic, managed care company, or any other area in which a nurse might be employed to practice professional nursing. Legal and ethical issues are a critical component of leadership, although it is not within the scope of this chapter to discuss these issues. The reader is encouraged to review Chapter 8 regarding legal issues and Chapter 9 regarding ethical issues.

LEADERSHIP AND MANAGEMENT: DIFFERENT BUT RELATED

Leadership and management are intertwined and it is difficult to discuss one without the other. However, the two terms are actually different, with each having its own defining characteristics as noted in the following discussion.

Leadership Defined

Leadership occurs any time a person attempts to influence the beliefs, opinions, or actions of a person or group (Hersey & Blanchard, 1988). Leadership is a combination of intrinsic personality traits, learned leadership skills, and characteristics of the situation. The function of a leader is to guide people and groups to accomplish common goals. For example, an effective nurse leader is able to inspire others to make patient-centered care an important aspect of all care activities.

It is important to note that even though leaders may not have formal authority granted by the organization, they are still able to influence others. The job title "nurse manager" does not make a nurse a leader. Today's complex health care environment requires that *every* nurse—regardless of their role or setting—provide leadership to advance excellence in nursing practice and patient care.

Management Defined

Management refers to the activities involved in coordinating people, time, and supplies to achieve desired outcomes and involves problem-solving and decision-making processes. Managers maintain control of the day-to-day operations of a defined area of responsibility. Managers plan and organize what is to be done, who is to do it, and how it is to be done. A manager has:

- An appointed management position within the organization with responsibilities to perform administrative

tasks, such as managing staffing, employee performance reviews, supply usage, and budget and productivity goals
- A formal line of authority and accountability to ensure that safe and effective patient care is delivered in a manner that meets the organization's goals and standards

Leadership vs Management

Leadership is the ability to guide or influence others, whereas management is the coordination of resources (time, people, and supplies) to achieve outcomes. People are led, whereas activities and things are managed. Leaders are able to motivate and inspire others, whereas managers have assigned responsibility for accomplishing goals. A good manager should also be a good leader, but this may not always be the case. A person with good management skills may not have leadership ability. Similarly, a person with leadership abilities may not have good management skills. Leadership and management skills are complementary; both can be learned and developed through experience, and improving skills in one area will enhance abilities in the other.

Power and Authority

Leadership and management require power and authority to motivate people to act in a certain way. Authority is the legitimate right to direct others and is given to a person by the organization through an official position, such as nurse manager. For example, a nurse manager has the authority to direct staff nurses to work a specific schedule. Power is the ability to motivate people to get things done with or without the legitimate right granted by the organization. The classic sources of power identified by Hersey and colleagues in 1979 are still relevant today:
- *Reward power* comes from the ability to reward others for complying and may include rewards such as salary, desired assignments, and acknowledgment of accomplishments.
- *Coercive power*, the opposite of reward power, is based on fear of punishment for failure to comply. Sources of coercive power include withholding of pay increases, undesired assignments, verbal and written warnings, and termination.
- *Legitimate power* is based on an official position in the organization. Through legitimate power, the manager has the right to direct staff members to perform tasks and assignments.

- *Referent power* comes from followers' identification with the leader. The admired and respected nurse is able to influence other nurses because of their desire to emulate them.
- *Expert power* is based on knowledge, skills, and information. For example, nurses who have expertise in areas such as physical assessment or technical skills or who keep up with current information on important topics will gain respect from others.
- *Information power* is based on a person's possession of information that is needed by others.
- *Connection power* is based on a person's relationship or affiliation with other people who are perceived as being powerful.

An individual may also have informal power resulting from personal relationships, being in the right place at the right time, or unique personal characteristics, such as attractiveness, education, experience, drive, or decisiveness. By understanding the authority of an assigned position and the sources of formal and informal power, the nurse will be better able to influence others to accomplish goals.

Formal and Informal Leadership

Both formal and informal forms of leadership exist in every organization. Formal leadership is practiced by the nurse who is appointed to an approved position (e.g., nurse manager, supervisor, director) and given the authority to act by the organization. Informal leadership is exercised by the person who has no official or appointed authority to act but is able to persuade and influence others. Informal leaders are respected by their work team because of their expertise, skills, and ability to guide and influence others and can improve the overall work environment (Lawson & Fleshman, 2020). The informal leader, who may or may not be a professional nurse, may have considerable power in the work group and can influence the group's morale and significantly affect the efficiency and effectiveness of workflow, goal-setting, and problem-solving.

Nurses should learn to recognize and effectively work with informal leaders. Informal leadership may be positive if the informal leader's purpose is congruent with that of the nursing unit and organizational goals. For example, the informal leader of a patient care team may be highly supportive of a new nursing care delivery model being implemented on the unit, and as a result the other team members will be more willing to accept the change. However, an informal leader who is not supportive of the nursing unit's goals can create an uncomfortable work environment for the entire team. Following are some strategies a nurse manager can use to work with informal leaders:

- Recognize that informal leaders can have a positive impact on the work environment.
- Identify the informal leaders in the work team and seek to understand their source of power. (See sources of power in the previous section.)
- Involve the informal leaders and other staff members in decision-making and change-implementation processes.
- Clearly communicate the goals and work expectations to all staff members.
- Do not ignore an informal leader's attempt to undermine teamwork and change processes. Coaching and counseling the person and setting clear expectations may be required.

LEADERSHIP THEORY

Understanding the development and progression of leadership theory is a necessary building block for developing leadership and management skills. Researchers began to study leadership in the early 1900s to describe and understand the nature of leadership. The following sections briefly review a few key leadership theories. Readers are encouraged to learn more about leadership and management theories, especially as they advance in their nursing career.

Leadership Trait Theory

Early leadership theory centered on describing the qualities or traits of leaders and has been commonly referred to as *trait theory* (Stogdill, 1974). Leadership trait theory was based on the assumption that leaders were born with certain leadership characteristics. Traits found to be associated with leadership include intelligence, alertness, dependability, energy, drive, enthusiasm, ambition, decisiveness, self-confidence, cooperativeness, and technical mastery (Stogdill, 1974). Although trait theories have been important in identifying qualities that distinguish today's leaders, these theories have neglected the interaction between other elements of the leadership situation. Trait theories also failed to recognize that leadership traits can be learned and developed through experience. However, by keeping in mind these traits

associated with effective leadership the new nurse can identify areas in which they should improve and develop.

Transformational Leadership

In a contemporary concept of leadership Burns (1978) identified and defined transformational leadership. Burns contends that there are two types of leaders: (1) the transactional leader, who is concerned with day-to-day operations, and (2) the transformational leader, who is committed to organizational goals, has a vision, and is able to empower others with that vision. The transformational leader is able to guide employees to feel pride in their work and to inspire them to be actively engaged in achieving the mission and goals of the organization. Transformational leaders spend time teaching and coaching, seek differing perspectives when faced with problems to solve, have a passion for excellence, and seek new ways to improve the work environment. Box 17.1 compares characteristics of Burns (1978) transformational and transactional leadership styles.

Studies have reported that nurse leaders who demonstrate more transformational leadership characteristics are able to provide nurses what they need to positively impact the nursing work environment, feel more engaged in their work to provide quality care, and have improved job satisfaction (Kowalski et al., 2020; Hudson, 2020). Readers are encouraged to read more

BOX 17.1 **Comparison of Transformational and Transactional Leaders**	
Transformational Leaders	**Transactional Leaders**
• Identify and clearly communicate vision and direction	• Focus on day-to-day operations and are comfortable with the status quo
• Empower the work group to accomplish goals and achieve the vision	• Reward staff for desired work ("I'll do X in exchange for you doing Y.")
• Impart meaning and challenge to work	• Monitor work performance and correct as needed
• Garner admiration and emulation	• Wait until problems occur and then deal with them
• Provide mentoring to individual staff members based on need	

about transformational leadership and to seek out transformational leaders as mentors. However, it is important to note that even the most effective transformational leaders fail unless they possess day-to-day management skills.

Leadership Skills and Practices

Three major types of skills and practices are required for effective leadership (Hersey & Blanchard, 1988):

- *Technical skills*—for nurses, this type includes clinical expertise and nursing knowledge.
- *Human skills*—the ability and judgment to work with and lead people in a compassionate, caring way.
- *Conceptual skills*—the ability to understand the complexities of the overall organization and to recognize how and where one's own area of management fits into the overall organization.

At the staff nurse level of management a considerable amount of technical skill and clinical expertise is needed because the nurse generally is involved in direct supervision of patient care and may be required to help train and mentor nurses. As one advances from lower levels to higher levels in the organization more conceptual skills and practices are needed. Box 17.2 provides examples of technical, human, and conceptual practices required for nurse leaders.

MANAGEMENT AND ORGANIZATIONAL THEORY

Behavioral theories emerged to explain aspects of management based on behaviors of managers, leaders, and followers. Three prevalent management behavior styles were identified by Lewin (1951) and White and Lippit (1960): authoritarian, democratic, and laissez-faire. Box 17.3 presents characteristics of these management styles, which vary in the amount of control exhibited by the manager and the amount of involvement that the staff has in decision-making. At one extreme, the autocratic manager makes all decisions with no staff input and uses the authority of the position to accomplish goals. At the opposite extreme is the laissez-faire manager, who provides little direction or guidance and will forgo decision-making. Democratic management is also often referred to as *participative* management because of its basic premise of encouraging staff members to participate in decision-making.

> **BOX 17.2 Effective Leading and Managing: Technical, Human, and Conceptual Practices**
>
> **Technical Practices**
> - Keep your own clinical skills and knowledge current.
> - Act as a willing expert resource and teacher for clinical problems.
> - Use sound clinical judgment and critical thinking.
>
> **Human Practices**
> - Maintain honesty and integrity in work and relationships—trust is essential for effective leadership.
> - Create a teaching and learning environment—earn a reputation for exceptional teaching and mentoring.
> - Develop and role model a commitment to excellence.
> - Create an open, transparent environment—share information, keep staff informed, and encourage them to discuss issues.
> - Become a proactive problem solver—knowing how to solve problems is more important than knowing all the answers.
> - Maintain a confident, positive outlook—identify areas in which you are weak and seek help to learn and grow.
>
> **Conceptual Practices**
> - Make a commitment to support the mission, vision, and goals of the organization.
> - Accept the realities of complex health care systems, which are under pressure to improve the safety and quality of care while reducing costs.
> - Understand the needs of external customers (patients, families, physicians, referring facilities) and internal customers (staff, administrators, team members from other departments).

Depending on the situation, the nurse leader may need to use different types of management styles. For example, autocratic management might be appropriate in an emergency situation, such as treating a patient in cardiac arrest. However, in structuring the weekend call schedule for a home health agency a participative style of management would be more effective.

Today's health care system requires the use of a democratic or participative management style that involves the staff in patient safety, quality improvement, patient-centered care, and cost reductions. Staff directly involved in the challenges presented by patient care often can suggest the most workable, practical solutions.

BOX 17.3 Management Styles

Autocratic/Authoritative	Democratic/Participative	Laissez-Faire
Determines policy and makes all decisions	Encourages staff participation in decision-making	Does not provide guidance or direction
Ignores subordinates' ideas and suggestions	Involves staff in planning and developing new ideas and programs	Unable or unwilling to make decisions
Dictates the work with much control	Believes in the best in people	Does not provide feedback
Gives little feedback or recognition for work	Communicates effectively and provides regular feedback	Initiates little change
Makes fast decisions	Builds responsibility in people	Limits communication with the team
May be effective with employees who have minimal education or training	Works well with competent, highly motivated people	May work well with professional people

Organizational Theories

Just as leadership and management theories evolved to provide a framework for understanding leadership and management, organizational theory evolved to provide a framework for understanding complex organizations. A brief review of systems theory and chaos theory can provide readers with insight into the value of using organizational theory to understand management processes within today's dynamic, complex health care organizations.

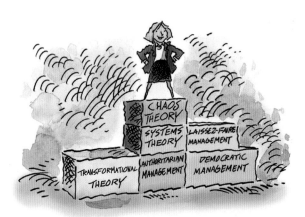

Leadership, management, and organizational theories provide the building blocks for effective nursing leadership and management practices.

Systems Theory. The systems theory views the organization as a set of interdependent parts that together form a whole (Thompson, 1967). Systems have been defined as "interdependent and interconnected people whose initial conditions create a ripple effect across an organization" (Weberg & Fuller, 2019, p. 23). The interdependent nature

of the parts of the organization (individuals, units, departments, community) suggests that anything that affects the functioning of one part of the organization will affect the other parts. Open systems theory suggests that the organization not only is affected by internal changes among any of its parts but also is directly influenced by external environmental forces, and vice versa—the internal forces will affect the external environment. In contrast to open systems theory, closed systems theory views the system as being totally independent of outside influences, which is an unrealistic view for health care organizations. To be successful today's health care organizations must be able to continually adapt to internal and external changes (Case Study 17.1).

CASE STUDY 17.1

The hospital in which Diego Rodriguez, RN, BSN, works has reduced the number of RNs employed by the hospital and now requires that the remaining RNs work overtime "at the request of administration." The quality of patient care, patient safety, and the individual nurses' professional practice and personal health have been negatively affected by this change. Diego and his fellow RNs seek advice from their state nurses association about their professional responsibility to work mandatory overtime. The state nurses association is responding to the situation, which is occurring more frequently across the state and nation, by proposing legislation to mandate hospitals to have effective staffing plans and to limit mandatory overtime. The state government may now require hospital administrators to respond to the need for increased staffing levels.

Consider the example in Case Study 17.1 to help explain systems theory. As internal forces in one department (hospital administration) mandated changes that affected another area (RNs and patient care), internal forces (RNs) pushed for changes from the external environment (state nurses association and state government). The external environment may now force changes to the organization (hospital administration). Systems theory has provided nurses with a framework to view nursing services as a subsystem of the larger organization and to realize the interrelatedness and interdependence of all the parts of the organization. The nurse will be wise to consider open systems theory and the effect a change in one area will have in another area, internal as well as external to the organization.

Chaos Theory. Chaos theory is a more recently developed organizational theory that attempts to account for the complexity and randomness in organizations. Despite the implications of the word *chaos*, the theory actually suggests that a degree of order can be attained by viewing complicated behaviors and situations as predictable (McGuire, 1999). Nurse managers may wish for balanced and steady work environments, but in reality they are dealing with what seems, at best, a chaotic system. Chaos theory says that variation is a normal part of managing health care systems. On the basis of chaos theory a nurse manager knows that staff absences due to illness, sick children, and family emergencies are a fact of life, which requires the nurse manager to have backup plans in the event that staff members "call in" and are unable to report for their assigned shifts. Other examples of variation in health care are cultural diversity, a constantly fluctuating patient census, and staffing shortages. Until nurses understand that these variations are a normal, predictable state in the organization that should be planned for, they may continue to experience excessive anxiety with the unplanned and unexpected events that occur daily.

MANAGEMENT FUNCTIONS

Classic theories of management suggest that the primary functions of managers are planning, organizing, and controlling (Stogdill, 1974). Leaders in nursing management have added two more functions to this list and now recognize five major management functions (Fig. 17.1) as necessary for the management of nursing organizations: (1) planning, (2) organizing, (3) staffing, (4) directing, and (5) controlling (Huston, 2024). These management functions are interrelated; different phases of the process occur simultaneously, and the processes should be circular, with the manager always working toward improving quality and patient safety, and creating healthy work environments. These five management functions, essential for success as a nurse leader, are discussed in further detail in the following sections.

Planning

Planning, the first management function, involves several steps: (1) identify goals and objectives to be achieved; (2) identify resources needed (e.g., people, supplies, equipment); (3) determine action steps; and (4) establish a timeline for the action steps and goal achievement. All management functions are based on planning. *Without effective planning, the management process will fail.* Effective planning requires the nurse to understand the organization's mission, philosophy, strategic plan, goals, and objectives.

Mission and Philosophy. The *mission* statement, the foundation of planning for any organization, describes the purpose of the organization and the reason it exists. Most health care organizations exist to provide high-quality patient care, but emphasis may be placed on different concepts, such as research, teaching, preventive care, spiritual care, or community service. The *philosophy* is the set of values and beliefs that guides the actions of the organization and thus serves as the basis of all planning. New nurses should be aware of the mission and philosophy of the employing organization and should understand the relationship between their own personal value system and that of the organization. You are encouraged to go online and review the mission and philosophy statement of the organization where you are doing your clinical training and/or where you work.

Strategic Planning. Strategic planning is long-range planning, extending 2 to 5 years into the future. It results from an in-depth analysis of (1) the business, community, regulatory, and political environment outside the organization; (2) customer and patient needs; (3) technology changes; and (4) strengths, problems,

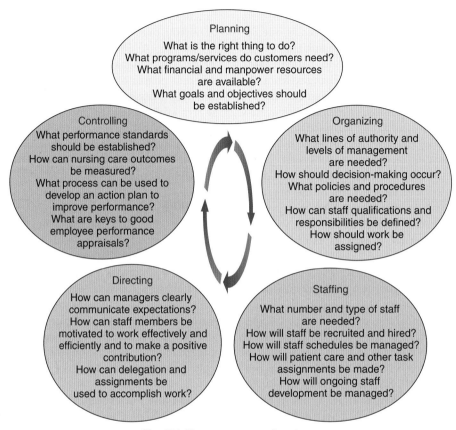

Fig. 17.1 Five management functions.

and weaknesses internal to the organization. The purposes of strategic planning are to:

- Identify strategies to respond to changes in customer needs, technology, health care legislation, the business environment, and the community.
- Dedicate resources to important services and new programs.
- Eliminate duplication, waste, and underused services.
- Establish a timeline for goal achievement.

The *strategic plan* is a written document that details organizational goals, allocates resources, assigns responsibilities, and determines time frames. Development of the strategic plan is generally coordinated by upper-level managers, who engage employees at all levels in the strategic-planning process. Consider the example in Case Study 17.2.

CASE STUDY 17.2

Susan Huff, RN, BSN, nurse manager for the Quality Care Home Health Agency, noticed that the office was receiving several calls per week for skilled nursing care for pediatric oncology patients. The agency did not provide services for pediatric patients. Susan reported the situation to the administrator. Susan soon was involved in gathering information about the number of home health agencies that offered pediatric oncology care, the standards of nursing care recommended for pediatric oncology patients, how pediatric oncology patients were receiving home care, how many pediatric patients in the area might need such services, and what reimbursement was available for such services. Within the next few months the management team for Quality Care Home Health Agency decided that as part of the agency's strategic plan a program for pediatric oncology services would be developed.

Goals and Objectives. Goals and objectives state the actions necessary to achieve the strategic plan and are central to the entire management process. Goals should be measurable, observable, and realistic. Objectives are more specific and detail how a goal will be accomplished with an established target date.

CASE STUDY 17.3

Michele Walker, RN, MSN, has recently been appointed as the Nurse Director in a 150-bed long-term care facility. The mission and philosophy of the organization are to "respect the dignity and worth of the individual and to provide care that will help restore individuals to the best possible state of physical, mental, and emotional health while maintaining their sense of spiritual and social well-being." Kenneth Cole, Administrator, has asked Michele to develop a set of goals that she views as priorities to accomplish in the next year. After gathering data about resident needs, costs, and staffing levels and meeting with the medical director, direct-care staff, and staff members in rehabilitation therapy, social services, dietary, and maintenance, Michele develops the following goals:

1. Increase by 25% over 12 months the level of satisfaction related to emotional well-being and socialization expressed by residents and family members on the quarterly quality of life satisfaction survey. This will be accomplished by improving coordination of care activities among nursing, therapy, and social services.
2. Reduce resident falls by 50% over 6 months through the implementation of an evidence-based guideline for falls prevention.
3. Increase by 30% over 12 months the number of nursing staff who achieve national certification as gerontologic nurses through the American Nurses Credentialing Center. To accomplish this goal the facility will offer certification review courses over the next 6 months.

Together Michele and Kenneth review the goals, agree that they fit with the overall organizational plan, and address the needs identified in Michele's facility assessment activities.

Goals and objectives serve as the manager's road map. Organization-wide goals are established in the strategic planning process, and then unit goals that support the organization-wide goals are developed. Nurse leaders should be able to clearly articulate the goals of both the organization and the nursing unit. Examples of goals for a medical-surgical unit in a hospital might include maintaining an overall patient-to-staff ratio of 5:1 with 70% RN staffing and reducing nurse turnover to less than 10% in the coming year. Additionally, goals and objectives must be communicated to everyone who is responsible for their attainment. Consider the example in Case Study 17.3 and think about how these goals need to be communicated to all employees throughout the organization.

Organizing

Organizing is the second management function. At the organizational level organizing is necessary to establish a formal structure that defines the lines of authority, communication, and decision-making within an organization. The organizational chart provides a visual picture of the organization and identifies lines of communication and authority. All nurses should be familiar with the organizational chart of their employing institution. Organizing also involves developing policies and procedures to help outline how work will be done and establishing position qualifications and job descriptions to define who will do the work.

At the unit level, nurses must determine how to best organize the work activities. Organizing involves:
- Using resources (e.g., staff, supplies, time) wisely.
- Assigning duties and responsibilities appropriately.
- Coordinating activities with other departments.
- Effectively communicating with subordinates and superiors to ensure a smooth workflow.

Models for staffing and organizing the delivery of patient care are discussed in Chapter 21.

Staffing

Staffing is the third management function. The provision of health care is labor intensive, with a workforce that is made up of people with a variety of education and skill levels (e.g., professional nurses, physicians, pharmacists, social workers, therapists, dietitians, licensed vocational or practical nurses, technicians, and assistive personnel). Hiring and managing staff to accomplish the work of the institution are important functions for all levels of managers. Following are key steps in the staffing function (Huston, 2024):

1. Determine the number and type of staff needed on the basis of goals, projected census, and budget requirements.
2. Recruit, interview, select, and assign personnel according to job description and performance standards.

3. Get new employees off to a good start by offering excellent orientation, training, and socialization programs.
4. Implement an ongoing staff-development program to ensure that employees at all levels have opportunities to develop personally and professionally and to enhance their knowledge and skill levels.
5. Implement creative and flexible scheduling based on patient care needs, employee needs, and *productivity* requirements.

The staffing process most likely will prove to be one of the most time-consuming and challenging functions for the nurse manager; however, it is probably the nurse manager's most important job. Little can be accomplished without the right people properly trained to do the work in an environment that promotes collegial, productive relationships among the health care team.

Nursing leaders are highly concerned with recruiting and retaining a talented RN workforce. Factors positively associated with RNs' work satisfaction are presented in Box 17.4. These factors are based on research studies and

provide leaders with information about how they can increase nurse satisfaction, reduce nursing turnover, and improve recruitment and retention efforts.

While meeting staff and patient scheduling needs the nurse manager must also accomplish organizational staffing and productivity goals. *Productivity* is the amount of work produced through the use of a specific amount of resources; it is measured as output divided by input. For example, the number of nursing hours worked over a 24-hour period divided by the patient census is a standard productivity measurement used by many hospitals. From a practical perspective the nurse caring for eight medical-surgical patients during one shift has a higher productivity ratio than the nurse caring for only five patients of similar acuity. Other examples of productivity measurements include number of home visits completed and number of procedures performed. Productivity is a method of measuring and tracking the amount of labor costs as compared with the amount of work produced and is a factor in staffing decisions (see Chapter 18 for more information on productivity).

BOX 17.4 Factors Influencing Nurses' Job Satisfaction and Dissatisfaction

Sources of Satisfaction	Sources of Dissatisfaction
• Realistic patient assignments/workload • Financial rewards (salary) appropriate for responsibilities and value of nursing • Supportive leaders who show appreciation for nursing staff and are available and present in the work setting • Flexible staffing options to promote work–life balance • Work environment that is physically and emotionally safe • Guidance, mentorship, and opportunities for professional development and advancement • Opportunity to be involved in change processes and problem-solving • Collegial and respectful relationships among nurses, physicians, peers, administrators, and those in other departments • Access to mental health and well-being support resources	• Inadequate staffing and resources to care for patients affecting quality and increasing stress • Uninvolved or unavailable supervisors • Tolerance for bullying and incivility • Poor communication and unclear expectations • Vague, inconsistent rules and regulations • Minimal thanks, appreciation, or recognition • Not being fully informed about changes or involved in the change process • No commitment to professional development • Inadequate feedback about performance or recognition that contributions are valued

Data from ANM Healthcare. (2023). *The Pandemic's consequences: 2023 Survey of Registered Nurses.* ANM Healthcare https://www.amnhealthcare.com/siteassets/amn-insights/surveys/amn-healthcare-rnsurvey-2023.pdf.; Gaffney, T. (2022). Retaining nurses to mitigate shortages. *American Nurse,* 17(1), 14–16; Gensimore, M.M., et al. (2020). The effect of nurse practice environment on retention and quality of care via burnout, work characteristics, and resilience. *The Journal of Nursing Administration, 50*(10), 546–553; Skillman, D., & Toms, R. (2022). Factors influencing nurse intent to leave acute care hospitals. *The Journal of Nursing Administration, 52*(12), 640–645; Sweeney, C.D., & Wiseman, R. (2023). Retaining the best: Recognizing what meaningful recognition is to nurses as a strategy for nurse leaders. *The Journal of Nursing Administration, 53*(2), 81–87.

Directing

Directing is the fourth management function. After managers have planned what to do, organized how to do it, and staffed positions to do the work, they must direct personnel and activities to accomplish goals. Directing involves issuing assignments and instructions that allow staff to clearly understand what is expected, in addition to guiding and coaching staff to achieve planned goals. Directing requires the nurse leader to:

- Clearly communicate performance expectations.
- Create a motivating climate and team spirit.
- Model expected behaviors.
- Facilitate feedback.

Communicating Performance Expectations. It is the nurse leader's responsibility to monitor how well staff are performing their jobs. The first step is to ensure that staff clearly understand job expectations. Consider the following:

- Does the staff member know what problems and issues should be reported to the supervisor and how and to whom to report?
- Does the staff member know how to perform clinical procedures correctly or how and where to seek help when necessary?
- Does the nurse clearly understand the expectations for documenting clinical care?
- Does the nurse know how and when to report to physicians and/or involve other members of the interprofessional team?
- Is the staff member able to meet patient care needs for the number of patients assigned during a typical shift?

These questions represent only a sample of issues that the nurse leader will consider when striving to communicate performance expectations.

Communicating performance expectations is an ongoing process that begins in new-employee orientation and continues throughout the term of employment. An important step in communicating expectations is to directly observe employees performing their jobs; through direct observation, the manager can identify strengths and weaknesses and determine areas where performance expectations need to be addressed. The next step is to communicate expectations in a respectful two-way process in which the manager seeks first to understand the staff member's perspective, feelings, and knowledge about the issue and then to clarify the expectations in a nonjudgmental, nonthreatening way. The final step is to determine issues that may be preventing the employee from meeting performance expectations and to work with that employee to develop a mutually agreed-upon plan so that they can achieve expectations.

Creating a Motivating Climate. Motivation is the inner drive that compels a person to act in a certain way. A great deal of research has been undertaken to better understand human motivation. Most researchers agree that motivation is complex and involves a combination of extrinsic, or external, rewards such as money, benefits, and working conditions, in addition to intrinsic, or internal, needs for recognition, self-esteem, and self-actualization. Box 17.4 summarizes factors that influence nurses' job satisfaction and dissatisfaction, which strongly influence motivation in the work setting.

Positive encouragement and support from nurse leaders are essential to create a motivating work climate. An effective method to demonstrate encouragement and support is a technique known as "management by walking around," in which the nurse manager/leader literally walks around the unit with the primary purpose of interacting positively with the staff. Just as it implies management by walking around allows the nurse leader to connect with many different staff on a day-to-day basis, be visible and accessible, promote quality patient care, and build positive relationships with not only staff but also patients, families, and the interprofessional team (Hedenstrom et al., 2022).

Personalized appreciation is also a powerful but often underused motivational resource that can foster a healthy work environment and productive staff committed to meeting job expectations (Prestia, 2018). Personalized appreciation is as simple as offering words of affirmation ("You did a very nice job working with that family member who was upset, thank you."); expressing kindness to the staff by smiling, making eye contact, and nodding; taking the opportunity to have a conversation and sincerely listen to the individual; and providing assistance without being asked (Prestia, 2018). To be effective appreciation must be specific, timely, accurate, and genuine. "Management by walking around" puts the manager in a position to observe and interact with employees and offer personalized appreciation for the work they do.

Role Modeling. Positive role modeling is another effective tool the nurse can use to create a positive team spirit and promote high-quality patient care. Positive role modeling simply means that the nurse performs the job in such a way that they demonstrate ideal performance as a professional nurse, with the hope that others will follow the example. Obviously, nurses must be role models for excellence in patient care; similarly, nurses must model caring and respectful relationships with the entire interprofessional health care team, along with an enthusiastic attitude to promote camaraderie and team spirit.

Several other skills are essential as nurses function in the directing role, including effective communication and conflict management skills (see Chapter 19), delegation skills (see Chapter 20), and team-building skills (discussed in section "Team Builder").

Controlling

The purpose of controlling, the fifth management function, is to ensure that employees accomplish goals while maintaining a high quality of performance. Controlling requires leaders to:

- Establish performance or outcome standards.
- Determine action plans to improve performance.
- Evaluate employee performance through performance appraisals and feedback.

Establishing Performance Standards. *Performance standards* describe a model of excellence for work activities and serve as the basis of comparison between actual and desired work performance. For example, performance standards in an ambulatory outpatient clinic might include that (1) every patient is informed about all laboratory results within 48 hours, whether normal or abnormal, and (2) all diabetic patients must remove their shoes and socks for a complete foot examination each time they come to the clinic. Nurses can draw on several resources for establishing performance standards, such as:

- Written organizational policies and procedures
- Standards for the practice of professional nursing developed by the ANA and published in *Nursing: Scope and Standards of Practice* (ANA, 2021)
- Standards for professional nursing specialty practices, such as *Public Health Nursing: Scope and Standards of Practice*, 3rd Edition (ANA, 2022); *Genetics/Genomics*

Nursing: Scope and Standards of Practice (ANA, 2016); and *Cardiovascular Nursing: Scope and Standards of Practice* (ANA, 2015a) (many other nursing specialty scope and standards are available on the ANA website www.nursingworld.org.)

- Evidence-based practice guidelines

Nurses should continually look for ways to improve individual, team, and organizational performance to achieve established standards of care. Chapter 22 provides more discussion about performance standards and presents an excellent process for measuring performance and planning for improvement.

Evaluating Employee Performance

Evaluating employee performance occurs through the formal annual evaluation process and through frequent feedback and coaching provided to employees. A manager should never wait until the annual performance review to discuss problems or deficiencies with a staff member. Consistent, ongoing feedback and coaching about job performance is required to clarify expectations, improve the quality of work, and allow the manager to correct problems before they become serious. Feedback and coaching can occur in brief, spontaneous interactions or in planned sessions with the employee. Box 17.5 presents useful tips for effective coaching.

Ongoing documentation about an employee's job performance is an essential management responsibility. Each health care organization has specific policies related to documentation of employee performance and annual performance evaluations. The result of routine performance evaluations should be mutual goal setting designed to meet the employees' training, educational, and professional development needs.

Balancing the Five Management Functions

The management functions of planning, organizing, staffing, directing, and controlling provide the nurse with a practical set of skills to guide the implementation of management activities. The new nurse will be challenged to maintain the different stages of management that occur in the span of just 1 day. In addition to managing different phases of the process that are occurring simultaneously, the nurse also must function in many different management and leadership roles described in the following section (Box 17.6).

BOX 17.5   Tips for Effective Coaching

- Discuss situations in a neutral way—avoid judgmental language that will put the employee on the defensive.
- Encourage the employee to provide their perspective about the situation (e.g., "What did you think about your exchange with Dr. Jones?").
- Encourage the employee to reflect on their performance through open-ended questions, such as:
  What are your main concerns?
  What can you learn from this situation?
  What is confusing to you?
  What are some things you could do differently next time?

- Be specific and provide clear examples when possible (e.g., "Next time you are dealing with a difficult family member, consider ...").
- Share your own experiences if they are relevant and might help.
- Be sincere. Provide coaching and feedback with the clear intent of helping the employee improve.
- Be realistic. Focus on factors that the person can control.
- Thank the employee for listening.
- Ask for feedback from your coworkers, subordinates, and peers about your own performance and listen when it is offered.

Data from Grensing-Pophal, L. (2000). Give-and-take feedback. *Nursing Management, 31*(2), 27–28; Harvard Business Essentials. (2004). *Manager's toolkit: The 13 skills managers need to succeed.* Harvard Business School Press.

BOX 17.6   Do You Aspire to Nursing Leadership as a Career Goal?

The nursing profession abounds with unique opportunities for nurses to move into formal leadership roles, regardless of age or experience. Following are some important considerations for professional development if you see yourself as a future nursing manager, nursing director, or in some other type of leader/manager role:

1. Be an active, engaged learner.
   - Keep up with current literature in your specialty field including reports from national and professional organizations.
   - Listen to leadership podcasts and read leadership books.
   - Take courses that will advance your leadership skills (e.g., finance, effective communication, conflict resolution, building teams, etc.).
2. Seek formal graduate education in nursing administration or leadership programs.
3. Develop your business and finance knowledge, as it will be key to success in advanced nursing leadership roles.

4. Develop self-awareness of your own strengths and areas that you need to improve as a leader.
5. Seek constructive feedback from peers, supervisors, and mentors about your leadership qualities and how you can grow and improve.
6. Develop your technical skills (e.g., Excel, PowerPoint, Microsoft Word).
7. Hone your skills in effective communication, conflict resolution, and negotiation.
8. Engage in a mentoring relationship with a respected and experienced nurse leader.
9. Seek opportunities to serve in roles with increasing responsibilities (e.g., committee leadership roles, governance council leadership, etc.).
10. When considering new leadership opportunities, look for positions with structured programs to ensure an effective transition to the new role.

Adapted from Tuttas, C. (2020). Professional discernment: Discover the leader in you. *Nurse Leader, 18*(4), 333–338; Warshawsky, N., et al. (2020). Organizational support for nurse manager role transition and onboarding: Strategies for success. *The Journal of Nursing Administration, 50*(5), 254–260.

ROLES OF THE NURSE LEADER AND MANAGER

Nurses assume various roles as they function in leadership and management positions. The first step to being an effective nurse leader is to clearly understand the job description, roles and responsibilities, and policies and procedures related to the position in which the nurse is employed or assigned. The following discussion presents information about roles that a nurse will assume in any position.

Patient Satisfaction and Customer Service Provider

Over the past few years patient satisfaction has moved to the forefront of the nurse's agenda. Nursing shortages, reduced length of stay, more complex patient needs, and national concerns about the quality and safety of patient care have contributed to this growing concern about patient satisfaction. With the advent of health care reform, patient satisfaction is now tied directly to financial rewards for hospitals. Medicare reimbursement rewards inpatient hospitals for providing quality care to include patient satisfaction based on the hospital's scores on the Hospital Consumer Assessment of Healthcare Providers and Systems (HCAHPS), a standardized patient satisfaction survey that addresses these seven core dimensions:

- Communication with nurses
- Communication with doctors
- Responsiveness of hospital staff
- Pain management
- Communication about medicines
- Cleanliness and quietness of hospital environment
- Discharge information

From how quickly call lights are answered to the extent of family support provided, nurses are challenged to meet a wide spectrum of patient needs to include promoting good communication with the health care team and the patient and family. The complex health care environment has created a competitive marketplace in which home health agencies, hospitals, ambulatory clinics, and even hospice agencies compete for patients. To survive and thrive in this competitive environment the nurse must keep patient satisfaction and customer service, which include safety and quality care, first and foremost as the motivator of all plans and activities.

Team Builder

A *team* is a group of people organized to accomplish the necessary work of an organization. Teams bring together a range of people with different knowledge, skills, and experiences to meet customer needs, accomplish tasks, and solve problems. Team members may be unit secretaries, nursing assistants, social workers, dietitians, therapists, physicians, licensed vocational or practical nurses, and RNs. Team building should create *synergy* (the ability of a group of people working together to accomplish significantly more than each person working individually).

Bringing people together to work as a group does not necessarily make them a team. To create synergy teams must have defined goals and objectives, a commitment to work together, good communication, and a willingness to cooperate. Team members should be encouraged

to communicate with one another to identify effective work division and solutions to problems so that synergy is accomplished. Teams need to know that their ideas and inputs are valued and included in decision-making at the next leadership level. Daily interactions, team huddles, and quick informal conversations can help to build team camaraderie (Weberg & Fuller, 2019).

The nurse leader, as team builder, must serve as a role model to encourage and help develop team principles of respect, cooperation, commitment, and a willingness to accomplish shared goals. As a role model for team members, the nurse leader should:

- Show respect for all members of the team, value their input, and ensure their input is communicated and used for decision-making.
- Clearly define team goals ("What do we want to accomplish?").
- Encourage team members to develop a sense of stewardship (or ownership) for the success of the team.
- Exhibit a personal commitment to team goals.
- Encourage team members to willingly help one another and exchange constructive feedback.
- Provide the resources necessary to accomplish goals (e.g., time for team meetings, information, supplies).
- Ask for feedback from team members while also providing relevant and timely feedback to the team.

The leader's behaviors have a significant effect on the behaviors of the team. The nurse as leader must have an astute self-awareness of their own emotional patterns and an understanding that negative moods can have a negative influence on relationships with staff members. Learning to recognize and manage one's emotional patterns and negative moods is an important step in team building. The nurse who is enthusiastic, caring, and supportive can generate those same feelings among all team members (Kostich et al., 2021).

Resource Manager

Resources include the personnel, time, and supplies needed to provide patient care and operate the organization. Resources cost money and are always in limited supply. Unfortunately, no health care organization can afford the luxury of an unlimited number of staff or supplies to accomplish the required work. With health care facilities' focus on cost containment, it is essential that nurses develop an understanding of and expertise in resource management.

Each of the management activities—planning, organizing, staffing, directing, and controlling—comes into play in the role of resource manager. The nurse leader needs to learn and develop skills in the following areas:

- Planning for the necessary resources (primarily staff and supplies) to manage the unit
- Organizing resources to meet identified goals
- Staffing appropriately as determined by patient needs and the budget plan
- Directing to maintain resource allocations within budgetary guidelines
- Controlling by analyzing financial reports and making adjustments where necessary

Budget and financial reports are the primary tools for resource management. Because budget and financial management is a minimal part of the nursing school curriculum, nurses must take initiative for on-the-job training about the organization's budget and financial management processes. Nurses are encouraged not to be unsettled by financial and budget reports and conversations and, instead, to get involved. They should not be afraid to say, "I don't understand. Please explain." Nurses should review budget and financial reports, ask questions, talk to seasoned nurse managers, talk to the organization's finance department staff, and even consider taking an accounting or finance course at the local college. Understanding financial and budget management is one of the most useful and powerful tools one can have as a nurse leader. Another resource is Chapter 18 of this text, which provides more detailed information about budgets.

Decision-Maker and Problem-Solver Using the Clinical Judgment Model

Problem-solving and decision-making are essential skills for professional nursing practice. Nurses make decisions and solve problems every day about ever-changing patient and family circumstances, as well as administrative decisions such as revising policies, planning for appropriate staffing for the unit, or effectively addressing a problem with a physician. The Clinical Judgment Model can be effective in managing the complex clinical, leadership, and management decisions required every day in nursing practice.

Recognize Cues. During this first stage the nurse begins to collect information about the issue of concern or the problem to be solved. It often is appropriate to involve others—especially those close to the situation—who may be able to provide a different viewpoint or

information the manager lacks. For example, the nurse manager who is concerned about increasingly high absenteeism among the staff needs to investigate the situation carefully. What is causing the absenteeism? Are there problems on the unit creating an unhappy work environment? Are several staff members coincidentally having personal problems? Are absentee policies being unfairly administered? Getting as much information as possible is important to fully understand the issue or problem.

Analyze Cues. During the analysis stage the decision-maker uses information gathered in the "recognize cues" stage to identify the specific problem to be solved. At this stage the manager must also decide whether the situation is important enough to require intervention and whether it is within their authority to intervene or if the next level of leadership needs to be involved.

Prioritize Hypotheses and Generate Solutions. During this stage the goal is to identify as many options as possible and then objectively weigh the options as to possible risks and consequences and positive and negative outcomes, including patient outcomes and staff satisfaction as key considerations. The decision-maker should be flexible, creative, and open to suggestions from other staff and peers when reviewing options. Preconceived ideas and rigid thinking, such as "There is only one way to do this job" or "That's the way we have always done it," should be avoided. It is also important to remember that decisions made with input from those who will be affected by the decision are more likely to result in positive outcomes. Cost, quality, and legal and ethical aspects of care should also be carefully considered.

Take Actions. Once the solution is determined then action is taken to implement the solution. This stage should include effective communication, delegation, and supervision. (See "Stages of Change" presented later in this chapter.) It is important for the nurse to show positive support for the decision outcome and to encourage cooperation and support among all staff. Persons higher in the organizational structure may mandate some decisions, and although not able to control that decision the nurse can influence a positive outcome.

Evaluate Outcomes. The evaluation stage is necessary to ensure that the implemented plan effectively resolved the problem or the decision situation. Considerable time and energy may be spent on identifying the problem, generating possible options, and selecting and implementing the best solution. However, time for follow-up evaluation must also be allocated. It is important to establish early how and what evaluation and monitoring will take place, who will be responsible, and when it will be accomplished.

Resources for Decision-Making and Problem-Solving.
Staff input should be included in each stage of the decision-making problem-solving process. Additionally, the nurse might seek help from others who are more experienced and knowledgeable in specific areas. Even the most experienced nurses will not be able to effectively solve every problem, nor will any nurse have all the answers. The key is to understand and incorporate the clinical judgment model into the decision-making problem-solving process; know when and how to access resources; and learn and improve as successes and failures are experienced.

Change Agent

This text frequently has referred to the changing health care environment, and true to that concept, change is an inevitable occurrence in health care. Whether working with individuals, groups, or the entire organization, the professional nurse is certain to be involved in managing change. The nurse as the change agent is responsible for guiding people through the change process. To successfully engage in change, the nurse must first be willing to confront the demand for change; staff cannot be expected to embrace change if their nurse leaders have not done so.

People often feel threatened by change and may react, especially at first, with resistance and hostility. Change that is carefully planned and implemented slowly, with all people continually informed and involved, will be more successful in reaching the desired outcome (or change). Change often creates a wide range of feelings among staff and managers, including fear, achievement, loss, pride, stress, and dissatisfaction. The successful change agent understands the very real nature of these emotions and manages the change process such that all involved experience at least some degree of success and pride in the outcome.

In his classic work on change Lewin (1951) identified the following rules that should be followed when change is necessary:
1. Change should be implemented only for good reason.
2. Change should always be planned and implemented gradually.

3. Change should never be unexpected or abrupt.
4. All people who may be affected by the change should be involved in planning for the change.

Change may be indicated for several reasons, such as solving an identified problem, implementing a new program, improving work efficiencies, and adjusting to new mandates from regulatory agencies. Even though a strong reason for change may exist it almost always is met with some resistance. Resistance is demonstrated by refusal to cooperate with a course of action or by active opposition to the change. The effective change agent recognizes that resistance is a natural response to change and does not waste time or energy attempting to eliminate it. Instead, the effective change agent identifies and implements effective change strategies to overcome resistance.

Stages of Change

Effective change strategies can be developed through the three classic stages of change identified by Lewin (1951). These stages are:
1. *Unfreezing stage*—The change agent promotes problem identification and encourages the awareness of the need for change. People must believe that improvement is possible before they are willing to consider change. The change agent's responsibilities are to:
   - Gather information about the problem.
   - Accurately assess the problem.
   - Decide whether change is necessary.
   - Make others aware of the need for change.
2. *Moving stage*—The change agent clarifies the need to change, explores alternatives, defines goals and objectives, plans the change, and implements the change plan. The change agent's responsibilities are to:
   - Identify areas of support and resistance.
   - Set goals and objectives.
   - Involve everyone affected in the planning.
   - Develop an appropriate change plan with target dates.
   - Plan for appropriate education and training to help staff understand and comply with new policies, procedures, work processes, duties, or responsibilities.
   - Consider how the change might impact other departments in the organization.
   - Implement the change plan.
   - Be available to help, support, and encourage others through the process.
   - Evaluate the change and make modifications if necessary.

3. *Refreezing stage*—The change agent integrates the change into the organization so that it becomes recognized as the status quo. If the refreezing stage is not completed, people may drift into old behaviors. The change agent's responsibilities are to:
   - Find ways to engage staff to support the change.
   - Adopt new policies that may be required to support the change.
   - Require compliance with the changed processes.
   - Support and encourage others until the change is viewed as part of the status quo and is well integrated into daily work.

In alignment with Lewin's (1951) three stages of change (i.e., unfreezing, moving, and refreezing) and as noted above, involvement and education are key to successful change.

Clinical Consultant

Staff members look to the nurse leader as a resource for clinical advice. For example, the nurse leader is frequently called on to assess difficult or unusual patient cases and guide the staff nurse to make appropriate nursing judgments. In this role the nurse serves as a role model for excellence in nursing care and clinical judgment and provides ongoing training and education.

Staff Developer

The nurse should be ever mindful of the need for learning and training opportunities to enhance professional and personal growth for all employees they supervise, as well as for themself. Accessing resources and planning staff development activities that meet the needs of individual staff members, including RNs, LPNs or LVNs, nursing assistants, and clerical staff, is a very important role for the nurse.

Mentor

As the nurse develops into an effective leader, they should accept the responsibility to act as a mentor to new nurses, helping them develop effective leadership and management skills. Mentorship is key to developing our future nurse leaders and managers.

CREATING JOY AND ENGAGEMENT IN THE WORKPLACE

Perhaps the most important responsibility for all nurses is to help create work environments where staff feel joy in the work they do and are engaged to ensure outstanding patient care and clinical outcomes. Decades of research have documented that high levels of staff satisfaction and engagement correlate to patient satisfaction and improved clinical and organizational outcomes. The Institute for Healthcare Improvement (IHI), in its seminal white paper entitled *IHI Framework for Improving Joy in Work* (Perlo et al., 2017), first identified that health care professionals need to experience joy in their work if we are to significantly improve care quality, improve each individual's care experience, and reduce the cost of care.

For nurses joy in the workplace is having (1) a fulfilling purpose as a nurse; (2) meaningful connections with patients, families, peers, students, and colleagues; (3) a positive impact on patients, families, or colleagues; (4) supportive relationships with colleagues and peers; (5) good leaders who are role models and openly value staff; and (6) opportunities for learning and growth (Galuska et al., 2018). Being engaged at work is reflective of the joy a nurse feels in the workplace. Being engaged in your work means that you have enthusiasm and energy for the work required of you and your team and you are willing to go above and beyond what is required to initiate innovative strategies to improve the work environment and patient care. Key components of the work environment required to promote joy and engagement in the workplace are (Clark, 2018; Collins, 2022; Haizlip et al., 2020):
- Highly visible, optimistic, and approachable leaders who foster meaningful relationships with staff
- Support for staff to engage in work that is meaningful to them at the personal, organizational, and societal level
- Trust in staff to work both independently and collaboratively to make sound decisions and be involved in unit and organizational governance
- Opportunities for staff to develop collegial and supportive relationships and to show appreciation through small acts of gratitude, recognition, and caring for each other
- Guidance and support for professional and personal growth
- Open, transparent communication to keep employees connected and informed
- Asking nurses to be part of the solution to challenging problems (e.g., "What can we do to make your work easier?")

- Embrace feedback and expressions of negative emotions and experiences, avoid delivering false reassurance, then after listening focus on how the problem can be solved

Staff members who feel that their work is valued and they are respected, listened to, involved in solutions to problems, and cared about as individuals are able to further contribute to a positive, joyful environment in which to provide excellent patient care. Creating a caring, joyful environment in the highly technical, fast-paced, and extremely stressful settings in which nurses work can be a significant challenge. However, it is a challenge that is at the heart of nursing if we are to promote joy in the work place and provide the very best in patient care.

Addressing and Preventing Bullying and Incivility

Unfortunately in today's workplace, bullying, lateral violence, or incivility are all too common among nurses, physicians, managers, and others. Bullying is defined as the "repeated, unreasonable actions of individuals directed toward an employee (or employees) which are intended to intimidate, degrade, humiliate or undermine; or which create a risk to the health or safety of the employees" (Washington State Department of Labor and Industries [WSDLI], 2011). Examples of bullying behaviors are unwarranted or invalid criticism, unjustified blame, profane or disrespectful language, being gossiped about or being the target of rumors, being yelled or shouted at in a hostile way, being sworn at or verbally abused, being assigned undesirable work differently from the rest of your colleagues, and being "put down" or humiliated in front of others (WSDLI, 2011). Bullying tends to be targeted toward an individual and is typically an ongoing pattern of behavior.

Incivility may be considered a milder form of bullying and, according to the ANA (2015b), "may take the form of rude and discourteous actions, of gossiping and spreading rumors, and of refusing to assist a coworker." Incivility is considered a precursor of bullying. These unacceptable behaviors may occur among coworkers or professional colleagues or may come from the manager against the employee or from other members of the health care team. *In today's workplace there should be absolutely no tolerance for any type of bullying, incivility, or violence from any source.*

The negative effects of bullying and incivility are significant. Nurses who are victims may have problems with their physical health (e.g., sleep disturbances, depression, musculoskeletal problems) and experience feelings of self-blame, reduced self-esteem, and work withdrawal (WSDLI, 2011). The extreme result of bullying for nurses is that they may leave the job or the profession completely (Sauer & McCoy, 2018). Bullying and incivility cause distress and low morale among other staff, result in lower productivity and higher costs for the organization, and may also lead to concern about patient safety and quality of care.

Nurses and other individuals who witness or experience workplace bullying, incivility, or violence and ignore it or who fail to report it are actually perpetuating these terrible behaviors (ANA, 2015b). In the same way, organizations that fail to promote policies that make it safe to report these actions and ensure the actions are addressed and stopped are also perpetuating these terrible behaviors. Nurses must be the leaders who *STOP* bullying and incivility in the workplace. Nurses, especially new nurses, must understand that under no circumstances should bullying or uncivil behaviors be tolerated. Health care leaders have the ultimate responsibility to ensure that such behaviors will not be tolerated and will be immediately addressed and stopped. Following are some important steps to address bullying and incivility from an individual level as an RN (ANA, 2015b):

- Develop and maintain healthy interpersonal relationships with all individuals in your work setting.
- Recognize that bullying or incivility is occurring and follow appropriate procedures to report it (remember that witnessing or experiencing workplace bullying, incivility, or violence and ignoring it leads to perpetuating these behaviors).
- Always be kind and polite, treat everyone with respect and dignity and apologize when indicated.
- Consider how your words and actions might negatively affect others.
- Avoid gossip and do not spread rumors.
- Offer help to your coworkers when needed.
- Know and follow the organization's policy on bullying and incivility in the workplace.
- Always uphold ANA's Code of Ethics, which states that nurses should "create an ethical environment and culture of civility and kindness, treating colleagues,

coworkers, employees, students, and others with dignity and respect" (ANA, 2015c).

Actions that employers MUST take to prevent bullying include (Sauer & McCoy, 2018):

- Implement and enforce zero-tolerance antibullying policies.
- Have robust training in place to ensure everyone is aware of what bullying and incivility are, how to appropriately respond, and how it must be reported.

- Create an environment where employees feel free to discuss their challenges related to incivility and bullying with their supervisors.
- Promote a culture of respect and an expectation of professional demeanor for all.

The reader is encouraged to learn more about bullying and incivility from articles in nursing journals and ANA's Position Statement, *Incivility, Bullying, and Workplace Violence*, available on the ANA website (http://www.nursingworld.org).

SUMMARY

To summarize this chapter let's return to Nancy's situation and questions in the opening Vignette in which she is learning about her new responsibilities for leadership and management expertise as a new RN. While the multifaceted set of theories, functions, roles, and skills presented in this chapter may at first seem overwhelming to the novice nurse like Nancy, she now understands that by learning the principles and concepts of leadership and management she can become a successful leader in her role as a staff nurse. Leadership, management, and organizational theories provide a framework on which to build effective nursing leadership and management practices. By understanding the mission and values of her work setting Nancy can support the mission and apply the values in her everyday work assignments. Additionally, by understanding the management functions of planning, organizing, staffing, directing, and controlling Nancy is better prepared to perform effectively in her various leadership and management roles (e.g., customer service provider, team builder, resource manager, change agent, clinical consultant, staff developer, mentor). She is excited to contribute to creating a work environment in which staff are engaged and feel joy in the work they do by being involved in working collaboratively with the other nurses and the interprofessional team to make sound decisions, by being involved in unit and organizational governance, by developing supportive relationships with her colleagues and showing appreciation to them through small acts of gratitude, and by seeking guidance and support for professional and personal growth from more seasoned nurses.

Nancy is eager to continue to develop effective leadership and management skills and knows this will be an ongoing process that continues throughout one's career as a professional nurse. Some of the ways Nancy will continue to develop her leadership and management skills are to engage in a mentoring relationship with a respected and experienced nurse leader, to seek opportunities to serve in roles with increasing responsibilities (e.g., committee leadership roles, governance council leadership, etc.), to develop advanced knowledge in her specific field of nursing (nephrology nursing), and to read relevant professional journal articles and leadership books. Management and leadership roles are challenging and exciting and present a wonderful opportunity to grow professionally and personally.

CLINICAL JUDGMENT AND NEXT-GENERATION NCLEX® EXAMINATION-STYLE QUESTIONS

Kevin Michaels, RN, BSN, has recently been appointed to be the new nurse manager for a 35-bed medical-surgical unit at a large academic medical center. Kevin is replacing a very experienced and highly respected nurse manager who had worked on the unit for more than 15 years and is now retiring. Kevin has been a nurse for only 2 years and this will be his first time to serve in a formal management position. He is concerned that some of the more seasoned nurses on the unit might begrudge him this opportunity and will feel like he is too inexperienced for the nurse manager role. However, he is also confident that he will work hard to be successful in this new role and knows he has the support of his supervisor and other nurse manager peers in the organization.

In thinking about ways to earn the trust of the nurses on his unit Kevin plans to create an environment where nurses feel more joy in the work they do and to spend more time learning about effective leadership and management practices. Consider the following actions that Kevin can take and select all that apply to him being successful as the new nurse manager.

Multiple Response: Select All That Apply

A. Be highly visible on the unit by making rounds routinely, interacting with the staff, and getting to know each on an individual level.

B. Encourage nurses to be involved in the unit council and allow them time away from their direct care duties to do the work required for the unit council to be successful.

C. Role model showing appreciation for the staff through small acts of gratitude and recognition.

D. Ignore minor instances of incivility between nurses and physicians since this is an expected part of working in health care.

E. Keep staff well-informed about unit operations, future change initiatives, and other important activities occurring in the organization.

F. Provide all staff with the opportunity to voice concerns and exchange ideas, then follow up on their concerns and ideas.

G. Plan the unit's work schedule and daily workload assignments without requesting input from the staff.

H. Do not involve staff in any change initiatives because it might cause them more stress.

I. Be available as a clinical consultant for staff when they are encountering difficult clinical situations.

J. Engage in a mentoring relationship with a respected and experienced nurse leader.

K. Begin to learn more about the budget and finance reports related to the unit's operations by seeking out advice from a finance officer and experienced nurse leader.

L. Read leadership books or listen to podcasts on leadership to help develop leadership skills.

REFERENCES

American Nurses Association (ANA) (2022). *Public Health Nursing: Scope and standards of practice* (3rd ed.) American Nurses Association.

American Nurses Association (ANA). (2021). *Nursing: Scope and standards of practice* (4th ed.) American Nurses Association.

American Nurses Association (ANA). (2016). *Genetics/genomics nursing: Scope and standards of practice* (2nd ed.) American Nurses Association.

American Nurses Association (ANA). (2015a). *Cardiovascular nursing: Scope and standards of practice* (3rd ed.) American Nurses Association.

American Nurses Association (ANA). (2015b). *Position statement: Incivility, bullying and workplace violence.* https://www.nursingworld.org/practice-policy/nursing-excellence/official-position-statements/id/incivility-bullying-and-workplace-violence

American Nurses Association (ANA). (2015c). Code of ethics for nurses with interpretive statements. American Nurses Association.

Burns, J. (1978). *Leadership.* Harper & Row.

Clark, C. (2018). 10 tips to boost employee engagement. *American Nurse Today, 13*(1), 12–14.

Collins, R. (2022). Leading forward: Embracing feedback and moving toward authentic positivity. *Nurse Leader, 20*(3), 270–272.

Galuska, L., Hahn, J., Polifroni, E.C., & Crow, G. (2018). A narrative analysis of nurses' experiences with meaning and joy in nursing practice. *Nursing Administration Quarterly, 42*(2), 154–163. https://doi.org/10.1097/naq.0000000000000280

Haizlip, J., McCluney, C., Hernandez, M., Quatrara, B., & Brashers, V. (2020). Mattering: How organizations, patients, and peers can affect nurse burnout and engagement. *Journal of Nursing Administration, 50*(5), 267–273. https://doi.org/10.1097/nna.0000000000000882

Hedenstrom, M., Harrilson, A., Heath, M., & Dyess, S. (2022). "What's old is new again": Innovative healthcare leader rounding—a strategy to foster connection. *Nurse Leader, 20*(4), 366–370.

Hersey, P., & Blanchard, K. (1988). *Management of organizational behavior: Utilizing human resources* (4th ed.). Prentice-Hall.

Hersey, P., Blanchard, K.H., & Natemeyer, W.E. (1979). Situational leadership, perception and impact of power. *Group & Organization Management, 4*(4), 418–428. https://doi.org/10.1177/105960117900400404

Hudson, M. L. (2020). Transformational leadership: An integrated evidence review. DNP Qualifying Manuscripts. https://repository.usfca.edu/dnp_qualifying/36

Huston, C.J. (2024). *Leadership roles and management functions in nursing: Theory and application* (11th ed.). Wolters Kluwer/Lippincott.

Kostich, K., Lasiter, S., Duffy, J.R., & George, V. (2021). The relationship between staff nurses' perceptions of nurse manager caring behaviors and patient experience: A correlational study. *Journal of Nursing Administration, 51*(9), 468–473. doi: 10.1097/NNA.0000000000001047

Kowalski, M.O. (2020). What do nurses need to practice effectively in the hospital environment? An integrative review with implications for nurse leaders. *Worldviews on Evidence Based Nursing, 17*(1), 60–70.

Lawson, D., & Fleshman, J.W. (2020). Informal leadership in health care. Clinics in Colon and Rectal Surgery, 33(4), 225–227. doi: 10.1055/s-0040-1709439

Lewin, K. (1951). *Field theory in social sciences.* Harper & Row.

McGuire, E. (1999). Chaos theory: Learning a new science. *Journal of Nursing Administration, 29*(2), 8–9.

Perlo, J., et al. (2017). *IHI framework for improving joy in work. IHI White Paper.* Institute for Healthcare Improvement. http://www.ihi.org/resources/Pages/IHIWhitePapers/Framework-Improving-Joy-in-Work.aspx

Prestia, A.S. (2018). Personalizing appreciation to attain the fourth aim. *Nurse Leader, 16*(4), 240–243. https://doi.org/10.1016/j.mnl.2018.05.012

Sauer, P.A., & McCoy, T.P. (2018). Nurse bullying and intent to leave. *Nursing Economics, 36*(5), 219–224.

Stogdill, R.M. (1974). *Handbook of leadership: A survey of theory and research.* The Free Press.

Thompson, J.D. (1967). *Organizations in action.* McGraw-Hill.

Washington State Department of Labor and Industries (WSDLI). (2011). *Workplace bullying and disruptive behavior: What everyone needs to know.* https://www.shrm.org/ResourcesAndTools/hr-topics/employee-relations/Documents/Bullying.pdf

Weberg, D.R., & Fuller, R.M. (2019). Toxic leadership: Three lessons from complexity science to identify and stop toxic teams. *Nurse Leader, 17*(1), 22–26. https://doi.org/10.1016/j.mnl.2018.09.006

White, R.K., & Lippit, R. (1960). *Autocracy and democracy: An experimental inquiry.* Harper & Row.

18

Budgeting Basics for Nurses

Barbara Cherry, DNSc, MBA, RN, NEA-BC

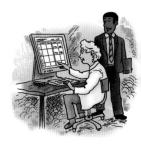

All nurses have a responsibility to ur stand budgeting processes and how can help reduce costs and improve qu

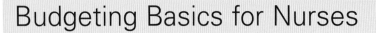

e Additional resources are available online at: http://evolve.elsevier.com/Cherry/

LEARNING OUTCOMES

After studying this chapter, the reader will be able to:

1. Understand the basic terminology of budgeting in health care settings.
2. Contribute to the budget development process for a nursing or clinical department.
3. Contribute to the capital budget development process for a nursing or clinical department.
4. Explain aspects of qualitative and quantitative variance analysis as a means to monitor an operational budget.
5. Articulate specific tools nurses can use to help reduce costs and improve quality in health care.

KEY TERMS

Budget Financial plan for the allocation of the organization's funds and a control for ensuring that results comply with the plan.

Budget assumptions Statements that reflect issues affecting the future performance of the organization; used as the framework for developing the budget; budget assumptions address questions such as: Are supply prices likely to increase or decrease? Is the patient census likely to increase or decrease over the next year?

Capital expenditures Amount spent on items that will have long-term (greater than 1 year) value to an organization; typically includes buildings and equipment.

Expense An event or item that requires the outlay of money for purchase or the incurrence of an obligation for future payment; major expenses for health care organizations include employee salaries, medical supplies and equipment, and facility maintenance.

Fiscal year A 12-month period used for calculating annual (yearly) financial reports in business; the fiscal year does not have to constitute the calendar year (January to December) but may be any 12-month period (e.g., August through July) established and maintained consistently by the business.

Full-time equivalent (FTE) The number of hours worked or paid that is equal to that expected of a full-time employee working a 40-hour workweek; annual work hours for 1 FTE equal 2080 hours, and monthly work hours equal 173.33 hours. One FTE position may be occupied by one employee working full time or shared by two or more employees working part time.

Incremental budgeting An approach to budget development that extrapolates from the prior period's budget and adjusts for future growth or decline in revenues or expenses to determine the budget for the next period.

Revenue Money that a health care organization receives in exchange for providing health care or other related services through normal business activities; synonymous with income. The sources of revenue are typically from commercial insurance, Medicare, Medicaid, and out-of-pocket payments from patients.

Salaries, wages, and benefits Budget category that typically includes direct payment for hours worked, bonuses, accrued paid time off, health benefits, employer portion of payroll taxes, and workers' compensation.

Supplies Materials used in performing tasks within the organization; typically includes clinical disposables, pharmaceuticals, and office supplies.

Variance The difference between the planned budget and the actual results.

Variance analysis The process of analyzing the differences in the planned budget results and the actual results; involves quantitative and qualitative analysis.

Zero-based budgeting An approach to budget development that begins as though the budget were being prepared for the first time.

PROFESSIONAL/ETHICAL ISSUE

Claire Ramsey, RN, works in the critical care unit of a large academic medical center. A new staffing policy for the hospital has been implemented and requires that either nurses are sent home or their shifts are cancelled in advance if the patient census is low. The nurse must either take paid time off to receive pay for the cancelled shift or can choose not to be paid for the cancelled shift. One of Claire's colleagues, Jonathan, is very vocal about his dislike of this policy and expresses to others that the hospital is "cheating" the nurses by cancelling shifts; he often remarks how unfair management is because, as he points out, the managers' shifts are never cancelled, and the hospital has "plenty of money" regardless of the number of patients on the unit. Claire is becoming uncomfortable with Jonathan's discussions because they seem to be leading to low morale and dissatisfaction among some of the nurses. She really likes her job and does not want to see the unit morale deteriorate over a policy that she herself does not understand and that she believes is not well understood by many other nurses, including Jonathan.

- Discuss the reasons from a budgeting perspective that the shift cancellation policy was implemented for this hospital.
- What steps can Claire take to help herself and her colleagues learn more about the staffing policy and why it was implemented?
- How should Claire respond to Jonathan when he begins to vocalize his objections about the policy to her?

VIGNETTE

Justine Scott, RN, sat in the staff meeting being led by the nurse manager for the cardiac telemetry unit where she has worked since graduating from nursing school 6 months ago. As Justine listened to the nurse manager discuss the unit's budget, she felt as if she were hearing a foreign language. The nurse manager discussed "variances for labor and supply costs that were most likely due to increased patient acuity and patient census above budgeted levels." The nurse manager explained the importance of accurately identifying reasons for the budget variances to ensure appropriate resources are allocated to their unit to support quality patient care. The nurse manager then requested input from the staff nurses regarding their observations about supply usage and overtime costs and how they might be better controlled. In the final topic for the staff meeting, the nurse manager requested input from the staff on "equipment needs to be considered as the unit's capital budget request is developed." As a new nurse, Justine noticed that staff meetings seemed to center more on discussions regarding the "budget" than on clinical issues. She realized that the budget must be extremely important to support patient care and resolved to learn more about budgets, the financial terminology used by her nurse manager, and what she could do as a staff nurse to support the nurse manager in this seemingly important area of nursing practice.

Questions to Consider While Reading This Chapter:

1. Who should be concerned about unit or departmental budgets?

2. What is the primary purpose of developing a unit or departmental budget?
3. How can nurses improve clinical care with a better understanding of the budget?
4. How can nurses help to reduce costs within the clinical setting?
5. What resources are available to help nurses learn more about budgets?

CHAPTER OVERVIEW

The budget serves as the financial guideline that enables a health care organization to achieve its goal of providing high-quality patient care services. Just as nurses learn about clinical guidelines for the care of patients with various diseases, it is also essential that nurses have a working knowledge of the guidelines that ensure the organization is able to operate in a stable financial environment through effective budget management. As nurses advance into management positions, they may have financial responsibility for a clinical unit and must be competent to serve as the bridge between the clinical setting and financial managers who have no clinical background. Additionally, the focus on cost and quality initiatives in today's health care settings requires that even staff nurses have a basic understanding of the budget. This chapter introduces the basic concepts of budgeting in health care organizations; for a deeper understanding of budgeting, nurses are encouraged to continue to build their knowledge by using a health care finance text and/or other resources noted on the Evolve site http://evolve.elsevier.com/Cherry/.

WHAT IS "THE BUDGET?"

As a nursing student, you are probably more aware of budget concepts than you realize. When you decided to become a registered nurse (RN), you had a goal to graduate from nursing school within a specified time period. You had to make a budget plan by predicting your expenses for that period, such as tuition, books, and living expenses. You also predicted your revenue from sources such as student loans, part-time jobs, savings, and financial support from family members. After predicting your expenses and your revenues, you most likely planned your budget for how much you could spend on a weekly or monthly basis during this time and eventually achieve your goal of graduating from nursing

school. Similarly, health care organizations develop budgets for a specified period by determining what goals they want to achieve, predicting expenses and revenues, then planning the annual budget and monitoring it on a monthly basis. For example, a hospital may plan its annual budget to maintain staffing and supplies to operate its current number of beds, provide a raise for all staff, and open a new outpatient surgical center.

The health care organization's budget is basically a document that details how financial resources will be allocated to ensure that the organization is able to conduct its daily business and achieve strategic goals. The budget itemizes the organization's predicted expenses and expected revenues (from sources such as commercial insurance, Medicare and Medicaid, and payments from individuals for services provided) for a given period of time. More important, budgets require ongoing attention to ensure that the organization's financial needs are met. Just as nursing students most likely have to make decisions to adjust their budgets during nursing school to meet unexpected changes in revenues or expenses, the health care organization invariably experiences the same challenges during the year. Thus the budget becomes a dynamic action plan that guides the allocation of resources and expenditures and influences the manager's decision-making on a day-to-day, week-to-week, or month-to-month basis.

Budgets perform four basic functions to make certain the organization can achieve its strategic goals and ensure continued operations from an economic point of view. The four budgeting functions, described in the following sections, are: (1) planning, (2) coordinating and communicating, (3) monitoring progress, and (4) evaluating performance.

Planning

Planning is the most important function of the budgeting process. During the planning phase, managers first decide on the goals to achieve for a specified period and identify resources (e.g., staff, supplies, equipment) needed to achieve those goals. Next, they predict revenues and expenses based on those goals and develop budget assumptions to use in planning the budget. Budget assumptions allow the managers to answer various questions that will have an effect on the budget, such as:

• What should nursing salaries be in the coming year to reward and retain nurses, and to remain competitive with other health care organizations in the area?

- How will new services being offered by other health care organizations in the area affect our organization?

Budgets are most often developed for a 1-year period on the basis of predicted amounts of services. For example, hospitals predict patient census and the related revenue that will be generated by providing services for those patients and then allocate funds for nursing salaries based on the predicted census.

Consider the following example: The hospital management team has decided to establish a chest pain center as part of the emergency department (ED). In planning the annual budget for the ED and its new chest pain center, the managers have developed the following assumptions:

- The chest pain center will see 12 patients every 24 hours. Of the 12 patients, 75% of the daily census (8 patients) are patients directed from the current ED census and 25% (4 patients) are patients new to this hospital.
- Four beds will be dedicated to the chest pain center and will require remodeling of an underused section of the current ED.
- The chest pain center will be staffed with RNs dedicated to the center.

The management team has planned to include the following expenses in the annual budget for the new chest pain center: salaries for nurses and support staff, supplies, monitoring equipment, equipment maintenance, funds for marketing the new program, and funds to remodel an area in the current ED for the program. Managers also need to think about the other areas that will be affected by the new chest pain center, such as the cardiac catheterization suite, echocardiography resources, laboratory, electrocardiography resources, and materials management, which all deserve budgetary consideration as a result of the wide-reaching effect of this seemingly small service expansion.

Historically, nursing has had limited input into fiscal (or financial) planning and development of the organization's budget. Administrators with no clinical background and little understanding of nursing values, beliefs, and care requirements traditionally made decisions about resource allocations related to nursing. Today participating in the budget process to determine resource allocation is a fundamental responsibility of nurse leaders. Involving staff nurses in the budget planning is also highly recommended. Managers and staff who participate in budget planning are more likely to be cost-conscious and to appreciate how their unit should function to meet the overall financial goals.

Coordinating and Communicating

Although not commonly associated with budgets, coordination and communication are very important functions of budgeting. The budget process, by necessity, requires that many different groups within an organization come together to discuss the resources necessary to accomplish the goals of a business unit. Therefore one can think of the budget process as the best opportunity to discuss concerns about resource allocation with the organization's leaders, who are capable of resolving issues.

Consider the new chest pain center described earlier. To plan how the center will establish itself as a center of excellence for emergency care of patients with chest pain, many groups must coordinate and communicate to ensure success for the new business unit:

- Nurses and physicians with experience in caring for patients with chest pain offer input about equipment and supply needs, room layout and design, staffing models, electronic health record needs, and support staff;
- Financial managers offer input about reimbursement rates and other financial considerations related to caring for this population;
- Marketing professionals offer input about how the program can be advertised to inform the community about the new service;
- Hospital administrators and department managers offer input as to how this new center will affect other areas of business both inside and outside the hospital.

Monitoring Progress

Monitoring progress is one of the most vital functions of the budget—and the function that the nurse manager is most involved with on a daily basis. It is through the comparison of actual financial performance against expected, or budgeted, performance that an organization measures the effectiveness of its budget. Ongoing monitoring of the budget allows timely corrective action or, if the budget plan is right on target, the knowledge that no adjustments are required.

Consider the chest pain center again. The budget was developed on an anticipated volume of 12 patients every 24 hours, and staffing was implemented to serve this volume of patients. At the end of its first month of operation, the nurse manager reviews the budget information and sees that the actual patient volume is averaging only eight patients per 24 hours, and the associated revenue for the center is approximately 70% of the planned revenue. The nurse manager has several issues to consider:

- Does staffing need to be reduced to better reflect the number of patients being treated?
- Are the patients being seen of higher acuity (i.e., sicker) and thus require a higher intensity of nursing care?
- Is the low volume a reflection of the newness of the program, which is not yet widely appreciated in the community, and so as its reputation grows will the volume also grow?
- If no immediate changes are made, how will the reduced revenue affect the financial status of the center?

Fortunately, the nurse manager can consult others involved in developing the budget to address these important issues and make decisions to ensure the success of the center.

The difference between the planned budget and the actual results is called a *variance*. A variance is favorable when the results are better than expected and unfavorable when the results are worse than expected. The lower-than-planned revenue in the chest pain center is an example of an unfavorable variance. *Variance analysis*, the process by which deviations from budgeted amounts are examined, is discussed in more detail later in the chapter.

Evaluating Performance

Budget results can also be used as part of the manager's performance evaluation, including the staff bonus structure for some health care organizations. Evaluating the manager's performance on the basis of budget results is becoming more widely used because of the growing trend toward accountability and compliance in the business world. By looking at the budget results for a given period an evaluator can determine the manager's overall success in achieving goals. Nurse managers are frequently evaluated according to their effectiveness in managing nursing overtime costs and supply use, both of which are reflected in the nursing unit's budget. Performance evaluations based on budget results can motivate managers to effectively control budgets and will serve as a basis for salary decisions and career advancement for these managers. Even though a manager is the captain of the unit and is ultimately accountable for the unit's

budgetary performance, a lack of staff ownership of and involvement in the unit's operation by the staff usually leads to problems for the manager.

TYPES OF BUDGETS

The three types of budgets for which a nurse manager typically has responsibility are operating, labor, and capital budgets (Jones et al., 2019). The components of these budgets are presented in Box 18.1 and are discussed in more detail in the following sections.

Operating Budget

The operational, or operating, budget represents revenues and expenses for an operational unit, such as a product line, unit, department, or overall organization. The chest pain center previously discussed is considered a product line; an example of a nursing unit is the intensive care unit or medical-surgical unit; an example of a department is dietary or human resources. The expenses in the operational budget are those necessary to operate on a daily basis (i.e., salaries and supplies), and the revenues are those paid to the organization from various payer sources (Box 18.2). (See Chapter 7 for more information about sources of payments for health care services.)

Labor Budget

The labor budget is a subset of the operating budget. Its purpose is to provide detailed documentation of salaries, wages, and benefits with respect to the operational unit.

BOX 18.1	Three Types of Budgets
Operating budget	Projects' expenses and revenues: funds for daily expenses, such as salaries, utilities, repairs, maintenance, and patient care supplies AND projects' revenues for health care services provided in the same time period
Labor budget	A subset of the operating budget; projects' funds for salaries, overtime, benefits, and staff development and training
Capital budget	Projects' funds for construction projects and/or long-life medical equipment, such as cardiac monitors, defibrillators, and computer hardware

BOX 18.2 Examples of Typical Expenses and Revenues for a Health Care Organization

Expenses	Revenues (Payments From)
• Salaries	• Medicare
• Benefits (paid time off; health insurance)	• Medicaid
	• Private insurance
• Patient care supplies	• Individuals (self-pay)
• Utilities	• Grants
• Administrative costs	• Charitable or philan-
• Maintenance	thropic donations
• Housekeeping	

Factors that affect the personnel budget include salary rates, overtime, benefits (e.g., paid time off, health insurance), staff development and training, and employee turnover. The labor budget is virtually always the largest expense item in an operational budget for a health care organization because salaries for nurses, other professional staff (pharmacists, physical therapists, etc.), and support staff (e.g., nursing assistants, unit secretaries, transportation staff) compose the greatest percentage of expenses in the budget. The labor budget is also used to provide managers with a *productivity metric*, which is the amount of work produced (i.e., hours of nursing care per patient-day) by a specific amount of input or resources (i.e., nursing hours worked).

The productivity metric is necessary to give managers a measurement of the number of nursing hours worked in comparison with the amount of patient care provided. Low productivity (high nursing hours worked with low patient census) is not desirable because it means higher staff salaries combined with lower revenues for patient care services. High productivity (high patient census with low nursing hours) means that there are fewer staff to take care of more patients, so the unit may not be able to provide safe, quality patient care. Most health care organizations have a recommended productivity measure that allows for a balance between financial efficiency and quality and safety of patient care. To achieve this balance, nurses must be at the table during budget planning to ensure that the patient quality and safety are discussed along with productivity and financial efficiency.

One of the primary difficulties encountered in managing the labor budget is accurately predicting future staffing needs. Because budgets are based on a *predicted* amount of services (i.e., patient census), variances between actual staffing levels and budget levels occur if the facility experiences an unanticipated increase or decrease in patient services. Another concern related to the budget and labor expense is balancing the patient acuity, or degree of patient illness, with the nurse-to-patient ratio. Can you imagine how difficult it might be to accurately predict how many patients a health care facility will treat over the next 12 months and how sick those patients might be? This is the challenge of budgeting!

An important aspect of labor budgeting is understanding the 12-month historical trend for labor hours and patient-days. As a general rule, organizations expect nurse managers to control the number of hours worked by staff and not the actual salary expense. Wage levels, benefit costs, and other related expenses are typically controlled at the leadership level with input from nursing leaders. The operational aspect of scheduling staff (measured in worked hours) to meet the needs of patient volume (measured by patient census) is best controlled and budgeted at the unit or departmental level.

Capital Budget

The capital budget represents funds allocated for construction projects and major equipment purchases (e.g., cardiac monitors, defibrillators, electronic health records, computer hardware) and are typically referred to as capital expenditures. The capital budget is developed separately from the operating budget because payments for capital purchases are spread out over multiple years. The main requirements for a purchase or acquisition to be considered as part of the capital budget is that it has a useful life expectancy of more than 1 year and it costs more than a minimum dollar amount established by the organization, typically $500 to $2000.

The term *capital* simply refers to the funds used to purchase long-term investments, such as major medical equipment, computer systems, and newly constructed buildings. A capital budget item is an expensive purchase that will be used by the organization for many years. Capital budget items are often referred to as *capital assets*, *long-term investments*, *capital investments*, or *capital acquisitions*. These capital assets are treated differently from the operating budget expense because of their multiyear value. Because capital purchases are often considered investments, they are scrutinized more carefully during the budgeting process.

Planning capital budget requests tests the nurse manager's long-range planning skills. The nurse manager must be able to look 1 year to several years into the future to identify capital budgeting needs. The unit or department need for a capital purchase must be weighed against the financial implications for the organization's entire capital budget. The nurse manager, along with input from the staff, has a critical role in helping to plan the capital budget, justify priorities, and ensure that the needs of the facility and patients are met. Staff nurses are vital to a successful capital planning process because their "frontline" equipment needs (e.g., beds, monitoring systems, patient lift equipment) must be made known to management for purchase consideration.

Budget Methods

There are two basic methods for budgeting: the *incremental* approach and the *zero-based* approach. Both approaches have particular strengths and weaknesses and both are sound approaches in most situations.

Incremental Budgeting. Incremental budgeting is the more commonly used method, primarily because it is relatively simple to apply to most circumstances. The incremental approach is simply a forward trend of recent performance, with adjustments for future growth or decline in revenues or expenses. For example, in this approach the nursing unit's budget is based on the actual costs from the previous budget period, with a small increase for planned salary raises and the higher cost of supplies. It is also possible that the incremental budget might include a decrease in all expenses.

Zero-Based Budgeting. Zero-based budgeting is used far less frequently than incremental budgeting. This method builds a budget starting from zero as though the budget were being prepared for the first time. Each budget cycle begins with a critical review of budget assumptions and proposed revenues and expenditures.

Again, consider the chest pain center. If the nurse manager were developing a zero-based budget, they would start each new budget planning cycle by:
- Determining the revenue and expenses for caring for one patient with chest pain.

- Predicting the average patient volume for the center.
- Calculating the total revenues and expenses for the budget period.

In developing the budget the nurse manager understands that whereas one nurse is necessary to care for one patient, that nurse may also be able to care for two or three other patients at the same time. Thus the cost of nursing salaries varies according to the volume of patients being treated in the center and the acuity of those patients.

The budget process works somewhat differently in support departments that do not provide a revenue-generating service such as patient treatment. Examples of departments that are necessary to support treatment and care delivery processes but are not revenue generating include administration and human resources. In such support departments expenses do not vary with patient volume. Thus these departments base their budgets not on a variable volume of patient visits but, rather, on a set core of expenses to run the department.

DEVELOPING A BUDGET

Developing a budget is actually a continual process. Organizations are constantly making projections for future budgets, implementing current budgets, and analyzing month-to-month variances in relation to the budget. The current budget usually covers a 12-month period, also known as the organization's *fiscal year*. The development of the budget for the new fiscal year occurs a few months ahead of the start of the new fiscal year so that the budget can be developed and approved at all levels before it becomes effective. For example, if the organization's fiscal year is from September 1 to August 31, then budget development for the new fiscal year will begin sometime in early summer—or perhaps even earlier depending on the size and complexity of the organization. Because of the number of approval layers, large health systems usually begin the budget process much earlier than smaller systems or single facilities.

Organizations usually have a defined procedure in place for budget development. This defined procedure tells managers whether the budget development will use the incremental method, zero-based method, or some other method defined by the organization. Organizations may also define whether they use a "top-down," "participatory," or "iterative" approach to budgeting (Box 18.3).

BOX 18.3 Approaches to Budget Development

Top-down approach: Upper management sets budget goals and imposes those goals on the rest of the organization.

Participatory approach: The people responsible for achieving the budget goals are included in goal setting.

Iterative approach: Combination of the top-down and the participatory approach, with upper management defining strategic goals and then unit leaders developing their operating budgets to incorporate their individual goals in conjunction with the organization's strategic goals.

One key to understanding budgets is to know the *unit of service* on which costs and revenues are based. "Patient-days" is the common unit of service for inpatient facilities; patient visits or visits by categories (short, intermediate, long) are the units of service for ambulatory clinics and home health agencies. Budgets are then developed on the basis of the units of service predicted for a given period. For example, the nurse manager in a hospital intensive care unit bases their budget on the average number of days that patients are expected to be on the unit over the course of 12 months. The director of the home health agency bases their budget on the number of home visits that will be made during a 12-month period. The unit of service may vary depending on the organization, setting, and financial policies; thus it is essential that the nurse understands the unit of service in the area in which they are employed.

Following are the basic steps for developing a budget:

1. Review the strategic plan to identify goals and objectives; the budget is developed to accomplish these goals and objectives.
2. Set budget assumptions on which to base budgeting decisions. Budget assumptions deal with issues that affect the future performance of the organization and address questions such as: Are supply prices likely to increase or decrease, and by what percentage? What salary range will ensure that the organization is able to recruit and retain quality employees? What will the cost of the health insurance plan be in the coming year? What are the competitors offering in terms of new services? Is the patient census likely to increase or decrease over the next year? Budget assumptions should be developed by a team of managers from different departments and areas of expertise to make certain that consideration is given to all issues that will affect the budget.
3. Gather information about past results, and use the information in combination with budget assumptions to set reasonable expectations about future performance.
4. Predict the units of service that will be provided during the budget period.
5. Project expected revenues on the basis of the units of service.
6. Project expenses on the basis of the units of service. Determine expenses for the labor budget first, based on the predicted units of service and the number of full-time equivalents (FTEs) needed to provide the predicted service volume. Each full-time employee is considered one FTE, or 2080 hours per year (40 hours per week). In some organizations, nurses are scheduled for three 12-hour shifts each week, 36 hours per week or 1872 hours per year, and each is considered 0.9 FTE. After determining units of service and related FTEs, other expenses are fairly straightforward to project.

Developing the budget is generally a process that involves many discussions among many different managers, from finance to nursing. It is important that nurses have a strong and knowledgeable voice in the budget process so that nursing and patient care needs are appropriately addressed (Jones et al., 2019). Box 18.4 lists hints to improve your budgeting skills.

VARIANCE ANALYSIS

One primary use of a budget is to evaluate the financial progress of the department or unit. Variance analysis is the process by which deviations from budgeted amounts are examined through comparison of actual financial performance results against expected, or budgeted, performance (Jones et al., 2019). Through this process, variances are evaluated on quantitative and qualitative bases. Quantitative analysis focuses on numerical variances to the budget. In other words, are you over or under budget for labor (employee salaries), supply usage, or revenue generated? See Table 18.1 for a sample budget and variance report.

Qualitative analysis of budget variances focuses on explaining how the current conditions in the clinical unit impact the budget that was previously developed. Often the daily operations for a department or unit change in ways that make the actual budget expenses

BOX 18.4 Hints to Improve Your Budgeting Skills

- Understand your organization's budgeting process. What guidelines do you need to follow? What key managers can serve as a resource to help you understand the budget process?
- Know the primary sources of revenue for your organization (Commercial insurance? Medicare? Medicaid? Private pay?).
- Learn your department's *unit of service* and exactly how it is defined.
- Build a relationship with a finance person in the organization and collaborate routinely on improvement projects; invite finance staff to your unit meetings and ask to participate in theirs; communicate regularly.
- Review financial reports with the finance person to make sure you are correctly interpreting the reports.
- Understand each line in your budget. If you do not know what something means or where a number comes from find out.
- Have ongoing discussions with your management team throughout the budgeting process. The more you participate in the planning process, the better you will understand the budget and your responsibilities related to it.
- Learn your organization's capital budgeting process and what qualifies a purchase as a capital expenditure.

and revenues different than what was originally planned in the budget. For example, a unit may be budgeted for nurse staffing at 4 hours per patient-day based on a given patient acuity level. Then the hospital's admission patterns change and a larger number of patients with significantly higher acuity levels are admitted to this unit. The nurse staffing increases to 6 hours per patient-day based on the new acuity level. This sort of qualitative change can make budgets difficult, if not impossible, to adhere to without modification. Nurse leaders in the clinical department or unit are best positioned to determine why variances have occurred because variances are almost always related to a clinical issue such as the one just described.

Variance information is presented by means of certain standard reports. Through such reports nurse managers are able to compare the budgeted amounts for expense items such as nurse salaries and patient supplies with what was actually spent for the items. From there the nurse manager can consider what is

occurring in the clinical setting to explain the variances in budgeted and actual expenditures. Nurses are encouraged to examine variance analysis reports and seek guidance from other managers or supervisors to learn more about reading the reports and becoming more comfortable with variance analysis.

COST CONCEPTS RELATED TO BUDGETING

When considering the budget one must have a basic understanding of how much health care services cost and how to predict changes in costs. Consider this question: How much does it cost to provide nursing care to one patient for one 12-hour shift? Unfortunately, the answer is not simple because many factors affect how much something costs. An important step to understanding costs is to review the primary types of costs that accountants consider when determining the cost of services in a health care setting; they are:

- *Service unit or unit of service:* The basic measure of the product or service being produced. The unit of service varies with the health care setting and type of service being provided. Examples include patient-days (hospital), home care visits (home health agency), patient visits (outpatient clinic), and operating room time (outpatient surgical center).
- *Direct costs:* Costs that can be traced directly to the production of the unit of service. Examples include nursing care and supplies to provide direct patient care. The important concept to remember about direct costs is that they vary with the volume of services. As the patient census rises, the need for additional nursing care and supplies increases.
- *Indirect costs:* Costs that are incurred as a result of the organization's operating expenses but are not directly related to providing the unit of service. Examples include salaries for administrative personnel and expenses for security, housekeeping, utilities, and building maintenance. Indirect costs are sometimes referred to as "overhead."
- *Full cost:* The total of all costs associated with a unit of service; it includes direct and indirect costs.
- *Fixed costs:* Costs that do not change as the unit of service volume changes. For example, administrative salaries do not change regardless of the patient census on the nursing units. The important point to remember about fixed costs is that they remain

TABLE 18.1 Sample Budget and Variance Report

Hometown General Hospital: Department Performance Analysis—Med-Surg for Period Ending 09/30/2023

	Prior Year Actual 9/2022	CURRENT MTD (MONTH-TO-DATE)			CURRENT YTD (YEAR-TO-DATE)			PRIOR YEAR	
		Actual 9/2023	Budget 9/2023	MTD Variance 9/2023	Actual 9/2023	Budget 9/2023	YTD Variance 9/2023	Prior Year 9/2022	Prior Year Variance
Gross Revenue									
Inpatient revenue	1,276,525	1,300,122	1,322,904	−22,782	11,087,012	12,575,946	−1,488,934	12,733,822	−1,646,810
Outpatient revenue	0	0	0	0	0	0	0	0	0
Other revenue	0	0	0	0	0	0	0	0	0
Total gross revenue	1,276,525	1,300,122	1,322,904	−22,782	11,087,012	12,575,946	−1,488,934	12,733,822	−1,646,810
Operating Expenses									
Total productive labor	241,270	293,541	257,954	35,587	2,375,340	2,419,097	−43,757	2,376,009	−669
Total nonproductive labor	29,012	40,031	37,352	2679	359,759	359,453	306	328,128	31,631
Employee benefits and taxes	40,372	38,483	41,133	−2650	366,203	401,616	−35,413	398,766	−32,563
Total SWB (salaries, wages, and benefits)	310,653	372,055	336,439	35,616	3,101,302	3,180,166	−78,864	3,102,903	−1601
Supplies	25,687	20,506	22,628	−2123	193,223	213,853	−20,630	219,267	−26,044
Medical and clinical fees	0	0	0	0	0	0	0	0	0
Contracted department and other fees	298	0	41	−41	506	371	135	929	−424

Continued

TABLE 18.1   Sample Budget and Variance Report—cont'd

Hometown General Hospital: Department Performance Analysis—Med-Surg for Period Ending 09/30/2023

	Prior Year Actual 9/2022	CURRENT MTD (MONTH-TO-DATE)			CURRENT YTD (YEAR-TO-DATE)			PRIOR YEAR	
		Actual 9/2023	Budget 9/2023	MTD Variance 9/2023	Actual 9/2023	Budget 9/2023	YTD Variance 9/2023	Prior Year 9/2022	Prior Year Variance
Repairs and maintenance	0	0	20	−20	0	184	−184	242	−242
Utilities and telephone	0	0	0	0	0	0	0	0	0
Rent, lease, and equipment rental	0	0	0	0	1485	0	1485	0	1485
Other controllable expenses	883	1232	953	279	8617	8741	−124	14,041	−5424
Other noncontrollable expenses	0	0	0	0	0	0	0	0	0
Total operating expenses	337,520	393,792	360,081	33,711	3,305,132	3,403,315	−98,183	3,337,382	−32,249
Gross margin	939,005	906,330	962,823	−56,493	7,781,880	9,172,631	−1,390,751	9,396,440	−1,614,561
Gross margin percentage	73.56	69.71	72.78	−3.07	70.19	72.94	−2.75	73.79	−3.6
Department patient-days	841	853	871	−18	7283	8280	−997	8384	−1101
Average daily census	28	28	29	−1	27	30	−4	31	−4
Observation days	1.67	3.5	5.5	−2	41.54	49.38	−7.83	48.17	−6.63
Total department patient-days	842.67	856.5	876.5	−20	7324.54	8329.38	−1,004.83	8432.17	−1,107.62

The budget report shows dollar performance, comparing actual revenues and expenses with budgeted revenues and expenses for the same month of the prior year, current month, and current YTD, and the annual totals and variances for the prior year. YTD is the totals for the prior months plus the current month in the fiscal year. The department has spent $33,711 (shaded in *green*) **more** than budgeted for expenses for the current month, but for the current YTD the department has spent $98,183 (shaded in *yellow*) **less** than budgeted for expenses.

steady regardless of the change in units of service (e.g., patient-days). As the units of service increase the greater the revenue to cover fixed costs. Conversely, as the units of service decrease the lower the revenue to cover fixed costs. An organization's finance leaders are always interested in increasing volume to provide additional revenue to help cover fixed costs.

- *Variable costs:* Costs that vary directly with changes in the volume of units of service. For example, in an ambulatory clinic the cost of immunizations varies directly with the number of patients who receive immunizations.

This list provides only a basic introduction to cost terminology; it does not provide a comprehensive range of cost accounting terminology and concepts. However, it does demonstrate the complexity of assessing and managing costs.

IMPROVING THE COST AND QUALITY OF CLINICAL CARE

Today's nurses face challenging situations given the nursing shortage, the strong focus on cost reductions while also improving quality, and the increasing acuity of patients in all settings from hospitals to home health agencies to nursing homes. At the same time, organizational leaders are faced with challenging economic times, with declining reimbursements that are tied to quality metrics and increasing costs in all areas, including salaries and supplies. It is imperative that nurses understand how health care reimbursement—specifically value-based reimbursement models (Chapter 7)—impacts the ability to provide cost-effective care for our patients and populations (Kerfoot & Buerhaus, 2023).

Changes to improve quality and reduce costs must be made! What tools can nurses use to make a difference and lower costs? In one example, a team of nurses in a large health care system implemented a video monitoring system to reduce patient falls while also reducing the cost of paying sitters to be with the

> **BOX 18.5 Tools to Help Nurses Reduce Costs and Improve Quality**
>
> - **Patient Education and Care Planning:** Ensure patients—especially those with chronic conditions such as congestive heart failure and diabetes—receive appropriate care planning, education, and follow-up so they have the resources needed to stay as healthy as possible and stay out of the hospital.
> - **Quality Improvement:** Engage in quality improvement projects to reduce the occurrence of complications such as pressure ulcers, falls, and central-line infections, which will improve patient outcomes and reduce costs.
> - **Value-based reimbursement:** Understand how new models of paying for health care are directly tied to specific outcomes of care provided by nurses. (See Chapter 7 for more information on value-based reimbursement.)
> - **Budget Knowledge:** Understand the staffing budget and how it relates to patient acuity to ensure that appropriate nursing resources are available to meet patient care needs.
> - **Supply Management:** Identify the most cost-effective patient care supplies to replace more expensive products, as well as identify ways to reduce waste and avoid the overuse or misuse of supplies.
> - **Evidence-Based Practice (EBP):** Promote the use of EBP to ensure the most cost-effective care is provided in the right setting at the right time.
> - **Patient-Centered Care:** Ensure that patients and families are fully informed about options in care decisions and have a voice in choosing the type of care they will receive.
> - **Governance Council Participation:** Actively engage in unit councils and/or shared governance councils to advocate for initiatives to promote staff retention, which is a significant cost savings for the organization.

patients (Kowalski et al., 2019). Box 18.5 summarizes key tools that are components of professional nursing practice and can be used to significantly lower costs and improve the quality of health care.

SUMMARY

To summarize this chapter let's revisit Justine and her questions about budgets. Justine learned that the financial well-being of health care organizations—and the value of health care—rests largely in the hands of the clinical team. The budget is the financial guideline that enables the clinical team to have the resources necessary to provide quality care, achieve goals, and pay its bills (like Justine's salary!). Thus all staff should be concerned with the budget and how to monitor costs and contribute to cost-effective care and services. By understanding the four major functions of the organization's budget—planning, communicating and coordinating, monitoring progress, and evaluating performance—Justine can better contribute to achieving budget goals for her unit. When nurses understand the basics of budgeting, costs, and reimbursement, they can promote more cost-effective care through actions such as reducing readmissions, lowering complication rates, reducing the length of stay, improving supply usage, improving nurse retention, and improving the overall quality of care.

The reader is cautioned that this chapter merely provides a general overview of budgeting basics to serve as a framework on which nurses can continue to build their knowledge of health care finance and budgeting. As nurses advance in their career, it is essential that they further develop their skills and knowledge in budgeting through personal study, working with mentors, attending classes or workshops, reading books and journals, and joining professional organizations that promote health care finance and budget knowledge.

REFERENCES

Jones, C.B., et al. (2019). *Financial management for nurse managers and executives* (5th ed.) Elsevier.

Kerfoot, K., & Buerhaus, P. (2023). The 'Not so hidden costs' associated with failing to educate nurses and researchers about health care economics, financing, and payment policies. *Nursing Economic$*, 41(3), 113–120.

Kowalski, S.L. (2019). Budgeting for a video monitoring system to reduce patient falls and sitter costs: A quality improvement project. *Nursing Economic$*, 36(6), 291–295.

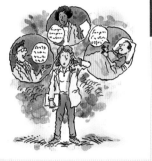

How is your message being received?

19

Effective Communication and Conflict Resolution

Anna Marie Sallee, PhD, RN, CCRN-K

ⓔ Additional resources are available online at: http://evolve.elsevier.com/Cherry/

LEARNING OUTCOMES

After studying this chapter, the reader will be able to:

1. Outline factors that can influence the communication process.
2. Communicate effectively with diverse intergenerational and interprofessional team members.
3. Apply positive communication techniques in diverse situations.
4. Recognize negative communication techniques.
5. Evaluate conflicting verbal and nonverbal communication cues.
6. Examine constructive methods of communicating in conflict situations.
7. Respond to inappropriate use of logical fallacies in communication.
8. Develop professional social media interaction behaviors.

KEY TERMS

Active listening The process of hearing what others are saying with a sense of seriousness and discrimination.
Conflict An experience in which there is simultaneous arousal of two or more incompatible motives.
Filtration Unconscious exclusion of extraneous stimuli.
Information The data that are meaningful and alter the receiver's understanding.

Interpretation Receiver's understanding of the meaning of the communication.
Negative communication Behaviors that block or impair effective communication.
Perception The manner in which one sees reality.
Positive communication Behaviors that enhance effective communication.

The greatest problem of communication is the illusion that it has been accomplished.
George Bernard Shaw

PROFESSIONAL/ETHICAL ISSUE

Naomi is a recent registered nurse (RN) graduate who works on an active medical-surgical floor in a large hospital in a university town. She has observed a colleague using the computer system to look up information on acquaintances who have been hospitalized at the facility—even from previous years. One night she observes the RN looking up personal health information on a hospitalized athlete who plays at the university and is a local celebrity. Naomi knows the nurse's actions are unethical and illegal. However, she recognizes the nurse is well liked by both their coworkers and the administrative personnel at the hospital. She is vibrant and friendly and has many years of experience. Naomi, however, is new to nursing and still on a high learning curve. As a single mother of two Naomi struggled to finish nursing school and support her family, accruing significant educational loans in the process. She is fearful that if the hospital administration feels forced to make a choice, she may lose her job. She struggles with whether to report the nurse or stay silent and hope that someone else will take action.

What ethical principles are in conflict here? Do you believe Naomi's fears regarding her job security are legitimate? What communication techniques will be important for Naomi to use in this situation? Discuss possible options for Naomi.

VIGNETTE

Stacy Shannon, RN, the charge nurse on 4-East, receives a telephone call from the secretary in the emergency department (ED) to inform Stacy that a patient is ready for transfer. Stacy was expecting this patient but had not anticipated the transfer would occur so soon and had not informed the nurse who would be assigned to the patient. The ED secretary explains that there are many patients waiting to be seen in the ED and it is becoming increasingly chaotic. Stacy replies that she will locate the nurse who will be assigned to the patient and facilitate the transfer as soon as possible. As Stacy goes down the hallway to locate this particular nurse, she learns that the nurse has left the unit on a short break and is expected back within 10 minutes.

Stacy calls the ED secretary to arrange for the transfer to occur in 20 minutes. To her surprise, she finds out that the patient has left the department and is being brought to 4-East immediately. Within a few moments the patient and ED nurse arrive. The ED nurse states that he wants to give report on this patient quickly because he needs to return to the ED right away. Stacy assists him in transferring the patient to a bed and making the patient as comfortable as possible.

As Stacy completes this process the nurse who was on break returns to the unit, learns that she has a new patient she did not expect, and immediately has to receive report from the ED nurse. Stacy notes through both body language and tone of voice that the interaction between the two nurses is less than cordial. Within 10 minutes Stacy receives a telephone call from the ED charge nurse, who wants to discuss this incident. Negative comments are made about the 4-East nurse who left the unit "unannounced" and that "there is a concern for patient safety." How can Stacy best facilitate a positive outcome in this situation?

Questions to Consider While Reading This Chapter:

1. What communication strategies should Stacy use to respond to the accusations being made by the ED charge nurse to resolve the conflict and build a trusting relationship with her?
2. What conflict resolution strategies should both the ED nurse transferring the patient and the 4E staff nurse have used to prevent this situation from occurring?
3. What important steps should Stacy, the staff nurse, the ED nurse, the ED charge nurse—and ALL nurses—be aware of to develop and promote a professional communication style?

CHAPTER OVERVIEW

Effective communication is a foundational component of professional nursing practice. The development of effective communication skills can only enhance each nurse's professional image while building strong relationships with both patients and colleagues. Understanding communication processes and principles is required for nurses to interact professionally with patients, families and significant others, nursing peers, managers, student nurses, physicians, other members of the interdisciplinary team, and the public. Nurses communicate through a variety of media, including the spoken and written word, demonstration, role modeling, and, on occasion, public appearances. The exchange of ideas and feelings is hardly limited to verbal communication. Many types of nonverbal communication are often as meaningful as, and in many instances more meaningful than, audible expression. Because communication is such a complex process, there are infinite opportunities for sending or receiving incorrect messages. All too frequently communication is faulty, resulting in misperceptions and misunderstandings. This chapter reviews the communication process and its components, communication styles, and principles of effective communication in professional nursing, including special communication issues.

OUR PROFESSION SPEAKS

Nurses must be as proficient in communication skills as they are in clinical skills.
American Association of Critical Care Nurses, Standard 1, in Standards for Establishing and Sustaining Healthy Work Environments (2023)

Open and candid communication with patients and their families is a key component of safe and effective health care.
The Joint Commission (2016)

The ability to communicate effectively is essential.
HIPAA (2023)

THE COMMUNICATION PROCESS

The human voice is the most beautiful instrument of all, but it is the most difficult to play.
Richard Strauss

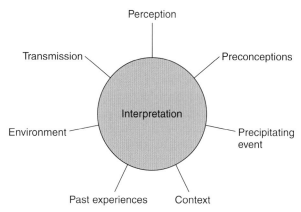

Fig. 19.1 Factors influencing interpretation of messages.

Communication is a process requiring certain components. There must be a sender, a receiver, and a message. Effective communication is a dynamic process: With a response (feedback) the sender becomes the receiver, the receiver becomes the sender, and the message changes. The method of delivery influences the effectiveness of communication. In addition, communication is affected by many subcomponents, both environmental and in the minds of the communicators. When communication with another person occurs, verbally or nonverbally, a typical pattern develops that includes the actual message being sent, the receiver's belief or interpretation of that message, and the reaction to the message.

Think about the communication activities that occur in the health care setting. There is often much to communicate in a limited time and sometimes during very high stress situations. In addition to the actual message, personal goals or hidden agendas can influence the way a message is delivered and/or received. For this reason it is very important to understand the many elements that influence the communication process.

Interpretation

Interpretation of information can be influenced by such factors as context, environment, precipitating event, preconceived ideas, personal perceptions, style of transmission, and past experiences. Because of the interaction of these factors, the sender's message may mean to the receiver something that was entirely unplanned or unexpected by the sender (Fig. 19.1).

Context and Environment. *Context* refers to the entire situation relevant to the communication, such as the environment, the background, and the particular

circumstances that lead to the discussion. *Environment* can denote physical surroundings and happenings and the emotional conditions involved in the communication.

Precipitating Event. *Precipitating event* refers specifically to the event or situation that prompted the communication. Precipitating event is a specific single event, whereas context describes the whole ambiance of the situation, with the inclusion of multiple circumstances that have led to the precipitating event.

Preconceived Ideas. *Preconceived ideas* are conceptions, opinions, or thoughts that the receiver has developed before the encounter. Such ideas can dramatically affect the receiver's acceptance and understanding of the message.

Style of Transmission. *Style of transmission* involves many aspects of the manner of conveyance of the message. Transmission styles include aspects such as open and closed statements and questions, body language, method of organizing the message, degree of attention to the topic and to the receiver, vocabulary chosen (professional jargon vs language a layperson could easily understand), and intonation.

Past Experiences. Each person comes to any type of communication—whether it is friendly conversation, informational lecture, staff meeting, performance evaluation, or any other possible scenario—with "baggage" in terms of past experiences. Because past experiences are a variety of positive, neutral, and negative events, the influence that the experiences can and will have on communication may be positive, neutral, or negative. *The importance of recognizing that any reaction from the receiver may be biased by previous experiences cannot be overstated.* An astute sender begins to investigate such a possibility if the receiver reacts in an unexpected or inappropriate manner to information that was not expected to produce such a response, which may range from nonresponse to overly vehement response.

Personal Perceptions. Personal perceptions can have a profound effect on the quality of communication. Perception is awareness through the excitation of all the senses. Perception can be described as all that the person knows about a situation or circumstance, based on what each of the senses—taste, smell, sight, sound, touch, and intuition—discover and interpret.

Filtration

The most concise delivery of information is subject to some amount of filtration. Think of the process as similar to washing vegetables in a colander. A large amount of water is poured over the produce. Some of the water comes quickly through the colander holes; some water drips through more slowly; and some water hangs on the contents or settles in the solid portions of the colander and never filters through. If people were not able to filter out a portion of the stimuli that bombard them daily, the clutter would be unmanageable! At the same time, however, it is possible to filter out some part of intended communication that is essential to understanding the communication.

Feedback

Feedback, simply put, is the response from the receiver. However, as with all communication feedback is a dynamic process. As the receiver interprets and responds to the original message the sender begins the same process of feedback to the receiver. Because of this circular property, the process frequently is referred to as the *communication loop* (Communication Theory, 2023). As with the original message feedback is not confined to verbal responses alone. Both communicants constantly assess nonverbal communication as well. Feedback is formed on the basis of all the components of interpretation and filtration.

VERBAL VS NONVERBAL COMMUNICATION

> *What you do speaks so loud that I cannot hear what you say.*
> **Ralph Waldo Emerson**

> *The most important thing in communication is hearing what isn't said.*
> **Peter F. Drucker**

Verbal Communication

Verbal communication, the most common form of interpersonal communication, involves talking and listening. Important clues to verbal communication are the tone or inflection with which the words are spoken and the general attitude the speaker uses. The key to the true meaning of a statement may be contained in the emphasis placed on a specific word. Consider how differently the following phrase could be perceived according to the inflection, or the emphasis on the wording:

- You are going to **bed**.
- **You** are going to bed.
- You **are going** to bed.

With an emphasis on *bed* the first phrase most likely will be perceived as an inquiry. The second phrase might imply that you are going to bed, but no one else is. The last phrase, an imperative (or command), gives the impression of increased emotion, such as anger or frustration.

Another element central to verbal interaction is the concept of attitude. Being aware of and learning to understand the concept of attitude is key to effective communication. Attitude involves a predisposition or tendency to respond in one way or another. Often the attitude that accompanies a verbal interaction, which can be positive or negative, is much more meaningful than the actual words spoken. Although we may hear "attitude" in a person's tone of voice, it is most often communicated "loud and clear" through nonverbal communication.

Nonverbal Communication

> *Oops! Did I just roll my eyes out loud?*
> **Facebook Posting**

Nonverbal communication involves many factors that either confirm or deny the spoken word. Facial expression, the presence or absence of eye contact, posture, and body movement all project a direct message. Indirect nonverbal messages might include dressing style, lifestyle, or material possessions. Never presume that external trappings and physical presentation do not influence the quality of communication. Preconceived ideas and expectations interpret input from all such sources, often on an almost subconscious level.

Consider the following scenario: Rhonda, a young wife and mother, was admitted to the ED with significant abdominal pain. As the nurse inquires about her symptoms Rhonda repeatedly glances at her husband, Tommy, before she answers. Although she denies any pain at this time, you observe that she guards her stomach, has a "clenched" jawline, and does not make eye contact with you. As you assess and question Rhonda, Tommy often interrupts with comments such as, "She's just fine. It was only a stomachache." Which message seems more likely to be true—the verbal or the nonverbal? How will you address the nonverbal cues? As you read the remainder of this chapter, consider strategies that you can use to enhance communication between this husband and wife.

The avoidance of eye contact may be construed to mean that the speaker is shy, scared, or not telling the truth. The judgment as to which condition is correct is based on all the factors that feed into the receiver's interpretation—perception, preconceptions, precipitating event, context, past experiences, environment, and transmission. Faced with the many opportunities for incorrect interpretation, is it any wonder that misunderstandings occur?

Disagreements between Verbal and Nonverbal Messages. An important concept to remember is that when the verbal and nonverbal messages do not agree, the receiver is more likely to believe the nonverbal message. In 1971 Albert Mehrabian (1981) conducted a seminal study on nonverbal communication in which he found that most communication is 55% nonverbal, 38% vocal signals (such as tone, pitch, and pace), and *only 7% the actual words we say*. Body language is often the most trusted indicator for conveying feelings, attitudes, and emotions (Borg, 2011) because it so often comes from our subconscious—which is much less likely to deceive! "Body language is a silent orchestra, as people constantly give clues to what they're thinking and feeling" (*Psychology Today*, 2023). Nonverbal language includes such things as dress, posture, facial expression, eye contact, body movements, body tension, spatial distance, touch, and voice. For nurses, body positioning toward the patient, a relaxed stance, a gentle touch, and an open face signal total presence.

An understanding of the importance ascribed to body language and other nonverbal clues to the intent of the message explains the advantage of face-to-face communication. Although a telephone conversation supplies verbal messages, intonation, and feedback, other signals are missing, such as facial expression, body position, and environmental clues. The perils inherent in written and electronic communication are discussed later in this chapter.

POSITIVE COMMUNICATION TECHNIQUES

To be a successful health care provider, clinical nurse, or nurse leader, you need exceptional communication skills—and you need to be able to use them during high-stress situations.
The University of St. Augustine for Health Sciences (2023)

Effective communication involves a positive exchange of ideas between or among individuals. The successful communicator strives to demonstrate openness, availability, and acceptance both verbally and nonverbally. Following are some of the many techniques that help achieve positive communication.

Developing Trust

Trust between the nurse and the patient is essential to good communication and often must be cultivated. Factors that enhance the development of trust include openness on the part of the nurse, honesty, integrity, and dependability. The nurse can demonstrate these factors by:
- Communicating clearly in language that laypersons can understand.
- Keeping promises.
- Protecting confidentiality.
- Avoiding negative communication techniques such as blocking and false reassurance.
- Being available to the patient.

The need for trust in the health care setting is not limited to the nurse–patient relationship but, rather, pervades all working relationships. Care is more effective when the nursing team and the interprofessional team share the essential element of trust.

Using "I" Messages

The use of "I" messages is a fundamental component in acceptable communication. Consider the following exchange.

Laura: "You make me so mad, Donald."

Donald: "I don't mean to make you mad."

Laura: "Well, you do. You never think about how I feel. You know I hate it when you leave a patient's room as cluttered as 103."

Donald: "You don't have the vaguest idea what went on here last night! That's what I hate about you—always so quick to judge. You are so critical. You must think that you are perfect!"

When a comment starts with "You," most commonly the receiver's defenses promptly go on alert. The use of "you" in such a context sounds—and most probably is meant to be—accusatory. Notice how the emotions quickly escalate to anger. Also notice that although the receiver initially tries to sound conciliatory, he soon begins to respond in a similar accusatory form. Instead of using accusatory and defensive language, the sender should frame the comment in terms of how it makes them feel. Consider this alternative:

Laura: "Donald, I feel so upset when I find a cluttered room like 103 at the beginning of my shift. I feel as if I am behind when I start."

The difference is obvious. When "I" messages are used they are less likely to sound accusatory. By using such an opening the sender allows the receiver to respond to the true message rather than start to mount a defense. It allows for more effective communication because the receiver is more likely to offer an explanation such as the following:

Donald: "I'm really sorry about room 103, Laura. I guess the wheel that doesn't squeak doesn't get oiled, as they say. Our shift started last night with a patient coding right after he arrived from the emergency department. There was no family here. It took forever to find them and then to support them through the shock. About the time things settled down, the patient in room 110 coded. It was quite a night."

In this instance the "I" message enhances communication by giving Donald the opportunity to address the real concern. In addition, if Laura is truly astute she has a wonderful opportunity to support her colleague by voicing appreciation for the working circumstances of his shift. Most people respond gratefully to recognition and commiseration. The exchange could build collegiality between the two coworkers and perhaps between the two shifts.

Establishing Eye Contact

As mentioned previously the avoidance of eye contact can be interpreted in a number of different ways. A person who does not make eye contact may be thought to be shy, scared, insecure, preoccupied, unprepared, or dishonest—the list could go on and on. None of these qualities is likely to be appreciated in a primary caregiver. By making direct eye contact the nurse gives undivided attention to the patient, and the patient is likely to feel valued and understood by the nurse. Eye contact is equally important in communication with coworkers and other members of the interprofessional team.

Keep in mind, however, that the use of direct eye contact is a Western value. In some cultures avoidance of eye contact is considered more appropriate social behavior. By careful observation the nurse will quickly recognize whether direct eye contact is interpreted as inappropriate or disrespectful. Nurses must make every effort to be sensitive to the cultural values of clients and their coworkers to enhance effective communication.

Keeping Promises

Little else can destroy the fragile trust developing in any interpersonal relationship as quickly as making and then breaking promises. Inherent in the concept of promise keeping are the qualities of honesty and integrity. Once a commitment is made every effort must be expended to fulfill the expectation. Sometimes the request is impossible to satisfy. If this happens the nurse must explain the situation or circumstances. The fact that the patient understands that the nurse has made an effort to meet their needs or desires is often more important than whether the goal is accomplished. If the nurse responds, "I'll check on that" and then finds the request impossible to fulfill but never returns with an explanation, the lack of dependability perceived by the patient (or colleague) will surely drive a wedge into the relationship.

Expressing Empathy

Empathy is the ability to mentally place oneself in another person's situation to better understand the person and to share the emotions or feelings of that person. Empathy is not feeling sorry for another; rather, it is understanding the experiences of the other person, and it is integral to the therapeutic relationship. The nurse is able to perceive and address the needs of the patient without becoming so emotionally involved as to become inappropriately immersed in the situation.

Using Open Communication

Certain styles of phrasing questions and statements lend themselves to obtaining more information. For example, suppose Chris asks Mr. Barrow, "Do you know where you are?" and Mr. Barrow responds, "Yes." Can Chris assume that Mr. Barrow knows he is in the hospital? Not necessarily. Chris may be surprised to hear a completely unexpected response if he rephrases the inquiry:

Chris: "Mr. Barrow, tell me where you are."

Mr. Barrow: "Why, I'm in the honeymoon cabin of the Titanic, of course. Have you seen my lovely bride?"

Using open-ended questions or statements that require more information than "Yes" or "No" responses can help gather enough facts to build a more complete picture of the circumstances. Questions or statements that are phrased to require only one- or two-word responses may miss the mark entirely.

Clarifying Information

Both communicants have a responsibility to clarify anything not understood. The sender should ask for feedback to be certain the receiver is correctly interpreting what is being said. The receiver should stop the sender any time the message becomes unclear and should provide feedback regularly so that misinterpretation can be identified quickly. Such phrases as "What I hear you saying is ..." and "I understand you to mean ..." help communicate to the sender what is being perceived. Other techniques of clarification include using easily understood language, giving examples, drawing a picture, making a list, and finding ways to stimulate all the senses to enhance the ability to understand.

Being Aware of Body Language

Body positioning and movement send loud messages to others. The nurse can imply openness that facilitates effective communication through awareness of body position and movement. In addition to eye contact effective communication is enriched through an open stance, such as holding one's arms at the sides or out toward the patient, rather than crossed, or leaning toward the patient as if to hear more clearly, rather than away from the patient.

Using Touch

Most people have a fairly well-defined personal space. It is important for the nurse to be sensitive to each patient's personal preference and cultural differences in terms of touch. However, for many people, a gentle touch can scale mountains in terms of demonstrating genuine interest and concern. A pat on the back, a hand held, a touch on the shoulder—these are all behaviors that indicate availability and accessibility on the part of the nurse.

NEGATIVE COMMUNICATION TECHNIQUES

Several negative communication techniques have been alluded to in the previous discussion. Closed communication styles, such as asking yes-or-no questions or making inquiries that require single-word answers, potentially limit the response and may prevent the discovery of pertinent facts. Closed body language can also hinder effective communication. Crossed arms, hands on the hips, avoidance of eye contact, turning away from the person, and moving away from the person all impose a sense of distance in the relationship. Three other techniques that are detrimental to good communication are termed *blocking*, *false assurances*, and *conflicting messages*.

Blocking

Blocking occurs when the nurse responds with noncommittal or generalized answers. For example:

"Nurse, I've never had surgery before. I'm afraid I might not ever wake up." Mr. Clayton is twisting the bed sheet as he speaks.

"Oh, Mr. Clayton, many people feel that way. It'll be okay." Makayla Butler, RN, smiles brightly, pats his hand, picks up the dirty linen bag, and bounces out of the room.

Does Mr. Clayton feel reassured? Not likely. Will he be inclined to broach the subject with Makayla again? Probably not. Makayla has incorporated some important aspects of positive communication into her response— cheerfulness and touch—but she has not truly communicated. She has effectively blocked Mr. Clayton's attempt to get the reassurance he wanted from her. He may be too intimidated to ask anyone else, assuming that his fear is invalid.

By generalizing in this way, Makayla has trivialized Mr. Clayton's concerns. He is not "many people." He needs to be validated as an individual experiencing a legitimate feeling. Makayla can validate his fear and put it into perspective at the same time with a different approach:

Makayla: "What makes you think you might not wake up, Mr. Clayton?"

Mr. Clayton: "Well, my wife's cousin's husband had surgery about 25 years ago, and he never woke up."

Makayla: "What kind of surgery did he have?"

Mr. Clayton: "Uh, it was some kind of heart surgery, and he had another heart attack on the table and died right there."

Makayla: "It sounds like his condition was critical going into surgery."

Mr. Clayton: "Yes, ma'am. He'd been sick for a long time."

Makayla: "It's not uncommon to feel afraid of having anesthesia, especially if you have never had surgery before. There are rare cases in which complications do occur during surgery. That's why we put the disclosures on the consent form, so that you will know just what the risks are. Thankfully, though, most surgeries are without such drastic problems. Although your gallbladder certainly has made you uncomfortable, you are otherwise in good health. The tests that were done before surgery, like the chest radiograph and the laboratory work, show that you are healthy and should do well with the anesthesia. That drastically decreases the chance for complications in your case. I will be glad to answer any other questions you have or to ask the anesthetist to come and talk with you some more."

Makayla has validated Mr. Clayton's feeling as legitimate, provided an explanation with reasonable reassurances, and offered to explore the issue with him further or to have someone else talk with him.

Some things are difficult to talk about with another person. The dying patient may want to talk about how they feel, ask questions, or perform a life review. A nurse who is uncomfortable with such topics may consciously or unconsciously block communication about them through generalizations or closed responses. Avoidance of the blocking technique requires a good understanding of oneself. If unable to provide the open communication the patient obviously needs, the nurse should access other personnel who are more comfortable in the situation.

False Assurances

False assurances are similar to blocking and have about the same effect. When someone is trying to get real answers or express serious concerns, an answer such as "Don't worry" or "It'll be okay" sends several unintended messages. Such answers can be interpreted by the patient as placating or showing a lack of concern or a lack of knowledge of the situation. The patient might even conclude that the nurse is being neglectful through trivialization of an issue that is important to them. At the very least the nurse has neither recognized the need the patient has expressed nor provided validation.

Conflicting Messages

If a person professes pleasure at seeing someone but draws back when that person extends a hand of greeting, the nonverbal message speaks more loudly than the words spoken. If a nurse enters a room and goes through the routine greeting by rote (even with a smiling face and a bouncing step), a patient can quickly perceive this and consider the nurse less approachable.

The nurse's statement that the patient's condition is important to the nurse followed by failing to answer the call bell in a timely manner or by forgetting to bring items promised sends a double message. Such behavior can leave the patient confused, frustrated, or angry. Carrying through with a commitment, no matter how unimportant it may seem, is a premier method of saying to the person, "You are important to me."

Logical Fallacies

Logical fallacies are related to an individual's culture, gender, background, and personal experiences and are barriers to meaningful communication. Individuals often cannot separate moods, thoughts, and perceptions. They become interconnected in one continuous evaluation process, involving feeling, thinking, and responding. In times of increased stress, as is common in health care settings, it is more likely that people will employ faulty thinking that affects the communication process. *Recognition of distortions and faulty logic will promote effective communication and reduce confusion or even prevent* conflict. Some commonly occurring logical fallacies in health care communication with examples are listed in Table 19.1.

LISTENING

Nature has given men one tongue and two ears, in token that we should listen twice as much as we speak.
Epictetus

Listening certainly is as important an element in clear and effective communication as any other component.

TABLE 19.1   Logical Fallacies That Trip Us Up, With Examples

Logical Fallacy	Example
Ad Hominen Abusive: *An argument that attacks the person instead of the issue.*	A nurse has a disagreement with a physician about lab results that were not properly reported. The nurse states to colleagues: "She thinks she's so smart just because she's a doctor." *The focus becomes the person rather than the issue.*
Appeal to Emotion: *An attempt to manipulate other people's emotions to avoid the real issue.*	Deb Engles, RN, has repeatedly failed to document patient care properly. She was called into the nurse manager's office to discuss the incidents and receives a written warning. She comes out tearful. She begins to discuss the problem and makes the following statements: "I am the first person in my family to even go to college. I'm a single parent, and I've worked so hard to get where I am. Our manager doesn't care anything about that. She just wants to pass out written warnings to cover herself. She doesn't care about us as individuals." *The nurse seeks an emotional response rather than facing the actual issue of poor documentation.*
Red Herring: *Introduction of an irrelevant topic to divert attention away from the real issue.*	Two nurses, Brian and Nikoah, are having an argument regarding Brian's failure to complete his assigned tasks. Brian states: "It's not my work that you're really mad about. It's that I'm a guy. You just don't like male nurses." *The issue is unfinished tasks, not nurse gender.*

Many distracters contribute to poor listening habits. Framing an answer while the other person is still talking interferes with receiving the entire message. Environmental disturbances can provide major disruption. A crying baby, a call light buzzing, and multiple concurrent conversations in a busy nurses' station are a few of the interruptions that jumble the simplest of instructions. Preexisting concerns or worries can block absorption of conversation because of the preoccupation. Attempts to continue work in progress leads to inattention. Ineffective engagement or peculiar mannerisms on the part of the speaker can be distracting. A person who does not make eye contact, shuffles through papers while talking, or overuses hand movements actually can deter communication. Active listening involves three steps: (1) listening carefully to know what was said; (2) processing the information you heard; and (3) making a decision about what you heard. Does it make sense? Do you believe it? How can you respond appropriately?

As the receiver, you can use a number of techniques to facilitate the ability to listen:

- Give undivided attention to the sender by moving to a quieter area to avoid distractions and clarifying any points you haven't understood.
- Provide feedback in terms of the perceived meaning of the message by rephrasing in your own words.
- Give attention to positioning so you are facing the sender and making eye contact.

- Note nonverbal messages, such as body language, and respond to them.
- Finish listening before you begin to speak.

If you have accomplished each of these steps, you have engaged in active listening. Active listening dramatically improves the likelihood of receiving the correct message. Equally important, active listening implies a respect for the speaker and communicates a regard for what the speaker has to offer. The nonverbal message that active listening delivers is, "I value you, and what you have to say is important to me."

WRITTEN AND ELECTRONIC COMMUNICATION

I admire machinery as much as any man, and am as thankful to it as any man can be for what it does for us. But, it will never be a substitute for the face of a man, with his soul in it, encouraging another man to be brave and true.

Charles Dickens

Charles Dickens referred to the brand-new telegraph when he admired machinery. Little could he imagine the advances of electronic communication over the decades. But his message is as appropriate today as in the late 1800s. Nothing quite replaces face-to-face communication and the accompanying nonverbal cues. However, written and electronic communications do open valuable new levels of connection and information exchange.

Electronic health records (EHR) are commonplace in health care organizations today to help promote higher-quality patient care. However, unique issues have impacted the transition to the EHR. Perhaps the most positive aspect is in improved communication among health care providers within the organization as well as between geographically distant sites. On the negative side is concern about maintaining patient confidentiality and privacy, an expectation that must be met with diligent attention to appropriate system management and careful individual protection of information, passwords, and other access sources for the EHR (see Chapter 15 for a more detailed discussion of EHRs and health information technology).

As communication moves into the cyber environment with the use of the EHR, e-mail and attachments, intranets, chat rooms for clinical discussions/meetings, and further into the realm of social media (see later discussion in this chapter), the style of health care documentation has changed. Nurses' electronic clinical notes often comprise detailed checklists designed to address a myriad of potential findings and streamline time spent charting. However, most checklist pages include a box for additional comments/explanations, and charting programs include some vehicle for a narrative entry. The following discussion is just as applicable to electronic charting as to pen-and-paper charting—perhaps even more so. By their very nature checklists do not allow for the unexpected or aberrant event. As tempting as it may be to confine the nursing record to the checklists, some occurrences simply cannot be adequately described without a narrative entry.

Accuracy

Absolute accuracy is paramount in recording legal documentation. For the nurse this statement most specifically applies to the nursing notes and any other entry the nurse makes in the patient's chart. Every effort should be made to report concisely, descriptively, and truthfully. To write "Patient walked today" is not adequate. A more concise and descriptive entry reads "Patient walked to the nurses' station and back three times this shift, a total distance of 96 yards" (many hospitals have distance measures marked in the hallway for this purpose).

Consider the following situation: Cody Johnson, RN, entered the patient's room and found her agitated and speaking loudly into the telephone as she twisted her hair with her free hand. She was crying and periodically pounded the bedside table with her fist. Later the patient told Cody that she had been talking with her mother. Would it be appropriate for Cody to chart "Patient became very angry with her mother while talking on the telephone"? No. The nurse must be diligent not to include personal judgments or quantify the patient's emotional state in such terms.

Attention to Detail

In addition to absolute accuracy, written documents should be descriptive. As mentioned previously information should be quantified whenever possible. How many feet did the patient walk? How many times was the patient out of bed? How many milliliters of fluid did the patient drink? Precisely what did the patient say?

Words can be used to depict a verbal picture of a wound, rash, bruise, or any type of injury or situation. Illustrative terms can create a mental image for the person reading the notes, memo, or other communication. Descriptive categories can include measurement, color, position, location, drainage, or condition when speaking of a physical condition; time, setting, people present, issues, or goals when reporting a discussion; and direct quotes when describing a meeting, conference, evaluation, or other interchange. Consider the differences between the following written communications:

- "1000: Dressing change completed. Site healthy."
- "1000: Dressing change completed. Edges of 4-inch surgical wound approximated, no drainage noted. Skin pink without any redness or edema."

The second entry allows the reader to "see" the wound mentally and follow the progress of healing, even when unable to be present at the time of the dressing change. A good rule when describing any kind of break in skin integrity—from a stabbing, a surgical wound, an intravenous line, and so on—is to describe color, drainage, and presence or absence of edema.

Consider the written communication in Box 19.1. What does this message really tell the nurse manager? Not much—only that there is some kind of perceived problem between Lucas and the students. The nurse manager cannot tell, from the information provided, whether the problem is "real," is based on a bias of Jessica's or a student, or has occurred more than once; whether an interpersonal communication problem or

---

BOX 19.1   Incomplete E-Mail Message

Date: 12/18/2020

To:	Bonnie Thompson, RN, BSN, Nurse Manager
From:	Jessica Lindsay, RN, BSN, Charge Nurse
Subject:	Student precepting

I have had lots of complaints about Lucas Alfred's treatment of students. I do not think he should be assigned as a preceptor anymore and do not plan to do so from now on.

BOX 19.2   Descriptive, Thorough E-Mail Message

Date: 12/18/2020

To:	Bonnie Thompson, RN, BSN, Nurse Manager
From:	Jessica Lindsay, RN, BSN, Charge Nurse
Subject:	Student precepting

Today (Monday, August 18) at 0710 I observed what appeared to be an animated conversation between Lucas Alfred, RN, and John Roberts, a student nurse from North Hills University. As I moved toward them I heard Lucas say loudly, "Well, you better stay with me because I am not going to come looking for you all day. I know how lazy students are." I asked Lucas, "Is there a problem?" He replied, "Oh, no problem. I just hate having students, that's all. They're more trouble than they're worth." I asked Lucas, "Would you prefer that I reassign the student?" He shrugged his shoulders and walked away. I suggested to the student that I assign him to another nurse for the day. He responded, "I'd really appreciate that. Mr. Alfred has let me know since I arrived that he didn't want to work with me."

Because this group of students has been on the unit 2 days per week for the past 3 weeks, I spoke with the other students who had worked with Lucas and asked them how things had gone. The other three students who have worked with him reported similar experiences.

I would like to arrange a time to meet with you and Lucas to address this problem.

---

misunderstanding exists; or whether obvious mistreatment of a student or students has occurred.

Now consider the written communication in Box 19.2. Carefully constructing a factual message of this length is more time-consuming initially, but it will save a lot of frustration in the long run. The nurse manager now has a clear picture of what has occurred and knows that an ongoing problem exists. Most appropriately, Jessica will speak to Bonnie about the problem, even if only briefly. However, a written account of the incident must be submitted and should be composed promptly while the facts are freshly remembered.

The skill of writing concisely yet descriptively must be developed. Over some time nurses build a repertoire of phrases and illustrative terminology that are useful and effective. Often, when a nurse is stumped as to how to express a situation, she or he will ask a colleague, "How would you write ...?" Accessing the experience and expertise of nursing peers is productive in terms of problem-solving, while also demonstrating respect for the colleague.

Thoroughness

The message examples in the previous section also illustrate the need for thoroughness. In addition to being descriptive in terms of the incident, Jessica's message in Box 19.2 reported her interview with other nursing students. By doing so Jessica is thorough in describing and reporting the extent of the problem she has discovered. Providing such completeness of information helps prevent communication breakdown. Anticipating and answering relevant questions before they are asked exemplifies thoroughness and clarifies communication.

Conciseness

Written communication must be concise. The message must state the necessary information as clearly and as briefly as possible. Consider the message written in Box 19.3. Whew! Extraneous details tend to confuse more than clarify. An inherent dilemma often develops as the nurse attempts to determine how to be descriptive and concise at the same time. One must determine what facts are pertinent to enable the reader to understand the true message. When in doubt and when appropriate, the writer can ask another party to read the message and provide feedback as to what the reader believes the message means. However, the right to confidentiality and privacy of the people involved must be observed. This basic principle applies to patients, families, students, members of the health care team—to all persons. Consequently, the nurse must be

---

BOX 19.3 Unclear, Rambling E-Mail Message

Date: 12/18/2020

To:	Bonnie Thompson, RN, BSN, Nurse Manager
From:	Jessica Lindsay, RN, BSN, Charge Nurse
Subject:	Student precepting

Today at about 0730 (it may have been earlier because I don't remember whether the breakfast trays had been served or not), I observed what appeared to be an animated conversation between Lucas Alfred, RN, and John Roberts, SN, a student nurse from North Hills University. I thought they might be arguing, but I couldn't tell for sure, so I decided to go over and see what the conversation was about. It really seemed like Lucas was angry because he was talking loudly and not smiling and neither was the student smiling, and I heard Lucas say, "Well, you better stay with me because I am not going to come looking for you all day. I know how lazy students are." Well I could just imagine how that made the student feel, so I asked, "Is there a problem?" even though it was pretty obvious that something was wrong. Lucas said, "Oh, no problem. I just hate having students, that's all. They're more trouble than they're worth." I asked Lucas, "Would you prefer that I reassign the student?" He shrugged his shoulders and walked away. Well I don't know for sure about the student, but I really thought that was rude. I suggested to the student that I assign him to another nurse for the day. He responded, "I'd really appreciate that. He has let me know since I arrived that he didn't want to work with me." Well I know how that would make me feel—to be a student and be treated that way.

The same group of students has been on the unit 2 days a week for the past 3 weeks (maybe a month, I'm not sure, and some of them may have been here on makeup days too), so I talked with other students who had worked with Lucas and asked them how things had been going. They said he'd acted the same way to them. We need to talk to him.

---

as judicious in handling written material in a confidential manner as with any other form of communication.

Electronic Communication

When speaking aloud you punctuate constantly— with body language. Your listener hears commas, dashes, question marks, exclamation points, [and] quotation marks as you shout, whisper, pause, wave your arms, roll your eyes, wrinkle your brow. In writing, punctuation plays the role of body language. It helps the readers hear the way you want to be heard.
Russell Baker

More and more communication is computer-based, using e-mail, text messages, chat rooms, file attachments, and other electronic modes. The computer-based written record can be somewhat more transient than other written documents. For example, e-mails are often read and then deleted. However, remember that communication via the computer can be saved and is often retrievable even after deletion. As with any form of written communication computer-based interaction loses nonverbal cues. Therefore it is important for the sender to elicit feedback and/or for the receiver to ask for clarification if the meaning of the communication is not clear.

HAND-OFF REPORT

A hand-off is a transfer and acceptance of patient care responsibility achieved through effective communication.
The Joint Commission (2017)

A hand-off report occurs any time the primary care of a patient is transferred from one health care provider to another. Examples include end of shift, relocation to another unit or another facility, and transfer to the operating room, radiology, dialysis, or other areas for testing or shorter periods of care. Every time patient care is transferred represents a potential for patient harm related to lack of adequate information about the patient and their care needs. Information can be insufficient, inaccurate, untimely, misinterpreted, or undergo any number of other missteps that result in minor to severe harm to the patient. Once again the sender–receiver dichotomy with all the associated communication skills is of primary importance.

Perhaps the most important condition of hand-off reporting is that it must be real-time, face-to-face. Recording the report or providing it in written or electronic form leaves too many opportunities for missed data and misunderstanding. Give and take between the sender and receiver must occur so that clarification and feedback are possible. Certainly written reinforcement of a verbal face-to-face report is essential. Reports should also be given in situations free from interruptions.

Many facilities use a standardized format or mnemonic for a systematic approach to end-of-shift and other hand-off reports. In the absence of formal report formatting individuals can certainly develop their own style of reporting that covers all aspects of the patient's condition and care. Following a systematic approach every time enhances the quality of the report, thereby protecting the patient.

Essentials of an effective report include the basic SBAR: situation, background, assessment, and recommendation (The Joint Commission, 2017) as well as pertinent information regarding patient events during the shift. Information should promote continuity of care.

Always give the receiver an opportunity to ask questions and clarify information. Clear, concise, and organized communication is also essential when reporting a change of condition to a provider or another clinician. Regardless of conducting a hand-off or reporting a change of condition, consistently be aware that it is the sender's responsibility to relay sufficient information to move the provision of quality care forward. See Table 19.2 for an example of communication with a provider regarding a patient's status using the SBAR technique.

COMMUNICATION STYLES

Communication also includes intentionality, mutuality, partnerships, trust, and presence.
American Association of College of Nursing (2023)

Communication is influenced by a myriad of individual characteristics learned over a lifetime. However, communication specialists generally recognize four basic communication styles: (1) assertive, (2) aggressive, (3) passive, and (4) passive–aggressive.

Assertive Communication

The healthiest form of communication is the assertive style. Assertive individuals pronounce their basic rights without violating the rights of others. Assertive communicators are honest and direct while valuing and respecting other individuals' views and seeking a win–win solution without the use of manipulation or game playing. Assertiveness includes active listening and reflective feedback so that other individuals recognize that their opinions are valued as the assertive communicator seeks to find an acceptable solution without compromising' their own needs.

Assertive communication requires self-confidence and the ability to set limits rather than to succumb to pressure to avoid disappointing or hurting others at the expense of one's own needs and expectations. Although it is the most effective style of communication, healthy assertiveness is difficult for many people to develop. Therefore assertive communication is typically the style most people use least.

Aggressive Communication

Aggressive communicators make decisions for themselves and others with the intent of always coming out

TABLE 19.2 **SBAR Example**	
Situation: Clearly and briefly describe the current situation.	"Dr. Merrill, this is Sandy Harper, RN. I am calling from University Hospital about your patient David Hodges. Here's the situation: Mr. Hodges is complaining of shortness of breath and chest pain and is having increasing diaphoresis with a rapid heart rate."
Background: Provide clear, relevant background information on the patient.	"The supporting background information is that Mr. Hodges had a total hip replacement 2 days ago for severe osteoarthritis. About 10 minutes ago he began complaining of sudden onset of chest pain and shortness of breath and perspiring profusely. His pulse is 126 and his blood pressure is 110 over 62. He is restless and appears to be short of breath and anxious."
Assessment: State your professional conclusion, based on the situation and background.	"My assessment of the situation is that he may be having a cardiac event or a pulmonary embolism."
Recommendation: Tell the person with whom you're communicating what you need from them, in a clear and relevant way.	"I recommend that you see him immediately and that we start him on O_2 stat. Do you agree? What other orders would you like to initiate?"

"the winner." Aggressive individuals want their needs met exclusively and immediately, using guilt, hurt, anger, and a repertoire of other manipulation tools. Aggressiveness may use honesty but in a hurtful, manipulative way. Aggressive individuals commonly feel superior to others and behave in very controlling ways. Persons with whom they communicate often feel humiliated, defensive, resentful, and hurt. Aggressive behavior often leads to, and certainly escalates, conflict.

Passive Communication

Passive communicators are the polar opposite of aggressive communicators. They allow others to make decisions for them in the hope of avoiding confrontation or difficult situations. Passive communicators are typically inhibited, indirect, and self-denying because they feel those characteristics make for the safe route. If they win in a situation it is purely by chance, typically because they happen to share the opinion of the more aggressive person in the exchange. Passive individuals are dishonest because they would rather succumb than state their true feelings or needs.

Passive–Aggressive Communication

Passive–aggressive communicators combine the worst of both styles. These individuals avoid direct confrontation while manipulating others to achieve their personal goals. They appear to be honest but "come in the back door" by undermining other individuals through gossip, pouting, playing the victim, and other manipulative behaviors that create or escalate conflict. They win in situations by making other individuals look bad.

SPECIAL INFLUENCES ON COMMUNICATION

Development of truly effective communication necessitates understanding various circumstances that influence communication. In addition to the concepts discussed up to this point, characteristics exist that might impede efficacious exchange of information. Issues such as gender differences, generational differences, cultural diversity, physical and intellectual disabilities, and dissimilarities in the professional approach of the various health care disciplines all contribute to disparate understandings and interpretations.

Communication and Gender Differences

A significant clarification must be made regarding communication between men and women. The information about gender differences resulting from socialization (although based on research and many years of observations and writings) consists of generalizations and should be viewed from that perspective. Attributes described do not necessarily apply to all persons or all the time. Nevertheless a plethora of observations indicate that men and women solve problems, make decisions, and communicate from different perspectives on the basis of socialization that begins shortly after birth. Typically boys are taught to be tough and competitive; girls are taught to be nice and avoid conflict.

For the most part women work toward compromise, even when it means relinquishing some of the original goal. Often women use indirect channels such as questions to guide a conversation toward the point they want to make. Preserving relationships is usually of paramount importance to women. The role of peacemaker and nurturer has been a traditional expectation of women throughout the ages.

Traditional role expectations of men have included provider and protector. Men learn early in life how to focus on goals and move aggressively toward accomplishment. Consequently men have been socialized to behave assertively when such performance is needed in pursuit of the goal and then move on without loss of friendships. Women have been socialized to believe that assertive behavior will endanger relationships and that conflict should be avoided to preserve friendships.

Men typically use communication as a tool to deliver information, whereas women value the process of communication itself as an important part of the relationship. Therefore in an effort to improve communication men might try spending more time in discussion, and women might try to phrase comments more succinctly.

Progress has been made over the years as women move into more lateral working situations, but the problem of gender communication style differences persists. Booher (2020) echoes these thoughts in light of today's work environment: "Little did we know that the communication differences we experienced as children on the playground would move from the classroom to the boardroom. Neither men nor women are better communicators. They're just different." Awareness of this difference supports effective communication in the health care environment, where effective transfer of information is essential.

Individuals With Physical or Intellectual Disabilities

Approximately 6.5 million people in the US have an intellectual disability ... [they] report difficulty finding appropriately trained and willing healthcare providers.

CDC (2019)

Sadly, health care literature indicates that individuals with disabilities, particularly adults, have deficits in health care interactions (Stransky & Morris, 2019). Reasons are multifaceted, including a misconception that individuals with mobility and/or speaking problems are also intellectually delayed. Persons with limited mobility or speech deficits often take more time to form and communicate a response, whether verbal, written, or via device. Allowing for processing time is one of the most important considerations for communication with the disabled. Individuals with intellectual disabilities have varying levels of understanding and communication skills. Every effort should be made to address the individual at the level and in the manner with which they can understand. Table 19.3 presents a list of the most common problems encountered by disabled individuals along with appropriate and inappropriate responses.

Communication and Generational Differences

In recent years much attention has been focused on the fact that our society has at least five distinct generational groups. They are variously described as follows:

- Silents/Traditionalists/Veterans—born before the mid-1940s
- Baby Boomers—born between the mid-1940s and the mid-1960s
- Generation X (Gen Xers)—born between the mid-1960s and 1980
- Generation Y/Millennials—born between 1981 and 2000
- Homeland Generation or Homelanders/Generation Z—variously described as born since 9/11/01 or 2000 (CBS News, 2010; Nurse Educator, 2009).

TABLE 19.3 **Communication With Individuals Who Have Disabilities**
Speak directly to the patient using a normal tone of voice and inflection. **DO:** Make eye contact when culturally acceptable. **DO NOT:** Look over the patient and talk to the accompanying significant other or caregiver.
Communication difficulties associated with physical or intellectual disabilities <ins>cannot</ins> be equated with complete lack of cognitive understanding. **DO:** Confirm the intellectual level of the patient's understanding prior to interacting. Use lay language to explain just as you would with any patient, modified only according to the known language level of the patient. **DO NOT:** Speak in "baby talk" or "talk down" to the patient.
Use modalities of communication that are familiar to the patient. **DO:** Use any devices the patient/caregiver brings to the health care setting. Allow the patient to write if that is more comfortable for them. Respond in writing if it is their preference. Consider visuals, letter boards, digital notepads, or other types of communication boards. Allow the patient plenty of time to consider information and respond. Establish gestures that can relay information such as eye blinks and hand gestures depending on the mobility level of the patient. Consider learning some basic American Sign Language signs for health-care–related topics (i.e., pain, hunger). **DO NOT:** Rush the patient, appear impatient, or commit other negative blocking techniques through verbal or body language.
Allow as much physical movement as needed/possible. **DO:** Make room for voluntary and involuntary movements. Recognize that movement is helpful for some patients to process. **DO NOT:** Constrain the patient with limited ability to achieve desired movement associated with communication.
Reduce outside stimulation—less is more. **DO:** Provide a calming environment—dim lighting, limited noise, fewer team members present. Present concise, clear information in as few words as possible, especially when giving directions. **DO NOT:** Overwhelm the patient with huge teams of caregivers, multiple simultaneous tasks, and rapid speech.

(Adapted from C. Hernandez, personal communication, May 10, 2020).

Awareness of generational differences and the accompanying differences in communication styles is important to nurses from two perspectives—communication with the patients/families and communication with one another.

Traditionalists. Generally members of this oldest surviving generation follow the rules, valuing authority, formality, and the chain-of-command. They take pride in accomplishment, are strong decision-makers, and have a good sense of self. Tradition is important to them, making them more likely to make decisions according to what has or has not worked in the past. Appearance and respect are important to them. Therefore they appreciate communication in a more formal style, appropriate dress, and displays of respect.

Baby Boomers. Baby Boomers grew up in an era of prosperity that formed their worldview, values, and work ethic. Although they questioned political policy, authority, and social mores, they ultimately embraced work as a definition of self-worth, adopting a strong work ethic, becoming goal-directed, and experiencing the accompanying struggle with work–personal life balance. These attributes lead to an expectation of similar commitment from younger generations. Effective communication with Baby Boomers includes direct information in a personable approach, a formal plan, and acknowledgment of value, purpose, and respect.

Generation X. The milieu that Gen Xers experienced during their formative years was fraught with insecurity. The breakdown in many of the traditional security sources helped create a generation of independent problem-solvers. The increase in divorces; the prevalence of acquired immunodeficiency syndrome, gangs, and abortions; and the exposure of corrupt government officials and policies created an unstable societal environment in which individuals who could meet challenges, recognize and respond to opportunity, and become comfortable with diversity excelled. Xers value autonomy in their work, decision-making, and life choices, but at the same time value the team and teamwork. Although they may appear to move too quickly and to be insensitive, having grown up in a technology-based society, they are capable of fierce commitment to tasks they value. These individuals should be allowed to be highly involved in decision-making about health care—whether they are the providers or the recipients.

Millennials. Millennials are the most diverse and most globally thinking generation in the workforce, in large part because of technology, which provides unfettered access to global issues and occurrences. Many come from or are close to "nontraditional" families and have witnessed unparalleled violence within the borders of our country. Their comfort with technology and diversity are hallmark characteristics. They value inclusion, team effort, and collective action, and they are quite adaptable to rapid change. Because they are focused on cohesiveness and peer orientation they value immediate feedback. Such activities as "huddles"—periodic and end-of-shift briefings that allow the team to stay informed and make plans work well with this group of communicators.

Homelanders/Generation Z. The line between Millennials and Homelanders/Generation Z is blurry, starting with the choice of years for transition from one to the other. Influences on Homelanders/Generation Z include the cascade of occurrences within our borders starting with 9/11, as well as continuously burgeoning technology. Like Traditionalists this generational group is growing up in a time of financial and political insecurity at home and globally. They are comfortable with multitasking, diversity, and technology like no one before them. Homelanders/Generation Z are expected to pursue college education as a matter of necessity as the gap between those who are financially sound and those who are not continues to widen. It remains to be seen how they will relate in the workplace or in the role of health care recipient, but we can expect articulate, motivated, tech-savvy individuals coming of age in the near future.

Communication and Cultural Diversity

Although Chapter 10 is devoted to cultural and social issues, it is important to highlight cultural issues specific to communication. Sensitivity to cultural differences is an integral part of the nurse's responsibility. Many cultural beliefs are tightly interwoven with strong religious convictions. Societies throughout the world depend on a variety of alternative healing sources as strongly as or even more strongly than on medical science. Some people rarely have an opportunity to interface with medical science as it is known in developed countries.

The obvious difficulty is a potential language barrier. Even if the person speaks English as a second language the preponderance of slang terms and colloquialisms can confound a literal translation. Additionally, the stress associated with illness and possibly hospitalization only adds to the potential for misunderstanding and frustration. Fortunately most communities have interpreters willing to translate in the health care setting. The variety of language interpreters (including sign language for the deaf) available even in smaller communities is surprising.

Many forms of communication do not carry the same meanings in various cultures. In some instances direct eye contact is to be avoided if possible. Touch, also considered a positive communication technique in Western culture, may be perceived as a serious invasion of privacy. Some gestures considered innocuous in one culture may represent vulgarity in another. Some cultures strictly adhere to paternalism; unless the male head of the family agrees to a procedure or treatment the family member will refuse under any circumstance. Although many people share a sense of modesty, some cultures experience a greater feeling of violation at having to expose certain body parts than do others. The consumption of certain foods, the use of blood or blood products—the possibilities of culturally diverse practices are endless. The prudent nurse must become knowledgeable about the specific cultural practices in the region of their employment. (See Chapter 10 for further discussion of communication issues related to culture.)

Interprofessional Team Communication

The *interprofessional team* is composed of people from a variety of disciplines who approach health care from the unique perspectives of the theories and therapies of their individual professions. Consider the variety represented by nurses, physicians, dietitians, respiratory therapists, pharmacists, occupational therapists, physical therapists, psychologists, and social workers. Then add to the mosaic the sublevel of specialists: cardiologists, endocrinologists, oncologists, orthopedists, clinical nurse specialists, recreational therapists, nurse anesthetists, nurse practitioners, and nurse scientists. RNs with varied educational backgrounds (diploma, associate degree, Bachelor or Master of Science in Nursing) and licensed vocational nurses are often found in the same unit with similar assignments. Now add managers, administrators, unlicensed assistive personnel, clerical staff, accountants, and housekeeping, to name a few. Also consider cultural and generational differences among health care professionals and workers. Is it any wonder that communication disasters occur?

All of the positive communication techniques previously discussed must be used to clearly understand another's perception. Listening is an essential tool for determination of the intended message as seen from the unique perspective of the other discipline. Frequent clarification and a sense of "safety" are paramount as people explore the meanings that each person attributes to the situation and the discipline-specific suggested solutions. Realization that the fundamental goal of all health care professionals and of ancillary staff is to provide quality patient care should facilitate positive communication.

Confidentiality and Privacy

No discussion of communication is complete without reference to issues of confidentiality and privacy. Breach of confidentiality and the patient's right to privacy through careless gossip has ethical and legal ramifications. Thoughtless conversation in the elevator, the cafeteria, the parking lot, or any other public place has created heartache for the patient and the health care provider alike.

Other sites where communication about confidential or personal patient issues needs to be controlled include the nurses' station, any desks or tables along the halls, and the utility rooms. Such locations are not often viewed as "public" places but many people pass by these areas and overhear information. Exchange of patient information should occur only between persons with the need and right to know and should take place in private areas.

SOCIAL MEDIA—WARNING! WARNING! WARNING!

Ongoing advances in technology ... have increased the likelihood of potential and unintentional breaches of private/confidential health information.
American Nurses Association (2015a)

Social Media: Good and Bad

Social media sites have burgeoned in the last decade, connecting health care professionals across the country and globally. Health care–related sites, chat rooms, blogs, forums, and video sites provide an unparalleled opportunity to network, share, and problem-solve health care issues. But the professional value of social media comes with a very serious caveat. The patient retains their right to confidentiality and privacy in every medium. Not only must nurses be very careful in not using a patient's name, but also they must be thorough in avoiding any other type of identifying information. Such information may include geographical location, facility name, room number, or the patient's age, gender, and diagnosis combined with any of these data.

Nurses, like most of our society, are connected in their personal lives to multiple online social media sources such as Facebook, Twitter, and various blogs. Sitting at home alone with a computer may create a sense of privacy, but nothing could be further from the truth. Postings intended for immediate family or friends and protected by the site's privacy policy are not infallible. Anything posted online exists forever on a server somewhere, even if it is deleted from the site. This information is forever discoverable in a court of law and can be used in a trial (NCSBN, 2018). Friends might find your story so touching or endearing that they repost to their friends, and the story takes on a life of its own with no available control of dissemination on your part.

A good example of the unintended outcome of a moment's misjudgement is presented in NCSBN's (2018) social media guidelines. A nursing student took a picture of a minor child (with permission) and posted it to her Facebook page with a comment about his bravery during his illness and how much she loved her chosen profession. Although she did not identify the patient by name, the patient's room number was visible in the photo. The patient and his hospital were identified by others viewing the post. Ultimately the hospital was charged with a violation of the Health Information Portability and Accountability Act (HIPAA), the nursing program was barred from the clinical site, and the student was expelled. Nursing board actions against a student who makes inappropriate disclosures on a social media site could include the following:

- Unprofessional conduct
- Unethical conduct
- Moral turpitude
- Mismanagement of patient records
- Revealing a privileged communication
- Breach of confidentiality (NCSBN, 2018)

The nursing student's actions in this example also violated state and federal law, putting her at jeopardy of "both criminal and civil penalties, including fines and possible jail time" (NCSBN, 2018).

Certainly it was never the student's intent to behave unethically but her actions created this cascade of events. As a profession we are held to a very high ethical standard to protect our clients' confidentiality. We must be very attentive to our actions.

Another issue that has appeared is the use of texting for communication of patient information among health care providers. Anything that is sent electronically has the potential to be inadvertently misdirected and/or intercepted. The use of secure texting has become a reality in many health care organizations; nurses are encouraged to learn about and understand policies regarding texting in the health care organizations where they practice.

Proper use of social media can open venues of learning, career advancement, mentoring, and networking, enhancing the global perspective in your nursing career. Use this opportunity wisely and with consideration of the permanence, wide visibility (beyond anything you may intend), and potential impact of your postings.

Online Etiquette

Interactions online are guided by the same sense of decency that any other style of communication dictates. Here are some simple rules:

- Be nice. Be ethical. Don't say anything to someone online that you wouldn't say in a face-to-face conversation, and certainly don't fan the flame of conflict or anger.
- Remember the TMI (too much information) concept. Don't give more personal information than others want to hear.
- Write with clarity. Reread what you've written to determine whether it is clear or whether it might be interpreted differently from what you intended.
- Respect others, including their privacy.
- Use discretion. Online postings live forevermore in cyberspace.
- Obey copyright laws.

UNDERSTANDING AND MANAGING CONFLICT

Nurses maintain professional, respectful, and caring relationships with colleagues and are committed to fair treatment, transparency, integrity-preserving compromise, and the best resolution of conflicts.
American Nurses Association, Code of Ethics for Nurses with Interpretive Statements (2015b)

The Nature of Conflict

A major goal of communication is to establish understanding and cooperation with others. However, much of our social environment is characterized by interactions that involve conflict, misunderstanding, and a failure to communicate. When more than one person is involved in the interaction, a potential exists for disagreement and misunderstanding. When the interaction becomes stressful, taking on a competitive, hostile, or oppositional nature, it can be classified as conflict (Mayer, 2012). Despite the discomfort disparate points of view can result in constructive behavior and positive outcomes or they can have detrimental consequences. Some of the benefits that may arise from conflict include: (1) recognize talents and innovative abilities; (2) identify an outlet for expression of aggressive urges; (3) introduce innovation and change; (4) diagnose problems or areas of concern; and (5) establish unity (Mayer, 2012). Harmful consequences of conflict include a negative effect on emotional and physical well-being, an emphasis on one's own welfare over that of the group, a diversion of time and energy from important goals, financial and emotional costs, and personal fatigue.

Most of us experience abundant opportunities for conflict, which may be related to the fact that we bring to our relationships an accumulation of attitudes, beliefs, opinions, and habits. Thus conflict is normal and is not necessarily something to avoid. Maintaining an environment supportive of professional, clear, and sensitive communication enables individuals to disagree more productively, with less hurt, and with a greater chance of resolving differences and disagreements. Characteristics that support professional communication are (Gibb, 1961):

- *Empathy:* Feeling what the other person is feeling and seeing the situation as they see it; believing that the other person's feelings are valid, legitimate, and justified.
- *Equality:* All participants in the process are equal; respect for individual differences is apparent, and people are comfortable expressing themselves freely and openly.
- *Openness:* Feelings and thoughts are stated directly and honestly; no attempt is made to hide or disguise the real object of disagreement.
- *Positivity:* Capitalizing on agreements and using them as a basis for approaching disagreements; conflict is viewed as positive, and individuals involved express positive feelings for one another and the relationship.
- *Supportiveness:* Feelings are expressed with spontaneity rather than with strategy; requires flexibility and a willingness to change personal opinions and positions.

Adopting these communication attitudes and using the positive communication strategies previously discussed can prevent most episodes of conflict in the workplace. However, situations are bound to arise in which the nurse will need to know how to handle a conflict situation and achieve a positive resolution.

Conflict Resolution

People's ability to connect with one another, especially during times of conflict, depends on their capacity to tune into the subtle messages that reveal how a message is actually being received. We seldom create conflict intentionally. Rather, it occurs because we may not be aware of how our own behavior contributes to interpersonal problems. Successful resolution to conflict begins to occur when people are aware of their own and others' feelings and emotions and believe that these concerns are relevant and respected.

The first step in conflict resolution is to recognize how individuals manage conflict. The most common conflict resolution styles are:

- *Avoidance:* One person uses passive behaviors and withdraws from the conflict; neither person is able to pursue goals.
- *Accommodation:* One person puts aside their goals to satisfy the other person's desires.
- *Force:* One person achieves their own goals at the expense of the other person.
- *Compromise:* Both people give up something to get partial goal attainment.
- *Collaboration:* Both people actively try to find solutions that will satisfy them both.

Awareness of one's usual conflict resolution style will go far in understanding how one's own behavior contributes to disagreements. For example, if an individual nurse recognizes avoidance as their common style of dealing with conflict then it would be important for that nurse to review the communication strategies presented in this chapter to identify specific techniques that can be used to develop a more collaborative style of conflict resolution.

Important points to remember: Don't make it personal or take it personally. Use "I" rather than "you" messages to avoid defensive responses. Keep the focus on the issue, not personalities. Do not create an environment in

BOX 19.4   Professional Response to Verbal Conflict

1. Maintain an open and empathetic tone of voice.
2. Maintain eye contact (keeping cultural differences in mind). This may be difficult but it conveys to the other party that you are confident and competent.
3. Maintain an open body stance with your hands at your sides or open toward the person (but not invading the other person's space). Do not cross your arms, tap your foot, wag your finger, or perform any body language that is commonly associated with anger.
4. Do not physically back away unless you perceive you actually are in physical danger. By standing your ground you will convey the message of assurance through your carriage.
5. Be aware of your own values, beliefs, and cultural perspectives.
6. When a conversation is obviously escalating move to a more private location.
7. Listen actively and carefully without criticizing or being defensive.
8. Focus on the problem or issue, not the person(s) involved.
9. Use "I" messages that state your thoughts, feelings, and beliefs in an open and clear manner.
10. Establish ground rules to maintain a safe environment for dialogue, such as that only one person speaks at a time while the other listens.
11. Offer explanations but do not make excuses.
12. Try to understand the intended meaning of what other people are saying.
13. Identify ideas that clarify your own issues and concerns and that are helpful to find solutions.
14. Avoid unhelpful responses to conflict, such as arguing, sarcasm, moralizing, disbelief, contradiction, criticism, ridicule, and threats.
15. Use metaphors and analogies as gentle ways to create and maintain rapport.
16. Maintain a positive context by stating what you want and avoid stating what you do not want.
17. Repeat, or play back, what you believe you are hearing.
18. In more difficult situations consider using a neutral facilitator who understands their role.

which other individuals respond defensively to protect themselves. Do not respond to a conflictive situation as a personal attack—even if it feels like one. Focus and refocus on the issue or behavior rather than the individual.

Another—and very important—step in conflict resolution is active listening (previously discussed in the chapter). Many of us are apprehensive or reticent when communicating during times of conflict, but active listening can reduce the emotional charge from the situation so that both parties can deal with their differences and assist in resolving the conflict.

Finally, the principle that underscores all successful conflict resolution is that all people involved must view their conflict as a problem to be solved mutually so that each has a sense of winning or discovering options that are acceptable to all. Although this is an easy principle to understand, it can be challenging to put into practice. If both people can remain open, honest, and respectful of each other's positions, feelings of resentment may be minimized. Box 19.4 presents some basic strategies that can augment a professional response to conflict. The principles listed are remarkably effective in cases of conflict and will help the nurse present herself or himself as a confident and competent professional who will not react to inappropriate behavior in like form but also will not withdraw from the issues.

■ SUMMARY

To summarize this chapter let's return to the questions posed following the opening Vignette in which a conflict develops during the transfer of a patient from the ED to the nursing unit.

1. What communication strategies should Stacy, 4E charge nurse, use to respond to the accusations being made by the ED charge nurse to resolve the conflict and build a trusting relationship with her?

Stacy must use some of the positive communication techniques discussed in the chapter: apologize for the situation and assure the ED charge nurse that the patient received safe, quality care during the transition (developing trust), relay empathy for the overcrowding in the ED (expressing empathy), clarify that the 4E nurse did not leave the unit unannounced but was on an approved break (clarifying information), and that she would like to meet for coffee to discuss how they can improve the communication between their two departments to prevent such a situation from occurring in the future (keeping promises). In today's health care environment, where high stress levels and overwhelming workloads are all too common, it is easy for communication challenges to occur.

2. What conflict resolution strategies should both the ED nurse transferring the patient and the 4E staff nurse have used to prevent this situation from occurring?

Both nurses involved in the hand-off for the ED patient needed to focus on the importance of the hand-off report to patient safety and quality care. The two nurses need to be aware of their feelings of frustration and possibly anger but move past them by focusing on conflict resolution strategies such as using "I" rather than "you" messages (ED nurse: "I'm sorry to be so rushed but the ED is really crazy right now!"); keep the focus on the issue (4E nurse: "I'm sorry to be a little flustered but I was just returning from my break when I learned I had a new patient and I do want to get a good hand-off report."). Once feelings are acknowledged and each nurse understands the other's situation, they can move forward with a productive hand-off conversation. With each nurse viewing the potential conflict as a problem to be solved

mutually, they could both be honest and respectful of each other's positions.

3. What important steps should Stacy, the staff nurse, the ED nurse, the ED charge nurse—and ALL nurses—be aware of to develop and promote a professional communication style?

The first step toward developing a professional communication style is understanding the many complex and varied factors that influence the communication process, such as gender, cultural, generational, and interdisciplinary differences, each of which presents many challenges for the nurse who must strive to understand and to be understood. The second step is adopting positive communication techniques such as developing trust, using "I" messages, feeling empathy, clarifying information, and being aware of body language. The third step is for each nurse to reflect on their use of negative communication techniques, such as blocking, false assurances, conflicting messages, and logical fallacies. The next step in developing a professional communication style is learning to address and resolve conflict in a positive way. Demonstrating a professional, clear, and sensitive communication style is an essential component of the professional nursing skill set. As the foundation for effective, supportive work environments and excellent patient care, professional communication must be one goal every nurse strives to achieve.

CLINICAL JUDGMENT AND NEXT-GENERATION NCLEX® EXAMINATION-STYLE QUESTIONS

Carlos Montelongo, RN, BSN, charge nurse working on the cardiac step-down unit, was notified by one of the staff nurses that she had put in a call for Dr. Nugent, a cardiologist who frequently admitted patients to the unit, to notify him about a critical lab value and Dr. Nugent had not returned her call. The staff nurse reported calling Dr. Nugent's office twice over the last 45 minutes with no return call. Carlos said he would call the office himself and see if he could get a response. Approximately 5 minutes after leaving a message with Dr. Nugent's office, Carlos received a call from Dr. Nugent talking in a loud voice and demeaning tone: "Don't you know I have patients to see in my office and I cannot just drop everything when you call?! What is so important that you have

to leave me three messages?" Carlos was uncomfortable with the tone and volume of the response from Dr. Nugent, but using a calm voice and SBAR communication he reported the patient's abnormal lab value. Dr. Nugent said he would enter new orders in the EHR to treat the patient, and then abruptly ended the call. Carlos knew this type of communication was unprofessional and should not be ignored, especially because Dr. Nugent had a pattern of being slow to respond to calls and then speaking to nurses in a loud and demeaning tone when he did respond. Many nurses on the unit were anxious when having to contact Dr. Nugent about a patient issue.

As charge nurse for the unit Carlos feels he should address Dr. Nugent's unprofessional behavior and attempt to create a better communication pattern in the future. Considering the communication strategies discussed in the chapter, for each potential action step noted use an X to indicate if it would be Effective (help to meet expected outcomes), Ineffective (would not help meet expected outcomes), or Unrelated (not related to the expected outcomes) to improving communication.

Action	Effective	Ineffective	Unrelated
When Dr. Nugent is on the unit, ask to speak to him in a private location; maintaining eye contact, calmly express concern about his communication style in phone conversations.			
Keep the conversation with Dr. Nugent focused on providing quality care to his patients.			
Use "I" messages to explain to Dr. Nugent how his tone of communication makes Carlos and other nurses feel disrespected.			
Tell Dr. Nugent that he is known as a difficult physician with whom none of the nurses like to interact.			
State a desired goal for this conversation.			
Acknowledge the staff nurse for providing excellent patient care and staying alert to abnormal lab values.			
Respectfully ask Dr. Nugent to clarify his preferred method to be contacted when nurses have a concern about one of his patients.			
Tell Dr. Nugent that if his behavior does not improve, you will report him to the nursing director.			
Confirm that the orders for the patient were received in the EHR and acted on.			
Tell the next shift about the difficult phone call with Dr. Nugent.			

REFERENCES

American Association of Critical Care Nurses. (2023). *Skilled Communication.* https://www.aacn.org/nursing-excellence/healthy-work-environments/skilled-communication

American Association of Colleges of Nursing. (2023). *Communication Concept.* https://www.aacnnursing.org/essentials/tool-kit/domains-concepts/communication

American Nurses Association. (2015a). *Privacy and confidentiality.* https://www.nursingworld.org/practice-policy/nursing-excellence/official-position-statements/id/privacy-and-confidentiality/

American Nurses Association. (2015b). Code of ethics for nurses with interpretive statements. http://nursingworld.org/DocumentVault/Ethics-1/Code-of-Ethics-for-Nurses.html

Booher, D. (2020). *Gender communication style differences: Women in negotiations.* https://www.negotiations.com/articles/gender-bender/

Borg, J. (2011). *Body language: How to know what's really being said.* Dorset Press.

CBS News. (2010). *Generation X (and Y) are history: What's next?* https://www.cbsnews.com/news/generation-x-and-y-are-history-whats-next/

Centers for Disease Control and Prevention (CDC). (2019). Addressing gaps in health care for individuals with intellectual disabilities. *Public Health Grand Rounds.* https://www.cdc.gov/grand-rounds/pp/2019/20191015-intellectual-disabilities.html

Communication Theory. (2023). *Communication loop / The process of communication.* https://www.communicationtheory.org/communication-loop-the-process-of-communication/

Gibb, J. (1961). Defensive communication. *Journal of Communication, 11,* 141–148.

HIPAA. (2023). Communication in nursing. *The HIPAA Journal.* https://www.hipaajournal.com/communication-in-nursing/

Mayer, B. (2012). *The dynamics of conflict resolution* (2nd ed.) Jossey-Bass.

Mehrabian, A. (1981). *Silent messages: Implicit communication of emotions and attitudes.* Wadsworth.

National Council of State Boards of Nursing (NCSBN). (2018). *A nurse's guide to the use of social media.* https://www.ncsbn.org/brochures-and-posters/nurses-guide-to-the-use-of-social-media

Nurse Educator. (2009). Generational conflict in nursing: How to relate to colleagues from multiple generations. *Nurse Educator, 34*(1):28. *DOI:* 10.1097/01.NNE.0000343404.13234.6c http://journals.lww.com/nurseeducatoronline/Fulltext/2009/01000/Generational_Conflict_in_Nursing__How_to_Relate_to.12.aspx

Psychology Today. (2023). *Body Language.* https://www.psychologytoday.com/us/basics/body-language

The Joint Commission. (2017). *Sentinel event alert: Inadequate hand-off communication.* https://www.jointcommission.org/-/media/tjc/documents/resources/patient-safety-topics/sentinel-event/sea_58_hand_off_comms_9_6_17_final_(1).pdf?db=web&hash=5642D63C1A5017BD214701514DA00139

The Joint Commission. (2016). *Busting the myths about engaging patients and families in patient safety.* https://www.jointcommission.org/resources/news-and-multimedia/podcasts/take-5-busting-the-myths-about-engaging-patients-and-families-in-patient-safety/

The University of St. Augustine for Health Sciences. (2023). *The Importance of Effective Communication in Nursing.* https://www.usa.edu/blog/communication-in-nursing/

Stransky, M.L., & Morris, M.A. (2019). Adults with communication disabilities face health care obstacles. *The ASHA Leader, 24*(3), 46–55. https://leader.pubs.asha.org/doi/full/10.1044/leader.FTR1.24032019.46

20

Effective Delegation and Supervision

Barbara Cherry, DNSc, MBA, RN, NEA-BC, and
Terri Stewart, MSN, RN

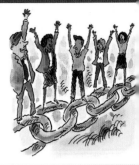

Delegation—linking together for b[...]
care and lower costs.

Ⓔ Additional resources are available online at: http://evolve.elsevier.com/Cherry/

LEARNING OUTCOMES

After studying this chapter, the reader will be able to:

1. Evaluate the effect of changes in the current health care system on nurse staffing patterns and responsibilities.
2. Outline six topic areas that the professional nurse should consider when making delegation decisions.
3. List seven essential requirements for safe and effective delegation.
4. Incorporate principles of delegation and supervision into professional nursing practice to ensure safe and legal patient care.

KEY TERMS

Accountability "To be answerable to oneself and others or one's own choices, decisions and actions ..." (American Nurses Association [ANA], 2015).

Assignment The distribution of work that each staff member is responsible for during a given work period; includes routine care, activities, and procedures that are within the licensed staff member's authorized scope of practice or part of the routine functions for assistive personnel (AP) (National Council of State Boards of Nursing [NCSBN] and ANA, 2019).

Assistive personnel (AP) Individuals who are trained to function in an assistive role to the RN by performing patient care activities as delegated by the nurse; may include nursing assistants, patient care technicians, clinical assistants, orderlies, health aides, and those with other titles designated within the work setting (NCSBN and ANA, 2019).

Competency The ability of an individual to perform defined actions proficiently by demonstrating the appropriate knowledge, skills, attitudes, and professional judgment required for a specific role or setting.

Delegation Transferring to a staff member (delegatee) the authority and responsibility to perform a selected nursing task that is outside the basic responsibilities of the delegatee's current job; the delegatee has the education, training, and validated competence to perform the task; the RN delegator retains accountability for the patient but the delegatee is responsible for the delegated task (NCSBN and ANA, 2019).

Supervision The active process of directing, guiding, and influencing the outcome of an individual's performance of an activity or task (ANA, 2012).

PROFESSIONAL/ETHICAL ISSUE

Nicole Adams, registered nurse (RN), has taken a position as the new charge nurse for a 24-bed medical-surgical unit at a long-term acute care and rehabilitation hospital. Nicole is excited about this new opportunity but is apprehensive because this is her first position as a charge nurse. After completing the hospital's orientation program Nicole reports to her unit for her first official day as charge nurse. She is immediately approached by a licensed practical nurse (LPN) who says, "I've worked here for 8 years and I always can take care of everything. I'll complete all patient assessments and let you know about anything you might need to follow up with." Nicole is alarmed about this statement but knows she must handle the situation carefully to ensure she follows safe delegation practices while also developing a good working relationship with the LPN. Discuss what elements of delegation Nicole should consider in this situation and what the best approach with the LPN might be.

VIGNETTE

Glenda Miller, BSN (Bachelor of Science in Nursing), RN, is the charge nurse on a medical-surgical floor of a hospital. She has received report from the 7 PM to 7 AM shift and is about to make assignments for the 7 AM to 7 PM shift. The philosophy of the unit is that the RN coordinates all patient care. Today on this 12-bed unit there are 8 patients and 4 empty beds. The nursing staff consists of Ms. Miller, two RNs, one LPN, one nursing assistant, and one unit secretary. The following interprofessional team members are available for specific patient care needs: respiratory therapist, physical therapist, occupational therapist, speech therapist, medical social worker, and chaplain. The patients are medically complex with extensive nursing care needs, including psychosocial and emotional support. The patients are described to Ms. Miller as follows:

502: Mr. A. is ventilator dependent with an infection that requires intravenous (IV) antibiotics every 12 hours. He needs to be out of bed in a chair twice a day. He has a stage I sacral decubitus ulcer and a percutaneous endoscopic gastrostomy (PEG) tube with bolus feedings. He is very hard of hearing, tries to speak, and becomes very frustrated and uncooperative.

503: Mrs. B., age 77, is on day 2 of 40 days of antibiotics for osteomyelitis. She is dehydrated with a central line

in her right subclavian and on total parenteral nutrition (TPN). She needs to be out of bed and ambulated in the room. She receives a respiratory treatment every 4 hours and needs assistance with AM care. Her daughter is at her bedside and is very upset that her mother may need to go to a nursing home.

504: Mr. C., age 52, is to be discharged to a rehabilitation hospital today. Discharge records need to be prepared for the transfer. The family is at his bedside and is extremely anxious.

507: Mr. D., age 64, has TPN infusing into a left subclavian catheter and is on multiple antibiotics. He has vancomycin-resistant *Enterococcus* in his urine and a stasis ulcer on his left leg that requires Pulsavac treatment every day.

508: Mr. E., age 72, is a ventilator-dependent patient who will start weaning this AM. He is on continuous tube feedings and IV antibiotics and needs to be assessed for a peripherally inserted central catheter (PICC) line. He is to begin ambulation in the hall twice a day per physician's orders. He also needs to have a pharyngeal speech evaluation scheduled.

509: Mrs. F., age 66, is 3 days post cerebrovascular accident (CVA) and unable to move her right extremities. She has an IV infusing via her left arm. Her blood pressure is 170/100. She needs total care with personal hygiene and feeding. The physician ordered new antihypertensive medication and range-of-motion exercises every day. Her husband is at her bedside, crying continually and asking, "What am I going to do now?"

510: Mr. G., age 72, has been off the ventilator for the past 24 hours and is doing very well. He continues on respiratory treatments every 4 hours. His TPN is being decreased, and his PEG feedings are increasing. Glucose monitoring has been ordered every 4 hours and IV antibiotics every 12 hours. He has an indwelling urinary catheter to gravity drainage. He needs to be out of bed, ambulating in the hall with assistance. If he stays off the ventilator, he will be discharged in 5 days. The family needs to find a nursing home for him; however, the family has not visited Mr. G. since his admission 18 days ago.

511: Mr. H., age 49, is a new admission who will be coming from the intensive care unit (ICU) sometime during the shift.

In addition to the tasks mentioned routine activities of taking vital signs, giving scheduled medications, updating care plans, and answering call lights must be assigned. When reviewing the tasks to be accomplished Ms. Miller must consider several issues to make safe and effective assignment and delegation decisions.

Questions to Consider While Reading This Chapter:

1. Which of the tasks listed in the vignette must the RN perform as required by your state's nurse practice act?
2. Which of these tasks can be delegated to the nursing assistant?
3. How can the training, skills, and competencies of the LPN or licensed vocational nurse (LVN) and nursing assistant be determined?
4. How can other members of the interprofessional health care team contribute most effectively to meet patients' needs?

CHAPTER OVERVIEW

The safe and effective delivery of patient care is the fundamental goal of every health care organization. To accomplish this goal cost effectively, teams of diverse professionals and assistants are used to deliver care. Because the RN is most often responsible for coordinating care provided by the various team members, they must clearly understand and be able to effectively use the management processes of delegation and supervision to ensure high-quality, safe patient care. This chapter highlights issues that influence staffing patterns and the delegation and supervision processes. The chapter also discusses the RN's role and responsibility in delegating to and supervising staff members, including assistive personnel (AP) and LPNs or LVNs, and provides useful guidelines for establishing a safe and effective delegation and supervision practice. Please note that another term for assistive personnel (AP) is unlicensed assistive personnel (UAP); while UAP and AP can be used interchangeably, this chapter will use the term AP.

DELEGATION AND SUPERVISION IN THE HEALTH CARE SYSTEM

Why Delegation and Supervision are Important

In today's complex health care environment it is critical that nurses are competent in their abilities to appropriately delegate, assign, and supervise staff members, including

AP. All health care settings from hospitals to home health to long-term care are focused on improving quality and reducing costs. Thus there will always be a need for competent, appropriately supervised AP, such as nursing assistants and patient care technicians, as one strategy to increase the cost-effectiveness of providing patient care.

Because the use of AP is common in most health care settings, the RN may be delegating tasks to individuals who do not have clearly defined parameters for education, training, job responsibilities, and role limitations. Therefore it is critical that the RN understand the components of safe delegation practice as discussed in this chapter. The RN must know that the profession defines the scope and standards of nursing practice (ANA, 2021) and that the state nurse practice acts define the legal parameters for nursing practice (NCSBN and ANA, 2019), both of which are important components of safe delegation. Supervision is another important component of professional nursing practice that requires an understanding of the activities that a staff member is responsible for performing as a condition of employment, consistent with the staff member's job position and description, legal scope of practice, and training and educational background.

Key Components of Delegation

Delegation is a legal and management concept that involves assessment, planning, intervention, and evaluation. Delegation is "allowing a delegatee to perform a specific nursing activity, skill, or procedure that is beyond the delegatee's traditional role and not routinely performed" (NCSBN and ANA, 2019). Although RNs can transfer the responsibility and authority for the performance of an activity, they remain accountable for the overall nursing care. When delegating tasks, the nurse should understand the delegatee's competencies, communicate succinctly, offer clear guidelines in advance, monitor progress, and remain accountable for the final outcomes of care.

Delegation is a three-way process that involves (1) the employer and designated nurse leader, (2) the RN who may be delegating activities, and (3) a delegatee who is a qualified staff member, such as AP. Each of these groups or individuals is accountable for safe delegation practices as follows (NCSBN and ANA, 2019):

The employer and designated nurse leader are responsible for:

- Performing a thorough assessment of the organization to understand the appropriate delegation needs and processes that should be considered in delegation practices.

- Determining nursing responsibilities that can be delegated, to whom they can be delegated, and under what circumstances they can be delegated.
- Developing delegation policies and procedures.
- Evaluating delegation policies and processes on a routine basis.
- Promoting a positive work environment and culture. The RN delegator is responsible for:
- Understanding the delegation guidelines and policies established by the employer and nursing leaders.
- Determining patient needs and when to delegate.
- Being available to the delegatee.
- Evaluating outcomes and being accountable for the delegated task.
- Any intervention or corrective actions that may be required to ensure safe and effective care. The delegatee is responsible for:
- Accepting delegation within the parameters of their competency level.
- Maintaining competence and accountability for performing the delegated task.
- Completing the task and communicating appropriate information to the delegator.

Delegation is a management strategy that when used appropriately can ensure the accomplishment of safe and effective patient care while also ensuring the most appropriate and effective use of resources within the health care setting.

WHAT SHOULD AND SHOULD NOT BE DELEGATED?

Unfortunately there is no easy answer to the question of what can and cannot be delegated. The answer varies depending on the (1) nurse practice acts and other applicable state laws, (2) patient needs, (3) job descriptions and competencies of staff members, (4) policies and procedures of the health care organization, (5) the clinical situation, and (6) professional standards of nursing practice. To establish a safe, effective delegation practice the RN must seek guidance and integrate information regarding each of these areas as discussed in the following paragraphs.

State Nurse Practice Acts

Each state's nurse practice act provides the legal authority for nursing practice, including delegation. However, each

state's nurse practice act expresses delegation criteria differently, and the criteria often are not clearly spelled out in the act, or they may be presented in various parts of the act. It is essential that every RN be familiar with their state nurse practice act and know the delegation criteria contained within it. Box 20.1 presents policies common to many nurse practice acts.

If the nurse practice act does not provide clear direction regarding delegation the state board of nursing may be able to offer guidance. The board of nursing may have developed definitions, rulings, advisory opinions, or interpretations of the law to provide guidance regarding delegation activities.

Most states also have a practice act to govern practice by LPNs or LVNs. Because the practice of LPNs or LVNs varies significantly from state to state, RNs should know the LPN or LVN practice act in the state in which they

---

BOX 20.1 Policies Common to Many State Nurse Practice Acts

- Only nursing tasks can be delegated, not nursing practice.
- The RN must perform the patient assessment to determine what can be delegated.
- The LPN or LVN and AP do not practice professional nursing.
- The RN can delegate only what is within the scope of nursing practice.
- The LPN or LVN works under the direction and supervision of the RN.
- The RN delegates based on the knowledge and skill of the person selected to perform the delegated tasks.
- The RN cannot delegate an activity that requires the RN's professional skill and knowledge.
- The RN is accountable and responsible for the delegated task.
- The RN must evaluate patient outcomes resulting from the delegated activity.
- Health care facilities should develop specific delegation policies in compliance with the state board delegation guidelines.
- Delegation requires critical thinking by the RN.

AP, Assistive personnel; *LPN,* licensed practical nurse; *LVN,* licensed vocational nurse; *RN,* registered nurse.
From Johnson, S. H. (1996). Teaching nursing delegation: Analyzing nurse practice acts. *Journal of Continuing Education in Nursing, 27*(2), 52–58.

practice and understand the LPN's or LVN's legal scope of practice. State law generally does not define practice by AP, although such practice should be governed by the health care organization's policies.

Patient Needs

When deciding to delegate the RN must remember that tasks can be delegated but nursing practice cannot. The functions of assessment, planning, evaluation, and nursing judgment cannot be delegated. Patient needs are key to safe delegation. In general the more stable the patient, the more likely delegation is to be safe. However, it also is important to remember that many tasks that can be delegated may also carry with them a nursing responsibility. Taking vital signs on a physiologically stable patient after a CVA could be delegated to the AP, but the task presents an opportunity for the RN to assess the patient's cognitive functioning. In the vignette presented at the opening of this chapter, Ms. Miller should not delegate any care for the newly admitted patient until the nursing assessment is complete.

Job Descriptions and Competencies

The RN who is delegating has the responsibility of knowing the background, skill level, training received, and job requirements of each person to whom tasks are delegated. The job description provides important information about what a staff member is allowed to do and delineates the specific tasks, duties, and responsibilities required of the person as a condition of employment. Job descriptions generally comply with state laws and the health care organization's standards of care. However, in all cases legal requirements related to delegation supersede any organizational requirement or policy.

The RN should be aware of what type of education and training the person received to function as described in the job description. The RN should also know what kind of orientation is provided to new employees. In the opening vignette the LPN's job description most likely would include duties such as "perform dressing changes" and "administer oral medications," but Ms. Miller also should know the LPN's knowledge and skill level for the population of patients on the unit.

In addition to requiring job descriptions for care providers health care organizations require employees to demonstrate that they are competent to perform certain technical procedures and to apply specific knowledge to safely care for patients. Written documentation of those skills and knowledge for which the employee has demonstrated competency is maintained in the employee's personnel file. Health care organizations require employees to undergo competency training for aspects of care unique to the population of patients generally being cared for in the nursing unit. Box 20.2 provides an example of competencies to be demonstrated by nurses in a family practice ambulatory care clinic. Various regulatory and accrediting agencies, such as The Joint Commission (TJC), require written documentation of staff competencies.

Organizational Policies and Procedures

When delegating the RN should comply with the specific skill requirements designated in the organization's written policies and procedures, which usually describe the supervision required for a specific task and how problems or incidents should be reported and documented. It is important for the nurse to remember that the legal requirements related to delegation supersede any organizational requirement or policy. The RN should also know the organization's general standards of care, such as infection control, and should ensure that the delegatee has the necessary knowledge and skills to comply with the standards. In the opening vignette, Ms. Miller should be aware of the hospital's policy regarding the orientation process. All clinical staff members should have received training about the unit's infection control as well as its emergency and safety procedures.

BOX 20.2 Competencies to Be Demonstrated by Registered Nurses and Licensed Vocational Nurses in a Family Practice Ambulatory Care Clinic

- Safety rules and regulations
- Health Insurance Portability and Accountability Act (HIPAA) policies and procedures
- Patient safety goals
- Infection control
- Telephone triage
- Glucose testing
- Patient education and health literacy
- Medication reconciliation
- Reporting abuse and neglect
- Documentation in the medical record
- Handling emergencies in the outpatient setting

Clinical Situation

Each delegation opportunity presents the RN with a variety of considerations, including the delegatee's current workload and the complexity of the task in relationship to the patient.

- Does the staff member realistically have time to accomplish the task based on their assignment?
- Is the staff member familiar with characteristics of the patient population (e.g., pediatric or geriatric) and with the task to be performed?
- Is the RN able to provide the appropriate level of supervision?

Other considerations include the availability of resources, such as supplies and equipment.

Professional Standards of Nursing Practice

Professional standards of nursing practice, as established by professional nursing organizations, exist to guide the RN in providing patient care. According to the ANA (2021), "The Standards of Professional Nursing Practice are authoritative statements of the duties that all registered nurses, regardless of role, population, or specialty, are expected to perform competently. The standards are subject to change with the dynamics of the nursing profession, as new patterns of professional practice are developed and accepted by the nursing profession and the public." To practice safe delegation the RN should be familiar with the standards of practice outlined in the ANA's *Nursing: Scope and Standards of Practice* (2021) and with the standards for any specialty area in which the RN practices (e.g., geriatric, pediatric, nursing administration, public health).

As an accepted standard of care the RN should use professional judgment to determine activities that are appropriate to delegate based on providing safe and effective patient care and protecting the public. In delegation the RN considers:

- Assessment of patient condition
- Capabilities of the nursing and unlicensed assistive staff
- Complexity of the task to be delegated
- Amount of clinical oversight (supervision) the RN will be able to provide
- Staff workload

Responsibilities related to making nursing judgments cannot be delegated except to another qualified RN. Examples of responsibilities that cannot be delegated include:

- Initial nursing assessment and any subsequent assessment that requires professional nursing knowledge, judgment, and skill.

- Determination of nursing diagnoses, establishment of nursing care goals, development of the patient plan of care, and evaluation of the patient's progress with the plan of care.
- Any nursing intervention that requires professional knowledge, judgment, critical thinking, and skill.

Box 20.3 presents a list of questions to assist the nurse in making delegation decisions.

DEVELOPING SAFE DELEGATION PRACTICES

For the RN to make safe, effective delegation decisions a good understanding of what should and should not be delegated on the basis of the previous discussion is required. However, safe delegation decisions require more! The RN also must know the patient, the staff members to whom they are delegating, and the tasks to be performed. The RN must provide for effective outcomes by clearly communicating expectations, supporting and appropriately supervising the delegatee, evaluating the outcomes, and reassessing the patient after the delegated task is completed. Following is a brief discussion of these essential requirements for safe and effective delegation.

Know the Patient

A nursing assessment must be completed before delegation—the RN must know the level of care required by the patient, considering their clinical, physiologic, emotional, cognitive, and spiritual status. Is the patient's condition considered stable? Generally the more stable the patient the more likely delegation of care is to be safe. What is the potential for change in the patient's condition as a result of the delegated task? If there is moderate to high risk that the task will result in a change in the patient's condition delegation should not be considered. Can the patient's safety be maintained with delegated care? The answer to this question must be a firm "yes" for delegation to be considered.

Know the Staff Member

Before the task is delegated the delegatee must have the skills and knowledge necessary to perform the task, as evidenced by the person's job description, education, and documented competencies. Experience and past job performance should also be taken into account. Is the staff member knowledgeable about and trained to

---

BOX 20.3   **Questions to Guide Decision-Making in Delegation**

A. State nurse practice act:
  1. Is the task within the RN's scope of practice?
  2. Does the nurse practice act address delegation of the task?
  3. Does the task to be delegated require the exercising of nursing judgment?
  4. Is the RN delegator willing to accept accountability for the performance of the delegated task?
B. Job description and competencies:
  1. Does the RN delegator understand the nature of the task and have the knowledge, skills, and competency required to perform the task?
  2. Does the delegatee have the appropriate education, training, skills, and experience to perform the task?
  3. Is there documented or demonstrated evidence that the delegatee is competent to perform the task?
  4. Does the delegatee perform the task on a routine basis?
  5. Is the delegatee familiar with the patient population?
C. Organizational policies and procedures:
  1. What skill level and level of supervision are required for the task as stated in the organization's policy/procedure manual?
  2. What is the policy or procedure for documenting tasks and reporting results, observations, problems, or unusual incidents?

3. Does the delegatee have the necessary knowledge and skills to comply with general standards of care, such as infection control?
D. Clinical situation and task:
  1. Is adequate supervision by the delegator available?
  2. Are adequate resources available, including supplies and equipment, for the delegatee?
  3. What is the delegatee's current workload? Does the person realistically have time to perform the task?
  4. How complex is the task? Does it frequently recur in the daily care of patients? Does it follow a standard and unchanging procedure?
E. Patient needs:
  1. Has the nursing assessment and plan of care been completed by the RN?
  2. What is the patient's clinical, physiologic, emotional, cognitive, and spiritual status?
  3. Is the patient's condition considered stable?
  4. What is the potential for change in the patient's condition as a result of the delegated task?
  5. Can the patient's safety be maintained with delegated care?
F. Professional standards of nursing practice:
  1. What specific standards of nursing practice apply to the specific situation?
  2. Does the delegated task include health counseling, teaching, or other activities that require specialized nursing knowledge, skill, or judgment?

---

perform the task? Does the staff member perform the task routinely? The right person must be selected for the right task. It is helpful for the RN to be involved in development of job descriptions, training programs, and competency documentation for staff members.

Know the Task(s) to Be Delegated

The RN delegator must be competent and skilled in performing any task they are considering delegating, and the task must be within the RN's scope of practice. Routine, standardized tasks that are performed according to a standard and unchanging procedure and have predictable outcomes are the safest to delegate. These routine tasks are most likely to have been documented in the staff member's competencies and may require fewer directions and less supervision. Complex tasks or activities that pose a high risk for patient complications or unpredictable outcomes should not be delegated.

Explain the Task and Expected Outcomes

The RN should explain the delegated task, what must be done, and the expected outcomes. If necessary the task should be outlined in writing. Failure to effectively communicate what is expected may result in unsatisfactory performance, errors, and possible harm to the patient. Directions should be provided clearly and concisely. Demonstration and return demonstration by the delegatee or other inservice education may be required. Delegation of the task is acceptable only if the staff member understands the task and is adequately prepared to carry it out.

Expect Responsible Action from the Delegatee

When the staff member accepts and understands the task they should then be allowed to perform the task. The staff member becomes responsible for their own actions and is obligated to complete the task as mutually agreed. It is important to note that the delegatee cannot delegate the task to another person; for example, if the RN delegates a task to an AP, that AP cannot ask another AP to perform the task. The RN should provide appropriate supervision but should not intervene in task performance unless assistance is requested or an unsafe situation is recognized. Interfering with the delegatee's task will negate their responsibility and obligation. The RN should expect responsible actions, give authority, and retain accountability.

Assess and Supervise Job Performance

Supervising job performance provides a mechanism for feedback and control. The RN assesses job performance by making frequent rounds, observing, and communicating (e.g., asking about progress and determining whether there are any questions or concerns). The appropriate level of supervision should be determined. The RN should be available to the delegatee in case there are any questions or unexpected problems. Supervision should be performed in a positive and supportive manner to reassure the staff member that their work is important and appreciated. The RN should intervene immediately if the task is **not** being performed in a safe and appropriate manner. Poor performance must be documented and reported to the nurse manager. Poor performance should never be ignored. When a mistake is made it should be used as a learning opportunity for all staff involved.

Evaluate and Follow-Up

Once the task is complete, the RN should evaluate the staff member's performance and reassess the patient to ensure that the expected outcomes were achieved. If the patient's care outcomes or the delegatee's job performance necessitate it, the RN should follow up with required interventions. Appropriate evaluation and follow-up will ensure a positive outcome for both patient and staff member. Box 20.4 presents some important steps to remember after the decision to delegate has been made.

The Five Rights of Delegation

The RN often expresses concern about legal liability—"putting my license on the line"—when delegating to unlicensed staff members. How does the RN know whether they might be at risk when delegating? One method to avoid high-risk delegation and simplify the

---

BOX 20.4 From Deciding to Delegate to Actual Delegation: Steps to Remember

A. Communicate effectively.
  1. The delegatee accepts the delegation and accountability for carrying out the task correctly.
  2. The RN delegator provides clear directions to the delegatee, including which specific task is to be performed, for whom the task is to be done, when the task is to be done, how the task is to be performed, which data are to be collected, any patient-specific instructions, and what information is to be communicated back to the RN.
  3. The RN delegator clearly communicates expected outcomes and time lines for reporting results.
B. Provide appropriate supervision.
  1. Monitor performance to ensure compliance with established standards of practice and organizational policies and procedures.
  2. Obtain and provide feedback.
  3. Intervene if necessary.
  4. Ensure proper documentation.
C. Evaluate and reassess.
  1. Reassess the patient.
  2. Evaluate the performance of the task and the delegatee's experience.
  3. Reassess and adjust the overall plan of care as needed.

---

delegation process is referred to as the Five Rights of Delegation (NCSBN and ANA, 2019):

1. The **right task:** Ensure that delegated tasks conform to the organization's established policies and procedures for performing the particular task.
2. The **right circumstances:** The clinical condition of the patient should be stable and delegated tasks should not require independent nursing judgment. Any change in the patient's condition must be reported immediately to the RN.
3. The **right person**: Delegate to someone who has the appropriate knowledge and skills to perform the activity.
4. The **right direction and communication:** Give clear explanation about the task, data to be collected, and expected outcomes; allow the delegatee to ask clarifying questions; and indicate when and what the delegatee should report back to the RN. The delegatee should also understand that they cannot make

any modifications in carrying out the task without first consulting with the RN.

5. *The **right supervision and evaluation:*** The RN delegator is responsible for following up with the delegatee when the activity is completed and evaluating the patient outcomes. Invite feedback to assess how the delegation process is working and how to improve the process.

RNs can prevent being placed into unsafe, risky delegation situations by adhering to the safe delegation practices recommended in this chapter. Consider the legal case in which an elderly patient was admitted to the hospital and died shortly after admission by aspiration of food after the nursing assistant left a turkey sandwich on the table for the patient to eat (Legal Eagle Eye, 2010). The patient's family sued the hospital for wrongful death, the nurse was ruled negligent, and the family won the case. In this situation the nurse was informed by the admitting physician that the patient had dysphagia, a swallowing disorder, and needed to be supervised while eating. Unfortunately the nurse failed to meet the standards of nursing care by not supervising the patient's eating herself or ensuring that the nursing assistant clearly understood the risk involved for a patient with dysphagia and had the skills necessary to respond to an emergency. This legal case could have been prevented had the nurse practiced the principles and strategies for safe delegation presented in this chapter. For an example demonstrating excellence in delegation practice in a home health care setting see Case Study 20.1. To further develop your clinical judgment regarding delegation please review Clinical Judgment Scenarios: Delegation.

CASE STUDY 20.1   Excellence in Delegation Practice

Amy Laurence, RN, works for a home health care agency. Ms. Laurence manages a caseload of 35 patients and makes between 6 and 8 skilled nursing visits a day. Several of Ms. Laurence's patients need assistance with activities of daily living, such as personal hygiene and mobility. Ms. Laurence assigns these tasks to the home health aides (HHAs) with whom she has worked with over the past 6 to 12 months. From her ongoing evaluation of patient outcomes and supervision of these aides she knows they are skilled and proficient in performing their assigned tasks.

Five of Ms. Laurence's patients are newly diagnosed with diabetes and need extensive assistance with monitoring blood glucose levels and administering insulin. The home health care agency where Ms. Laurence works recently adopted a diabetic delegation policy. This policy allows HHAs that have been specifically trained and certified to perform glucose testing and give insulin from prefilled, labeled syringes. Ms. Laurence actively participates in the training classes to certify HHAs in diabetic care.

In caring for her patients with diabetes Ms. Laurence does extensive diabetic teaching with each of her patients and sees them weekly to assess their learning, monitor their physiologic status, evaluate and adjust their individualized plans of care, and provide ongoing education and support as needed. During the weekly visits Ms. Laurence fills and labels the exact number of insulin syringes with the correct doses of insulin to last the week. Ms. Laurence is then able to delegate the daily insulin administration and glucose monitoring to the HHAs certified in diabetic care. During the initial delegation process Ms. Laurence makes supervisory visits to each patient's home to ensure that the HHA is performing the tasks correctly and has been carrying them out according to the patient's plan of care. To provide appropriate supervision of these delegated tasks Ms. Laurence plans her weekly skilled nursing visits to coincide with the HHAs' daily visits. During these visits Ms. Laurence observes each HHA perform the glucose testing and insulin administration and reinforces any specific training needed. Following these supervisory visits Ms. Laurence is confident that the HHAs are competent to perform the delegated tasks.

In this case Ms. Laurence is following all of the criteria essential for safe delegation in her state. She is adhering to the agency's policy, which also is in line with the state board of nursing rules for delegation in a home health care setting. She has actively participated in the training programs for the HHAs and provided clear direction during the initial delegation process. Ms. Laurence provides ongoing patient assessment, care evaluation, and supervision of the HHAs. In performing appropriate delegation Ms. Laurence is able to focus her energy on skilled nursing services, such as providing patient education, assessing and monitoring patients' physiologic condition, and coordinating the care for the interprofessional home health care team.

SUPERVISION

Supervision is defined by ANA (2012) as "the active process of directing, guiding and influencing the outcome of an individual's performance of a task." Supervision may be categorized as on-site, in which the nurse is physically present or immediately available while the activity is being performed, or off-site, in which the nurse has the ability to provide direction through various means of written, verbal, and electronic communication. On-site supervision generally occurs in the acute care or ambulatory care settings where the RN is immediately available. Off-site supervision may occur in home health care practice, community settings, and long-term care facilities.

Various levels of supervision may be required on the basis of the task delegated and the education, experience, competency, and working relationship of the people involved (Hansten & Jackson, 2009):

- *Unsupervised*: One RN is working with another RN in a collegial relationship and neither RN is in the position of supervising the other. Each RN is responsible and accountable for their own practice. However, the RN in a supervisory or management position (e.g., team leader, charge nurse, nurse manager), as defined by the health care organization, will be in a position to supervise other RNs.
- *Initial direction and/or periodic inspection*: The RN supervises a licensed caregiver or AP, knows the person's training and competencies, and has developed a working relationship with the staff member. For example, the RN has been working with the nursing assistant for 6 months and is comfortable in giving initial directions for a delegated task and following up with the assistant once during the shift.
- *Continuous supervision*: The RN has determined that the delegatee needs frequent to continual support and assistance. This level of supervision is required when the working relationship is new, the task is complex, or the delegatee is inexperienced or has not demonstrated an acceptable level of competence.

ASSIGNING VS DELEGATING

Assigning tasks is not the same as delegating tasks. Assignment is "the routine care, activities and procedures that are within the authorized scope of practice of the RN or LPN/VN or part of the routine functions of the AP" (NCSBN and ANA, 2019). An assignment designates those activities that a staff member is responsible for performing as a condition of employment and is consistent with the staff member's job position and description, legal scope of practice, and training and educational background. The staff member assumes responsibility and is accountable for completing the assignment. Assignments can vary based on the type of unit or clinical setting.

Assignment Considerations

Assigning groups of patients to various care providers, including AP and LPNs or LVNs, is not appropriate. For example, AP cannot be assigned to a patient or group of patients, but rather should be assigned to an RN. Typical assignments for AP include passing trays, assisting patients with activities of daily living, transporting patients, stocking supplies, and completing delegated tasks for the RN. The LPN or LVN may be assigned specific patients for whom to perform care, but the RN remains responsible for all nursing practice activities, including patient assessment, care planning, and patient teaching.

The RN is also responsible for assignments made to personnel in the clinical setting. Several factors should be considered when making assignments:

- *Patient's physiologic status and complexity of care*: Are vital signs unstable? Is the patient's condition changing rapidly? Does the patient have multisystem involvement? Does the patient need extensive health education? Does the patient need extensive emotional support? What technology is involved in the care (e.g., cardiac monitor, IV pump, patient-controlled analgesia pump)? Patients with more unstable physiologic status or complex care requirements need a higher level of skilled care.
- *Infection control*: To what extent are isolation procedures required? Which patients could be adversely affected as a result of cross-contamination? For example, a new patient is admitted with a history of night sweats and chronic cough. The results of a sputum culture are pending. Another patient on the unit was admitted with complications resulting from chemotherapy. The same caregiver should not be assigned to a potentially infectious patient and an immunocompromised patient.
- *Degree of supervision*: What level of supervision, direct or indirect, is required on the basis of staff members' education, experience, skill level, and competence?

Is the appropriate supervision available? The on-call RN who works an occasional weekend may require more supervision than the LPN who has worked in the unit full time and has demonstrated competence in caring for the patient population on the unit.

Note that the most experienced skilled staff members should not be exclusively assigned to the most complex, difficult cases. Assignments should be used as a staff development tool. Assigning a less-experienced nurse to a more complex patient while at the same time increasing the level of supervision increases that nurse's skill level, competence, and confidence while maintaining safe, effective patient care.

Working With Interprofessional Health Care Team Members

Other health professionals, including respiratory therapists, physical therapists, occupational therapists, speech therapists, nutritionists, medical social workers, and chaplains, are very valuable in helping meet patient care needs. In the vignette for this chapter Ms. Miller will need to coordinate the efforts of each of the interprofessional team members available to her unit to accomplish the many and varied tasks needed by the patients for whom she is responsible and accountable. For example, the respiratory therapist monitors all patients on ventilators and assists in the weaning process. The medical social worker provides valuable assistance to identify family support and assists with nursing home placement for Mr. G. The speech therapist can work on communication techniques with Mr. A., the ventilator-dependent patient who becomes very frustrated when he tries to speak.

To further develop your clinical judgment regarding supervision please review Clinical Judgment Scenarios: Supervision.

BUILDING DELEGATION AND SUPERVISION SKILLS

Effective delegation and supervision are underlying qualities for the success of working with others efficiently and being able to provide safe, cost-effective care to patients. Delegating can be very difficult, especially for the novice nurse. Some of the struggles the nurse has are the fear of being disliked; fear of making a mistake; inexperience in working with AP, LPNs, or LVNs; lack of confidence; and lack of knowledge of the delegation

process itself. Because delegation and supervision involve interactions between two people, the RN needs to develop strong interpersonal skills and a supportive work environment to guarantee effective delegation and supervision situations. Following are management skills RNs need to develop to become proficient at delegation and supervision.

Communicate Effectively

Clear communication is the key to successful delegation and supervision. The first step toward effective communication is for the RN to know exactly what needs to be done and what outcomes are expected. What is the specific task to be done? For whom is the task to be done? When is the task to be done? How is the task to be performed? What data need to be collected? What is the expected outcome? What feedback is expected? Why does the task need to be done in a certain way?

Maintaining self-control and confidence is an important communication skill. New RNs often have expressed concern about delegating to more seasoned LPNs or LVNs, or AP. "I have been working here for 12 years, and I do not need you telling me what to do" might be a typical response directed to the new RN. The RN's correct response is to maintain composure and confidence and remain positive. "I really appreciate your experience and knowledge, and I need you to help our team and patients by . . . [describe the task clearly]."

It also is important to listen carefully to the delegatee's response. Did the delegatee appear to listen and understand the directions? Did they appear hesitant to accept the task? Angry? Uninterested? Frustrated? If a delegation action elicits a negative response from the delegatee the RN should ask for feedback using open-ended, nonthreatening statements such as "You seem unsure about performing this task." The RN should always provide an opportunity for the delegatee to ask questions. The positive communication techniques discussed in Chapter 19 provide additional guidelines to enhance delegation skills.

Create an Environment of Trust and Cooperation

Staff members will report problems more quickly if they know that the reaction from the supervisor will be supportive, nonthreatening, and nonjudgmental. When mistakes occur the person making it should not be blamed or criticized; rather, the supervisor should look for root causes and system issues, such as inadequate training or an excessive workload. Encouraging staff members to report and discuss problems is an excellent method of improving patient care and maintaining a helpful, supportive attitude. Just as the RN establishes trust and rapport with patients they should strive for the same type of supportive relationships with staff members.

Provide Feedback and Follow-Up Evaluation

The delegation process is not complete until the RN reassesses the patient and adjusts the plan of care as indicated. The RN should also provide honest feedback to the delegatee about their performance. An easy, although often overlooked, delegation skill is to praise good performance. Often more difficult for the RN, and sometimes ignored, is the duty to address poor job performance.

The RN should tell the staff member about mistakes in a supportive manner—in private—with a focus on "learning from mistakes." However, if the staff member performs in an inappropriate, unsafe, or incompetent manner, the RN must intervene immediately and stop the unsafe activity, document the facts of the performance, and report to the nurse manager. In addition, the RN should request additional training or other appropriate action for the staff member to ensure that patient safety is protected. The RN has a professional responsibility to intervene appropriately when poor performance is observed.

SUMMARY

To summarize this chapter let's return to Ms. Miller, RN, in the opening Vingette as she makes assignments and delegation decisions for the day. She understands the use of AP and LVNs or LPNs is common in acute care settings, thus she has developed expertise with her delegation and assignment skills, as all nurses should do. She knows she cannot delegate the initial nursing assessment or any subsequent assessment that requires professional nursing knowledge, judgment, or critical thinking and that the RN is always responsible for determining nursing diagnoses, establishing nursing care goals, developing the patient's care plan, and evaluating the patient's progress with the plan of care.

Ms. Miller is guided to safe, effective delegation and supervision through an assessment of (1) the clinical situation; (2) patient needs; (3) the job descriptions and competencies of the assistive and vocational or practical nursing personnel; (4) the health care organization's policies and procedures; (5) nurse practice acts and other regulations and applicable state laws; and (6) professional standards of nursing practice. She understands appropriate assignment strategies such as assigning AP to an RN and how she can use the knowledge and skills of the interprofessional team to address specific patient care needs. Most importantly, Ms. Miller understands the value of effective communication, creating an environment of trust and cooperation, and providing feedback and follow-up evaluation. These activities and skills provided in this chapter are the tools all RNs need to provide safe and legal delegation in practice.

CLINICAL JUDGMENT AND NEXT-GENERATION NCLEX® EXAMINATION-STYLE QUESTIONS

1. Carol Gibson, BSN, RN, who has been a nurse for 2 years, arrived on the unit at 0645 to receive report from the night shift RN who was caring for five patients. The medical unit houses patients who are on dialysis (peritoneal and hemodialysis) experiencing acute health issues.
   - Patient 1 needs to be taken to the dialysis unit at 1000. He needs to be weighed, vital signs checked, and help with bathing.
   - Patient 2 has peritonitis and needs to have the dialysate changed at 0900. She needs vital signs taken, weighed when the dialysate is drained, medications given, and a specimen of dialysate sent to the lab.
   - Patient 3 was admitted for fluid overload due to missing two dialysis treatments. The patient was dialyzed during the night and will be sent home later today. He needs to be educated regarding his plan of care and the importance of not missing

dialysis. He also needs vital signs and weight taken and medications given.

- Patient 4 was just brought to the unit to start on peritoneal dialysis. The full admission process must occur.
- Patient 5 was admitted 2 days ago with fever of unknown origin (FUO) and has been treated. She is to be in dialysis at 0800 and then will be discharged to continue on home dialysis. She needs reinforced teaching on the new medications she is taking.

Carol wants to delegate some of the tasks to Thomas, nursing assistant, who is assigned to work with her today. To delegate tasks to Thomas Carol must know the following about him:

Multiple Response: Select All That Apply:
A. Skill level
B. Training received
C. Job description
D. The kind of orientation Thomas received
E. Thomas' experience in working with this patient population
F. Rules and laws in place that support delegation
G. Hospital policies related to delegation

2. Carol, BSN, RN, received report from the night nurse for the dialysis patients she will be caring for and is making rounds with Thomas, nursing assistant. Carol will give report to Thomas and then delegate to Thomas what she wants him to do. Carol knows that nursing practice cannot be delegated, only tasks can be delegated. Carol also knows that delegation is a two-way process and the RN is accountable for completion of the tasks. Carol delegates the following tasks to Thomas.

Multiple Response: Select All That Apply:
A. Taking vital signs
B. Passing medications
C. Conducting discharge teaching
D. Weighing the patient
E. Collecting the dialysate specimen
F. Taking the patient to dialysis
G. Taking the patient to discharge area
H. Doing the initial assessment on the patient being admitted

3. When Carol, BSN, RN, was a new graduate she had many questions regarding delegation and what she could and could not delegate to the assistive personnel. To use assistive personnel most efficiently Carol reviewed the state's nurse practice act regarding

delegation and then made a list of items that she could *not* delegate. Which choices should be on Carol's list?

Multiple Response: Select All That Apply:
A. Initial nursing assessment
B. Establishment of nursing diagnosis and nursing care goals
C. Routine tasks such as passing meal trays and taking vital signs
D. Development of the patient plan of care
E. Evaluation of patient care outcomes
F. Complex tasks or activities that pose a high risk for patient complications

4. Carol, BSN, RN, has been asked by the nursing director to give an inservice on delegation at the next unit staff meeting. As Carol prepares for the inservice she identifies some key points that should be included in the inservice. Identify the correct key points from the options provided.

Multiple Response: Select All That Apply:
A. The RN delegates based on the knowledge and skill of the person selected to perform the delegated task.
B. The RN can only delegate activities that are within the scope of nursing practice.
C. The RN is accountable and responsible for the delegated task.
D. The RN can choose whether or not to evaluate patient outcomes from the delegated activity based on the LPN/LVN or assistive personnel report.
E. The RN must clearly communicate to the delegatee what needs to be done and the expected outcomes.
F. The RN should intervene when poor performance is observed but be sure to maintain a helpful, supportive attitude to correct the poor performance.
G. Routine, standardized tasks that are performed according to a standard and unchanging procedure and have predictable outcomes are the safest to delegate.

5. Carol continues preparing for the inservice review, noting that delegation is a skill that requires the nurse to think critically and be intimately familiar with the board of nursing rules and regulations related to delegation and the agency policy related to delegation. She plans to ask staff attending the inservice review to identify which of the following nursing actions can be delegated.

Use an X for the nursing actions listed below that can or cannot be delegated. Only one selection can be made for each nursing action.

Nursing Actions	Can Be Delegated	Cannot Be Delegated
Perform patient assessments		
Conduct patient teaching		
Obtain vital signs		
Perform AM care		
Collect daily weight		
Collect urine specimen from Foley		
Hang blood for infusion		
Transport patient to discharge area		
Evaluate outcome of a delegated task		

6. Mary Aberdeen, RN, has been a nurse for more than 2 years and has been the charge nurse many times. Mary is accustomed to making assignments. Today she has a new nurse working on the unit so she is going to spend some time reviewing what supervision entails. Mary reminds the new nurse that, according to the American Nurses Association, supervision is defined as directing, guiding, and influencing the outcomes of the staff member's performance. Mary goes on to review that there are various levels of supervision required when delegating a task. Mary asks the nurse to name some items on which to base a decision about what level of supervision is needed. The nurse identifies the following items that should be considered on the basis of the task delegated.
Multiple Response: Select All That Apply:
A. Patient's clinical condition
B. Family members present
C. Delegatee's experience
D. Delegatee's competency
E. If the delegatee likes doing the task
7. Mary, RN, shifts to discussing supervision in terms of making work assignments, which entails distributing work to staff members who are responsible for getting the work done in a given time frame. Each staff member assumes responsibility and accountability for completing their given assignment. Assignments are based on the job description, what the person was hired to do as a condition of employment, and the staff member's legal scope of practice and educational background. The nurse making assignments has several issues to consider.

Use an X for the item a nurse will consider when making assignments that are Indicated (appropriate or necessary), Contraindicated (could be harmful), or Nonessential (makes no difference or is not necessary). Only one selection can be made for each nursing action.

Considerations a Nurse Will Use When Making Assignments	Indicated	Contraindicated	Nonessential
AP should be assigned to a nurse			
LPNs or LVNs are assigned specific patients but the RN remains responsible for nursing practice activities, including patient assessment, care planning, and patient teaching for these patients			
Patient's physiologic status			
Complexity of care			
Infection control needs			
Staff members' meal break preference			
Layout of the unit			
Degree of supervision required			
Most experienced staff should get the most complex patients			

REFERENCES

American Nurses Association. (2012). *Principles for delegation.* American Nurses Association.

American Nurses Association. (2015). *Code of ethics for nurses with interpretive statements.* American Nurses Association.

American Nurses Association. (2021). *Nursing: Scope and standards of practice* (4th ed.). American Nurses Association.

Hansten, R.I., & Jackson, M. (2009). *Clinical delegation skills: A handbook for professional practice* (4th ed.). Jones and Bartlett.

Johnson, S.H. (1996). Teaching nursing delegation: Analyzing nurse practice acts. *Journal of Continuing Education in Nursing, 27*(2), 52–58. https://doi.org/10.3928/0022-0124-19960301-04

Legal Eagle Eye: Newsletter for the Nursing Profession. (2010). *Patient chokes, dies: Nurse ruled negligent, delegated supervision of patient to aide. 18*(1). http://www.nursinglaw.com/jan10ang7.pdf

National Council of State Boards of Nursing and American Nurses Association. (2019). *National Guidelines for Nursing Delegation.* https://www.nursingworld.org/,4962ca/globalassets/practiceandpolicy/nursing-excellence/ana-position-statements/nursing-practice/ana-ncsbn-joint-statement-on-delegation.pdf

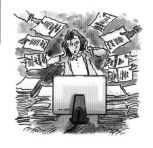

Staffing and assigning work are two vital but challenging roles for nurses.

21

Staffing and Nursing Care Delivery Models

Barbara Cherry, DNSc, MBA, RN, NEA-BC

ⓔ Additional resources are available online at: http://evolve.elsevier.com/Cherry/

LEARNING OUTCOMES

After studying this chapter, the reader will be able to:

1. Outline key issues surrounding staffing for a health care organization.
2. Evaluate how nurse competencies and patient care needs become critical components of all nursing care delivery models.
3. Analyze the advantages and disadvantages of nursing care delivery models in relation to patient care in various settings.
4. Differentiate among several nursing care delivery models by evaluating their defining characteristics.
5. Explain the purpose and components of nursing case management and related models.
6. Differentiate the use of clinical pathways and clinical practice guidelines in the clinical setting.
7. Summarize factors important when considering future models of nursing care delivery.

KEY TERMS

Assistive personnel (AP) Individuals who are trained to function in an assistive role to the RN by performing patient care activities as delegated by the nurse; may include nursing assistants, patient care technicians, clinical assistants, orderlies, health aides, and those with other titles designated within the work setting (National Council of State Boards of Nursing [NCSBN] and American Nurses Association [ANA], 2019).

Clinical pathway Clinical management plans that specify the optimal timing and sequencing of major patient care activities and interventions, based on evidence, by the interprofessional team for a particular diagnosis, procedure, or health condition (Case Management Institute, 2023); clinical pathways are designed to standardize care delivery, reduce unnecessary variation in care, and improve patient outcomes; they may also be called critical paths, practice protocols, or care maps.

Clinical practice guidelines (CPGs) Recommendations for appropriate treatment and care for specific clinical circumstances; they are developed through a systematic process to integrate the best evidence for treating specific medical conditions and while they are not meant to replace judgment by the clinician, they do assist health care providers to make decisions about appropriate treatment (Case Management Institute, 2023).

Nursing care delivery model Also called care delivery system or patient care delivery model; details the way work assignments, responsibility, and authority are structured to accomplish patient care; depicts which health care worker is going to perform what tasks, who is responsible, and who has the authority to make decisions.

Patient acuity Indication of the severity of the patient's illness and the amount and complexity of nursing care required; high acuity indicates a need for more intense, complex nursing care, and lower acuity indicates a need for moderate, less-complex nursing care.

Patient classification system Method used to group or categorize patients according to specific criteria and care requirements and thus help quantify the patient acuity, or amount and level of nursing care needed.

Patient outcome A measurable condition that results from interventions by the health care team; a change in a person's health after treatment; outcomes may be positive, such as better mobility or improved laboratory values, or negative, such as infection, fall, or death.

Staff mix Combination of categories of workers employed to provide patient care (e.g., RNs, LPNs or LVNs, and AP).

Staffing Ensuring that an adequate number and mix of health care team members (e.g., RNs, LPNs or LVNs, AP, interprofessional team members such as respiratory and physical therapists, clerical support) are available to provide safe, quality patient care.

PROFESSIONAL/ETHICAL ISSUE

LaMicha Hopkins, registered nurse (RN), staff nurse in a pediatric unit, is concerned about quality-of-care issues on her unit. When she first came to work in this unit 18 months ago she was very impressed with the quality of care the patients received and the camaraderie among the nurses. Team nursing was fully implemented and all nurses supported one another and the families to ensure that the pediatric patients received the best care possible. LaMicha was thrilled to have become part of such a great team and to be able to provide excellent care to her patients. Over the last few months patient acuity and patient census have increased but the number of nurses on the unit has not changed. In response to the higher workload charge nurses have started making patient care assignments on the basis of tasks rather than the team nursing model, explaining to the staff nurses that assignments by task are a more efficient way to get the work done. Some of LaMicha's colleagues have expressed dissatisfaction with their ability to provide good nursing care, and they are also noticing more complaints from family members. LaMicha believes that the shift away from the team nursing model, along with the higher patient volume and acuity, has led to fragmented care and a loss of the team spirit once so prevalent among the nurses.

What can LaMicha do as a staff nurse to help find a resolution to the staffing concerns? What data might be available to staff nurses to help them assess patient outcomes and patient and nurse satisfaction for a quantifiable analysis of the staffing situation? Who should be involved in evaluating and making decisions about staffing and nursing care delivery models? How can LaMicha approach the charge nurses and/or the nurse manager to help address the situation?

VIGNETTE

As a student nurse, Johnathan Knox noticed during rotations through the different clinical areas that the RNs had various types of responsibilities and duties. On the medical-surgical units, RNs supervised a group of licensed practical nurses (LPNs) and nursing assistants who provided direct patient care, and the RNs performed patient assessments, care planning, and education. In the critical care unit, RNs provided all the care required by the patient with little help from any other caregivers. In the obstetric unit, two RNs worked as a team to provide care to laboring mothers. In the outpatient health clinic, each RN was assigned to perform specific tasks; one nurse was assigned to do all diabetic teaching, and another was assigned to triage all telephone calls from patients. Some of the clinical areas used a mostly RN staff, whereas other clinical units had a variety of staff, from RNs to nursing assistants. Johnathan had many questions about why care delivery was very different in the various clinical sites.

Questions to Consider While Reading This Chapter:

1. Why is the RN's work assignment different in various units—obstetrics, critical care, medical-surgical, and the outpatient clinic?
2. What are key considerations when making staffing and patient care assignment decisions?
3. How do nurse managers or other nursing leaders decide which type of nursing care delivery model will be used?

CHAPTER OVERVIEW

Of all the nurse's varied and complex roles, staffing and assigning work are probably the most challenging and certainly the most important to the delivery of safe, quality patient care. Charge nurses spend a significant amount of time on staffing issues. *Staffing* ensures that an appropriate number of competently trained staff members are available to provide care; *assigning* is the method used to divide work tasks among the various staff members. This chapter presents a brief introduction to staffing and its surrounding issues, such as acuity levels and staff satisfaction. A description follows of various nursing care delivery models, which detail how work assignments are structured. Also discussed are case management and its related models, in addition to the use of clinical pathways and clinical practice guidelines (CPGs).

STAFFING—THE KEY TO QUALITY CARE

Staffing can be defined as the activities required to ensure that an adequate number and mix of health care team members (e.g., RNs, licensed vocational nurses [LVNs] or LPNs, assistive personnel [AP], clerical support) are available to meet patient needs and provide safe, quality care. Through the past two decades, research has validated the contribution and value of RNs to a multitude of benefits, including improved patient outcomes, reduced rates of complications and length of hospital stays, reduced errors and the potential for errors, prevention of premature mortality, improved patient satisfaction, and reduced readmissions. Two landmark reports—*Keeping Patients Safe: Transforming the Work Environment of Nurses* (Institute of Medicine [IOM], 2004) and *The Future of Nursing: Leading Change, Advancing Health* (IOM, 2011)—have strongly affirmed nurses' essential roles in achieving quality patient care and safety.

Appropriate nurse staffing is not just about the number of nurses present to provide care for patients—it is much more complex. According to the ANA (2020), "Appropriate nurse staffing is defined as a match of registered nurse expertise with the needs of the recipient of nursing care services in the context of the practice setting and situation" (p. 6). For nurses to have the greatest opportunity to achieve safe, quality

care, staffing systems must address the following five principles (ANA, n.d.,a):

1. *Health Care Consumer*: Staffing is based on the needs of the individuals, families, groups, communities, and populations served.
2. *Interprofessional Teams*: The needs of the population being cared for determine the appropriate competencies for the RN and the other members of the interprofessional team; staffing systems monitor and address vital issues important to nurses such as job satisfaction, burnout, turnover and retention, and workplace safety.
3. *Workplace Culture*: Reflects the value of RNs as vitally important to the organization and patient care while also balancing quality and safety with the overall costs of nursing resources and maintaining a culture of respect, trust, and collaboration among the health care team.
4. *Practice Environment*: Staffing processes ensure the safety of patients and nurses; recognize that appropriate nurse staffing is vital to achieving patient safety and quality goals; and provide nurses with control over their nursing practice and autonomy in the workplace.
5. *Evaluation*: Ongoing evaluation of staffing plans occur with adjustments as needed to meet patient/population needs and the evaluation plan addresses both patient outcomes and nurse-specific indicators such as turnover, nurse satisfaction, and patient satisfaction.

The following sections will discuss key elements of staffing related to (1) patient needs, (2) nursing characteristics, and (3) organizational needs.

Staffing and Patient Needs

Primary considerations for staffing a specific nursing unit are the number of patients; the level of intensity of care required by those patients (commonly referred to as patient acuity); contextual issues, such as the architecture and geography of the environment and the available technology; level of preparation and experience of the staff members providing the care; and the quality of the nurses' work life (ANA, 2020). Using only the number of patients who require care is an ineffective way to plan staffing because of the wide range of care requirements needed by individual patients. To account for the diverse care needs and quantify the intensity of care required by a group of patients, nurses use various patient classification systems.

Patient Classification Systems. Patient classification systems group or categorize patients according to specific criteria and care needs and thus help quantify the amount and level of care needed, referred to as the *acuity level*. The higher the acuity level, the more intense and complex the patient's nursing care needs. For example, patients may be grouped in such categories as "uncomplicated postpartum" or "ventilator dependent." These two groups of patients require very different levels and amounts of care and therefore are categorized at different acuity levels. Other considerations for the acuity level include the frequency of required medications, intravenous drips, patient's self-care requirements, and complex treatments such as continuous renal replacement therapy. Imagine the many different kinds of patients treated by a health care facility, and you can begin to picture the complexity of patient classification systems. Electronic patient classification systems that extract data from the electronic health record and determine patient acuity scores are now available to streamline the method of managing patient acuity.

Because of this complexity and the differences in patient populations across different health care facilities, patient classification systems vary from organization to organization. However, the ANA (2020) has recommended that the following physical and psychosocial factors be considered in the determination of the intensity of care required for any group of patients:

- Age and functional ability
- Complexity of care needs
- Communication skills
- Cultural and linguistic diversities
- Existence and severity of comorbid conditions
- Scheduled procedures or treatments
- Ability to meet health care requisites
- Psychosocial and family support needs
- Other specific needs identified by the patient and by the RN

Understanding the intensity of care required by individual patients and groups of patients on the basis of these factors is the first step in developing effective patient classification systems and planning for appropriate staffing levels. The second step is knowing the level of preparation, skill, and experience of the staff members who are available to provide patient care.

Staffing and Nursing Characteristics

It is of critical importance that the staff members available to provide patient care have the educational preparation, skill, clinical judgment, and experience necessary to meet patient care needs. Another consideration in staffing is the clinical competencies that are required to care for the population being served, as well as the nurse's competency with technology and clinical interventions (ANA, 2020). In recognition of the importance of nurse competencies in staffing the American Association of Critical Care Nurses (AACN) recommends the *AACN Synergy Model for Patient Care* (AACN, n.d.). Staffing systems based on the *Synergy Model* match patient needs and nurse competencies to achieve ideal patient outcomes. The *Synergy Model* also urges nurses to advance their competencies to meet specific patient care needs. For more information on the *Synergy Model* visit the AACN website at www.aacn.org. The nurse leader responsible for making staffing decisions must be aware of each staff member's educational level, competencies, experience, skill, and training. Ideally, clinical support from experienced RNs should be available to support and advance the skills of those RNs and other staff members with less experience.

Nursing Satisfaction. Nurses who are satisfied with their work generally provide higher quality, more cost-effective care. Staffing systems must address the quality of work life for the nursing staff as equal in importance to the quality of patient outcomes. Attention to staff schedules is a major responsibility for the nurse leader, especially in light of the 24-hour/day, 365-day/year staffing needs in many health care facilities. Many creative staffing options are available to meet the varied needs of staff members and patient care such as:

- 9- or 10-hour shifts, 4 days per week
- 12-hour shifts, 3 days per week
- Combination of 8-hour and 12-hour shifts
- Premium pay or part-time staff for weekend work
- Job sharing, flextime, and/or staff self-scheduling

The many and varied staffing options have various advantages and disadvantages. For example, long shifts over consecutive days may result in clinical errors when nurses become fatigued. Self-scheduling is a popular staffing technique in which the responsibility for staffing the unit is delegated to the employees on the unit, who work collectively to design the schedule according to preestablished staffing criteria and some guidance from the manager. No one scheduling system has proven to be best overall for staff satisfaction. However, staffing methods that allow nurses to be fully engaged in the design of their work schedules is key to staff satisfaction and nurse retention (Bradley, 2023).

Staffing and Organizational Needs

The three basic organizational needs that are significantly affected by staffing are: (1) financial resources, (2) licensing regulations and The Joint Commission (TJC) or other accreditation standards, and (3) customer satisfaction.

Financial Resources. Productivity, the ratio of the amount of outputs produced (e.g., home visits) to the specific amount of input (nursing hours worked), is the measure of staffing efficiency. Because staff salaries are by far the largest expense for any health care organization, productivity—or the efficient use of staff—has a direct effect on the organization's bottom line. Fortunately, even though RNs typically represent the highest-paid staff in a facility they are also the key to improved quality outcomes and reduced costs, thus representing a very good investment for the health care organization (Kerfoot, 2019). It is important to remember that most health care organizations operate under tight financial constraints, making efficient management of staff essential to ensure the organizations' financial solvency. The nurse leader is accountable for appropriately managing staffing to stay within budgetary guidelines for:

- Numbers of staff working at any given time to provide care to a given number of patients
- Staff mix, the combination of types of workers present to provide patient care (e.g., RNs, LVNs or LPNs, and AP)

Licensing Regulations and Accreditation. Health care facility licensing agencies, such as a state health department, and accreditation agencies, such as TJC, address minimum staffing levels. However, TJC and most state licensing agencies do not impose mandatory staffing ratios. These agencies look for evidence that patients receive adequate care, which can occur only with adequate staffing. They also require documentation of staff training and competency to care for the organization's specific patient population. Licensing regulations for long-term care facilities stipulate minimum RN coverage for the facility but do not mandate specific nurse-to-patient ratios.

State legislative bodies and professional organizations have addressed staffing in various ways. In 1999 California became the first state to enact legislation mandating specific nurse-to-patient ratios in every hospital unit and continues in 2023 as the only state with this legislative mandate for nurse staffing (Davidson, 2023); Massachusetts enacted legislation mandating staffing ratios only for intensive care units (ICU) while some states require staffing committees with at least 50% clinical nurses to address the staffing plan (Davidson, 2023). Rather than mandating staffing ratios the ANA (n.d.,b) recommends staffing committees composed of at least 55% direct-care RNs to develop unit-specific staffing plans to encourage flexible staffing levels considering various factors including: (1) nurse experience and expertise, (2) physical space and layout of the nursing unit, (3) numbers of admissions, discharges, and transfers, (4) patient complexity and acuity, (5) patient outcomes, and (6) availability of ancillary support and other resources. Such staffing committees, which empower nurses to articulate the resources they need for safe, high-quality patient care, have shown positive outcomes on the nurses' perceptions of a health work environment (Skarbek et al., 2022). Other key recommendations for effective staffing plans include (Dawson, 2014):

- Staff nurses must be fully engaged in creating work schedules.
- Work schedules must be predictable so that nurses can plan for family and personal responsibilities.
- Nurses should have 10 consecutive hours off duty to allow for 7 to 9 hours of sleep.
- Uninterrupted rest breaks must be provided during the work shift.
- Nurse-sensitive patient outcome data should be used to support appropriate staffing.

The National Database of Nursing Quality Indicators (NDNQI) serves as a resource for data on nurse-sensitive outcomes, including patient falls, catheter-associated urinary tract infections, and nurse turnover and job satisfaction. Such data can serve as a powerful influence for nurses to advocate for safe staffing.

Customer/Patient Satisfaction. Perhaps most critical to an organization's success in a competitive health care environment is customer (patient) satisfaction. The key to customer satisfaction is the patient's and family's personal interaction with the organization's employees. Positive and therapeutic interactions between clinicians and their patients and families can play a very significant role in improving patient health and clinical outcomes. With the advent of health care reform, patient satisfaction is now tied directly to financial rewards for hospitals. Medicare reimbursement, known as Value-Based Purchasing, rewards inpatient hospitals for providing quality care to include patient satisfaction (see Chapter 7 for a more detailed discussion of Value-Based Purchasing). Appropriate staffing with well-trained, competent, professional nurses is essential to ensure patient satisfaction and allow hospitals to gain the financial rewards of high patient satisfaction.

Further Study of Staffing

This section has provided the reader with a brief introduction to staffing issues, such as scheduling options, patient classification systems, productivity and staff mix, and the RN's contribution to improved patient outcomes. These issues related to staffing in a health care organization are much more complex than may appear from this introduction. The reader, especially the person interested in entering nursing management, is encouraged to learn more about staffing and these related issues.

NURSING CARE DELIVERY MODELS

Nursing care delivery models, also called *care delivery systems* and *patient care delivery models*, detail the way task assignments, responsibility, and authority are structured to accomplish patient care. The nursing care delivery model describes which health care worker is going to perform what tasks, who is responsible, and who has the authority to make decisions. The basic premise of nursing care delivery models is that the number and type of caregivers are closely matched to patient care needs to provide safe, quality care in the most cost-effective manner possible.

The four classic nursing care delivery models used during the past six decades are: (1) total patient care, (2) functional nursing, (3) team nursing, and (4) primary nursing. Efforts to continually improve both the quality and cost-effectiveness of patient care have resulted in variations to these four classic models with hospitals and clinical settings continually looking for improved methods for delivering nursing care. Other types of nursing care models include patient-centered care and case management. As the health care system continues to evolve in the 21st century—with a focus on rapid patient turnover in acute care settings, growing use of outpatient and community-based settings, and evidence of the RN's valuable role in patient safety and improved outcomes—new models of nursing care delivery are continually emerging. Thus considerations for future care delivery models are also presented.

Total Patient Care

The oldest method of organizing patient care is total patient care, sometimes referred to as *case nursing*. In total patient care nurses are responsible for planning, organizing, and performing all care, including personal hygiene, medications, treatments, emotional support, and education, required for their assigned group of patients during the assigned shift. A diagram of the total patient care model is shown in Fig. 21.1.

Advantages of the total patient care model are:
- The patient receives holistic, unfragmented care by only one nurse per shift.
- At shift change the RN who has provided care and the RN assuming care can easily communicate about the patient's condition and collaborate about the plan of care.
- The nurse maintains a high degree of practice autonomy.
- Lines of responsibility and accountability are clear.

The disadvantages of the total patient care model are that the number of RNs required to provide total patient care may simply not be available because of nursing shortages or financial constraints and the RN performs many tasks that could be performed by a caregiver with less training at a lower cost.

Today the total patient care method is commonly used in the hospital's critical care areas, such as ICU and postanesthesia care units, where continuous assessment and a high degree of clinical expertise are required at all times. This method is less widely used in other patient care settings as health care organizations move to more efficient, interprofessional team approaches to patient care, allowing RNs to concentrate on aspects of care essential to good patient outcomes, such as providing patient teaching and evaluating the patient's response to the plan of care.

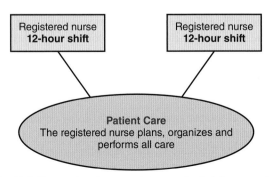

Fig. 21.1 The total patient care (case method) delivery model.

Functional Nursing

In the functional nursing method of patient care delivery, staff members are assigned to complete certain tasks for a group of patients rather than care for specific patients. For example, the RN performs all assessments and care planning, and administers all intravenous medications; the LVN or LPN gives all oral medications; and the assistant performs hygiene tasks and takes vital signs. An RN makes the assignments and coordinates the care. A diagram of the functional nursing care model is shown in Fig. 21.2.

Advantages of the functional nursing model are:
- Patient care is provided in an economic and efficient manner because less-skilled, lower-cost workers are used in areas where task completion is the focus.
- A minimum number of RNs is required to supervise and to perform strictly nursing duties.
- Tasks are completed quickly, and there is little confusion about job responsibilities.

The disadvantages of the functional nursing model include the potential for fragmented care and the possibility of overlooking priority patient needs because several different workers focus only on performing specific patient care tasks. Additionally, the patient may feel confused because of the many different individuals providing different aspects of care.

Although the functional nursing model is considered efficient and economical, the patient is treated by many caregivers who may not be focused on giving personalized care because they are focused on performing a task. This model may not fit well in the new health care system, which emphasizes customer service. However, functional nursing care delivery is still appropriate in some care settings, such as the operating room.

Team Nursing

In team nursing the RN functions as a team leader and coordinates a small group (generally no more than four or five) of ancillary personnel to provide care to a small group of patients. As coordinator of the team the RN must know the condition and needs of all the patients assigned to the team and must plan for individualized care for each patient. The team leader is also responsible for encouraging a cooperative environment and maintaining clear communication among all team members. The team leader's duties include assessing patients and planning care, assigning duties, directing and assisting team members, giving direct patient care, teaching, and coordinating patient activities. A diagram of the team nursing model is shown in Fig. 21.3.

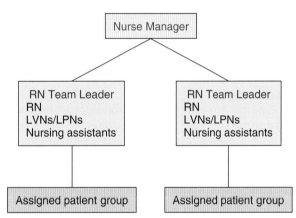

Fig. 21.3 The team nursing model. *LPNs,* licensed practical nurses; *LVNs,* licensed vocational nurses; *RN,* registered nurse.

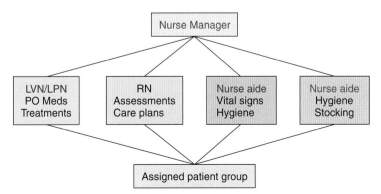

Fig. 21.2 The functional nursing care delivery model. *LPN,* Licensed practical nurse; *LVN,* licensed vocational nurse; *PO,* oral; *RN,* registered nurse.

Advantages of the team nursing model are:

- High-quality, safe, and effective care can be provided with a relatively high proportion of support staff and/or AP.
- Each team member participates in decision-making and contributes their own special expertise in caring for patients.

Disadvantages of the team nursing model include the challenge to maintain continuity of care if the daily team assignments vary and the potential for insufficient time for care planning and communication, leading to unclear goals or fragmented care.

Team nursing is an effective, efficient method of patient care delivery and has been used in most inpatient and outpatient health care settings. However, for team nursing to succeed the team leader must have strong clinical skills, good communication skills, delegation ability, decision-making ability, and the ability to create a cooperative working environment. In an attempt to overcome some of its disadvantages the team nursing design has been modified many times since its original inception, and variations of the model are evident in other methods of nursing care delivery being implemented in clinical settings.

Especially since the Covid-19 pandemic and the resulting nursing shortage, health care settings are implementing unique models of team nursing such as combinations of LPNs/LVNs and patient care technicians in unique roles to support patient care, having admission and discharge teams, sharing one charge nurse across two units, or using dedicated teams for wound care or CAUTI (catheter-associated urinary tract infections) rounds. The options for organizing care and using the full range of all team members' expertise is endless when nurses become creative and identify how to get the work done in the very best way for the very best patient outcomes.

Primary Nursing

In primary nursing, the RN, or "primary" nurse, assumes 24-hour responsibility for planning, directing, and evaluating the patient's care from admission through discharge. This model differs significantly from the total patient care model in that the "primary nurse" assumes 24-hour responsibility for directing the patient's plan of care. While on duty the primary nurse may provide total patient care or may delegate some patient care tasks to LPNs or LVNs, or AP. When the primary nurse is off duty care is provided by an associate nurse, who follows the care plan established by the primary nurse. The primary nurse, who has 24-hour responsibility, is notified if any problems or complications develop and directs alterations in the nursing plan of care. A fundamental responsibility for the nurse in the primary nursing model is to maintain clear communication among all members of the health care team, including the patient, family, physician, associate nurses, and any other members of the health care team. A diagram of the primary nursing model is shown in Fig. 21.4.

Advantages of the primary nursing model are:

- One-to-one relationships between nurse and patient support relationship-based care.
- Nurses practice using high levels of clinical judgement and excellent communication with the clinical team.

Disadvantages of the primary nursing model include the challenges of the RN willing to accept 24-hour responsibility for their primary care patients, and the number of nurses required for this method of care may be difficult to recruit and may prove to be more costly for the organization.

The primary care nursing model lends itself well to home health nursing, hospice nursing, oncology nursing, and long-term care settings in which the patient requires nursing care for an extended period. Primary

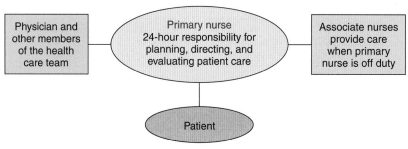

Fig. 21.4 The primary nursing model.

nursing may be more difficult to provide in acute care settings, where stays are short and the nurse may see each patient for only 1 or 2 days.

PATIENT-CENTERED CARE

Patient-centered care has been a core nursing value since the beginning of professional nursing; however, it is receiving renewed attention for all health professionals as a result of the IOM's focus on safety and quality in health care. The IOM (2001) defines *patient-centered care* as "providing care that is respectful of and responsive to individual patient preferences, needs, and values and ensuring that patient values guide all clinical decisions." Delivering patient-centered care means that nurses, physicians, and other health professionals partner with patients and families in shared decision-making to ensure that:

- Health care decisions respect patients' wants, needs, and preferences; and
- Patients have the education and support they need to make decisions about and participate in their own care.

To give patient-centered care means to support patients to live their best possible lives within their own unique experiences.

Patient-centered care is more a philosophy of care than a typical nursing care delivery model, as discussed in the previous sections. However, because patient-centered care has become a core focus in today's health care organizations, it must be incorporated as an essential component of any nursing care delivery model. Practical methods for engaging in patient-centered care are to include patients, families, and significant others in:

- Developing care plans and discharge plans that address the uniqueness of the individual and their life and family circumstances.
- Participating in shift-change or other handoff reports.
- Sharing decision-making by providing education when and how the individual needs it to make informed decisions.
- Establishing family or consumer advisory councils to engage former patients and families to advise organizational leaders in ways to involve patients and families in decision-making and care improvements.

The Agency for Healthcare Research and Quality (AHRQ) recommends the SHARE Approach to guide nurses and other health care professionals to support patients and families to make informed decisions regarding their health care. The health care team can use the following five steps to implement the SHARE Approach and ensure patients and families are fully engaged in their health care decision-making (AHRQ, 2016).

1. **S**eek the patient's participation.
2. **H**elp the patient explore and compare treatment options.
3. **A**ssess the patient's values and preferences.
4. **R**each a decision with the patient.
5. **E**valuate the patient's decision.

For more information on the SHARE Approach, visit the AHRQ website at www.ahrq.gov/shareddecision-making.

The nurse is responsible for making the patient and family an integral part of the team, keeping the patient involved in decision-making, and promoting an environment respectful of the patient's wants, needs, and preferences.

CASE MANAGEMENT

Case management is a model of care in which an RN case manager coordinates patient care with the goal of focusing attention on the quality, outcomes, and cost of care throughout an episode of illness and helping the patient move through the continuum of care. Case managers may be employed by health insurance companies to guide care for health plan members, or they may be employed by hospitals to coordinate individual patients' care throughout the course of illnesses. Hospital nurse case managers manage a caseload of patients from preadmission (or onset of illness) to discharge (or resolution of illness). Although case managers generally do not perform direct-care duties, they assume a planning and evaluative role and collaborate with the interprofessional health care team to ensure that goals are met, quality is maintained, and progress toward discharge is made. For example, the nurse case manager coordinates arrangements to move the patient from acute care to rehabilitation to home health to independent living as determined by patient needs. See Case Study 21.1 for an example of case management.

CASE STUDY 21.1   Case Management

The following is a case study demonstrating the roles and responsibilities of a nurse case manager:

Mr. Smith, 58 years of age, was diagnosed with lung cancer 1 year ago. He has been in Medical Center Hospital with multiple complications for more than 3 weeks. Debra Welch, RN, the case manager assigned to Mr. Smith's case, is working with the patient, family, physician, other members of the health care team, and the insurance company to determine a timely, cost-effective discharge plan. Debra has performed a comprehensive health assessment and understands the patient's condition and the available support systems. The physician, patient, family, and health care team agree that Mr. Smith's prognosis is grave and that the treatment plan should be for palliative care only. Pain management is most important at this stage of the disease. Mr. Smith has a strong desire to go home, and his wife and adult daughter are willing to share the responsibility for home care. Debra also has identified the family's need for emotional support to deal effectively with the terminal illness.

After contacting Mr. Smith's insurance company Debra learns that the company does not provide home health care or hospice benefits, but that the patient could be transferred to a subacute facility for continued care. Knowing Mr. Smith's strong desire to go home and the support systems in place, Debra identifies all the costs for home care (hospital bed, bedside commode, oxygen, wheelchair, and hospice support with pain management) and reports the comparative costs of home care and subacute care to the insurance company. By demonstrating that home care is less expensive than inpatient subacute care Debra is able to successfully negotiate a payment for home care from Mr. Smith's insurance company.

Debra's next responsibilities as case manager are to coordinate Mr. Smith's discharge and to arrange for home services needed, including hospice care and medical equipment. The home plan of care is developed by the health care team. Debra communicates the plan of care to the home care providers to ensure unfragmented care. As a result of case management Mr. Smith and his family are able to go home with continued support and a smooth transition of care.

Case Management Related to Other Nursing Care Delivery Models

Nursing case management in a health care facility supplements nursing care and does not take the place of the nursing care delivery model in place to provide direct patient care. For example, if a hospital's medical-surgical unit uses a team nursing approach to patient care, a system of case management might also be in place to assist with coordinating the patient's total care through discharge. Case management is not needed for every patient in a health care facility and generally is reserved for chronically ill, seriously ill or injured, and long-term, high-cost patients.

Newer Models of Case Management

Health care reform is guiding health care to move from expensive acute care settings to less costly community and home settings. Along with this movement to lower cost care settings there is a growing need to improve care for individuals with multiple chronic diseases who may also struggle with issues related to social determinants of health, such as a lack of safe housing, nutritious food, and other social supports that enable good self-care. Thus new care models with a foundation in case management are emerging to help better support these individuals. The first such model is the use of *patient navigators*. First conceptualized in cancer treatment, patient navigators help patients maneuver through the maze of medical appointments, treatments and procedures, insurance and payment systems, patient-support services, educational resources, and multiple other components of the health care system. The use of patient navigators has been expanded to better manage patients with chronic diseases such as diabetes and heart failure and to coordinate support from the interprofessional team, including pharmacists, dietitians, and social workers. Patient navigator responsibilities, in conjunction with the interprofessional team, include helping patients access resources such as the community food bank and free medication programs, making home visits to assess the home environment and implications for chronic disease management, and communicating with other members of the health care team to support appropriate care decisions.

A second model, *transitional care*, has provided a new role for the RN. As patients with complex care needs move through different levels of care and between multiple providers, communication may be rushed and inadequate, resulting in medication errors, lack of follow-through on key referrals, duplicative testing, inconsistent patient monitoring, and overall poorer patient outcomes. Health care systems are recognizing the value of nurses to facilitate safe and effective transitions for chronically ill patients. Box 21.1 lists some typical responsibilities of a transitional care nurse.

Nurse case managers, patient navigators, and transitional care nurses all have similar goals—to work throughout the maze of health care entities to ensure that patients receive the best care possible at the lowest cost in the most appropriate setting with the resources they need to be successful in managing their own care to the extent possible.

CLINICAL PATHWAYS

Clinical pathways, also called *critical paths*, *practice protocols*, *patient care protocols*, and *care maps*, are clinical management plans that specify major patient care activities, interprofessional interventions, and desired outcomes within a specified time for a particular diagnosis or health condition. The advantage of the clinical pathway is that it provides a means of standardizing care for patients with similar diagnoses and defines key processes and patient goals in the day-to-day management of care. For example, a patient with a total-knee replacement would follow a specified clinical pathway through their recovery.

A similar but different term, clinical practice guidelines (CPGs), focus on the decisions to perform a procedure or service. For example, a CPG would be used to determine whether, on the basis of their specific cancer diagnosis, age, and other comorbidities, a patient diagnosed with prostate cancer should undergo radiation treatment while the clinical pathway would guide the care provided to a cancer patient currently undergoing radiation therapy.

In essence the clinical pathway can be viewed as a road map the patient and health care team should follow to guide the patient's care management and recovery. Clinical pathways were developed in response to the need to identify quality, cost-effective care plans to reduce the patient's length of stay in the hospital. In one study a large hospital developed 30 clinical pathways for the care of pediatric patients being admitted with various diagnoses such as bronchiolitis, which resulted in improved parent and patient satisfaction and decreased nursing turnover (Johnson-Salerno et al., 2020). Accreditation agencies such as TJC may stipulate that certain health care facilities use clinical pathways or CPGs to meet accreditation standards. It is important to be knowledgeable about any CPGs and/or clinical pathways used in your work or clinical setting; to get this information, visit with a nurse leader or case manager in your organization.

BOX 21.1   Typical Responsibilities for a Transition Care RN

- Ensure good communication among the patient, significant others, providers, and caregivers as transitions across different levels of care occur; facilitate timely transfer of important information.
- Coordinate appropriate follow-up with appointments and other necessary care treatments (e.g., chemotherapy, appointments with medical specialists).
- Educate the patient and significant others on their prescribed medication regimen, ensure the safe use and storage of medications, and enlist the assistance of a pharmacist to assist with medication management.
- Ensure the patient has the resources to obtain required medications.
- Coordinate support from the interprofessional team, including pharmacists, dietitians, and social workers.
- Coordinate needed services, such as home health or physical therapy.
- Assist with referrals for needed resources, such as transportation, food, and possibly a safe living environment.
- Educate and counsel patients to be active participants in their own care and make informed decisions.
- Support patients and families to develop effective self-care management skills.

For more information, visit the National Transition of Care Coalition at www.ntocc.org.

CHOOSING A NURSING CARE DELIVERY MODEL

The nursing care delivery models presented in this chapter can be integrated into a variety of health care settings, including acute care, long-term care, ambulatory care, home care, and hospice. The organizational structure, patient needs, and staff availability influence which delivery system will be used.

Acute care settings may use different types of care delivery models for various patient care units. Emergency departments often use functional approaches to care because emphasis is on efficient assessment and immediate treatment. Team nursing is frequently used in medical-surgical units, whereas total patient care is common in critical care units.

In long-term care settings, such as nursing homes, skilled nursing facilities, and rehabilitation settings, patients remain in the care settings for extended periods. Therefore the care delivery models may be structured differently from those in the acute setting. Because of its economy and efficiency, functional nursing may be used for daily care tasks, whereas a form of primary care nursing is used for assessment, care planning, and evaluation.

The variety of ambulatory care settings continues to grow as health care moves out of the more expensive inpatient settings to the less-costly outpatient settings. Outpatient surgery centers, minor emergency clinics, outpatient cancer centers, outpatient dialysis units, outpatient birthing centers, health clinics, and physicians' offices are examples of ambulatory care settings. The nursing care delivery model used in ambulatory settings varies widely, depending on the type of patients being treated and their particular needs. For example, in outpatient dialysis units a combination of functional and primary care nursing usually works well. Patient care technicians are assigned to perform specific patient care functions such as dialysis machine setup and treatment initiation, whereas the RN is assigned primary nurse responsibilities for a group of patients to ensure effective assessment, care planning, and care coordination with the interprofessional team. Home health care agencies often use a variation of the primary care model. Although in home care the RN does not provide 24-hour care, they are responsible for the patient's needs for a 24-hour period and will coordinate intermittent care provided by others, including the home health aide and therapists involved in the patient's care. In the home health care setting the RN may also function in the role of case manager for their assigned patients.

In every care setting nurses should carefully evaluate the nursing care delivery model to ensure safe, efficient, and effective patient care. In the evaluation of any nursing care delivery model the following questions should be asked:

- Is patient safety ensured while optimal patient satisfaction and patient outcomes are achieved in a timely, cost-effective manner?
- Is patient-centered care being provided with significant involvement of the patient and their family or significant other?

- Are nurses, physicians, and other health care team members satisfied with the safety and quality of care they are able to provide?
- Does the system allow for implementation of the clinic judgment model in a timely and efficient manner?
- Does the system facilitate communication among all members of the health care team?

THE FUTURE IS HERE: EVOLVING NURSING CARE DELIVERY MODELS

Without a doubt the ways in which nursing care is delivered is changing dramatically as a result of the following factors:

- Unprecedented stress placed on hospitals to care for complex patients amid a serious nursing shortage
- Fast-paced patient turnover in acute care settings with rapid discharge and admission cycles
- Need to address the mental health and work–life balance for nurses and all members of the health care team
- Social determinants of health recognized as playing a strong role in an individual's overall health
- Strong focus on patient satisfaction, safety, outcomes of care, and reducing costs
- Need to engage patients and families to become active partners to make informed decisions and manage their health needs

Because acute care settings now admit only the most seriously ill or injured individuals with a focus on stabilization and transition, the traditional models of nursing care may no longer apply. In the past, nurses provided care on the basis of comprehensive knowledge of the patients' needs, which were learned by caring for the patients over an extended period. Now nurses may have an entirely new group of patients to care for every shift or even more than once during a shift. Identifying effective models of care to support the rapid transition of patients from one setting to another will be a continuing challenge for nurses and health care organizations.

Innovation in care delivery models has become vitally important to provide care in our changing health care systems. Health care leaders are using advanced data and analytics to develop dashboards to aggregate patient care needs and nurse characteristics to match patient needs with nurse expertise in care delivery models that create optimal patient and nurse outcomes (Ruppel, et al., 2023). Even a standard as simple as allowing nurses time to take an uninterrupted break during their workday has become a challenge that must be addressed by nurses and their leaders (Sagherian, Cho, & Steege, 2023). Nursing care delivery models that provide for adequate rest breaks must be a standard to promote nurse satisfaction and mental health. Nurses in outpatient and community-based settings are challenged with similar problems in attempting to address (1) patients' demands for instant access to care and information and (2) patients' needs for support and education to address lifestyle and personal choices that may affect their health.

Relationship-based care must also be considered part of the care delivery model in high-tech, fast-paced environments where nurses struggle to provide care that is consistent with nursing values of compassion, caring, and healing. Therapeutic relationships to promote optimum health for our patients and communities are the essence of nursing practice and must be accepted as a primary responsibility by every RN. Innovative models of care will continue to be developed and implemented by nurses to ensure that safe, high quality care is delivered in even the most challenging circumstances.

SUMMARY

All nurses must be concerned that patient care is delivered in the most efficient and cost-effective method possible and that staffing is appropriate to ensure safe, high-quality care and contributes to staff satisfaction. To help summarize this chapter, let's revisit the questions posed following the opening Vignette.

1. Why is the RN's work assignment different in various units—obstetrics, critical care, medical-surgical, and the outpatient clinic?

   The structure of the work setting, patient needs, and staff availability will all influence the type of nursing care delivery system used. For example, acute care settings will have different care delivery models for various patient care units with team nursing frequently used in medical-surgical units and total patient care common in critical care units. In long-term care settings where patients remain for extended periods functional nursing may be used for daily care tasks, whereas a form of primary care nursing is used for assessment, care planning, and evaluation.

2. What are key considerations when making staffing and patient care assignment decisions?

   Primary considerations for staffing are the number of patients; the level of intensity of care required by those patients; architecture and geography of the environment and available technology; level of preparation and experience of the staff members; and the quality of the nurses' work life (ANA, 2020). The primary key to safe staffing and

patient care assignments is matching the patient needs with the nurse's expertise.

3. How do nurse managers or other nursing leaders decide which type of nursing care delivery model will be used?

   Ideally, nursing leaders will fully engage staff nurses to help design care delivery models that ensure optimal patient satisfaction and patient outcomes are achieved in a cost-effective manner; patient-centered care is provided with significant involvement of the patient and their family or significant other; nurses and other health care team members have high job satisfaction; and the model allows for effective communication among all members of the health care team.

   Nursing care delivery models have undergone tremendous change throughout the past decade and will continue to evolve as organizations look for ways to improve patient safety and outcomes in complex health care systems that are challenged by the need to reduce costs, shortage of RNs, rapidly advancing technology, high patient turnover, and consumer demand for instant access and information. Regardless of changes that are certain to occur, the RN will retain responsibility for evaluating nursing care delivery models to ensure that patient care is delivered safely and efficiently, that caregivers are competent and legally qualified to perform the duties they have been assigned, and that high-quality, safe, patient-centered care and staff satisfaction are maintained.

REFERENCES

Agency for Healthcare Research and Quality. (2016). *The SHARE approach: A model for shared decision making.* https://www.ahrq.gov/sites/default/files/publications/files/share-approach_factsheet.pdf

American Association of Critical Care Nurses. (n.d.). *The AACN synergy model for patient care.* https://www.aacn.org/nursing-excellence/aacn-standards/synergy-model

American Nurses Association (2020). *Principles for nurse staffing* (3rd ed.) American Nurses Association.

American Nurses Association (n.d.,a). Principles for nurse staffing. https://www.nursingworld.org/practice-policy/nurse-staffing/staffing-principles

American Nurses Association. (n.d.,b). Advocating for safe staffing. https://www.nursingworld.org/practice-policy/nurse-staffing/nurse-staffing-advocacy/

Bradley, C. (2023). Designing a system for safe staffing. *Nurse Leader, 21*(4), 485–488.

Case Management Institute. (2023). Case management study guide: Clinical pathways, standards of care, practice guidelines. https://casemanagementstudyguide.com

Davidson, A. (2023). Nurse-to-patient staffing ratio laws and regulations by state. *Nurse Journal.* https://nursejournal.org/articles/nurse-to-patient-staffing-ratio-laws-by-state/#:,:text=California%20is%20the%20only%20state,ratio%20in%20every%20hospital%20unit

Dawson, J.M. (2014). Nursing practice and work environment. *American Nurse Today, 10*(1), 16.

Institute of Medicine. (2001). *Crossing the quality chasm: A new health system for the 21st century.* National Academies Press.

Institute of Medicine. (2004). *Keeping patients safe: Transforming the work environment of nurses.* National Academies Press.

Institute of Medicine. (2011). *The future of nursing: Leading change, advancing health.* National Academies Press.

Johnson-Salerno, E. (2020). Evaluation of an innovative model of care for a limited-stay pediatric unit. *The Journal of Nursing Administration, 50*(6), 328–334. https://doi.org/10.1097/NNA.0000000000000893

Kerfoot, K. (2019). Patient-centered staffing as the path forward. *American Nurse Today, 14*(9), 87–90.

National Council of State Boards of Nursing and American Nurses Association. (2019). *National guidelines for nursing delegation.* https://www.ncsbn.org/public-files/NGND-PosPaper_06.pdf

Ruppel, H., et al. (2023). Developing a nursing dashboard to align nursing care delivery with patient and family needs. *The Journal of Nursing Administration, 53*(4), 197–203.

Sagherian, K., Cho, H.L., & Steege, L.M. (2023). The state of rest break practices among 12-hour shift hospital nurses in the United States. *The Journal of Nursing Administration, 53*(5), 277–283.

Skarbek, A., et al. (2022). Nursing work environment staffing councils. *Journal of Nursing Administration, 52*(7/8), 419–426.

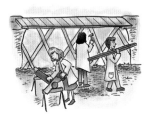

22

Nurses are building bridges to patient safety and quality care.

Quality Improvement and Patient Safety

Cindy Acton, DNP, RN, NEA-BC*

ℯ Additional resources are available online at: http://evolve.elsevier.com/Cherry/

LEARNING OUTCOMES

After studying this chapter, the reader will be able to:

1. Apply principles of quality improvement to the role of the professional nurse.
2. Analyze the basis for the increasing emphasis on health care quality and medical errors.
3. Analyze the role of health care regulatory agencies and how they have embodied the principles of quality improvement.
4. Discuss the role that quality improvement can play in ensuring patient safety and improving quality in the health care system.
5. Describe the tools and skills necessary for successful quality improvement activities.
6. Discuss the professional nurse's role in promoting patient safety.

KEY TERMS

Cause-and-effect diagram Tool that is used for identifying and organizing possible causes of a problem in a structured format. It is sometimes called a fishbone diagram because it looks like the skeleton of a fish.

Clinical indicators Measurable items that reflect the quality of care provided and demonstrate the degree to which desired clinical outcomes are accomplished.

Customer Individual or group who relies on an organization to provide a product or service to meet some need or expectation. It is these customer needs and expectations that determine quality. Patients are considered customers.

Failure mode and effects analysis (FMEA) A systematic process for identifying potential design and process failures before they occur, with the intent to eliminate them or minimize the risk associated with them.

Flowchart Picture of the sequence of steps in a process. Different steps or actions are represented by boxes or other symbols.

Hospital-acquired condition (HAC) A term used to indicate an unintended and typically adverse patient-acquired condition occurring as a result of being cared for in a hospital.

National Academy of Medicine (NAM) A nonprofit organization (formerly known as the National Institute of Medicine [IOM]) that is one of three academies that make up the National Academies of Sciences, Engineering, and Medicine, collectively known as the National Academies, in the United States. Its mission is "to improve health for all by advancing science, accelerating health equity, and providing independent, authoritative, and trusted advice nationally and globally" (NAM, 2020). The NAM provides objective, timely, authoritative information and advice concerning health and science policy to the government, the corporate sector, the professions, and the public.

*We would like to thank Kathleen M. Werner, MS, BSN, RN, CPHQ, for her contributions to this chapter in Editions 1–8.

403

Never events Serious adverse events during an inpatient stay that should never occur or are reasonably preventable through adherence to evidence-based guidelines. The Centers for Medicare and Medicaid Services, through revisions in coverage and payment policies, provide hospitals with financial incentives to reduce the occurrence of never events.

Pareto chart A graphic tool that helps break down a big problem into its parts and then identify which parts are the most important.

Process A series of linked steps necessary to accomplish work. A process turns inputs, such as information or raw materials, into outputs, such as products, services, and reports. Clinical processes are a series of linked steps necessary for the provision of patient care.

Process variation The differences in how the steps in a work process might be accomplished and/or the variables that may affect each step in the process. Variation results from the lack of perfect uniformity in the performance of any process. Understanding variation in a process is necessary to determine the direction that improvement efforts must take.

Quality improvement (QI) Framework for taking action to systematically make changes that lead to measurable improvements in health care services for patients, staff, and organizations; quality is determined by the needs, expectations, and desired health outcomes of individuals and populations.

Root cause analyses and actions, or RCA^2 (RCA "squared") Method of problem-solving that identifies how and why an event occurred, determines causal factors, and develops improvements to eliminate further occurrences while emphasizing the importance of an organization's need "to act" to prevent future harm. Formerly known simply as "root cause analysis," the uptake of RCA^2 is prevailing in many organizations. Both the Institute for Healthcare Improvement (IHI) and The Joint Commission (TJC) developed tools to help clinicians address RCA^2. For more information, visit the IHI website (www.ihi.org), location: Resources > Tools > All Tools > View All > RCA^2: Improving Root Cause Analyses and Actions to Prevent Harm.

Run chart Graph of data in time order that helps identify any changes that occur over time; also called a *time plot*. A run chart to which a centerline and statistical control limits have been added is known as a *control chart*.

Sentinel event Defined by TJC (2023a) as a patient safety event that reaches a patient and results in death, permanent harm, or severe temporary harm, and intervention is required to sustain life. Such events are called "sentinel" because they signal the need for immediate investigation and response.

Standardization Approach to process improvement that involves developing and adhering to best known methods and repeating key tasks in the same way, time and time again, until a better way is found, thereby creating exceptional service with maximal efficiency.

The Joint Commission (TJC) A national agency that conducts surveys of inpatient and ambulatory facilities and certifies their compliance with established quality standards.

PROFESSIONAL/ETHICAL ISSUE

Christine Nguyen, RN, works in the cardiac step-down unit at a large teaching hospital. Christine graduated from nursing school 6 months ago. She has been managing her own patient assignment for the last few months but she continues to work closely with her mentor, an experienced RN who has worked on the unit for 15 years. Recently Christine has become concerned about a pattern on the unit in which the nurses ignore alarms on medical devices. She knows that the purpose of the alarms is to alert caregivers about changes in patient conditions, but she also knows improperly set alarms can be a nuisance and pull nurses away from other important work. Her greatest concern is that ignoring alarms might result in patient harm. To make the situation more complicated, Christine does not feel comfortable discussing her concerns with her mentor because she has overheard her mentor tell other nurses that there are times when it is okay to ignore alarms. How should Christine begin to address this situation with her colleagues or supervisor? Discuss how this safety concern might be addressed through the quality improvement process.

VIGNETTE

It was the third postoperative day for Mrs. Hernandez in room 918 on the general surgical unit of Metro Hospital. As he arrived for his day shift Jaheem Harper, RN, was eager to care for this patient. Jaheem had been with Mrs. Hernandez every day since her admission and was looking forward to helping her prepare for discharge. Jaheem carried out the routine morning care and did a thorough assessment of Mrs. Hernandez. Much to Jaheem's dismay, Mrs. Hernandez was not her usual, upbeat self and was less cooperative than normal, stating, "I just don't have much energy. I know I should get up and walk, but I just don't feel like it." Jaheem also noted that Mrs. Hernandez's temperature was higher than normal, so he alerted the surgical house staff during rounds. Mrs. Hernandez's blood was drawn for a complete blood count (CBC) and a urine sample was collected. Within the hour, the answer to Mrs. Hernandez's sudden lack of energy and enthusiasm became known—she had a urinary tract infection (UTI), most likely as the result of the indwelling catheter that had been placed during surgery and still remained. Mrs. Hernandez would not be going home until the catheter was removed and treatment of the infection was well under way. Jaheem experienced the wisdom of "hindsight" by noting that the catheter should have been removed by postoperative day 2. Owing to the surgeon's failure to write an order to discontinue the indwelling catheter in a timely manner—as well as Jaheem's failure to bring this to the provider's attention—Mrs. Hernandez was now experiencing a setback in her recovery.

Jaheem began to reflect on the number of times this may have occurred with other patients. He also began to consider the implications of the lack of a consistent and standardized way to track the dwell time of urinary catheters. As in Mrs. Hernandez's situation, the development of a UTI could cost $12,000 to $20,000 in additional expenses for the hospital; it would mean additional care and treatment with an extended length of stay that would not be paid by the patient's insurance company because the catheter-associated UTI would be deemed an event that should have been prevented (a "never event"). Multiplying this cost by just 10 additional patients makes catheter-associated UTIs

a significant financial burden for the organization. More importantly, patients who experience discomfort and increased fatigue risk developing even more complications because of their decreased willingness or ability to cooperate with their postoperative care.

The next week Jaheem approached his nurse manager and expressed concern about the delays in discontinuing indwelling urinary catheters that create the potential for catheter-associated UTIs. Jaheem's nurse manager thanked him for the feedback and expressed similar interest in resolving this problem. Infection prevention staff members had already been in preliminary conversations with Jaheem's manager about the increased risk of infection and were willing to work collaboratively with the nursing staff and physicians to find a solution to this problem. Jaheem eagerly volunteered to participate in a quality improvement team that was charged with standardizing the care processes for discontinuation of urinary catheters to ensure compliance with removal by postoperative day 2 for 100% of all patients.

The team met regularly for several weeks and gained a clear understanding of why both physicians and nurses "lost track of time" with respect to removal of these catheters. A better understanding was accomplished by creating a "documentation" flow chart detailing what typically occurred for postoperative orders by the surgical staff and the routine care implemented by nursing personnel. Breakdowns in this process for ensuring completeness of all necessary orders were identified, and the team began working on constructive ways to prevent these breakdowns in the future. The team worked with information technology experts to incorporate the indwelling catheter discontinuation order in an electronic order set easily accessible for all prescribing health care providers. Furthermore, if the discontinuation order was not documented an electronic alert would be sent to the attending surgeon to remind them to either complete the order or document the rationale for not doing so. Likewise, nursing staff would receive an electronic "best practice alert" reminding them to check the orders for this purpose.

Over time, with ongoing monitoring of the ordering practices and the catheter-associated UTI rates, significant progress was made, to the point that infection rates are now nearly zero. Jaheem knows that the proper steps are in place to guarantee that this successful infection reduction effort will be sustained through the thoughtful process that was developed. When his patients are ready for discharge there will be no setbacks caused by situations that could have been prevented. Jaheem feels that he is a vested part of this success.

Questions to Consider While Reading This Chapter:

1. What key principles of quality improvement are demonstrated in the Vignette?
2. What quality improvement tools did Jaheem and the team most likely use to identify the causes of catheter-associated UTIs?
3. What resources are available to help Jaheem and others in his organization learn more about improving the quality of health care?

CHAPTER OVERVIEW

Although Jaheem Harper's story depicted in the Vignette seems credible and would be a logical way for any organization to begin addressing customer concerns, far too often this has not been the case. Hospitals and other health care organizations have been slow to recognize the necessity of a true customer perspective and to emphasize quality and safety in a proactive manner. The intention of this chapter is to make the reader aware of the pressing nature of the nation's quality health care crisis and to address the following questions:

- What is quality in health care?
- Who determines the degree to which quality and safety are evident in our health care system?
- How can work processes be redesigned to improve quality and safety?
- What do the potential answers to the first three questions mean for professional nursing accountability?

The responses to these questions provide the elements of hope for determining and implementing sustainable, positive improvements in the design and delivery of health care, particularly as they relate to nursing's commitment to lead and facilitate quality improvement efforts.

THE URGENT CASE FOR QUALITY IMPROVEMENT IN THE US HEALTH CARE SYSTEM

In an alarming 2000 report by the Institute of Medicine (IOM), *To Err Is Human: Building a Safer Health System,*

the writers extrapolated and summarized data from two major studies and concluded that up to 98,000 patients die each year from preventable medical errors, confirming that poor quality of care is a major problem in the United States (IOM, 2000). Contributing factors cited in this original IOM report include:

- Overuse of expensive, invasive technology
- Underuse of inexpensive care services
- Error-prone implementation of care that could harm patients and waste money

Following this report the IOM released *Crossing the Quality Chasm: A New Health System for the 21st Century* (2001) to define a vision for improving the quality of our nation's health care. Although this report was released more than two decades ago, its main premise still holds true today: "The U.S. health care delivery system does not provide consistent, high-quality medical care to all people. Americans should be able to count on receiving care that meets their needs and is based on the best scientific knowledge—yet this frequently is not the case. Health care harms too frequently and routinely fails to deliver its potential benefits. Indeed, between the health care that we now have and the health care that we could have lies not just a gap, but a chasm."

Over the past 20 years these two major reports created persistent and unrelenting national attention on patient safety and quality in the US health care system, with hospitals and health systems across the country working to improve the quality and safety of the care provided. As a result there have been improvements, yet after many years patient safety and quality care continue to be a significant problem. For example, an estimated 25% of hospitalized Medicare patients experienced some type of harm from events including adverse drug events, pressure injuries, and infections (Grimm, 2022). As one can see, there is still much work to be done in our health care systems to promote patient safety!

Today's nurses must be the leaders who will continue the improvements started more than 20 years ago by following some of the basic tenets recommended in the *Quality Chasm* report, which offers six guiding aims for improvement, calling for health care to be (IOM, 2001):

- *Safe:* Preventing injuries to patients from the care that is intended to help them
- *Timely:* Reducing waits and sometimes harmful delays for both those who receive and those who give care

- *Effective:* Providing services based on scientific knowledge to all who could benefit, and refraining from providing services to those not likely to benefit
- *Efficient:* Preventing waste, including waste of equipment, supplies, ideas, and energy
- *Equitable:* Providing care that does not vary in quality because of personal characteristics, such as gender, ethnicity, geographic location, and socioeconomic status
- *Patient centered:* Providing care that is respectful of and responsive to individual patient preferences, needs, and values and ensuring that patient values guide all clinical decisions

These six guiding aims are collectively referred to by the acronym STEEEP and should be adopted by every individual and group involved in the provision of health care, including health care professionals, public and private health care organizations, purchasers of health care, regulatory agencies and organizations, and state and federal policymakers.

To help establish a framework for accomplishing the significant redesign of the health care system, the writers of the *Quality Chasm* report formulated a set of 10 simple rules to guide improvement initiatives. Professional nurses must serve as role models for all health care professionals, caregivers, and administrators in practicing the following 10 rules (IOM, 2001):

1. *Care is based on continuous healing relationships.* Patients should receive care whenever they need it and in many forms, including face-to-face visits, via the Internet, by telephone, and other means as needed.
2. *Care is customized according to patient needs and values.* The system should be designed to meet the most common needs but should also be responsive to individual choices and preferences.
3. *The patient is the source of control.* Patients should be given the necessary information and opportunity to exercise the degree of control they choose over health care decisions that affect them.
4. *Knowledge is shared, and information flows freely.* Patients should have unfettered access to their own medical information and to clinical knowledge, with clinicians communicating effectively and sharing information.
5. *Decision-making is evidence based.* Patients should receive care based on the best available scientific knowledge, and care should not vary illogically from clinician to clinician or place to place.

6. *Safety is a system property.* Patients should be safe; reducing risk and ensuring safety require greater attention to systems that help prevent and mitigate errors.
7. *Transparency is necessary.* The system should make available to patients and families information that allows them to make informed decisions, including information describing the system's performance on safety, evidence-based practice, and patient satisfaction.
8. *Needs are anticipated.* The system should anticipate patient needs rather than simply react to events.
9. *Waste is continually decreased.* The system should not waste resources (e.g., supplies, health professionals' time and energy) or patient time.
10. *Cooperation among clinicians is a priority.* Clinicians should actively engage in collaboration and communication to ensure an appropriate exchange of information and coordination of care.

As the IOM led the promotion of safer health care systems it has transitioned to the National Academy of Medicine and continues its strong focus on using science to improve health for all.

The remainder of this chapter provides the reader with a set of principles and skills necessary to implement improvements and move toward a system of health care that is safe, timely, effective, efficient, equitable, and patient centered.

PRINCIPLES OF QUALITY IMPROVEMENT

Many buzzwords describe activities associated with quality improvement (QI). The most prevalent are total quality management (TQM), continuous quality improvement (CQI), continuous process improvement, statistical process control, and performance improvement (PI). The terms themselves are not as important as the principles they embody: assessing and improving work processes while focusing on what customers want and need. In the example of Jaheem and his patient, the work process is completing postoperative orders that include timely removal of an indwelling urinary catheter. The customer in this situation would be Jaheem's patient, who wants to recover from surgery without complications so that she can go home as soon as possible. Essentially the cornerstones of QI are quality, scientific approach, and "all one team" (Joiner, 1994).

Quality

To provide a better appreciation of the importance of these three QI cornerstones, a customer's perspective of quality must be considered, including the personal interactions experienced with an organization's personnel in addition to the products or services they receive. The products or services provided to the customer are not made up of just the physical items or a one-time experience that the customer encounters, but rather of all the services that go with it. Organizations actually provide a "bundle" of products and services to customers to satisfy some needs. If the service and product or outcomes together are perceived as a good value, a loyal customer following will be established. Or, as in the case presented in the Vignette, Jaheem's patient might view the entire hospital stay negatively because of the delay in discharge due to a preventable complication. Recognizing the value of the customer's perspective of quality, the Centers for Medicare and Medicaid Services (CMS) surveys patients on their experience and uses a scoring system to reward providers through its Value-Based Program, discussed later in this chapter. For more information on patient experience surveys, Consumer Assessment of Healthcare Providers & Systems, visit the CMS website at www.cms.gov, location: Medicare > Quality > Quality Initiatives > Hospital Quality Initiative > HCAHPS: Patients' Perspectives of Care Survey.

Scientific Approach

The scientific approach, the second cornerstone of QI, emphasizes that to make significant improvements in an organization's processes, decisions must be based on sound, valid data, and the people managing the processes must have a clear understanding of the nature of variation in processes. Remember that a process is a series of linked steps necessary to accomplish work. For example, the steps necessary to complete a new medication order, from the time the order is received until the medication is administered to a patient, is a process. Understanding process variation—the differences in how the steps in the process might be accomplished and/or the variables that may affect each step—is necessary to identify the direction that improvement efforts must take.

Two types of variation in processes can occur: common cause variation and special cause variation. Processes that demonstrate common cause variation are stable, predictable, and statistically in control. Processes that demonstrate both common cause and special cause variation are unstable, unpredictable, and not in statistical control. The actions that should be taken to implement improvements under each type of variation are significantly different.

The best way to understand common cause and special cause variations is to use Jaheem's example again. Jaheem's team members collected data over time regarding the number of times surgeons failed to write postoperative orders that included discontinuation of urinary catheters. Overall, the number of missed orders showed variability because of numerous factors associated with this process, one example being the total number of patients with postoperative orders on any given day. The team recognized the total number of postoperative patients as common cause variation and realized that to decrease the occurrence of missing elements within these orders, the overall process would need to be studied to determine the best ways to change the postoperative care processes, regardless of the total volume of patients.

The team was also aware of a significant physician learning curve associated with the automation of electronic order sets, with two surgeons who had not completed the required training session before the system went "live." The failure to document the catheter discontinuation order under these circumstances was considered to be special cause process variation, one of extreme impact but related to a clearly identified single source. If the team had modified the overall documentation process solely on the basis of the special cause factor, the underlying problem most likely would not have been improved for the long term.

"All One Team"

Effective team functioning is the third QI cornerstone, which embodies the principles of believing in people; treating everyone in the workplace with dignity, trust, and respect; and working toward win–win situations for all customers, employees, shareholders, suppliers, and perhaps even the broader community as a whole. For people to work this way they must believe it is in their best interest to cooperate; they need to be more concerned with how the system as a whole operates rather than optimizing their own contributing area. In other words, all team members must rely more on cooperation and less on competition.

Example

Jaheem's example is one that demonstrates the following three principles of QI:

Quality: Jaheem began to consider the patient as the one who would define the quality of her hospital stay. The nurse recognized that the perceived quality of the entire hospital stay could suffer if the prevention of complications could not be improved.

Scientific approach: Jaheem was supported organizationally by his manager, who provided the opportunity for Jaheem to collaborate with other key members of the health care team to better comprehend the current status of catheter-associated UTIs through analyzing data and examining variations in the process. This group's work led to a clearer understanding of the interrelationship of the processes across multiple health care professionals, which together affected the overall timeliness of urinary catheter discontinuation and enabled the group to make the necessary improvements to achieve the desired result.

"All one team": Managers in Jaheem's hospital had faith in the people who were working on the catheter-associated UTI team. They were recognized as the people who had the best understanding of how the postoperative care processes were happening and where the system was breaking down.

ADVANCING QUALITY THROUGH REGULATION AND ACCREDITATION

Today almost all health care regulatory and voluntary accrediting agencies require QI in some form. The Centers for Medicare and Medicaid Services (CMS), which administers the US Medicare program, has "conditions of participation" for its quality foundation, and most state licensing authorities also have required QI standards. The Joint Commission (TJC), an organization that offers voluntary accreditation for health care settings, has a strong focus on quality standards, as discussed in the following sections.

The Joint Commission

The Joint Commission was one of the first accreditation agencies to embrace QI principles as an accreditation requirement in hospital-based settings. TJC accredits and certifies more than 22,000 health care organizations and programs in the United States, including hospitals and health care organizations that provide ambulatory and office-based surgery, behavioral health, home care, laboratory, and nursing care center services (TJC, 2023b). Health care organizations voluntarily seek TJC accreditation to demonstrate that they have achieved a "gold seal of approval" by following the quality and safety standards established by TJC. TJC standards address the organization's level of performance in key functional areas such as patient safety, patient rights, patient treatment, and infection control. The TJC accreditation system not only focuses on an organization's ability to provide safe high-quality care but also requires evidence of actual performance and continued improvement. Health care organizations that are accredited by TJC receive "deemed status" to automatically meet foundational approval from CMS. Although TJC is the most recognized CMS-approved accreditation agency, other organizations have entered the field. For a current list of CMS-Approved Accrediting Organizations visit www.cms.gov, location: Medicare > Health and safety standards > Accreditations programs > Downloads > Accrediting Organizations Contacts for Prospective Clients.

Core Measures: National Hospital Quality Measures

In 2002 TJC-accredited hospitals began collecting data on standardized "core" performance measures, and by 2003 TJC and CMS were working together to align current and future measures common to both organizations. Examples of core measures are related to treatment of acute myocardial infarction, childhood asthma, and stroke, among many others. These standardized measures are now referred to as National Hospital Inpatient Quality Measures and can be found on TJC's website: www.jointcommission.org, location: Measurement > Specifications Manual > Chart Abstracted Measures. The performance data for hospitals across the country are now publicly reported on TJC's website Quality Check (www.quality-check.org) and through the CMS Hospital Compare website (www.medicare.gov/hospitalcompare).

The National Hospital Inpatient Quality Measures now have an added level of significance beyond the public reporting aspect. These measures, in concert with patient feedback and other select clinical outcome measures, are being used increasingly in programs designed to "pay for performance" in moving health care payments away from simply paying for the provision of services to paying on the basis of the quality and outcomes associated with those services.

As part of the Patient Protection and Affordable Care Act of 2010 CMS was authorized to begin its *Value-Based Purchasing Program*, whereby hospital inpatient Medicare payments are reduced annually (from 1% in the first program fiscal year of 2012 up to a maximum of 2% by fiscal year 2017 and beyond). Through the Value-Based Program, hospitals may earn back the reduced payments or even exceed the original payment amount on the basis of their performance results. The Value-Based Program gauges hospitals on outcome measures such as: mortality and complications; health-care associated infections (HAI); patient safety; patient experience; and efficiency and cost reduction. Similar payment programs have expanded to home health, skilled nursing facilities, and physician offices. Other commercial insurance carriers and state agencies are beginning to deploy similar strategies in their payment agreements. For more on Value-Based Programs, visit the CMS website: www.cms.gov, location: Medicare > Quality > Value-Based Programs.

It is especially important for nurses to be knowledgeable about the *National Hospital Inpatient Quality Measures and Value-Based Purchasing Program* because they are in the unique position of leading the overall management of patient care, working collaboratively with other health care professionals to initiate changes, and monitoring ongoing effectiveness of the care and follow-up provided.

CLINICAL INDICATORS AND PROCESS IMPROVEMENT TOOLS AND SKILLS

The basic foundation of the monitoring and evaluation process required by QI principles is in the use of clinical indicators, measurable items that reflect the quality of care. Just like the National Hospital Inpatient Quality Measures previously referenced, clinical indicators are aspects of clinical care that can be measured to show the extent to which care is or is not being implemented as it should be. Indicators focus on clinical actions or outcomes of clinical care; indicators should not focus on procedures that support clinical care. For example, replacing the intravenous (IV) solutions on the IV supply cart as they are used is a procedure that supports clinical care. Administering the correct IV solution at the correct rate as prescribed is appropriate clinical care. Both items are measurable but only the latter is truly a clinical indicator. Indicators are meant not to define quality but, rather, to point the way to assessment of areas in which quality issues may be present.

How do process improvement skills and tools fit with clinical indicators? Clinical indicators help identify the goals of QI, whereas process improvement skills and tools support the quantitative understanding of key work processes. Several different methods are used by health care facilities for QI and process improvement, including Lean methodology, Lean Six Sigma, and failure mode and effects analysis (FMEA). The tools described within this section (e.g., flowcharts, Pareto charts) are all used in each of these various methods of QI. Addressing these specific improvement strategies is not within the scope of this chapter, but it is important to note that all improvement models generally have the following activities in common:

- Analyzing and clearly understanding the process
- Selecting key aspects of the process to improve
- Establishing "trial" targets to guide improvement measures
- Collecting and plotting data
- Interpreting results
- Implementing improvement actions and evaluating effectiveness

Various tools, such as flowcharts, Pareto charts, cause-and-effect diagrams, and run charts, may be used to accomplish each of these six steps. Through use of these tools, results can be analyzed with interpretations subsequently guiding appropriate improvement actions. Once improvements are initiated, ongoing monitoring is initiated to evaluate the effectiveness of the changes implemented. It is becoming increasingly necessary for professional nurses to understand improvement models and develop the ability to apply these tools.

Flowchart

The analysis of a work process is usually initiated through construction of some sort of flowchart or flow diagram. These are indispensable tools in mapping out what actually occurs during the process vs what is intended. There are several different types of flowcharts, each of which is valuable in its own way. A top-down flowchart simply lists the main steps and substeps of a process in a linear fashion (Fig. 22.1). A deployment flowchart maps out the steps of a process under headings that designate the people or departments carrying out each step. This type is especially helpful to deal with processes that involve multiple areas or caregivers and when there is a need for common understanding of what the process is doing as a whole (Fig. 22.2). As

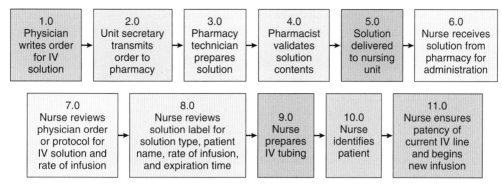

Fig. 22.1 Top-down flowchart of process for administering intravenous solutions.

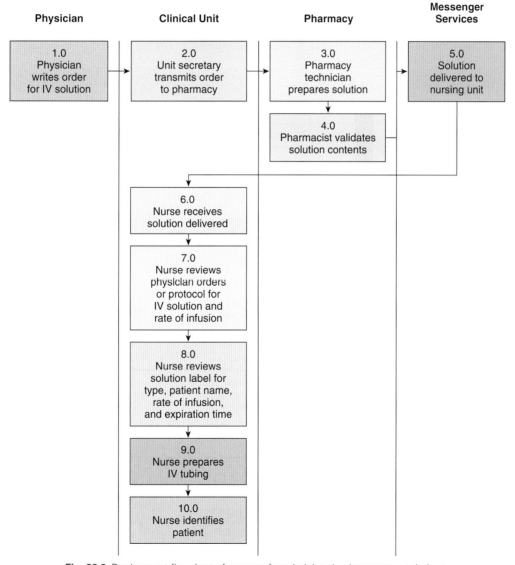

Fig. 22.2 Deployment flowchart of process for administering intravenous solutions.

illustrated in Figs. 22.1 and 22.2, top-down and deployment flowcharts can be used to view the process of administering the correct IV solution at the correct rate.

Pareto Chart

For selecting key aspects on which to focus within the process, a Pareto chart may be an appropriate tool. Collecting data on presumed or known problems in a given process can identify areas of focus or concentration. This tool itself is a type of bar graph, with the height of bars reflecting the frequency with which events occur or the effect events have on a process problem. The bars are arranged in descending order so that the most commonly occurring problems are readily visible. Fig. 22.3 is based on the Pareto principle, which proposes that 80% of process or system problems are generated from only 20% of the possible causal factors. Therefore focusing on the significant few causes can achieve a much broader effect on improvement efforts.

Cause-and-Effect Diagram

The cause-and-effect diagram is another worthy tool that can help determine potential sources of a problem. Such a diagram is a list of potential causes arranged by categories to show their potential effect on a problem. The categories are usually broad, with subsequent levels of detail to illustrate what "might cause" the effect in question. This diagram is sometimes referred to as a "fishbone diagram" because it resembles a fish skeleton when complete (Fig. 22.4). Cause-and-effect diagrams are helpful when the major problem areas have been localized through the use of the Pareto chart.

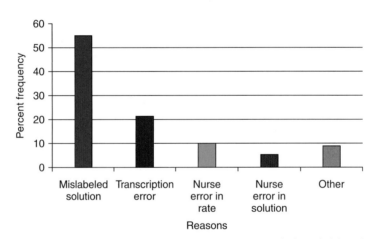

Fig. 22.3 Pareto chart of reasons for incorrect intravenous solution administration.

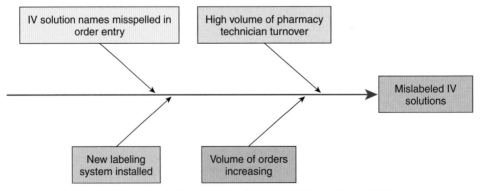

Fig. 22.4 Cause-and-effect diagram of mislabeled intravenous solutions.

Run Chart

Measuring data over time to evaluate patterns in process variation typically is suited for tools such as the run chart and the control chart. Run charts, also known as time plots, are graphs of data points as they occur over time (Fig. 22.5). Valuable information can be obtained regarding process variation through study of the trends in the run chart. A control chart is a slightly more sophisticated tool to help distinguish between common cause and special cause variations. A control chart is basically a run chart with statistical control limits added.

UNDERSTANDING, IMPROVING, AND STANDARDIZING CARE PROCESSES

Standardized processes, otherwise referred to as "best known methods" or "best practices," when effectively managed, have been shown to be the foundation for improvements in all areas of business today, but especially in the clinical care setting. There is a typical resistance to standardizing practices, especially when they involve providing patient care, but the realistic effect of care without standardization must be considered in the following context as described by Joiner (1994):

- Employees may receive little training on how to do their jobs. Instead the majority are left to learn by watching a more experienced employee.
- Most employees have developed their own unique versions of any general procedures they witnessed or were taught. They think, "My way is the best way."
- Changes to procedures happen haphazardly; individuals constantly change details to counteract problems that arise or in hopes of discovering a better method. Tampering is rampant.

Each of the QI cornerstones could easily be applied to caregiver situations. At first glance it would be assumed that all care practices are based on scientific evidence and research, and although many are, others exist simply because that was how the practitioner originally was educated. Those practices that are research based, even though they represent best known methods, may still not be widely practiced, thereby resulting in lack of standardization.

During the past few years a number of methods have been used in health care settings for the purpose of supporting standardization of care processes. Clinical guidelines, critical pathways, and clinical protocols or algorithms are standardization methods that are more prevalent and familiar. Although these terms sometimes are used interchangeably, the following is offered as a context in which to understand their potential differences.

Clinical Pathways or Critical Pathways

Clinical pathway or *critical pathway* typically defines the optimal sequencing and timing of interventions by physicians, nurses, and other interprofessional team members when providing care for a patient with a particular diagnosis or procedure, such as a patient who is hospitalized for a coronary artery bypass graft. These pathways are usually developed through collaborative efforts of the interprofessional team, which includes physicians, nurses, pharmacists, and others, to improve the quality and value of the patient care provided. Among the most obvious benefits of using clinical pathways are (1) reduction in variation of the care provided, (2) facilitation and achievement of expected clinical outcomes, (3) reduction in care delays and lengths of stay

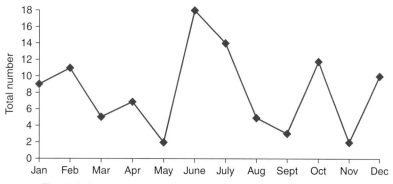

Fig. 22.5 Run chart of number of mislabeled intravenous solutions.

in the inpatient setting, and (4) improvements in cost-effectiveness of the care delivered while maintaining or increasing patient and family satisfaction.

Clinical Protocols or Algorithms

Clinical protocols or algorithms are different from clinical pathways because they represent more of a decision path that a practitioner might take during a particular episode or need. For example, common algorithms exist for treatment of hypertension, provision of both basic and advanced life support, and general diagnostic screening (Fig. 22.6).

BREAKTHROUGH THINKING TO IMPROVE QUALITY

Just as standardization is critical to the foundation of health care improvement, so is the notion of breakthrough thinking and swift application of best known methods for practice. The premise behind breakthrough thinking and its resulting action is threefold: (1) substantial knowledge exists about how to achieve better performance but it may not be applied in practice; (2) strong examples already exist of organizations that have applied that knowledge and broken through to substantial improvements; and (3) the stakes are high and relevant to the most crucial strategic needs of health care (Berwick, 1997).

The Institute for Healthcare Improvement (IHI), a voluntary organization formed to assist leaders in all health care settings actively involved in improving quality, recommends the Model of Improvement, developed by Langley and colleagues (2009) and composed of two parts. Part one asks three fundamental questions:
1. What are we trying to accomplish?
2. How will we know that a change is an improvement?
3. What changes can we make that will result in improvement?

Part two uses a sequence of steps, starting with developing an action plan based on the three questions and going on to taking actions to test the plan, making refinements as needed, and implementing the resulting changes in real work settings. This is known as a plan–do–study–act (PDSA) cycle (Fig. 22.7). For more in-depth information, visit the IHI website: www.ihi.org, location: How to Improve (see Case Study on Applying the IHI Model in Practice).

To support QI initiatives and breakthrough to improved care, AHRQ's *Making Healthcare Safer* report provides an excellent resource to support the implementation of evidence-based patient safety improvement practices across all health care settings, including acute care, ambulatory care, and long-term care. Since 2001 AHRQ has released three editions of the report, with the fourth report released in 2023 providing health care leaders, clinicians, researchers, and policymakers with more timely updates and protocols on important harm areas such as handoff protocols, opioid stewardship, sepsis recognition and intervention, and engaging family caregivers, among many others; this report also provides the review of the potential harms that may be associated with telehealth. Nurses can use this excellent resource to guide QI actions and improve patient safety regardless of the health care setting in which they practice. The report is available on the AHRQ website: www.ahrq.gov, location: Research > Research Findings & Reports > Making Healthcare Safer Reports.

PATIENT SAFETY INITIATIVES

Nowhere is the need for QI more evident than in the area of health care errors. As discussed previously the IOM report *To Err Is Human: Building a Safer Health System* (2000) placed the issue of medical mistakes and patient safety on the pages of many national newspapers, on the agendas of health care governing boards, and at the forefront of federal government legislation. In response to the focus on patient safety and the need for data to better understand the priority concerns, several national initiatives were implemented and are discussed in the following sections.

Institute for Safe Medication Practices

An outcome of the patient safety and QI movement was establishment of the Institute for Safe Medication Practices (ISMP), a nonprofit organization that is now well known as an education resource for the prevention of medication errors. The ISMP provides independent, multidisciplinary, expert review of errors reported through the ISMP Medication Errors Reporting Program (MERP). Through MERP health care professionals across the nation voluntarily and confidentially report medication errors and hazardous conditions that could lead to errors. The reporting process is simple and easily accessible by clinicians. All resulting information

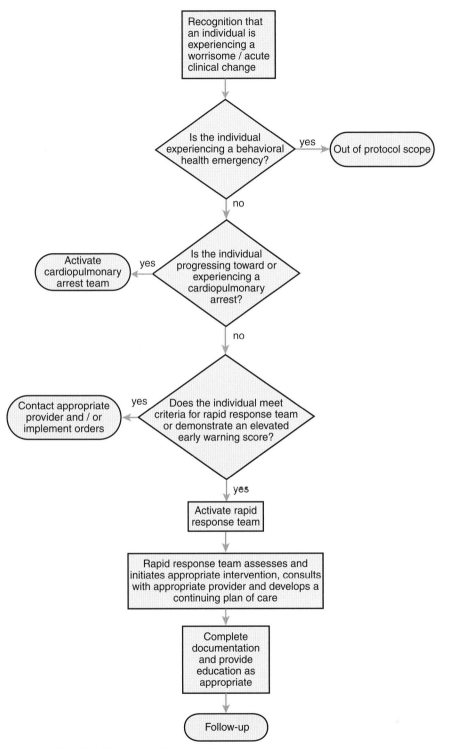

Fig. 22.6 Clinical algorithm—health care protocol: rapid response team.

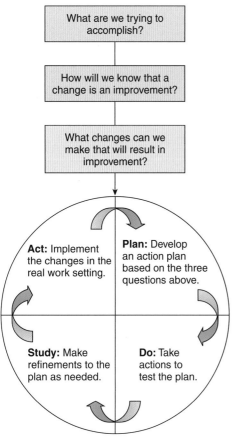

Fig. 22.7 Model of Improvement.

and programs to promote patient safety. Three such programs are discussed in the following sections.

Sentinel Event Standard. As one response to the increasing emphasis on patient safety, TJC established its sentinel event standard in 1996. This standard, which continues today, requires organizations to carry out designated steps to fully understand the factors and systems associated with adverse patient events. The steps revolve around a "root cause analyses and action plan" (RCA²), which is a direct application of the QI principles and methods defined earlier in this chapter. The intention behind the RCA² is to understand the systems at fault within the organization so that improvements can be determined and implemented to prevent any future occurrences. TJC allows organizations some latitude in determining the policy for disclosure of these events to the commission.

National Patient Safety Goals. The purpose of TJC's national patient safety goals is to help accredited organizations address specific areas of concern in regard to patient safety. These goals are based on ongoing analyses of reported sentinel events and the identified root causes of these events. An annual review of these goals generally results in modification of existing goals and the creation of new ones (Box 22.1).

Never Events. In 2006 CMS began to investigate ways that Medicare could help decrease or eliminate the occurrence of never events—serious and costly errors in health care delivery that should never happen. Examples of such events include wrong site surgery and mismatched blood transfusions, which can cause serious patient injury or death and can result in increased costs to Medicare. CMS worked with the National Quality Forum (NQF) to identify hospital-acquired conditions (HACs) determined to be reasonably preventable and for which the additional cost of hospitalization for treating these conditions should not be paid. Box 22.2 presents the most current list of HACs for which Medicare will no longer make additional payments for treatment.

Beginning in the CMS fiscal year 2015 and still in place today, reimbursement penalties are applied to hospitals scoring in the 75th percentile or greater of all total HAC scores (worst-performing quartile). The

and error-prevention strategies are shared with the US Food and Drug Administration (FDA).

The ISMP has also developed *Medication Safety Self-Assessments* to allow nurses and other health care professionals to assess the medication safety practices in their work setting. These tools contain items that address the use of medications in the clinical setting, use of high-alert medications, and system improvements and safeguards that the ISMP has recommended in response to analysis of medication errors (ISMP, 2023). The assessments are publicly available on the ISMP website: www.ismp.org/self-assessments.

Role of Regulatory and Accrediting Agencies in Promoting Patient Safety

The leaders of regulatory agencies (e.g., CMS) and accrediting agencies (e.g., TJC) have developed standards

---

BOX 22.1 2023 Hospital National Patient Safety Goals

1. Identify patients correctly
   - Use at least two ways to identify patients. For example, use the patient's name and date of birth. This is done to make sure that each patient gets the correct medicine and treatment.
2. Improve staff communication
   - Get important test results to the right staff person on time.
3. Use medicines safely
   - Before a procedure, label medicines that are not labeled. For example, medicines in syringes, cups, and basins. Do this in the area where medicines and supplies are set up.
   - Take extra care with patients who take medicines to thin their blood.
   - Record and pass along correct information about a patient's medicines. Find out what medicines the patient is taking. Compare those medicines with new medicines given to the patient. Give the patient written information about the medicines they need to

take. Tell the patient it is important to bring their up-to-date list of medicines every time they visit a doctor.
4. Use alarms safely
   - Make improvements to ensure that alarms on medical equipment are heard and responded to on time.
5. Prevent infection
   - Use the hand cleaning guidelines from the Centers for Disease Control and Prevention or the World Health Organization. Set goals for improving hand cleaning. Use the goals to improve hand cleaning.
6. Identify patient safety risks
   - Reduce the risk for suicide.
7. Prevent mistakes in surgery
   - Make sure that the correct surgery is done on the correct patient and at the correct place on the patient's body.
   - Mark the correct place on the patient's body where the surgery is to be done.
   - Pause before the surgery to make sure that a mistake is not being made.

The Joint Commission. (2023). *National patient safety goals.* Simplified version effective July 2023. https://www.jointcommission.org/-/media/tjc/documents/standards/national-patient-safety-goals/2023/hap-npsg-simplified-2023-july.pdf

---

BOX 22.2 Never Events: The Centers for Medicare and Medicaid Services Listing of Hospital-Acquired Conditions

Pressure ulcer rate
Iatrogenic pneumothorax rate
In hospital fall with hip fracture rate
Perioperative hemorrhage or hematoma rate
Postoperative acute kidney injury requiring dialysis rate
Postoperative respiratory failure rate
Perioperative pulmonary embolism or deep vein thrombosis rate
Postoperative sepsis rate
Postoperative wound dehiscence rate
Abdominopelvic accidental puncture/laceration rate
Central line–associated bloodstream infection (CLABSI)
Catheter-associated urinary tract infection (CAUTI)
Colon and abdominal hysterectomy surgical site infection (SSI)
Methicillin-resistant *Staphylococcus aureus* (MRSA) bacteremia
Clostridium difficile infection (CDI)

From the Centers for Medicare and Medicaid Services. (2023). *Hospital-acquired conditions.* https://www.cms.gov/Medicare/Quality-Initiatives-Patient-Assessment-Instruments/Value-Based-Programs/HAC/Hospital-Acquired-Conditions

penalty consists of a 1% deduction of an organization's baseline annual Diagnosis-Related Group (DRG) Medicare reimbursement. Like value-based purchasing this program is a result of the Patient Protection and Affordability Act of 2010. In the case presented in the vignette, if other patients have similar experiences like Mrs. Hernandez and Jaheem's team fails to improve the postoperative process, reductions in Medicare reimbursement to the hospital will occur. Possible deductions include the 2% hospital value-based purchasing, discussed earlier in this chapter, and 1% for the HAC (catheter-associated UTI). Plus, Medicare would not pay for the days related to the catheter-associated UTI. Due to patients' negative feedback about their experience on the Hospital Consumer Assessment of Healthcare Providers and Systems (HCAHPS) survey, a standardized patient satisfaction survey, financial incentives would go unrewarded. The total adjustments for the harmful postoperative process could severely impact the hospital's financial status. Visit the CMS website for more information on HACs and how adjustments are calculated, www.cms.gov, location: Medicare > Quality > Value-based programs > Hospital-acquired condition reduction program.

THE PROFESSIONAL NURSE AND SAFETY IMPROVEMENT

For nurses the challenge starts with making patient safety improvement and error reduction not just an organizational priority but a personal one as well. This means adopting a state of mind that recognizes the complexity and high-risk nature of modern health care, implementing standardized best practices, and working to eliminate never events. Two significant nursing functions that most closely affect patient safety, quality of care, and resulting outcomes are:

- Monitoring for early recognition of adverse events, complications, and errors.
- Initiating deployment of appropriate care providers for timely intervention, response, and rescue of patients in these situations.

A critical factor in supporting a nurse's ability to carry out these two functions is nurse staffing. Although defining the appropriate level of staffing is a matter of debate, there is significant research that has demonstrated a strong linkage between patient outcomes and nurse staffing. Chapter 13 presents a thorough discussion of strategies nurses can use to promote quality care and a safe work environment.

Nursing Quality Indicators

The governing body of the American Nurses Association (ANA) established the National Database of Nursing Quality Indicators (NDNQI) in 1998 as part of the ANA's safety and quality initiative. In 2014 the NDNQI database was acquired by Press Ganey, a national provider of patient satisfaction surveys and other strategic resources for health care organizations. This national database program collects information on designated indicators that strongly affect patient clinical outcomes for two major purposes: (1) to provide comparative data to health care organizations to support QI activities and (2) to develop national data to better understand the link between nurse staffing and patient outcomes (Box 22.3).

The NDNQI is unique in that it is the only national nursing quality measurement program that allows comparison measures of nursing quality among national, regional, and state hospitals of similar type and size, from the unit-level perspective. Quarterly reports are provided to hospitals that participate in the NDNQI

BOX 22.3 Nursing-Sensitive Quality Indicators

Clinical Indicators

Structure
- Nurse turnover
- Patient volume and flow
- Patient contacts
- RN education/specialty certification
- Staffing and skill mix
- Workforce characteristics

Process
- Advance care planning
- Body mass index (BMI) screening and follow-up
- Care coordination
- Depression screening and follow-up
- Diabetes care
- Hypertension screening and follow-up
- Pain impairing function
- Patient falls
- Pressure injuries
- Pediatric pain assessment/intervention/reassessment (AIR) cycle
- Restraints
- Suicide risk screening and follow-up

Outcome
- Assaults by psychiatric patients
- Assaults on nursing personnel
- Catheter-associated urinary tract infections (CAUTI)
- Central line catheter–associated bloodstream infections (CLABSI)
- Multidrug-resistant organisms (MDRO) (such as *C. difficile* infections and MRSA infections)
- Pain impairing function
- Patient falls
- Pediatric peripheral intravenous infiltrations
- Perioperative clinical measure set (PCMS) (patient burns, surgical errors, unplanned postoperative transfers/admissions)
- Pressure injuries
- Ventilator-associated events (VAEs)
- Ventilator-associated pneumonia (VAP)

RN Survey Options
- RN Survey with job satisfaction scales
- RN survey with practice environment scale (PES)

Press Ganey. (2023). https://info.pressganey.com/press-ganey-blog-healthcare-experience-insights/your-comprehensive-guide-to-the-press-ganey-national-database-of-nursing-quality-indicators-ndnqi

measurement and reporting program for analysis of their own care processes and support systems as related to nurse staffing (Press Ganey, 2023).

Interprofessional Teamwork

Equally critical in its effect on patient safety is the work environment that supports the interdependence and effective communication among nurses and other health care professionals. Most nurses and other clinical staff assume they already work in teams; however, teamwork concepts are infrequently taught in health professional educational programs. Patient care depends on effective interprofessional communication to support the coordination of activities that promote efficiency and safety. One strategy to improve interprofessional teamwork is TeamSTEPPS (Team Strategies and Tools to Enhance Performance and Patient Safety). TeamSTEPPS was developed by the AHRQ and the US Department of Defense as an evidence-based teamwork system aimed at optimizing patient outcomes by improving communication and teamwork skills among health care professionals. Comprehensive information about Team-STEPPS, including readiness assessments and training materials, is available on its website: https://www.ahrq.gov/teamstepps-program/index.html.

ROLE OF PROFESSIONAL NURSES IN QUALITY IMPROVEMENT

The value of quality improvement in the role of the RN is recognized by the American Association for Colleges of Nurses (AACN) in its new publication, *The Essentials: Core Competencies for Professional Nursing Education,* which outlines the expected competencies of graduates from baccalaureate, masters, and Doctor of Nursing Practice programs (AACN, 2021). Although the AACN Essentials are noted for baccalaureate and higher education, students from all types of nursing programs need these same competencies to build their expertise for improving the safety and quality of health care. Following are the major competencies related to patient safety and quality recommended by AACN (2021):

- Apply quality improvement principles in care delivery
- Contribute to a culture of patient safety.
- Contribute to a culture of provider and work environment safety

There are many sub-competencies under each of these major categories. Readers are encouraged to visit the AACN website to review the entire list of competencies: www.aacnnursing.org > Initiatives > Essentials.

Additionally, there are lessons for all nurses from one of the original patient safety and QI mentors, Florence Nightingale. Nightingale used data to support her efforts to reduce the incidence and spread of infections in the patient wards she was accountable for during the Crimean War. What resulted from her work was a broader shift in the culture of health care at that time. What can result from the current emphasis on quality and patient safety is a new cultural shift in health care, with "building health care systems that do no harm" increasingly being the shared value and goal of all those involved in health care delivery. Nurses are in the perfect position to lead this cultural change. QI should be considered not a separate function within the role of care provider but, rather, an ongoing part of the professional role for all health care professionals.

SUMMARY

For today's graduating nurses the challenge is to find whatever means are available to refine the knowledge and skills fundamentally necessary to enter a partnership with all other interprofessional team members in the ongoing improvement of health care. Just as essential to professional nursing practice as knowing, for instance, the symptoms of diabetic ketoacidosis or how to give an injection, are understanding the basic principles of QI, process improvement, and variation; using clinical indicators, process improvement tools, and standardized care processes; and addressing patient safety in every aspect of care. Every nurse should enter practice accepting accountability for the quality of care provided by the health care organization and taking a leadership role to implement improvements to achieve health care that is safe, timely, effective, efficient, equitable, and patient centered.

CLINICAL JUDGMENT AND NEXT-GENERATION NCLEX® EXAMINATION-STYLE QUESTIONS

Krista Watson, RN, has been the charge nurse for the night shift in a rehabilitation facility for 2 years. She was recently appointed to the facility's committee that routinely reviews quality reports on patient outcomes including the frequency of patient falls, infections, and weight loss. After reviewing the reports, members of the committee recognize that the number of falls resulting in injury is increasing. Krista reports that the facility has a falls' risk assessment program in place, but she is concerned that staff may not be consistently adhering to all components of the program. She also questions if there might be additional evidence-based practices related to the prevention of falls that could be implemented. After

discussion, the committee agrees that a focused QI project is needed to reduce patient falls and prevent injury. The aim of the QI project will be to reduce falls by 80% from the current rate. Krista volunteers to serve as the chair for the QI team. The team will use the Model of Improvement to guide this improvement initiative.

Krista understands there are several actions required to achieve a successful QI project. For each action step use an X to indicate if it is Indicated (will eventually help to meet expected outcomes), Not Indicated (will not eventually help to meet expected outcomes), or Unrelated (not related to the expected outcome).

Action	Indicated	Not Indicated	Unrelated
Appoint an interprofessional QI team that includes direct care staff, nursing supervisor, pharmacist, physical therapist, and physician.			
Use the available data to understand the current rate of falls as the baseline and answer the question from the Model of Improvement: What are we trying to accomplish?			
Assess each patient who has a fall for injury.			
Assess the reasons patient falls have increased using a cause-and-effect diagram.			
Do not rely on feedback from direct care staff because they do not understand quality improvement.			
Identify changes that can be made using evidence-based recommendations for preventing falls and answer the question from the Model of Improvement: What change can we make that will result in improvements?			
When a patient has a fall, call the patient's family to inform them about the fall.			
As Chair of the QI Team, Margaret will develop the plan and then tell the team what they are responsible for doing.			
Understand how falls are defined and measured in the facility to answer the question from the Model of Improvement: How will we know that a change is an improvement?			
Use available data to understand when falls are most frequently occurring and which patients are most susceptible to falling.			
Ask the medical director to dictate the actions that should be taken to reduce falls.			

REFERENCES

Agency for Healthcare Research and Quality (AHRQ). (2023). *AHRQ's making healthcare safer reports: Shaping patient safety efforts in the 21st century.* https://www.ahrq.gov/research/findings/making-healthcare-safer/index.html

American Association of Colleges of Nursing. (2021). *The essentials: Core competencies for professional nursing education.* https://www.aacnnursing.org/essentials

Berwick, D. (1997). The breakthrough series. *Quality Connection,* 6(2), 11.

Grimm, C.A. (2022). Adverse events in hospitals: A quarter of Medicare patients experienced harm in October 2018. US Department of Health and Human Services Office of Inspector General. https://oig.hhs.gov/oei/reports/OEI-06-18-00400.pdf

Institute of Medicine (IOM). (2000). *To err is human: Building a safer health system.* National Academies Press.

Institute of Medicine (IOM). (2001). *Crossing the quality chasm: A new health system for the 21st century.* National Academy Press.

Institute for Safe Medication Practices (ISMP). (2023). *ISMP self assessments.* http://www.ismp.org/selfassessments

Joiner, B.L. (1994). *Fourth generation management.* McGraw-Hill.

Langley, G.J., et al. (2009). *The improvement guide: A practical approach to enhancing organizational performance* (2nd ed.) Jossey-Bass.

National Academy of Medicine (NAM). (2020). *About.* https://nam.edu/about-the-nam.

Press Ganey. (2023). *Nursing excellence made simple (NDNQI).* https://www.pressganey.com/platform/ndnqi/

The Joint Commission (TJC). (2023a). *Sentinel events policy.* https://www.jointcommission.org/resources/sentinel-event/sentinel-event-policy-and-procedures/

The Joint Commission (TJC). (2023b). *Facts about the Joint Commission.* https://www.jointcommission.org/who-we-are/facts-about-the-joint-commission/

23

Health Policy and Politics: Get Involved!

Barbara Cherry, DNSc, MBA, RN, NEA-BC, and
Carole R. Myers, PhD, RN, FAAN

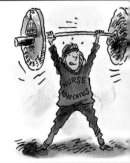

Nurses must be powerful, informe[d] [advo]cates for health policy that improve[s] for all!

e Additional resources are available online at: http://evolve.elsevier.com/Cherry/

LEARNING OUTCOMES

After studying this chapter, the reader will be able to:
1. Differentiate between policy and politics.
2. Discuss roles of the legislative, executive, and judicial branches of government.
3. Differentiate among federal, state, and local governments and their roles in governing and influencing health care and nursing.
4. Identify three policy issues of significant consequence to nurses and nursing.
5. Demonstrate the knowledge needed to be a responsible and informed, politically active nurse.
6. Use diverse technologic resources to obtain information about current health policy developments and political issues.

KEY TERMS

Constituent A citizen who has the opportunity to vote for candidates in elections for representation at the local, state, and federal levels.

Constituent/State Nurses Association (C/SNA) The professional organizational unit member of the American Nurses Association that represents all professional nurses within a state or territory or other defined organizational entity or boundary—also known as the state nurses association (SNA).

Grassroots lobbying Personal advocacy by individual constituents—everyday citizens—in support of a problem/position/option related to a policy issue.

Health policy A set course of action(s) undertaken by governments or health care organizations to impact the health of individuals and populations. Private health policy is made by health care organizations, such as hospitals, whereas public health policy refers to local, state, and federal legislation, regulations, and court rulings that govern health care within a certain arena.

Lobbying Acting to persuade or educate policymakers to respond positively to a particular position on an issue or to follow a particular course of legislative, regulatory, or funding activity.

Platform The statement of principles and policies of a political party, candidate, or elected official.

Policymaker A local, state, or federally elected or appointed official who can propose and directly affect legislation, regulations, or programs that can be put into practice.

Regulations Rules used to implement legislation and translate concepts into actions that can be put into practice.

Stakeholders Individuals, groups, or organizations who have a vested interest in and may be affected by policy decisions and actions being taken, and thus may attempt to influence those decisions and actions.

PROFESSIONAL/ETHICAL ISSUE

Tashauna Banks works in a very busy outpatient surgical center where the nurses often stay past the end of their shifts to care for patients who are not yet stable enough to go home. Tashauna and other nurses in the center typically work more than 50 hours per week. Although the pay is very good, Tashauna is often so fatigued, especially at the end of the week, that she is concerned about making mistakes that might harm her patients. Tashauna also knows that two of her colleagues work as agency nurses on their days off from the surgical center, which means they may be working up to 65 to 70 hours per week. Tashauna has begun to notice that nurse fatigue is a problem in their surgery center, negatively affecting the nurses' motivation and energy levels. She also notices lapses in attention to detail and what sometimes seem to be slow reactions to urgent situations. She becomes very concerned as she realizes that fatigue could have extremely serious legal ramifications if a medical error caused by fatigue were to lead to patient harm.

When visiting with some of her nurse friends who work at the local medical center Tashauna learns that nurse fatigue is a concern there as well. Tashauna and her nurse friends discuss their responsibility to make good decisions when agreeing to work overtime and using the *Code of Ethics for Nurses* as a guide. After the discussion with her friends Tashauna is motivated to take action to address the problem of nurse fatigue in her own work setting, as well as at a broader level through her state nurses association. She understands that together nurses can have a powerful voice to effect change both in the work setting and at state and national policy levels.

- What resources are available for Tashauna and her colleagues to learn more about nurse fatigue?
- How can the *Code of Ethics for Nurses* guide nurses to make balanced decisions about their work hours?
- What responsibility do the managers in health care organizations have to implement policies to address nurse fatigue and keep nurses and patients safe?
- After reading the chapter discuss steps Tashauna can take to begin to address the problem of nurse fatigue as a policy issue in her own work setting and through the state nurses association (SNA).

VIGNETTE

Juan Hernandez is one of only four registered nurses (RNs) now staffing the 7:00 a.m. to 7:00 p.m. shift in a 12-bed medical intensive care unit (MICU); two RN colleagues just transferred to positions in the hospital's rapidly growing case management service. The chief nursing officer (CNO) and MICU nurse manager are actively recruiting permanent RNs for the vacant positions but have been unsuccessful. Temporary service RNs and nursing assistive personnel are filling in within the staffing mix. Juan is aware that all posted openings for RNs throughout his hospital system now include "BSN (Bachelor of Science in Nursing) preferred" as a descriptor, following the hospital's recently announced plans for achieving Magnet Hospital status.

When Juan begins to inquire about the issues in hiring BSN-prepared nurses he is both relieved and alarmed by what he hears. First, the hospital administrators clearly support his position that adequate numbers of permanently employed, well-educated RNs are essential to provide high-quality, safe patient care. The hospital's rapidly evolving care models and driving force to succeed on the Magnet journey require giving a preference to nurses with a BSN or higher degree. However, an underlying complicating issue for health care organizations in Juan's state and region is that the numbers of nurses with the needed education and credentials simply are not available to meet the demand, and hiring is taking much longer than in the past, further complicating issues of safety, quality, and continuity of care in the MICU, where Juan works, and probably across the hospital.

Juan calls his SNA to discuss his concerns and to learn more about the nursing workforce trends. Through that call he discovers that other nurses and hospitals across the state where he lives and across the United States are facing many of the same dilemmas. Meeting nurses' current professional responsibility to provide and advocate for safe care for patients is colliding with the larger national and employer issues of securing a higher number of better-educated, more broadly skilled nurses to meet the rapidly evolving expectations in complex care systems. Therefore Juan makes a commitment to engage in discussions about policy and political strategies that are needed now to promote and protect models of care that will facilitate professional nursing practice; promote development of a highly educated nursing workforce to meet his state's and region's needs;

and ensure his ability to grow in his own professional career.

Questions to Consider While Reading This Chapter:

1. What are the major steps in health policy development that Juan must understand to engage in policy improvements for the nursing workforce and his own professional career?
2. How can Juan relate his knowledge of the clinical judgment process to an effective plan for policy development related to improving the nursing workforce and his own professional career?
3. What types of grassroots political strategies can Juan use to ensure that policymakers hear his interests and concerns about quality, safe patient care, and the supply of professional nurses?

CHAPTER OVERVIEW

Perhaps at no other time in the history of the nursing profession has there been such an imperative for strong, involved, informed nursing leadership. The challenges currently faced by the US health care system—reducing disparities to achieve health equity; strengthening the nursing workforce; and transforming a fragmented health-care delivery system to be more accessible, higher quality, and lower cost—affect the health and well-being of patients, families, and communities across the country. According to the World Health Organization (WHO), social determinants of health are "the non-medical factors that influence health outcomes. They are the conditions in which people are born, grow, work, live, and age, and the wider set of forces and systems shaping the conditions of daily life" (WHO, 2023, para. 1). Frequently these critical issues can be understood, addressed, and resolved only through the policy process. Without a doubt, legislation, regulation, and health policy directly affect how health care is delivered and how health care leaders respond to the very real challenges and opportunities facing our country.

Decisions affecting health care systems, patient care, social determinants of health, and the nursing profession will be made with or without the input of nurses. As the reader will see from health policy examples provided throughout this chapter, health and nursing practice are highly political endeavors, with health policy determining the types of care systems in place and how

that care is paid for. Thus it is absolutely essential that nurses become actively engaged in the policy process and use effective political action to successfully achieve the development of health policies that are reflective of nursing's perspective on the preferred future for the profession and for the health of people in the United States. Nurses can no longer simply move forward and participate in the delivery of patient care without also addressing these larger issues that have a direct impact on the whole of the health care system and society.

This chapter explores the effect of governmental roles, structures, and actions on health care policy and demonstrates how nurses' participation in the policy process can shape the US health care system and nursing practice. The focus of local, state, and federal health policy is discussed. Nurses' very important role in the policy process including the involvement of professional nursing organizations in policy and politics is described. This chapter provides the reader with a basic understanding of policy development and political processes, tools to gain political savvy, and methods for getting politically involved.

WHAT IS HEALTH POLICY?

Health policy is a set course of action(s) undertaken by governments or organizations to impact the health of individuals and populations. Private health policy is made by health care organizations, such as hospitals, and includes those policies instituted to govern innumerable employer/employee practices and processes in the delivery of the health care services provided within the organization. A hospital's specific plan to report errors in patient care is an example of private health policy. *Public health policy* refers to local, state, and federal legislation, regulations, and resource allocation related to health, health care service delivery, coverage, workforce, and reimbursement. The mandatory requirement for licensure to practice professional nursing is an example of public health policy. There is a close link between private policy and public policy, in that the policies of health care organizations must conform to (and are actually frequently developed and implemented to comply with) a public policy. Although it is vital that the RN be an informed participant in policy development at their employing health care organization, this chapter focuses on the development of public or governmental health policy, which will be referred to simply as *health policy*.

Health Policy at the Local, State, and Federal Levels

Health policies may be developed and implemented at the local, state, or federal level, and they apply to all residents within the jurisdiction of the respective governmental authority. Local health policy applies only to those people who are residents of the local community, whereas health policy enacted at the federal level applies to all residents of the United States.

Local Health Policy. At the local level, many cities or counties offer a variety of health care services to meet the needs of their residents. Allocating funds to employ RNs as school nurses in public schools is an example of local health policy. Another local health policy is a community's requirement for tobacco-free public areas, such as restaurants and office buildings. Local health policy varies considerably across the United States, with some communities funding an extensive variety of health programs and others offering very limited health services or none at all. However, even the smallest communities are involved to some extent in health policy through partnerships with their state governments to provide public health programs, such as safe drinking water, enforcement for seat belt and child restraint laws, and emergency medical systems.

State Health Policy. Health policy at the state level has a powerful influence on the health and safety of each state's residents. In addition to its lead role in governing nursing and other health professions' scope, practice, and performance through the state's professional practice acts, each state also has innumerable health policies that may not be visible. These policies include maintaining a safe meat supply through livestock inspections; ensuring safe food storage, preparation, and serving in restaurants; monitoring infectious disease outbreaks; and ensuring that health care facilities provide safe, quality care through regulatory compliance. Only when these activities fall short of preventing problems—as in cases of *Escherichia coli (E. coli)* outbreaks—do most residents of the state realize the critical nature of these health policies.

State health policy also involves paying for some individual health care services. The Medicaid program, which is funded through a blend of state and federal funds, is a health insurance program for health care services for eligible people at (or below) a specific income level and other designated categories (as defined by a combination of federal and individual state standards). Most states also have a state Children's Health Insurance Program (CHIP) that provides health insurance coverage to uninsured children who do not qualify for the state Medicaid program. The CHIP is funded through a partnership between federal and state governments. State and federal governments are also the prime sources of funding for public mental health and substance abuse services, long-term care services for older adults and disabled persons, and health care services for prisoners.

A key piece of the Patient Protection and Affordable Care Act (ACA) of 2010 was the provision for states to implement State Health Insurance Exchanges (SHIEs). An SHIE is a set of state-regulated and standardized health care plans from which individuals may purchase health insurance eligible for federal subsidies; such plans offer affordable and credible coverage that meets national standards for covered services with individual state benchmarks.

Federal Health Policy. State government and state health policies have an enormous effect on people's health and safety. Likewise, the federal government plays a vitally important role in the health of Americans, including significant funding for health and disease prevention and research; supplemental funding for education for health professionals, such as nurses and physicians; and establishing reimbursement rules and paying for individual health care services through Medicare, Medicaid, CHIP, the Veterans Health Administration, and the Indian Health Service.

Federal health policies have played and continue to play a pivotal role in shaping nursing practice. The first federal policy to provide funding for nursing services was the Sheppard-Towner Act of 1921. This act, passed by Congress despite objections from the American Medical Association (AMA), provided states with matching funds to establish prenatal and child health centers staffed by public health nurses. The goal of the act was to reduce maternal and infant mortality rates by teaching women about personal hygiene and infant care. Eventually this highly successful program was discontinued when the AMA successfully persuaded Congress that physicians should perform these health activities (Starr, 1982), but these services were later reinstated (and continue today) within Title V of the Social Security Act of 1935.

Another example of federal legislation that has significantly influenced the context of nursing practice over the past seven decades was the Hill-Burton Act of 1946. This act provided federal funding to local communities for the construction of hospitals across the country. As a result of this federal funding the number of hospitals increased rapidly, as did the need for nurses to staff them. Thus the professional nurse's historic role shifted from community and public health settings to be predominantly hospital/acute care settings over the last seven decades. Other key federal legislation has affected nursing practice through expanding Medicare and Medicaid reimbursement directly to advanced practice nurses (APRNs) and implementing policies and programs to increase the supply of nurses through enhancing access to nursing education at all levels of nursing, from BSN to Doctor of Nursing Practice (DNP) and Doctor of Philosophy (PhD). Table 23.1 provides some historic examples of how health policy enacted at the federal level has affected nursing practice and health care. Current policy issues affecting nursing practice and health care are addressed later in this chapter.

HOW IS HEALTH POLICY DEVELOPED?

Health policy is developed to address societal problems that have a significant impact on the quality of life and health for large segments of the population. The development of health policy at the state or federal level is a complex, dynamic process that occurs primarily through the enactment of legislation and the accompanying rules and regulations. The enactment of the ACA is an example of one of the most significant pieces of legislation passed in the history of the United States (second only to the passage of Medicare and Medicaid in 1965) designed to improve access to health care for US residents. The ACA was developed in response to the significant societal problem of uninsured and underinsured individuals and their inability to access health care due to the lack of affordable health insurance.

Numerous players (individuals and groups) are involved in developing health policy, including: elected officials and their staffs; officials/staffs of executive branch governmental agencies; individual experts in a health-related area; citizens who may be affected by a health problem; stakeholders, such as corporate representatives, who may be affected by a health problem or policy; and representatives from special interest groups who have a

particular focused interest in one or more policy options. As a special interest group representing the interests of the approximately 4.3 million registered nurses throughout the United States, the American Nurses Association (ANA) carries a strong voice and high visibility in influencing health policy and nursing practice. At the state level the Constituent/State Nurses Associations (C/SNAs) of the ANA are the policy voices of the nursing profession with state governors and legislatures.

The development of health policy involves all three branches of government: executive, legislative, and judicial. A basic knowledge of the functions of the three branches of government is necessary to understand health policy development. Table 23.2 presents a brief review of the three branches of the federal government and their differing roles in health policy. Although most state governments parallel the structure and functions of the federal government, there are differences among states. Each nurse is encouraged to learn about the governmental structure of their state. In addition to understanding the branches of government, nurses also need to understand the influence of legislation and regulation on health policy as discussed in the following sections.

Legislation and Health Policy Development

The *development of health policy* refers to the steps through which a health issue moves from being a societal problem to becoming an actual health program that can be funded, implemented, and evaluated. The legislative process is fundamental to the movement from a public problem to a public solution: a public plan, program, or service. Although there are many problems related to health care and nursing practice, problems that attain policy solution status are those that are brought to the attention of a policymaker who is willing to take definitive action through legislative, regulatory, or funding processes.

Generally, interested individuals or citizens' groups approach policymakers either to present a problem to be solved or to suggest a policy option to a health problem that they have identified. However, policymakers may also become aware of problems through their personal experiences or that of their constituents and may take on development of policy solutions independently. At the federal level only members of Congress can introduce legislation. The congressional member who introduces a specific piece of legislation becomes the prime sponsor of that legislation. Legislation is

TABLE 23.1   Examples of Health Policies That Have Influenced Professional Nursing Practice

Legislation	Influence on Professional Nursing Practice
Nurse practice acts and registration of nurses were established (1910).	Established scope of practice and minimal educational requirements for nurses; implemented by most states.
Sheppard-Towner Act (1921) funded prenatal and child health centers staffed by public health nurses.	First federal policy to provide funding for nursing services.
Hill-Burton Act (1946), also known as the Hospital Survey and Construction Act, provided federal funding for hospital construction.	Caused a boom in hospital construction, shifting nurses' primary employment setting from public health to hospitals.
Nurse Training Act (1964), Public Law 88-581, provided enhanced funding for collegiate nursing programs.	Expanded university education for nurses and laid the groundwork for the development of advanced practice nurses (APRNs).
Medicare program (1965) provided funding for health care services for older adults and the disabled.	Led to an increased number of hospitalized older adults and a greater need for nurses in acute care settings.
Renal Disease Program (1972) provided funding for dialysis treatments and renal transplantation for individuals with kidney failure.	Led to the development of a new area of nursing practice that is now a recognized specialty—nephrology nursing.
Diagnosis-related groups (DRGs) (1983) changed Medicare reimbursement to hospitals from a fee-for-service method to a fixed-fee method.	Forced hospitals to reduce patients' lengths of stay, cut costs, and initially reduced staff, including nurses; led to the development of new nursing roles—nursing case management and utilization review.
Balanced Budget Amendment (1997), Title 42, provided for direct reimbursement of nurse practitioners (NPs) and clinical nurse specialists, regardless of geographic location, following state nurse practice act requirements for scope and practice.	Expanded practice opportunities for APRNs and further increased the importance of political action at the state level to remove barriers to APRN practice, such as medical supervision and other unwarranted limitations on scope and independence.
Medicare Modernization Act (Medicare Part D) (2003) added a prescription drug benefit for Medicare enrollees.	Provided needed access to medications for Medicare enrollees and called attention to cost-and-effectiveness outcome from policymakers, requiring nurses to stay alert to proposed legislation and to advocate for appropriate benefits for the nation's older adults.
Mental Health Parity and Addiction Equity Act (MHPAEA) (2008) removed discrimination in insurance coverage and benefits for mental illnesses and substance abuse disorders.	Greatly increased access to a continuum of mental health/substance abuse services and put pressure on development of a nursing workforce with sufficient numbers and knowledge to address these illnesses as integrated with other chronic illnesses and as specialty services.
Patient Protection and Affordable Care Act (2010), Public Law 111–148.	Comprehensive health care reform legislation providing a health insurance program requiring US citizens and legal residents to secure quality health insurance at reasonable rates with income-based subsidies while also providing for provisions to improve the quality of health care and reduce costs.

introduced by a member of Congress after careful analysis of the problem, which likely includes:
- Public perception of the problem
- Definition of the problem
- Societal consequences of action or inaction, the number of people affected by the problem, and options for resolution

- Levels of support and opposition from other members of Congress, special interest groups, business leaders, and the general public, especially the member's constituents

After the problem is thoroughly analyzed and a decision is made to move forward with a policy solution, the sponsoring congressperson drafts the legislation.

TABLE 23.2 The Three Branches of the Federal Government

	Executive	Legislative	Judicial
Composition	Office of the President and 15 executive departments (State, Treasury, Defense, Agriculture, Energy, Housing and Urban Development, Justice, Commerce, Education, Health and Human Services, Interior, Labor, Transportation, Veterans Affairs, and Homeland Security)	Senate and House of Representatives, known collectively as Congress, with 535 elected members	US Supreme Court, federal district courts, and US circuit courts of appeals
Role in health policy	Recommends legislation and promotes major policy initiatives. Implements laws and manages programs after they have been passed by Congress through regulation, oversight, and presidential funding priorities. Writes regulations that interpret statutes (laws). Has the power to veto legislation passed by Congress.	Possesses the sole federal power to enact legislation and to tax citizens and allocate federal spending. Able to originate and promote major policy initiatives. Has the power to override a presidential veto.	Judicial interpretations of the Constitution or various laws may have a policy effect. Resolves questions regarding agency regulations that may affect policy.
Restrictions to power	Unable to enact a law without the approval of Congress (legislative branch)	US Supreme Court may invalidate legislation as unconstitutional	Unable to recommend or promote legislative initiatives

Congressional staff translate the option into legal, technical, and constitutional language that the congressperson then introduces through the appropriate process. Only then does the health problem addressed by a policy option/solution become a bill—a proposed legislative policy solution. Visit https://votesmart.org/education/how-a-bill-becomes-law to review all the many steps in how a bill becomes law.

Although the legislative process to enact a new law appears to be simple and straightforward, it is actually very complex and convoluted, with only a fraction of introduced legislation actually making it through the final process to become law. In the 117th US Congress (2021 to 2023) 17,817 bills were introduced but only 365 of those actually became public law (Govtrack, 2023). In other words, only 2% of bills introduced in the 117th Congress actually became public law!

Once a bill becomes a law (a public policy) implementation falls to the jurisdiction of one of the departments under the executive branch of government (see Table 23.2). At the federal level most health-related policies fall under the jurisdiction of the US Department of Health and Human Services (DHHS) and its related agencies. The agency that will administer the law develops the regulations to implement the law. Implementation of new legislation can often be very different from what was originally intended when Congress debated and passed the bill. It is extremely important that supporters of any new law take steps to ensure that its advocates and the legislative policymakers implement the law as intended. This important caution leads us to the discussion about regulation and health policy.

Health Policy Through Regulation

The regulatory arena is an important but often overlooked area of policy that significantly affects nursing practice. An understanding of regulatory authority and processes provides nurses with the knowledge necessary to become involved and more successfully influence the future of nursing. Regulations refer to written sets of rules issued by an executive branch agency that has responsibility for administering a law. Because regulations carry the force of the law they directly shape the implementation of health policy. Thus it is very important that regulations reflect the intent of the law as enacted by the legislative body. Once the proposed regulations are developed they must be published and open to public comment for a specified time before being adopted as final rules.

As regulations are being developed by the government agency public hearings are held to allow interested individuals and groups to comment on the draft content of the regulations and to suggest amendments or substitutions. At this stage in the development of a health care law nurses can and must play an influential role in shaping the final regulations by writing to the regulatory agency or speaking at public hearings. Informed comments are critical for the development of administrative law. Each comment received must be considered and responded to before final regulations are issued. The time between the interim rules and final rules is critical for assessing the effect of the proposed rules and requires concerted nursing vigilance and action to react to the proposed rules either positively or negatively. Final published regulations carry the force of the law and will dictate how the law is actually implemented.

At the federal level the proposed (or interim) regulations are published in the *Federal Register*. The *Federal Register* (located online at https://www.federalregister.gov) is the best source of information about proposed new rules, as well as proposed changes to existing rules for federal programs. It is published each day and contains complete directions about where to send comments, in addition to the deadlines for the public comment period. Most states have a parallel publication (e.g., *Texas Register*) with information about proposed rules and regulations at the state level for state legislation. It cannot be overemphasized that supporters of any new law must be vigilant and involved in the development of rules and regulations long after the legislation has passed and been adopted as law to ensure its implementation as planned and supported.

HEALTH POLICY AND POLITICS: A KEY CONNECTION

Many people may view politics as somewhat questionable or ambiguous activities that occur in and around federal, state, and local governments to influence the outcomes of candidate elections and/or the passage of legislation. Mason et al. (2021) have defined politics as "the use of relationships and power . . . to influence policy and the allocation of scarce resources." Politics can also be defined as the process used to influence decisions and exert control over policy, circumstances, and events. As the reader will see "influence" is the common denominator in any definition of politics. Political influence can be achieved through many methods, including:
- campaign activity and contributions
- knowledge

- relationships
- information/data
- talent
- perceived control over large groups of votes

Florence Nightingale was the consummate political nurse. She understood how to use data and expert knowledge to influence the British Parliament to allocate funds to reform British military hospitals and substantially improved the health conditions for the troops through changes in sanitary practices (Nightingale, 1859).

Politics is a necessary part of the policy process. Multiple interest groups (such as government officials, special interest groups, and corporate leaders) are all competing to achieve their potentially different policy goals/outcomes. The process becomes even more interesting when the varied and increasingly polarized agendas of the Democratic, Republican, and emerging independent parties are added to the mix. Groups and individuals who have a stake in the fate of a piece of legislation or the election of a candidate use political strategies to obtain their desired outcome(s). Thus it is through *effective* political action that nurses can positively influence legislative and regulatory decisions and the development of health policies that will affect nursing practice and the health of Americans in a positive way. Following is a discussion of how nurses can get involved in the political process and use effective political strategies to influence health policy.

Health Policy and the Clinical Judgment Model

The first step for nurses to get involved in health policy development and politics is to learn to recognize nursing and health care issues that are amenable to and/or require policy action. During nursing school students learn the Clinical Judgment Model as the foundation for professional nursing practice. Once nursing students graduate they appreciate this model as the basis for making sound clinical judgments. As nurses commit to being more policy focused and politically active they will find that applying the Clinical Judgment Model is a natural and comfortable approach to identifying and taking on broader professional and health policy issues. See Table 23.3 for an example of using the Clinical Judgment Model to support health policy development. Policy work is challenging, important, and, in so many instances, fun and exciting and should become a part of the professional nurse's skill set.

TABLE 23.3   Using the Clinical Judgment Model to Promote Health Policy

	Steps	Example
1. Recognize cues	Collect and understand information about the issue of concern.	A recent state-wide staffing survey documented a serious shortage of RNs willing to work in long-term care (LTC) facilities.
2. Analyze cues	Analyze the information and identify the fundamental issue or underlying problem that needs to be addressed.	New graduate nurses prefer to work in acute care settings, including pediatrics, emergency room, and critical care. There are no incentives to encourage new RNs to look at LTC as a viable career option.
3. Prioritize hypotheses and generate solutions	Develop options for an effective policy plan with input from many sources and perspectives.	Options to address the lack of new RNs willing to work in LTC include (1) allow student nurses more opportunities to have clinical experiences in LTC during nursing school; (2) offer a student loan forgiveness program for nurses who work in LTC; and (3) ask LTC companies to offer scholarships to nursing students in exchange for a commitment to work in their facility for a specified time.
4. Take actions	Develop the policy plan and then use political action and a set of strategies and interventions to give the policy the best chance of becoming law.	The state nurses association and the professional organization for LTC providers both support legislative action to create a student loan forgiveness program for nurses who work in LTC; this option is moved forward through the legislative process and eventually becomes a bill to be voted on by the state legislature.
5. Evaluate outcomes	Assess evidence that determines if the policy plan was a success or not and why, then determine next steps. If the proposed policy plan has been passed as legislation, then the regulatory process is the next step to address; if the policy plan failed to become law, then evaluate how to develop a new plan.	The student loan forgiveness bill does not receive enough support in the legislature to be voted on and enacted as a new law; the nurses and other groups who supported and promoted this bill will assess the barriers to its passage, determine actions to overcome the barriers, and try again to get the bill passed in a new legislative session.

GRASSROOTS POLITICAL STRATEGIES

Grassroots lobbying, or political strategies, are actions taken at the local level to influence policymakers. Nurses as political constituents have a right (and a responsibility!) to petition, lobby, or persuade policymakers to ensure that their interests and concerns are heard. Such advocacy actions (frequently referred to as *lobbying*) offer individuals and groups who are stakeholders in a particular issue an opportunity to be heard. The lobbying process also provides policymakers with needed information from health experts upon which to base their decisions. Following are various methods through which nurses can be effective grassroots participants/players:

- Registering to vote and voting in *all* elections

- Joining professional nursing organizations with policy advocacy agendas
- Working on political candidates' campaigns
- Meeting with policymakers or their staff members
- Attending and speaking up at "meet-the-candidates" town hall meetings
- Communicating with policymakers by e-mail, fax, and telephone

Register to Vote and Vote in All Elections

Voting is a must for *every* nurse. However, voting is not enough. *Informed voting* is necessary to enhance nurses' political power to ultimately improve the health of patients and the care that they receive. Becoming informed involves reading legislative newsletters and finding out about policymakers' backgrounds, voting records, and current party and candidate platforms. Discussing your findings on these issues with nurse colleagues and others in the community enhances everyone's understanding of candidates and their positions and facilitates informed voting. Nurses must participate in identifying and electing "nurse-friendly" candidates and then must become candidates and policymakers themselves.

Join a Professional Nursing Organization

Another must for the professional nurse seeking to make a policy difference is to join a professional nursing organization. The value of the ANA, its C/SNAs, and its organizational affiliates is that, *together*, the nursing profession is much more powerful than any individual RN speaking alone. Within a professional collective nurses know more, have more resources, and are able to pool their strengths and direct resources toward "winning" the health policy competition and thus ensuring a more "nurse-friendly" public policy.

The ANA is the foremost recognized professional nursing organization for federal health and nursing public policy. The ANA speaks for all professional nurses, regardless of specialty. All nurses should consider ANA membership as one of their fundamental professional investments. The nurse who chooses to also be a member in a specialty organization that represents their focus arena of nursing practice has the additional advantage of receiving clinical and health policy information related to that specialty.

Because professional nursing organizations monitor public policy and offer avenues for their members to learn about health policy, they serve as invaluable resources for reliable information related to policy issues and policymakers. Joining a professional nursing organization that has a political action committee (PAC) can help nurses develop the necessary skills to understand and participate in political issues and elections and can give nurses increased access to policymakers. A PAC is an arm of a corporation, association, or union formed to provide support and resources either to work toward the election or reelection of policymakers who support the organization's overall goals or to persuade a policymaker to support a certain policy.

Not all professional nursing organizations have PACs, but those that do may choose to endorse a specific candidate for office. Endorsement simply means that, in a particular political race, the nursing organization selects a particular candidate to support because of that candidate's platform or record supporting specific issues or policy goals. Although endorsement does not mean that everyone in the organization *must* vote for the selected person, it does mean that the organization has carefully screened the candidate, and the nurse can be reasonably sure that, if elected, the candidate will support the organization's preferred outcomes and interests. Nursing organizations are looking for health-friendly and nurse-friendly candidates who will champion laws and programs to improve health and nursing.

Work in Political Candidates' Campaigns

Most political candidates are not health professionals and do not fully understand health-related issues. By becoming involved in political campaigns nurses can (and should) educate and inform candidates about health care issues. Other activities that the nurse may undertake on behalf of the candidates include assisting in writing health care position statements; working in campaign offices; attending local debates; displaying the candidates' political buttons, signs, and stickers; and participating in fundraising events. Nurse supporters may also write letters/e-mails to and/or call other nurses in the region to tell them about their support of the candidate and to ask for their vote. Having nurse-friendly candidates win and become nurse-friendly policymaking officials is critical to achieving nursing's policy agenda.

Visit With Policymakers and Their Staff Members

Personal visits to policymakers and their staff members can be one of the most effective methods of advocacy for or against a health care policy. Nothing is more effective in communicating nursing's position on an issue than face-to-face contact between a group of well-informed nurses and a policymaker and their staff. Face-to-face meetings provide a great opportunity for nurses to educate policymakers about health care issues while enhancing the image of the nurse as an informed, trustworthy constituent.

Many state nurses' associations sponsor a "Nurse Day at the Capital" where they organize opportunities for nurses to meet with state policymakers; this special day is a great way for nurses to meet with policymakers, learn to be more involved in the policy process, and educate policymakers about health-related issues.

Policymakers are very interested in information that will increase their knowledge about health care and help them develop options for future health care policy. For more information, visit the ANA's *Practice and Advocacy* section on their website (https://www.nursingworld.org) to learn about the most current federal policy initiatives related to nursing and health care and ways that nurses can get involved to support important policy initiatives.

Participate in "Meet-the-Candidates" Town Hall Meetings

A strategy that nursing associations can use to determine which candidate(s) to endorse is to invite all candidates running for a particular office to a town hall meeting to discuss their positions and platforms directly with nurses. Town hall gatherings with nurses allow the candidates to talk about their platform to a group of interested likely voters and afford nurses an opportunity to voice their experiences, opinions, and concerns about health care issues and assess the candidates' views. Box 23.1 provides the correct titles to use when addressing state elected officials.

Communicate with Policymakers Through E-mail, Fax, and Telephone

Contacting policymakers through letters, e-mail, fax, and telephone can be effective if properly planned and implemented. The timing of the communication is important; it should be made early, before policymakers publicly commit to a certain policy option. It is easier to persuade an undecided policymaker than to get them to switch positions. A second, very effective step is to send a follow-up communication immediately before the vote on a particular bill is scheduled. Information about voting schedules can be obtained online in most states

and certainly from your C/SNA. Using e-mail or sending a fax is the best way to make sure your voice will be heard in a timely way to make a difference. Suggestions for communicating effectively with policymakers include:

1. *Be brief.* Short, direct e-mail and faxes are the most effective.
2. *Be specific.* Deal with just one subject or issue in the communication; state your topic clearly in the first sentence. The subject of an e-mail message should contain the number of the bill to which you are referring in the message. For example, "In Opposition to Senate Bill 123." The message itself should be just a few short lines to relay a clear and strong message related to the issue. Brief examples of how the issue/policy affects people in the policymaker's district are often most persuasive.
3. *Be personal.* Communication is most effective when it reflects your personal experiences and presents your views in your own words; mass-produced letters, e-mails, and faxes do not carry as much weight as a communication that you have written/modified in your own words.
4. *Provide your name and address.* Policymakers pay most attention to communications that come from their constituents—the very people who may be voting for or against them in their next election. So it is important to let them know whether you are from their district. Include contact information so that the elected official may respond to your concerns.
5. *Be persistent.* Communicate often, especially if the policymaker is undecided on an issue.

Telephone calls are usually taken by a staff member; ask to speak to the staff person assigned to the bill or issue for which the call is being made. After introducing yourself give a brief and simple message such as "Please tell Senator or Representative [name] that I support/oppose [bill number]." You may briefly state your reasons for supporting or opposing the bill and ask for the policymaker's position on the bill. Conclude the call by leaving your name, telephone number, and address; if appropriate ask for a written response to your telephone call.

Rosters of state legislators can be found online in most states. The roster contains contact information for each policymaker and usually includes information about their committee memberships. Contact information for members of the US House of Representatives is available online (https://www.house.gov). This site shows committee memberships and has links to individual

---

BOX 23.1   How to Address the Governor, Lieutenant Governor, Legislators, or Staff

Governor: Governor (last name)
Lieutenant Governor: Lt. Governor (last name)
Speaker of the House: Mr. Speaker or Madam Speaker
Senator: Senator (last name)
Representative: Representative (last name) or Mr. or Ms. (last name)
Staff: Mr. or Ms. (last name)

representatives' websites. Similar information for US senators is also available online (https://www.senate.gov).

THE AMERICAN NURSES ASSOCIATION

The ANA is the professional nursing organization representing the nation's entire RN population—approximately 4.3 million RNs (as of 2023) and is the strongest voice for advancing the nursing profession and transforming health and health care in the United States. The ANA is composed of Constituent/State Nurses Association (C/SNA) from the majority of states in the United States plus other direct membership categories that represent state and US territory nursing associations. Subsidiaries of ANA are the American Academy of Nursing, the American Nurses Credentialing Center (ANCC), and the American Nurses Foundation (ANF). The ANA has more than 35 affiliated specialty organizations, such as the American Psychiatric Nurses Association and the American Association of Critical-Care Nurses. A complete list of ANA-affiliated organizations and links to their websites can be found on the ANA website.

Through legislative, regulatory, and political activities the ANA has taken firm and visible positions on a large variety of health policy issues of great importance to the nation and to the profession. A few of these are passage of Medicare and Medicaid bills and then significant reforms of these programs over time, including APRNs' direct reimbursement in the plans; patients' rights; the importance of safe workplaces and safe health devices and practices, such as safe needles, safe patient handling, and whistle-blower protection for health care workers; and comprehensive health care reform.

Just as important, it is the ANA members—the SNAs—that carry forward on the policy and political activities for health policy and nursing practice, roles, and reimbursement within a given state. A tremendous amount of health policy development and implementation occurs within state boundaries, and in order for the nursing profession's voice to be heard SNA membership and participation are a must, because very few of the specialty nursing organizations have an individual state presence for policy and political activity. Students are encouraged to spend time browsing the ANA website and to learn more about this nursing organization so important to us all.

Students are also encouraged to visit ANA's Action Center and sign up to receive legislative updates and action alerts important to nurses and health care (www.rnaction.org). Through action alerts, members are informed about when e-mails, telephone calls, and faxes will have the most effect. Being connected through the ANA Action Center website makes the political process less intimidating by keeping nurses informed of political issues and providing strategies for making their opinions known.

NATIONAL STUDENT NURSES ASSOCIATION (NSNA)

Becoming involved as a nurse policy advocate can start during your time as a student nurse by becoming involved with the NSNA. The NSNA is a national association representing student nurses in all 50 states and US territories. The mission of the NSNA is *"to mentor students preparing for initial licensure as registered nurses, and to convey the standards, ethics, and skills that students will need as responsible and accountable leaders and members of the profession"* (NSNA, 2023). Most states have an affiliated state student nurses association, and individual nursing schools may also have a school chapter of the NSNA. Students are encouraged to visit the NSNA website (nsna.org) to learn more about this national organization and the chapter or association affiliated with your state and school.

CURRENT HEALTH POLICY ISSUES

A variety of factors or influences shape policy issues. Factors include political, demographic, economic, social, technological, cultural, ecological, and legal influences (Meacham, 2021). The COVID-19 pandemic has significantly influenced policy in the United States, and this is expected to continue at least in the near future. Similarly, the 2022 Supreme Court decision on Roe vs Wade and climate change will have effects for years. Public policy is a government's response to a societal problem. Health-related priority problems that drive policy decisions in the United States include relatively poor health status, persistent health and health care disparities, unsustainable health care costs, nursing work, workforce, and well-being issues. Several interconnected policy topics bear watching over the next several years:

1. Rethinking health by reducing disparities to achieve health equity

2. Strengthening nursing capacity, expertise, and leadership
3. Transforming the delivery of health care services

Rethinking Health: Reducing Disparities to Achieve Health Equity

Disparities in health and health care refer to "differences between groups that stem from broader social inequities" (Ndugga & Artiga, 2023, paragraph 2) and are therefore avoidable (Centers for Disease Control [CDC], 2023; Ndugga & Artiga, 2023). Disparities include the "unequal distribution of social, political, economic, and environmental resources" (CDC, 2023, paragraph 3). In 2014 the Robert Wood Johnson Foundation (RWJF) launched a new initiative, *Culture of Health*. A Culture of Health recognizes health as inextricably linked to all aspects of a person's and community's life, including where people live, work, play, and their choices. At the center of the grand vision of a Culture of Health is the certainty that "everyone deserves to live the healthiest life possible" and that "we must [as a nation] ensure all people have equal opportunity to make healthy choices" (RWJF, n.d.).

The Culture of Health initiative transcends the idea that health is equated with health care. Health care is necessary for health; however, it is insufficient alone. The evidence-based County Health Rankings Model (Fig. 23.1) depicts health outcomes as a composite of several health factors and determines the contribution of each factor to overall health. Clinical care (health care) accounts for 20% of overall health outcomes, social and economic factors for 40%, health behaviors for 30%, and physical environment for 10%. These factors can improve individual health outcomes and make communities healthier (University of Wisconsin Population Health Institute [UWPHI], 2021). Part of the call to action to nurture a Culture of Health is recognizing that the US health care system must change fundamentally to be more community-oriented and patient- and population-centered, all representing a major transition.

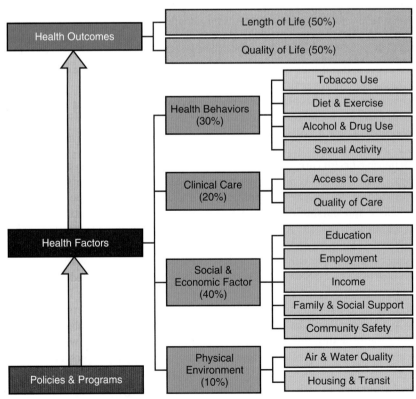

Fig 23.1 County Health Rankings Model.

Nurses are uniquely qualified to be leaders in promoting health equity. Nurses' holistic perspective of health is congruent with a focus on social factors that influence health outcomes (these are sometimes called "social determinants" or "drivers of health"). Nursing has a rich historical legacy of working with diverse and often disadvantaged populations. Nurses have long understood how environmental and other social factors can enable or constrain choices available to people. They have worked to improve circumstances that impact health and empower people to take better care of themselves. Examples of nurse leaders known for addressing social determinants or drivers of health include Florence Nightingale, Lilian Wald, Clara Barton, and Mary Breckenridge. Florence Nightingale is remembered for her attention to improving the environment to promote healing among wounded soldiers of the Crimean War in the 1850s. Lillian Wald started the Visiting Nurses Service in 1893 to serve poor immigrants in New York City. Wald was also the founder of the Henry Street Settlement, which provided community-based nursing services and worked to improve neighborhood conditions. Mary Breckenridge established the Frontier Nursing Service in eastern Kentucky in 1920, which provided services to the rural, poor, and isolated communities and included a system of community-based clinics, central monitoring of patients, and home visitation. Today's nurses have innumerable opportunities to advocate for and promote a Culture of Health in their own communities. Visit the Robert Wood Johnson Foundation website (www.rwjf.org) for information and ideas about how to make a difference.

Transforming the Delivery of Health Care

Health care reform is the general term used to refer to health policy initiatives to effect significant changes in how health is promoted, and health care is accessed, delivered, and paid for in the United States. Health care costs, quality, and outcomes are major policy concerns. In addition, significant economic implications are related to the performance of the US health-care delivery system and outcomes. According to a 2023 report (Organization for Economic Co-Operation & Development, [OECD]) the United States has the highest per capita health care costs across similar wealthy, democratic countries. The estimated $12,914 per person spent on health care in the United States compares with $8049 in Switzerland, the second-highest spending

country, and an average of $6414 among the comparator countries.

The dollars spent on health care in the United States do not result in better outcomes. People in the United States have the lowest life expectancy, highest death rates for avoidable or treatable conditions, most chronic health conditions, high suicide rates, and the highest maternal and infant mortality as compared to other industrialized nations (Gunja, Gumas, & Williams II, 2023). Many Americans, consumer groups, health care organizations such as the ANA, and vocal individuals, including many professional nurses, have long supported bold and comprehensive health care reforms to address critical issues facing our nation and its citizens. These issues include high health care costs that are not sustainable at the individual and societal levels, barriers in access to care, health care disparities, concerns about quality and safety, and a system that is focused on illness care rather than one that promotes health and wellness.

The ACA, passed in 2010, is a complex, far-reaching, and initially phased plan to address some of the issues plaguing our nation's health care system and approach to health care. The passage and the course of the ACA was contentious. However, there is growing evidence regarding the positive impact of the ACA and increased public acceptance (see Chapter 7 for more information about the ACA). Provisions in the ACA provided for the creation of the Centers for Medicare & Medicaid Innovation Center to support the development and testing of innovative health care payment and delivery system models. At the center of developing and testing innovative health care payment and delivery system models is the concept of value and migration to value-based reimbursement, where improved outcomes at lower costs are emphasized. Value reflects "the quality and safety outcomes achieved for a patient relative to the cost of resources used to produce those outcomes" (Yakusheva et al., 2022). The Hospital Value-Based Purchasing program increasingly emphasizes efficiency and cost-reduction, safety, clinical outcomes, and personal and community engagement and de-emphasizes the volume of services delivered.

Medicare has three programs to incentivize hospital-based, value-based performance (good outcomes at low cost):
1. Hospital Value-Based Purchasing Program in which hospitals are paid based on their performance on quality measures, including patient satisfaction.

2. Hospital-Acquired Conditions Reduction program where payments to some hospitals are reduced or eliminated for treating hospital-acquired, preventable conditions, such as falls, decubitus ulcers, and infections.
3. Hospital Readmissions Reduction Performance program resulting in reduced Medicare payments to hospitals for preventable hospital readmissions.

Hospitals may see up to $300 extra per Medicare discharge (+2%) or lose up to $900 per discharge across the three programs (−9%).

Value-informed nursing is not only an economic imperative and a means to improve outcomes but also an ethical one consistent with nurses' social contract (Yakusheva, Rambur, & Buerhaus, 2021). Nurses are critically important in influencing Medicare payments by preventing hospital-acquired conditions, promoting patient satisfaction and other quality measures, and reducing preventable hospital readmissions through appropriate care transitions and discharge planning. Students are encouraged to visit the CMS Innovation Center to learn more about these new care delivery models, which will require active, engaged nursing practice to be successful (https://innovation.cms.gov/).

Pivoting to value-informed nursing practice requires changes in attitudes and practices. Despite the required changes in thinking and actions nurses are uniquely positioned to thrive and elevate the profession. Historically, nurses have been innovative in facing health and health care challenges and demonstrated the profession's value in promoting patient satisfaction and engagement, quality, safety, and improved health outcomes. Nurses now have the opportunity (and social mandate) to generate value for the good of society and the profession.

Nurses must pay particular attention to evolving developments regarding the ACA and other national and state health care reforms. The ANA/SNAs provide the professional venue for nurses to stay current—and become involved—as health care reform moves forward. Comprehensive health system change will not be smooth or seamless or without continuing controversy but it is critical. Through informed participation in health care reform initiatives nurses can advocate for their profession and the safety, quality, value, and availability of health and nursing care for all Americans.

Strengthening Nursing Capacity, Expertise, and Leadership

Besides revealing and exacerbating long-standing disparities among various population groups in the United States, the COVID-19 pandemic (2020–2022) compounded nursing work and workforce problems of increased demand, decreased supply, and workload and workplace problems. The *2022 National Nursing Workforce Study* (Smiley, et al., 2023) revealed an exodus from the nursing workforce precipitated by the pandemic, resulting in a major drain of experienced nurses. High workloads, stress, and burnout are factors in attrition and are prevalent among working nurses. Approximately 20% of the RN workforce reported they will likely leave the profession in the coming years (Smiley, et al., 2023). However, there is a bright future for nurses and the nursing profession if we stay involved and use our leaderships skills and expertise to focus on solutions for healthier work environments. The *Future of Nursing* reports discussed in the following sections provide us with specific recommendations for policy initiatives to address these serious challenges and strengthen our profession for improved health for all.

The Future of Nursing Report 2010–2020. In 2010 the Institute of Medicine (IOM) issued a landmark report, *The Future of Nursing: Leading Change, Advancing Health*, calling attention to the essentiality of nursing in the success of reforming the US health care system. In this report the IOM had four major recommendations:

1. Nurses should practice to the full extent of their education and training.
2. Nurses should achieve higher levels of education and training through an improved education system that promotes seamless academic progression, with a goal that 80% of nurses in the United States hold at least a bachelor's degree by 2020.
3. Nurses should be full partners with physicians and other health care professionals in redesigning health care in the United States.
4. Effective workforce planning and policymaking require better data collection and information infrastructure.

The Future of Nursing 2020–2030 Report. The 2010 *Future of Nursing* report was primarily directed at the capacity of the nursing profession. The *Future of*

Nursing 2020–2030 report focuses on the role of nurses in creating a culture of health, reducing health disparities, and improving the health and well-being of the US population (National Academy of Medicine [NAM], 2020). Several priorities with major policy implications are identified in the report. These priorities include:
1. Building a stronger, more diversified workforce;
2. Promoting health and well-being among individuals, communities, and nurses; and
3. Addressing systemic inequities at the root of persistent disparities.

Examples of recommended actions consist of (National Academies of Science, Engineering, and Medicine (NASEM), 2021):
1. Substantial increases in the number, type, distribution, and diversity of nurses
2. Increase in nursing knowledge and skills addressing social drivers of health
3. Eliminating restrictions that prevent Registered Nurses and Advanced Practice Registered Nurses to practice at the full extent of their education and experiences
4. Designing payment mechanisms to support nurses in improving patient outcomes while reducing costs and addressing social drivers of health
5. Building capacity of nurses by including educational content and experiences that promote health equity, reduce health disparities, and improve health
6. Fostering collaborative leadership that promotes nurses' involvement at every level and across settings
7. A mandate for nurses to address structural racism and discrimination based on identity, place, and circumstances within the nursing profession and at the societal level.

SUMMARY

To summarize this chapter let's return to the opening Vignette and the questions posed about Juan's concerns with his nursing practice environment.
1. What are the major steps in health policy development that Juan must understand to engage in policy improvements for the nursing workforce and his own professional career?
   Health policy development is a complex process involving many stakeholders including one or more policymakers who are willing to take definitive action through legislative, regulatory, or funding processes. Juan can be most effectively involved in health policy development and regulation by working with his state nurses association and being an active, engaged member of nursing professional organizations, which have the knowledge and expertise to guide effective health policy initiatives. Much thoughtful, focused effort goes into the development of health policy—from the time a public health problem is identified through when a legislative solution is conceived, a bill is passed, and a health policy is actually implemented through regulation and funding. By understanding and becoming involved in these processes nurses can protect and influence nursing practice and create and shape positive change throughout the health care system and our own communities.
2. How can Juan relate his knowledge of the clinical judgment process to an effective plan for policy development related to improving the nursing workforce and his own professional career?
   As Juan commits to being more policy focused and politically active he will find that applying the Clinical Judgment Model is a natural approach to identifying and taking on broader professional and health policy issues. By working through the five steps in the Clinical Judgement Model Juan can learn to recognize nursing and health care issues that are amenable to and/or require policy action and what steps are necessary to move toward policy action.
3. What types of grassroots political strategies can Juan use to ensure that policymakers hear his interests and concerns about quality, safe patient care, and the supply of professional nurses?
   Nurses can effectively influence health policy action by participating in various grassroots initiatives including registering to vote, being a well-informed voter, and voting in *all* elections; joining and actively participating in professional nursing organizations; working on political candidates' campaigns; meeting with policymakers or their staff members; attending and speaking up at "meet-the-candidates" town hall meetings; and

communicating with policymakers by e-mail, fax, and telephone.

Nurses can significantly contribute to developing health policies that promote a healthier society and healthier work environments by understanding the policy and political processes presented in this chapter. Just as the first politically active nurse, Florence Nightingale, used expert knowledge to shape health policy to make a difference, so can *we make a difference* in the lives of people we care for, our own lives, and the future of our profession by being powerful advocates for better health for all and better health for the nursing profession.

CLINICAL JUDGMENT AND NEXT-GENERATION NCLEX® EXAMINATION-STYLE QUESTIONS

Silas Everett, RN, BSN, is starting his third year as the school nurse for a large elementary school with more than 600 students aged 5 to 11 years. As Silas sits in his office and observes the children as they walk into the building on the first day of school in August, he is troubled about the number of children he observes who are overweight. He wonders if this is a problem just at his school because it is located in a lower socioeconomic area of the city and many of the students and their families live in poverty or near the poverty level. Or is this a more widespread trend? He does an Internet search and learns that, according to the Centers for Disease Control, 18.5% of children and adolescents are obese. Silas continues to review reputable studies and reports about childhood obesity and learns many key facts about childhood obesity. Lower socioeconomic status plays a significant role in childhood obesity, which may explain the rates of obesity in the community served by his school. Obesity in children is associated with several health issues including high blood pressure, high cholesterol, asthma, sleep disturbances, poor self-esteem, behavior problems, and even difficulty in being successful in the learning environment. Obese children are much more likely to become obese adults with all the health consequences that accompany being overweight. Health care spending for an individual with obesity is approximately 150% more than that for a person of average weight.

Silas remembers learning about the social determinants of health in nursing school and realizes that he is seeing social determinants in action! Silas feels compelled to take up the cause of childhood obesity and identify some ways to address the problem in his community. Using the Clinical Judgment Model applied to health policy development (as demonstrated in the chapter), determine actions that Silas can take to develop a health policy solution for childhood obesity.

Multiple Response Select All That Apply
1. Select actions related to "Recognize cues"
   A. Collect and understand information about the issue of concern.
   B. Summarize facts about childhood obesity in the local school.
   C. Report your own experience that you think childhood obesity is a problem in your community.
   D. Summarize facts from reputable reports and literature about childhood obesity in the local community, state, and nation.
   E. Plan solutions to the problem of childhood obesity.
2. Select actions related to "Analyze cues"
   A. Analyze the information collected about childhood obesity.
   B. Engage other stakeholders (e.g., teachers, community leaders, parents, health care providers, and students) to help to analyze the information collected and understand the problem.
   C. Continue to collect data from national reports about the problem of childhood obesity.
   D. Assume that a lack of access to healthy foods is the primary contributing factor in childhood obesity.
   E. Identify the fundamental issues or underlying problems that need to be addressed.
3. Select actions related to "Prioritize hypotheses and generate solutions"
   A. Develop options for an effective policy plan to address childhood obesity with input from many sources and perspectives.
   B. Promote the one solution that you think will be most beneficial to reduce childhood obesity.
   C. Discuss potential options with many stakeholders including teachers, community leaders, parents, health care providers, and students.
   D. Identify options that flow from the data collected, analyzed, and supported by stakeholders.

E. Identify options that have the potential to be well received by the community.
4. Select actions related to "Take actions"
   A. Develop the policy plan.
   B. Use political strategies and interventions to give the policy plan the best chance of becoming law or regulation.
   C. Engage community and state education leaders to support the new policy plan to address childhood obesity.
   D. Engage with one or more state legislators to support legislation mandating the new policy to address childhood obesity.

E. Develop a brief, clear, and strong message about childhood obesity and the proposed policy plan.
5. Select actions related to "Evaluate outcomes"
   A. Assess evidence and metrics that determine if the policy plan was a success or not and why.
   B. Determine next steps if the policy plan was not successful.
   C. If the proposed policy plan has been passed as legislation, then no further action is needed.
   D. If the policy plan failed to become law, then evaluate how to develop a new plan.
   E. Develop a new action plan to continue to address additional actions to reduce childhood obesity.

REFERENCES

Centers for Disease Control & Prevention (CDC). (2023). *Health disparities.* https://www.cdc.gov/healthyyouth/disparities/index.htm

Govtrack. (2023). Statistics and historical comparison. https://www.govtrack.us/congress/bills/statistics

Gunja, M.Z., Gumas, E.D., & Wiliams II, R.D. (2023). *U.S. health care from a global perspective, 2022: Accelerating spending, worsening Outcomes.* Commonwealth Fund Issue Brief. https://www.commonwealthfund.org/publications/issue-briefs/2023/jan/us-health-care-global-perspective-2022

Institute of Medicine (IOM) (2010). *The future of nursing: Leading change, advancing health.* National Academies Press.

Mason, D.J., et al. (2021). *Frameworks for action in policy and politics.* In D.J. Mason, E.L. Dickson, G.A. Perez, M.R. (Eds.), Policy and Politics in Nursing and Healthcare, 8th Ed., St. Louis: Saunders.

Meachum, M. (2021). Longest's Health policymaking in the United States. (7th ed.). Washington D.C.: Health Administration Press.

National Academy of Medicine (NAM). (2020). *The future of nursing 2020–2030: A consensus study from the National Academy of Medicine.* https://nam.edu/publications/the-future-of-nursing-2020-2030

National Academies of Science, Engineering, and Medicine (NASEM), (2021). *The future of nursing 2020–2030.* https://www.nationalacademies.org/our-work/the-future-of-nursing-2020-2030

National Student Nurses Association (NSNA). (2023). *NSNA mission at a glance.* https://www.nsna.org/about-nsna.html

Nightingale, F. (1859). *Notes on hospital.* John W. Parker and Sons.

Ndugga, N., & Artiga, S. (April 21, 2023). *Disparities in health & health care: 5 key questions & answers.* Kaiser Family Foundation. https://www.kff.org/racial-equity-and-health-policy/issue-brief/disparities-in-health-and-health-care-5-key-question-and-answers/

Organisation of Economic Co-Operation & Development (2023). *OECD health statistics.* https://www.oecd.org/els/health-systems/health-data.htm

Robert Wood Johnson Foundation (RWJF). (n.d.). *Why we need a culture of health.* https://www.rwjf.org/en/cultureofhealth/about/why-we-need-a-culture-of-health.html

Smiley, R.A., Allgeyer, R.L., Shobo, Y., Lyoms, K.C., Letourneau, R., Zhong, E., Kaminsk-Ozturk, N., & Alexander, M. (2023). 2022 National Nursing Workforce Survey. *Journal of Nursing Regulation, 14,* Supplement 2, S10S90. https://www.journalofnursingregulation.com/issue/S2155-8256(23)X0004-0

Starr, P. (1982). *The social transformation of American medicine: The rise of a sovereign profession and the making of a vast industry.* Basic Books.

University of Wisconsin Population Health Institute (UWPHI). (2021). *County Health Rankings Model.* https://www.countyhealthrankings.org/cxplore-health-rankings/county-health-rankings-model

World Health Organization (WHO). (2023). *Social determinants of health.* https://www.who.int/health-topics/social-determinants-of-health#tab=tab_1

Yakusheva, O., Rambur, B., O'Reilly-Jacob, M., & Buerhaus, P. (2022). Value-based payment promotes better patient care, incentivizes health care delivery organizations to improve outcomes & lower costs, & can empower nurses. *Nursing Outlook, 70,* 215–218. https://doi.org/10.1016/j.outlook.2021.12.012

Yakusheva, O., Rambur, B., & Buerhaus, P. (2021). The ethical foundations of value-informed nursing practice. *Nursing Outlook, 69,* 539–541. https://doi.org/10.1016/j.outlook.2021.03.014

24

Clinical Judgment

Keevia Y. Porter, DNP, APRN, NP-C, PMHNP-BC

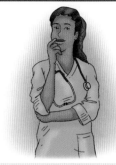

Professional nurses use clinical judgn skills to provide safe, effective care.

Ⓔ Additional resources are available online at: http://evolve.elsevier.com/Cherry/

LEARNING OUTCOMES

After studying this chapter, the reader will be able to:
1. Demonstrate clinical judgment skills needed for professional nursing practice.
2. Describe processes to formulate a clinical judgment.
3. Explore ways of demonstrating clinical judgment in nursing practice.
4. Compare the stages of Tanner's clinical judgment model, the nursing process, and the National Council of State Boards of Nursing-Clinical Judgment Measurement Model (NCSBN-CJMM).

KEY TERMS

Clinical judgment An interpretation or conclusion about a patient's needs, concerns, or health problems, and/or the decision to take action (or not), use or modify standard approaches, or improvise new ones as deemed appropriate by the patient's response (Tanner, 2006).

Clinical reasoning The processes by which nurses and other clinicians make their judgments, which includes the deliberate process of generating alternatives, weighing them against the evidence, and choosing the most appropriate, and those patterns that might be characterized as engaged, practical reasoning (Tanner, 2006).

Critical thinking The mental process of active and skillful perception, analysis, synthesis, and evaluation of collected information through observation, experience, and communication that leads to a decision for action (Papathansiou et al., 2014).

Interpreting The process of analyzing data to determine the patient's problem (Ignatavicius, 2021).

Noticing The nurse's perception of a situation or encounter (Ignatavicius, 2021).

Nursing process A scientific, clinical reasoning approach to patient care that includes assessment, analysis, planning, implementation, and evaluation (NCSBN, 2021).

Reflecting The process of the nurse thinking about what they learned from a patient situation that may be applied to a future patient situation (Ignatavicius, 2021).

Responding To monitor a patient or act on current evidence to prevent, detect early, or resolve patient problems (Ignatavicius, 2021).

PROFESSIONAL/ETHICAL ISSUE

Bradley is a recent Bachelor of Science in Nursing (BSN) graduate working in the medical-surgical intensive care unit in an urban hospital. He receives a postoperative patient from surgery. The patient is recovering from a partial colectomy. The Post Anesthesia Care Unit (PACU) nurse reports to Bradley the following vital signs: B/P 110/65 mm Hg, HR 60 bpm, RR 12 bpm, SaO2 93 % on 2L BNC, and a pain level of 6 on a scale of 1 to 10. Upon arrival to the unit the patient is difficult to arouse.

Bradley begins his postoperative care by assessing the patient's postoperative vitals. Bradley connects the patient to a point-of-care (POC) monitoring device. After several attempts to obtain a blood pressure reading the POC device displays the blood pressure as undetectable. Bradley shifts his attention from the patient and tries to fix the monitoring device. He assumes the device is having trouble assessing the patient's blood pressure due to a technical issue. As Bradley continues to fumble with the monitor, the patient's level of consciousness is deteriorating. Without noticing the patient's declining condition, Bradley uses the patient's call button to ask for assistance from the charge nurse.

After the charge nurse enters the room, Bradley gives the charge nurse a briefing on the situation. The charge nurse responds by firmly asking Bradley, "Did you think to assess the patient before troubleshooting the equipment?" Immediately the charge nurse manually assesses the postoperative patient's vital signs. The results are B/P 60/44, HR 130, and RR 8. The charge nurse places an emergency call to the rapid-response team.

As Bradley reflects upon this situation he should ask himself the following questions:

What went well? What went poorly? What should he do differently if he ever encounters a comparable situation? Reflection will allow Bradley to think about and process his own thoughts and feelings about his clinical judgment while caring for this patient.

VIGNETTE

I am a new nursing student in a first-semester clinical course. My clinical instructor shared with my clinical group that we will use simulations and case studies to improve our clinical judgment and critical thinking skills. However, I do not think this is best for new nursing students. We need hands-on experience in the clinical setting. What is the benefit of reading case studies or simulating with mannequins instead of hands-on-training with real patients?

Questions to Consider While Reading This Chapter:

1. Why should nursing faculty, within nursing education programs, introduce clinical judgment to beginning nursing students?
2. Why is it important for the professional nurse to develop and become proficient in clinical judgment?
3. What is the relationship between critical thinking, clinical reasoning, and clinical judgment?
4. How do skills in clinical judgment set the professional nurse apart from unlicensed assistive personnel?
5. Why is self-reflection important for nursing students and the professional nurse?

CHAPTER OVERVIEW

Today professional nurses are practicing in ever-changing and complex care environments. For this reason professional nurses' proficiency in clinical judgment is foundational to the quality of the nursing care provided. Clinical judgment is the conclusion (clinical decision-making) of the thinking process (clinical reasoning) nurses use when caring for patients. Clinical judgment is ongoing. Nurses will develop their clinical judgment through nursing knowledge, practice, and experience within and outside of the clinical setting.

Supporting and sustaining high-quality care practices is essential for nurses to learn and constantly develop the skill of clinical judgment. To arrive at a clinical judgment, initially the nurse is presented with a situation. The nurse uses a decision-making process, including the nursing process, to assess, identify, prioritize, and decide on an evidence-based solution to deliver high-quality and safe patient care.

Nursing students should begin to develop clinical judgment while enrolled in their education programs. Clinical reasoning includes the thinking process related to patient situations and experiences. Nursing students can practice the skill of clinical reasoning to make clinical judgments through various learning modalities such as nursing theory, clinical case studies, clinical simulations with pre- and post-briefings, and hands-on clinical experiences. Using a combination of theoretical and practical learning experiences, students will begin their transition from novice to expert nurse clinicians.

Clinical reasoning and critical thinking skills in combination with nursing experience support nurses making sound clinical judgments in care delivery. This chapter will introduce the concept of clinical judgment in nursing. It will also provide an overview of the correlation between clinical judgment and the nursing process, the steps to arrive at a clinical judgment, and implications for nursing practice.

CLINICAL JUDGMENT AND THE NURSING PROCESS

Over time clinical judgment has become interrelated to the nursing process. Like clinical judgment is the act of clinical decision-making, the nursing process is also an inductive form of decision-making or problem-solving. The nursing process consists of five stages: assessment, nursing diagnosis, planning, implementation, and evaluation. Outcomes of decision-making guided by the nursing process may be affected by the nurse's personal and professional experiences (Ignatavicius, 2021; Ignatavicius & Silvestri, n.d; Toney-Butler & Thayer, 2023).

As a function of the nurse's role the nurse will collect, analyze, and interpret data related to a patient's condition. The nurse will then use the information to formulate one or more nursing diagnoses. It is important for the nurse to identify actual and potential patient problems. Based on the nursing diagnosis assigned, the nurse will decide which evidence-based actions or interventions are needed to achieve mutually set patient outcomes (Gonçalves et al., 2019). The nurse will conduct an evaluation of the patient's plan of care. During this evaluation the nurse examines, evaluates, and modifies the patient's plan of care (Toney-Butler & Thayer, 2023). The nursing process is an effective and efficient method to organize the nurse's thought processes needed for clinical decision-making (Gonçalves et al., 2019) (Fig. 24.1).

Clinical Judgment: The Decision-Making Process

Clinical judgment is an essential skill for a professional nurse. It is a skill that separates professional nurses from assistive personnel. In today's clinical environment

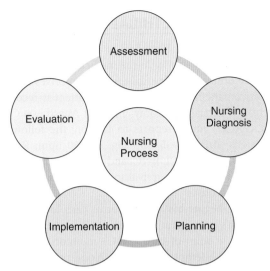

Fig. 24.1 Nursing process.

nurses are faced with caring for patients who have complex issues. Nurses must be able to decide the best course of action when dealing with these complexities in patient care (Karam et al., 2021).

In 2006 Dr. Christine Tanner developed a model for clinical judgment. Tanner (2006) defined clinical judgment as "an interpretation or conclusion about a patient's needs, concerns or health problems, and/or the judgment to take action (or not), use or modify standard approaches, or improvise new ones as deemed appropriate by the patient's response" (p. 204). Clinical judgment is not a linear but a fluid process. During a nurse's educational programs it is important for the nursing student to "learn to think like a nurse" (Tanner, 2006). Based on Tanner's (2006) research and review of the literature related to clinical judgment, it was concluded:

- Clinical judgments are most influenced by what nurses bring to the situation rather than the objective data at hand.
- Sound clinical judgment rests on the nurse knowing the patient and their typical or atypical responses. This includes engaging with the patient about their concerns.
- Clinical judgments are influenced by the context in which the situation is and the culture of the unit where the situation is occurring.
- Nurses use a variety of reasoning patterns.
- Reflection is critical for improving clinical knowledge and clinical reasoning skills.

Clinical Judgment Model: Overview

Tanner's (2006) clinical judgment model (TCJM) includes four phases: noticing, interpreting, responding, and reflecting. The clinical judgment model was derived from and based on the judgments of experienced nurses. This model purposefully includes reflective nursing practice to guide and develop clinical judgment skills. The use of reflective practice by nursing students and novice nurses will enhance their clinical judgment in future clinical situations (Tanner, 2006).

In overview, noticing is a nurse's perception of the situation or encounter. The nurse develops an understanding of the situation to respond; this act is defined as interpreting. The nurse decides on a suitable action or no action at all, which is termed as responding. After responding the nurse reflects (reflecting) on the patient's response to the nurse's action (Tanner, 2006) (Fig. 24.2).

Clinical Judgment Model: Noticing

The noticing phase of the clinical judgment model consists of remarkably similar skills that are used during the assessment phase of the nursing process. These skills include assessment techniques such as physical assessment and subjective and objective data collection. During this phase, the nurse may internally notice that something does not seem right (Caputi, 2021; Tanner, 2006). The noticing phase is based on the nurses' knowledge of the patient and their patterns of responses. The nurse uses earlier knowledge, clinical and practical, from similar or past patient experiences and theoretical knowledge from textbooks. Noticing is shaped by the context and background relationship, expectations, and the first grasp of the situation (Tanner, 2006).

As mentioned the noticing phase aligns with the nursing process assessment phase. During assessment and noticing the nurse identifies signs and symptoms. The nurse collects this data systematically in a comprehensive manner. The nurse gathers the most accurate information to detect or predict complications (Caputi, 2021).

In the clinical setting, when noticing, a nurse compares normal with abnormal findings (Caputi, 2021). Effective noticing involves focused observations, recognizing deviations from expected findings, and seeking information. During noticing the nurse observes and monitors subjective and objective data. The nurse will recognize any subtle changes and deviations from expected patterns in data based on the patient assessment. The assertive nurse seeks additional information from patient and family observations and interactions if needed (Marques 2022).

Assume a nurse in the emergency department is caring for a patient who has suffered a femur fracture from a motor vehicular accident. The nurse notices the patient is grimacing and moaning as if they are in extreme pain. In response the nurse conducts a pain assessment. The patient rates their pain level as a 10 on a 0 to 10 pain scale. The patient's pain level coincides with the nurse's observation.

Clinical Judgment Model: Interpreting

The interpreting phase of the clinical judgment model aligns with the planning phase of the nursing process. Interpreting requires the nurse to use the skill of clinical reasoning to analyze data related to the patient's status (Ignatavicius, 2021). During the interpreting phase the nurse begins to "make sense" of the data. The data

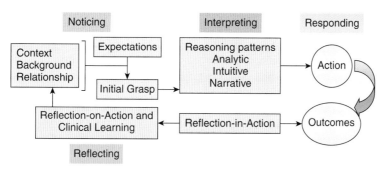

Fig. 24.2 Tanner's model of clinical judgment. (From Tanner, C.A. (2006). Thinking like a nurse: A research-based model of clinical judgment in nursing. *Journal of Nursing Education, 45*(6), 204–211. https://doi.org/10.3928/01484834-20060601-04)

collected is used to decide the next course of action (Caputi, 2021; Tanner, 2006). In the clinical setting the nurse uses their initial interpretation of the data to identify priorities in care (Glynn, 2012).

Based on what the nurse notices the nurse should decide what issues are emerging and what are the clear health problems. Even though formulating a nursing diagnosis is not required in the interpreting phase, the nurse's diagnosis will assist the nurse in communicating with the appropriate interdisciplinary team members (Ignatavicius, 2021). The nurse should focus on the most important and relevant data (Gonzalez, 2018). For effective interpretation to occur prioritization is a key component in the care planning for the patient. The nurse should use evidence-based practices and guidelines and organizational policies and procedures to plan care for the patient (Gonzalez, 2018).

While interpreting the nurse may encounter data that is complex, confusing, or conflicting. If this occurs, the nurse should notice patterns within the patient's data. The nurse may compare these patterns with previously known patterns that are based on theory and prior nursing knowledge and patient experiences (Marques et al., 2022).

For example, the nurse is caring for a patient with a diagnosis of diabetes mellitus type II. The patient is complaining of increased thirst, frequent urination, and blurred vision. The nurse interprets these findings and suspects the patient is experiencing hyperglycemia.

Clinical Judgment Model: Responding

During the responding phase the nurse implements and intervenes. The nurse decides on the best course of action based on the patient's situation. When responding the nurse may find to take immediate action or no action at all (Tanner, 2006; van Graan et al., 2016).

Responding includes clear communication, well-planned interventions, flexibility, and being skillful (Gonzalez, 2018). After assuming responsibility of patient care, the nurse effectively communicates and educates patients on what to expect with the proposed interventions (Lasater, 2011). The nurse identifies patient and family goals, determines if interdisciplinary collaborations are needed, and delegates tasks to appropriate team members (Caputi, 2021; Glynn, 2012; Lasater, 2011).

The nurse tailors the response and interventions to the individual patient's needs. The nurse monitors the patient's response to the interventions and adjusts

treatments accordingly. For skilled interventions to be successful the nurse must show ability in those skills that are necessary in the response efforts (Lasater, 2011).

As an illustration of responding, consider that a nurse working on a psychiatric nursing unit is confronted by a patient diagnosed with schizophrenia. The nurse notices that the patient appears delusional. The patient believes the news anchor on television is reading their mind. The patient is threatening to throw the television out of the window. After interpreting that their safety and that of the patient and others is at risk, the nurse responds by using skills and techniques learned in training to attempt to deescalate the situation.

Clinical Judgment Model: Reflection

In the final phase of TCJM (Tanner, 2006) the nurse reflects on the care provided for the patient and the nurse's actions during and after the care of the patient. This encompasses the two stages of the reflective phase, which include reflection-in-action and reflection-on-action with clinical learning. Reflection helps nursing students and nurses improve their thinking skills (Tanner, 2006).

The nurse engaging in reflection evaluates the care outcomes of their patient and conducts a self-analysis. The nurse must have an underlying commitment to improvement of process and patient care. The nurse transfers the learning and knowledge, gained through reflective practices, to the future care the nurse will provide (Gonzalez, 2018).

Reflection is an important practice. It encourages the nurse to delve deep into and understand their own thinking. Reflective practice allows the nurse to evaluate and foster professional growth. In response the nurse will improve their critical thinking and clinical judgment skills. Self-reflection will improve patient care outcomes in future clinical care situations (Bussard, 2015; Caputi, 2021).

For instance, during a nightshift a nurse is caring for a female patient with a right-sided mastectomy. The nurse enters the patient's room while the patient is asleep to obtain a blood pressure measurement. The nurse places the blood pressure cuff on the patient's right upper arm. The patient awakens to the tightening of the blood pressure cuff. The patient yells at the nurse and says, "My surgeon said no one is to ever take my blood pressure using my right arm." The nurse apologizes and immediately releases and removes the blood pressure cuff from the patient's arm. The nurse reflects on why this happened and what went wrong.

National Council of State Boards of Nursing

Using the Next-Generation® Examination (NGN) the National Council of State Boards of Nursing (NCSBN) will begin to implement its own method for assessing clinical judgment in nursing candidates who are testing to obtain state nursing licensure. The NGN exam will measure clinical judgment abilities "through innovative item types" (NCSBN, "The NGN Project," 2023; Ignatavicius, 2021). Candidates sitting for the NGN examination will be expected to have clinical judgment skills to ensure patient safety and quality.

The National Council of State Boards of Nursing-Clinical Judgment Model (NCSBN-CJM) has four layers, including observation (Layer 0), cognitive operations (Layers 1–3), and contextual factors (Layer 4). Layer 0 consists of *patient needs and patient decisions*. Layer 1 primarily focuses on *clinical judgment*. Layer 2 represents three cognitive operations: *form hypotheses, refine hypotheses, and evaluate hypotheses*. Lastly, Layer 4 includes *contextual factors, environmental factors, and individual* factors (Dickison et al., 2016, 2019).

The NCBSN model consists of six skills that are recommended for nurses to make sound clinical judgments. These six skills include: recognize cues, analyze cues, prioritize hypotheses, generate solutions, take actions, and evaluate outcomes. These skill recommendations are influenced by the nursing process and TCJM (Dickison et al., 2016, 2019, Ignatavicius, 2021) (Fig. 24.3).

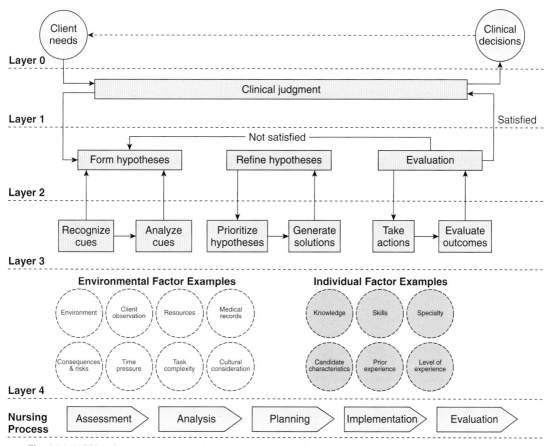

Fig. 24.3 NCSBN Clinical Judgment Measurement Model. (Copyright 2021. National Council of State Boards of Nursing, https://www.ncsbn.org/video/ngn-talks-the-clinical-judgment-measurement-model-and-action-model Accessed August 16, 2023.)

Comparison of the Nursing Process, Tanner's Clinical Judgment Model, and the National Council of State Boards of Nursing's Clinical Judgment Model

The nursing process's *assessment* aligns with TCJM's *noticing* and the NCSBN-CJM *recognizing cues* cognitive skills (Dickison et al., 2016, 2019; Ignatavicius, 2021; Tanner, 2006). While using these skills nurses collect patient data by performing various assessments. In addition to data collection the nurse is also organizing, validating, and documenting data (Berman et al., 2021). Nurses will notice small or significant changes in their patient's condition or recognize cues or alterations to the patient's health status.

Next the nurse will *analyze* the data by *interpreting* and *analyzing* cues. The nurse should identify the patient's strengths and weaknesses while recognizing potential health problems. Based on the nurse's primary area of concern for the patient the nurse will formulate and *prioritize hypotheses*. The act of TCJM's interpreting and using the NCSBN-CJM's cognitive skill of prioritizing hypotheses enables the nurse to utilize this information to determine *nursing diagnosis(es)*, the second stage of the nursing process (Dickison et al., 2016, 2019; Ignatavicius, 2021; Tanner, 2006). An appropriately developed nursing diagnosis should consist of a diagnostic label, etiology, and identifiable signs and symptoms if applicable. If more than one nursing diagnosis is needed the nurse should prioritize the diagnoses based on the seriousness or severity of the patient's problem(s) (Berman et al., 2021).

Planning and *implementation* correspond with Tanner's *responding* phase (Berman et al., 2021; Tanner, 2006). *Generating solutions* and *taking action* are the NCSBN-CJM's skills that are useful in completing the tasks of planning, implementing, and responding. The nurse is expected to set realistic patient's outcomes or goals based on the previously established priorities. The nurse aims to reduce or prevent any actual or potential complications. When the nurse takes action or implements interventions, the nurse is responding to what was deemed priority in the care of the patient. These components are all a part of planning and coordinating the patient's plan of care (Dickison et al., 2016, 2019).

Evaluation, evaluating outcomes, and *reflecting* are the final phases or skills needed for the nursing process, NCSBN-CJM, and TCJM. The nurse should evaluate and compare patient responses to the patient's set outcomes (Ignatavicius, 2021). The nurse should also evaluate the effectiveness of the patient's plan of care. This is the opportunity to continue, modify, or terminate the plan of care. The nurse should also evaluate the patient's overall quality of care provided. Quality improvement and quality assurance activities may be implemented to evaluate the quality of care provided for a patient population (Berman et al., 2021). During the final phases the nurse uses the clinical judgment skill of reflection. While evaluating the nurse can reflect on and learn from the experience. The knowledge gained from the reflective and evaluative period may be useful in future or similar patient encounters (Caputi, 2021; Tanner, 2006).

▮ SUMMARY

To summarize the chapter let's review the questions posed at the beginning of the chapter and see what you have learned.

1. Why should nursing faculty, within nursing education programs, introduce clinical judgment to beginning nursing students?

   Today professional nurses are practicing in ever-changing and complex care environments. For this reason professional nurses' proficiency in clinical judgment is foundational to the quality of the nursing care provided.

2. Why is it important for the professional nurse to develop and become proficient in clinical judgment?

   Clinical judgment is an essential skill for a professional nurse. It is a skill that separates professional nurses from assistive personnel. In today's clinical environment nurses are faced with caring for patients who have complex issues. Nurses must be able to decide the best course of action when dealing with these complexities in patient care.

3. What is the relationship between critical thinking, clinical reasoning, and clinical judgment?

   Clinical reasoning and critical thinking skills in combination with nursing experience support nurses making sound clinical judgments in care delivery.

Clinical judgment is the conclusion (clinical decision-making) of the thinking process (clinical reasoning) nurses use when caring for patients. Clinical judgment is ongoing. Nurses will develop their clinical judgment through nursing knowledge, practice, and experience within and outside of the clinical setting.

Supporting and sustaining high-quality care practices is essential for nurses to learn and constantly develop the skill of clinical judgment. To arrive at a clinical judgment, initially the nurse is presented with a situation. The nurse uses a decision-making process, including the nursing process, to assess, identify, prioritize, and decide on an evidence-based solution to deliver high-quality and safe patient care.

Nursing students should begin to develop clinical judgment while enrolled in their education programs. Clinical reasoning includes the thinking process related to patient situations and experiences. Nursing students can practice the skill of clinical reasoning to make clinical judgments through various learning modalities such as nursing theory, clinical case studies, clinical simulations with pre- and post-briefings, and hands-on clinical experiences. Using a combination of theoretical and practical learning experiences, students will begin their transition from novice to expert nurse clinicians.

4. How do skills in clinical judgment set the professional nurse apart from unlicensed assistive personnel?

Clinical judgment is acquired through experiential learning in the clinical environment and is what separates the professional nurse from unlicensed assistive personnel. The ability to make a clinical judgment is influenced by the nurse's knowledge, intuition, and experiences.

5. Why is self-reflection important for nursing students and the professional nurse?

Reflection is an important practice. It encourages the nurse to delve deep into and understand their own thinking. Reflective practice allows the nurse to evaluate and foster professional growth. In response the nurse will improve their critical thinking and clinical judgment skills. Self-reflection will improve patient care outcomes in future clinical care situations.

REFERENCES

Berman, A., Snyder, S., & Frandsen, G. (2021). Kozier & Erb's fundamentals of nursing: Concepts, process, and practice (11th ed.) Pearson Education.

Bussard, M. (2015). The nature of clinical judgment development in reflective journals. *Journal of Nursing Education, 54*(8), 451–454. https://doi.org/10.3928/01484834-20150717-05

Caputi, L. (2021). Think like a nurse: The Caputi method for learning clinical judgment. Windy City Publishers.

Dickison, P., et al. (2019). Integrating the national council of state boards of nursing clinical judgment model into nursing educational frameworks. *Journal of Nursing Education, 58*(2), 72–78. https://doi.org/10.3928/01484834-20190122-03

Dickison, P., et al. (2016). Assessing higher-order cognitive constructs by using an information-processing framework. *Journal of Applied Testing Technology, 17*, 1–19.

Glynn, D.M. (2012). Clinical judgment development using structured classroom reflective practice: A qualitative study. *Journal of Nursing Education, 51*(3), 134–139. https://doi.org/10.3928/01484834-20120127-06

Gonzalez, L. (2018). Teaching clinical reasoning piece by piece: A clinical reasoning concept-based learning method. *Journal of Nursing Education, 57*(12), 727–735. https://doi.org/10.3928/01484834-20181119-05

Gonçalves, P.D., et al. (2019). Data, diagnoses, and interventions addressing the nursing focus "delusion": A scoping review. *Perspectives in Psychiatric Care, 56*(1), 175–187. https://doi.org/10.1111/ppc.12401

Ignatavicius, D.D. (2021). *Developing clinical judgment for professional nursing and the next-generation NCLEX-RN® Examination.* Elsevier.

Ignatavicius, D., & Silvestri, L. (n.d.). *Getting Ready for the Next-Generation NCLEX® (NGN): How to Shift from the Nursing Process to Clinical Judgment in Nursing.* Elsevier. Retrieved June 21, 2023, from https://evolve.elsevier.com/education/expertise/next-generation-nclex/ngn-transitioning-from-the-nursing-process-to-clinical-judgment/

Karam, M., Chouinard, M. C., Poitras, M. E., Couturier, Y., Vedel, I., Grgurevic, N., & Hudon, C. (2021). Nursing care coordination for patients with complex needs in primary healthcare: A scoping review. *International Journal of Integrated Care, 21*(1), 16. https://HYPERLINK "http://doi.org/10.5334/ijic.5518"doi.org/10.5334/ijic.5518

Lasater, K. (2011). Clinical judgment: The last frontier for evaluation. *Nurse Education in Practice, 11*(2), 86–92. https://doi.org/10.1016/j.nepr.2010.11.013

Marques, F.M., Pinheiro, M.J., & Alves, P.V. (2022). Clinical judgment and decision-making of the undergraduate nursing students. O julgamento clínico e a tomada de decisão nos estudantes do Curso de Licenciatura em Enfermagem. *Ciencia & saude coletiva, 27*(5), 1731–1740. https://doi.org/10.1590/1413-81232022275.23142021

National Council of State Boards of Nursing. (2023). Next generation NCLEX: An enhanced NCLEX. Next Generation NCLEX. Retrieved June 22, 2023, from https://www.nclex.com/next-generation-nclex.page

National Council of State Boards of Nursing. (2021). *NCSBN clinical judgment measurement model. NCSBN.* https://www.ncsbn.org/14798.htm

Papathanasiou, I. V., Kleisiaris, C. F., Fradelos, E. C., Kakou, K., & Kourkouta, L. (2014). Critical thinking: The development of an essential skill for nursing students. *AIM: Journal of the Society for Medical Informatics of Bosnia & Herzegovina: casopis Drustva za medicinsku informatiku BiH, 22*(4), 283–286. https://doi.org/10.5455/aim.2014.22.283–286

Tanner, C.A. (2006). Thinking like a nurse: A research-based model of clinical judgment in nursing. *Journal of Nursing Education, 45*(6), 204–211.

Toney-Butler, T., & Thayer, J. (2023, April 10). Nursing Process. StatPearls. Retrieved June 27, 2023, from https://www.ncbi.nlm.nih.gov/books/NBK499937/

van Graan, A.C., et al. (2016). Professional nurses' understanding of clinical judgement: A contextual inquiry. *Health SA Gesondheid, 21*, 280–293. https://doi.org/10.4102/hsag.v21i0.967

25

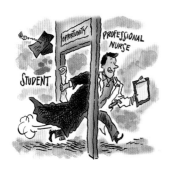

Moving from student to professional can be frightening; plan your strategies.

Making the Transition from Student to Professional Nurse

Tommie L. Norris, DNS, RN

ⓔ Additional resources are available online at: http://evolve.elsevier.com/Cherry/

LEARNING OUTCOMES

After studying this chapter, the reader will be able to:

1. Compare and contrast the phases of reality shock with the phases of transition shock.
2. Differentiate between the novice nurse and the expert professional nurse.
3. Design strategies to ease the transition from novice nurse to professional nurse.
4. Differentiate between compassion fatigue and burnout.
5. Make the transition from novice nurse to professional nurse.

KEY TERMS

Biculturalism The merging of school values with those of the workplace.

Compassion fatigue The gradual decline of compassion over time as caregivers are exposed to events that have traumatized their patients.

Horizontal violence (also known as lateral violence) The harmful or hostile nonphysical behavior occurring between coworkers. Bullying is another term used for this type of behavior (Glynn, 2022). Eye-rolling, badgering, belittling, and withholding information are examples.

Intuition Extracting clues from one's subconscious, so decisions are based on a holistic view of the patient and surroundings.

Mentoring A mutually interactive method of learning in which a knowledgeable nurse inspires and encourages a novice nurse.

Novice nurse A nurse who is entering the professional workplace for the first time; usually applies from the point of graduation until competencies required by the profession are achieved.

Preceptor An experienced professional nurse who serves as a mentor and assists with socialization of the novice nurse.

Reality shock Occurs when a person prepares for a profession, enters the profession, and then finds that they are not prepared.

Role model A person who serves as an example of what constitutes a competent professional nurse.

Socialization The nurturing, acceptance, and integration of a person into the profession of nursing; the identification of a person with the profession of nursing.

Transition Moving from one role, setting, or level of competency in nursing to another; change.

Transition shock The distress that a new nurse experiences upon moving from the familiarity of the student role to entering the "unpredictable and unfamiliar context" of the professional nurse. This period can last days or weeks and is commonly accompanied by feelings of intense doubt, loss, uncertainty, and unsettledness (Laskowski-Jones & Castner, 2022).

Trust Confidence that one's peers in the workplace have good intentions toward one.

Workplace violence Sexual harassment and abusive acts from patients or coworkers that can be physical, verbal, and emotional and can lead to a hostile work environment. It has been suggested that identifying workplace violence is difficult owing to its subjectivity (how it is seen by the recipient).

PROFESSIONAL/ETHICAL ISSUE

Lauren, a new nurse who just graduated with her bachelor of science in nursing (BSN), is interviewing with the nurse manager. She comes with questions and asks, "Can you tell me about the culture of your unit?" The nurse manager describes the culture as "accepting, diverse, and dynamic." Lauren decides to accept this position.

Lauren is excited to have such a culture to begin her nursing career. She attends new employee orientation for 3 days and looks forward to beginning her career on her first nursing unit. She arrives 30 minutes early and enters the nursing lounge. She scans the lockers to determine whether one is available. She notices several of the night shift nurses watching, so she asks, "Do we have assigned lockers or should I just choose one that is empty?"

One nurse rolls her eyes and mumbles, "New BSN nurses think they deserve what we have worked for."

Lauren hopes she didn't understand her correctly and waits for her preceptor to arrive. She shares with the preceptor her concern with choosing a locker and what she thought she heard from the night nurse.

Lauren's preceptor replies, "Never mind her. She is always like that. She doesn't like anyone, especially new nurses with a BSN."

Lauren takes report the following day from the night nurse and is told that the "patient is monitoring her own blood sugar" and that the nurse did not report lab values ordered at midnight. Lauren is surprised when she finds the results from the lab posted from the previous night showing that the patient's blood glucose was actually 400 mg/dL.

When she reports this second experience to her preceptor, she is told, "Sometimes the night nurse forgets to check lab results." Lauren feels anxious and wonders whether she can ever work under these conditions.

1. Was Lauren being targeted for horizontal violence?
2. Was information being purposefully withheld?
3. What are the signs of horizontal violence?
4. Should Lauren report the night nurse to the nurse manager?

VIGNETTE

Every nurse has experienced the transition from student to professional nurse. Why can't we learn from our experiences and help our future nurses have a positive first impression of nursing? The cost alone of the revolving door for new nurses should be enough for organizations to reconsider not only how novice nurses are orienting to the facility but also what proactive measures are in place to ensure that experienced nurses stay rather than leave due to violence or burnout.

Questions to Consider While Reading This Chapter:

1. What could educators incorporate into the curriculum to decrease the "reality shock" of transition from student to professional nurse?

2. What could employers of novice nurses do during the orientation phase to help nurses learn the ropes of their organization, which may differ somewhat from the learning environment?

3. What strategies should novice nurses use to gain self-esteem and prove themselves capable of having the required skills while still needing help with specific tasks and skills that come with experience?

4. Should professional nurses form official teams to look at the role of mentoring as one means of transitioning novice nurses into the profession?

5. What could orientation for new employees include to help novice nurses be proactive in preventing or reacting to violence at work?

CHAPTER OVERVIEW

According to *The Merriam-Webster Dictionary* (2020), *transition* is defined as "change" or the "passage from one state, stage, subject, or place to another" (https://www.merriam-webster.com/dictionary/transition). As nurses prepare to enter the profession and make the transition from student to registered nurse (RN), they move not only from one role to another but also from the school or university setting to the workplace. Transition is a complicated process during which many changes may be happening at once. The novice nurse tries to juggle all these changes while continuing a life outside of nursing (e.g., as mother, father, husband, wife, daughter, son, active church leader, or community volunteer).

To help students gain an understanding of the issues involved in the transition from the student role to that of the professional nurse, this chapter discusses the various stages of reality shock. Strategies that may alleviate this shock and ease the transition are also suggested.

REAL-LIFE SCENARIO

The first impression the novice nurse has of their chosen profession is valuable and sets the stage for entry into nursing. This first impression occurs during the transition phase from student to professional. Consider Case Study 25.1.

CASE STUDY 25.1

Rachel Stevens had wanted to be a nurse for as long as she could remember. As a child she donned a pretend laboratory jacket and set to work providing care to teddy bears and dolls. She softly spoke to her pretend patients, explaining that she was a nurse and would make everything better. After graduation from high school, Rachel entered nursing school and visualized her dream coming true. She was a high achiever and received comments from her instructors such as "shows evidence of applying the nursing process to the clinical environment," "psychomotor skills improving," and "becoming more autonomous." Her patients complimented her nursing abilities and caring attitude. Finally, Rachel graduated from nursing school, passed the national licensure examination, and accepted her first position as an RN. She proudly entered the hospital and felt confident that she would be a caring nurse and would help patients achieve their highest level of health.

The hospital provided a 2-month orientation period. The first week consisted of classes to explain benefits, safety education, Standard Precaution protocols, and computer skills. Rachel loved her new job. The next step in her employment was orientation to the medical-surgical unit where she would be working.

The nurse manager welcomed her to the unit and introduced her to the staff. Because all of the seasoned nurses wanted to transfer to the day shift, Rachel was hired to work the evening shift, which had a higher nurse–patient ratio than the day shift. Rachel proudly sat through the shift report, jotting down reminders that were stressed by the previous shift, such as "The patient in room 200 needs a blood glucose sample drawn at 6:00 p.m." and "The patient in room 215 is to receive a unit of blood." Rachel's assignment consisted of six patients. The charge nurse encouraged Rachel to ask if she had any questions. The nursing assistants hurried to complete their tasks.

Rachel reread her assignment and entered the first room, saying, "Hello, my name is Rachel Stevens, and I'll be your nurse tonight." She assessed each of her patients and reviewed their medication sheets. No medications were due until 6:00 p.m., so she began researching those medications with which she was not familiar. At 5:30 p.m. the charge nurse informed Rachel that the only other nurse on the floor would be going for dinner and that Rachel should respond to that nurse's patients during her absence. Rachel was a little nervous about the responsibility but positively acknowledged the assignment.

Moments later Rachel was paged to respond to a newly admitted patient who was assigned to the nurse on break. As soon as Rachel entered the room the patient complained of nausea and began vomiting. Rachel assessed and comforted

Continued

CASE STUDY 25.1—cont'd

the patient and reviewed the medication record for orders related to antiemetics. The physician had not ordered medication for nausea, so Rachel quickly telephoned his office to report the patient's condition. She received an order to insert a nasogastric tube and place to suction. Rachel was anxious; she had inserted only one such tube, and that with her instructor's assistance. She gathered supplies and reentered the patient's room. She measured for correct placement and was positioning the patient when she received a page that the blood had arrived for the other patient and that the laboratory assistant could not obtain a blood culture specimen ordered on yet another of Rachel's patients.

After numerous unsuccessful attempts to insert the nasogastric tube, Rachel became more anxious and requested assistance from the charge nurse. The charge nurse replied, "I'm admitting a new patient and can't help you. Don't you know how to insert the nasogastric tube?" Rachel explained that she had made numerous attempts, and the patient was continuing to vomit.

Rachel returned to the patient's room and attempted again to insert the tube. The nurse originally assigned to the patient returned to the floor; however, neither the secretary nor the charge nurse informed the returning RN of the new admission with orders. Not knowing this, Rachel proceeded to care for her other patients. Finally, Rachel again requested help, and the charge nurse inserted the tube to the relief of Rachel and the patient.

Now the medications were late, Rachel had forgotten to check the patient's blood sugar, and she had not completed the charts. "Where are my notes?" she asked herself. Oh, well, she would just have to remember.

Finally, at 10:00 p.m., 1 hour before the shift ended, Rachel sat down to chart. She took out scrap paper and began writing her notes; what time had she started the blood? She became more and more anxious. The clock continued to advance to 11:00 p.m., and Rachel was still charting.

"You need to give the shift report to the oncoming shift," said the charge nurse. Rachel complied and 15 minutes later returned to her charting. At 1:00 a.m., Rachel left the unit feeling depressed and incompetent.

IMPACT OF SHOCK IN NOVICE NURSES

Novice nurses describe feelings of being overwhelmed (Kleber, 2022) and lack self-confidence (Najafi & Nasiri, 2023). Novice nurses feel they have insufficient mastery for the work of nursing, described as "clogging" due to mental conflict brought on by self-doubt. The gap that exists between what was learned in the nursing program related to the conceptual context of lecture and limited clinical exposure left a shortcoming and low confidence (Najafi & Nasiri, 2023). When the expert student moves into the novice nurse role, uncertainty takes over, and the support of classmates and the nursing instructors is gone. This time marks the end of one era as a student and the beginning of a new era in a nursing career. The extra time needed to process and apply information to a new situation leads to excessive levels of anxiety and often feelings of defeat. These experiences can impact home life and lead to sleep disturbances and the need to process away from significant others.

The phases of transition into practice were first recognized by Kramer as *reality shock* in the 1960s, and Duchscher (2009) coined the term "transition shock" to reflect that transition in today's dynamic environment.

Kramer (1974) describes *reality shock* as the result of inconsistencies between the academic world and the world of work. Reality shock was believed to occur in novice nurses when they became aware of the inconsistency between the actual world of nursing and that of nursing school. The excitement of passing the licensure examination quickly fades in the struggle to move from the student to the staff nurse role. Both reality shock (Kramer, 1974) and transition shock (Duchscher, 2009) lead to stress, threatening the well-being of new nurses and resulting in decreased caring performances and quality of life (Babapour et al., 2022), anxiety, phobias, depression, change in mood and behavior, and physical illness. Stress also contributes to nurse turnover (Zhou et al., 2022).

The National Council of State Boards of Nursing (2023) cites that 25% of new nurses leave their positions within the first year, a fact that has a substantial impact on employers. Care of sicker patients and increased stress levels have led new nurses to report more practice errors and negative safety practices. The loss of these new nurses can negatively impact patient outcomes. New nurse turnover in the United States is estimated to cost a hospital $52,350 for a staff RN, with a national vacancy rate of

15.7% (Nursing Solutions Inc., 2023). Well-paid travel assignments and burnout felt by caring for COVID-19 patients resulted in nurses leaving the bedside at an even faster rate. Other reasons for leaving were education, salary, retirement, scheduling, and workload ratios. The American Nurses Association (n.d.) suggests the following retention strategies: provide wellness programs, competitive salaries, opportunities for autonomy, and create opportunities for professional advancement while removing mandatory overtime. Care of patients with serious illness including COVID-19, severe acute respiratory syndrome, and the comorbidity of our aging population may make transitioning to practice look different for today's graduates. Although most nursing programs have returned to planned clinical experiences with simulation being an important learning strategy, new graduates continue to face a dynamic health care system. The four phases of reality shock, *honeymoon, shock or rejection, recovery,* and *resolution,* first described by Kramer in 1974, continue to be recognized in novice nurses today (Casey, Oja, & Makic, 2021).

This chapter offers a brief tour of Kramer's reality shock theory to give a historical perspective on the "shock" phenomenon. Then it explores "transition shock" to help the reader understand the causes and how to be proactive to prevent it from happening or at least to reduce its effects.

REALITY SHOCK

Kramer describes the four phases of reality shock, from the honeymoon phase to the shock phase through recovery to the resolution phase, when the novice transitions into the role of "nurse."

Honeymoon Phase

During the honeymoon phase everything is just as the new graduate imagined. The new nurse is in orientation with former school friends or other new graduates who often have similarities. Many novice nurses in this phase are heard making the following comments: "Just think, now I'll get paid for making all those beds" and "I'm so glad I chose nursing; I will be a part of changing the future of health care." When asked, novice nurses today admit to calculating budgets on the basis of their anticipated salary.

Shock (Rejection) Phase

Then orientation is over and the novice nurse begins work on their assigned unit. This nurse receives daily assignments. "But wait. I've only observed other nurses hanging blood. Where is my instructor?" Now the shock or rejection phase comes into play. The nurse comes into contact with conflicting viewpoints and different ways of performing skills, but lacks the security of having an expert available to explain uncertain or gray areas. Kramer (1974) suggests that during this phase, novice nurses ask themselves two important questions:
1. What must I do to become the kind of nurse I want to be?
2. What must I do so that my nursing contributes to humankind and society?

Kramer described several approaches novice nurses take to deal with reality shock.

Natives. Many nurses choose to "go native" (Kramer, 1974). That is, they decide they cannot fight the experienced nurses or the administration so they adopt the ways of least resistance. These nurses may mimic other nurses on the unit and take shortcuts, such as administering medications without knowing their actions and side effects and the associated nursing responsibilities. Unfortunately, the NCSBN (2018) identified this shortcut as a current issue leading to errors.

Runaways. Others choose to "run away." They find the real world too difficult. These new nurses may choose another occupation or may return to graduate school to prepare for a career in nursing education to teach others their "values in nursing." The NCSBN (2018) reported that novice nurses continue to leave the workplace; however, residency programs have provided resources to reduce nurse turnover.

Rutters. Some adopt the attitude that "I'll just do what I have to do to get by" or "I'm just working until I can buy some new furniture." These nurses are called *rutters*. They consider nursing just a job. A focus on professionalism and involvement in professional organizations may prevent this behavior. Have you witnessed a "rutter" on any of the nursing units where you have had clinical experiences?

Burned Out. Some nurses bottle up conflict until they become burned out. Kramer (1974) describes the appearance of these nurses as having the look of being chronically constipated. In this situation patients may feel compelled to nurse their nurse. The majority of all nurses in the United States experience burnout, resulting in emotional fatigue and apathy (McLeod, 2019). With a focus on working as a team and not accepting horizontal violence, nurses have support to prevent or at least reduce burnout. Heavy workload assignments and complex patient situations continue to contribute to burnout. The Mayo Clinic, which is committed to recognizing and dealing effectively with nurse burnout, has developed the Well-Being Index to enable organizations to evaluate distress among their nurses and prevent burnout (https://www.mywellbeingindex.org/versions/nurse-well-being-index).

Compassion Fatigue. Not to be confused with burnout, compassion fatigue actually encompasses burnout. With compassion fatigue, mental, physical, and emotional exhaustion occur (MasterClass, 2022). Even Mother Teresa recognized compassion fatigue, recommending that her nuns take off an entire year every 4 to 5 years to recover from the care they provided. Burnout and compassion fatigue do share some of the same symptoms, such as emotional, mental, and physical exhaustion and lack of meaning from work. Loss of hope and self-worth and effects on well-being are common in compassion fatigue. The single greatest risk for compassion fatigue is sacrificing one's own self-care (AAPACN, 2020). Coping mechanisms for compassion fatigue include prevention—you must know the warning signs; work–life balance—create boundaries between home and work; self-care—exercise, sleep, nutrition, mindfulness meditation, and journaling; and step away from work—take time to better be able to

help others (MasterClass, 2022). The Minnesota Department of Education (n.d.) offers the Awareness, Balance, and Connection (ABCs) of prevention for compassion fatigue self-assessment (Handout 6 ABCs of Addressing Compassion Fatigue updated 082521 prod046220(2)). The compassion fatigue process is depicted in Fig. 25.1.

Loners. The nurses who react to reality shock by becoming loners create their own reality. They adopt the attitude "Just do the job and keep quiet." These nurses may prefer night shifts, during which they often are "left alone." Have you observed a loner on any nursing units?

New Nurse on the Block. Some nurses change jobs frequently. They go from the hospital setting to community health to the physician's office. They are always the new nurse on the block in their settings and therefore adopt the attitude "Teach me what you want; I'm new here." During orientation, you may meet some individuals who report being new but who have just completed a short stay at another health care facility.

Change Agents. Nurses who are called change agents care enough to work within the system to elicit change. They frequently visit the nurse manager or head nurse to suggest change or a better way. They keep the welfare of the patient at the forefront. Leaders, whether in formal or informal positions, are often adept at leading and/or supporting change. See whether you can identify the change agents on the units where you have had clinical experiences as a student or novice nurse.

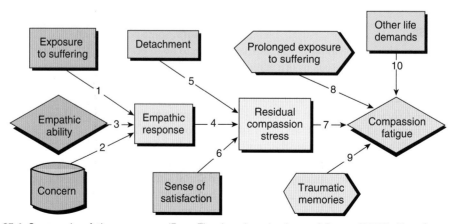

Fig. 25.1 Compassion fatigue process. (From The American Institute of Stress [2023]). The *Compassion fatigue Process (Figley, 2001)*. https://www.stress.org/military/for-practitionersleaders/compassion-fatigue)

Recovery Phase

Usually the first sign that a nurse has entered the recovery phase is the return of their sense of humor or desire to succeed. The novice nurse begins to understand the new culture to a certain degree, so feels less tension and anxiety, and healing begins. The nurse in this phase may comment, "I'll hang that blood, and I'll bet I can infuse it before 8 hours this time."

Resolution Phase

The resolution phase is the result of the shock phase combined with the novice nurse's ability to adjust to the new environment. If the nurse is able to positively work through the rejection phase, they grow more fully as a person and a professional nurse during the resolution phase. Work expectations are more easily met, and the nurse will have developed the ability to elicit change.

Individual Experiences of Reality Shock

Most novice nurses experience each phase of reality shock (honeymoon, shock or rejection, recovery, and resolution); however, the degree of shock is individualized. For example, the new graduates who complete their clinical rotation during school in the same institution as they choose to begin their career may suffer reality shock to a much lesser extent because they are already familiar with the environment, staff, and overall personality of the nursing unit. The staff in the institution where novice nurses were educated may continue to see them as only "student nurses," however, an attitude that simply presents another barrier for novice nurses to overcome. Many students choose another institution for various reasons, such as better hours, better pay, and less travel time to work.

Zerwekh and Garneau (2023) suggest that nurses complete a reality shock inventory to make them more aware of how they feel about themselves and the situation at present. The higher the score, the better the nurse's attitude. It might be helpful to take the test at different times throughout one's career or when one is trying to decide whether a career change would be advantageous (Box 25.1).

BOX 25.1 Reality Shock Inventory

Respond to the following statements with the appropriate number.

1—strongly agree
2—agree
3—slightly agree
4—slightly disagree
5—disagree
6—strongly disagree

1. I am still finding new challenges and interests in my work.
2. I think often about what I want from life.
3. My own personal future seems promising.
4. Nursing school or my work has brought stresses for which I was unprepared.
5. I would like the opportunity to start anew knowing what I know now.
6. I drink more than I should.
7. I often feel that I still belong in the place where I grew up.
8. Much of the time my mind is not as clear as it used to be.
9. I have no sense of regret concerning my major life decision of becoming a nurse.
10. My views on nursing are as positive as they ever were.
11. I have a strong sense of my own worth.
12. I am experiencing what would be called a crisis in my personal or work setting.
13. I cannot see myself as a nurse.
14. I must remain loyal to commitments even if they have not proven as rewarding as I had expected.
15. I wish I were different in many ways.
16. The way I present myself to the world is not the way I really am.
17. I often feel agitated or restless.
18. I have become more aware of my inadequacies and faults.
19. My sex life is as satisfactory as it has ever been.
20. I often think about students or friends who have dropped out of school or work.

To compute your score, reverse the number you assigned to statements 1, 3, 9, 10, 11, and 19. For example, 1 would become a 6, 2 would become a 5, 3 would become a 4, 4 would become a 3, 5 would become a 2, and 6 would become a 1. Total the number. The higher the score, the better your attitude. The range is 20 to 120.

From Zerwekh, J., & Garneau, A.Z. (2023). *Nursing today: Transition and trends* (11th ed.) Elsevier

TRANSITION SHOCK

Duchscher's *Transition Shock* (2009, 2012) built on Kramer's theory of reality shock in recognizing the following fundamental elements of transition of new nurses to the professional role (Duchscher & Windey, 2018):

- *Stability* is described as being "steady" or what is unlikely to change for you as a new nurse. Asking the following interview questions can help you judge the likelihood of stability on the unit: (1) How many nurses have left in the past year? (2) What are the staffing levels? (3) What are the acuity and average length of stay for patients? (4) Are any socialization activities planned? (5) Do people like working here? and (6) What does a routine day look like on this unit?
- *Predictability* is knowing with some certainty the types of patients you will encounter, who is staffing the unit, and what your work schedule will be.
- *Familiarity* is developing routines and becoming familiar with the staff and layout of the unit.
- *Consistency* can be described as "sameness"—whether you can expect similar types of patients and staff.

Duchscher stressed that it takes 6 months to find your "sea legs" as a novice nurse.

To help novice nurses deal with transition shock, Duchscher provides "need to know," "need to think about," and "need to do" approaches. The "need to know" concepts are the need to understand that although you are educationally prepared it is not possible to be a polished practitioner right away. Transition shock is intellectual, cultural, social, physical, emotional, and spiritual. The "need to think about" questions to ask yourself include "What is the SAFEST place for me to work that will allow me the environment needed for transition?" "Need to do" comprises understanding transition shock. You must know your capabilities and boundaries, and you must learn to say "no" if you do not feel comfortable with an assignment. Consider how you deal with stress, let your friends, family, and significant other know you will be under stress as you transition, and recognize how you deal with stress. Get plenty of sleep, make wise healthy decisions, and use positive coping strategies. The stages of transition according to Duchscher—doing, being, and knowing—are demonstrated in Fig. 25.2.

Wakefield (2018) married the concepts found in Duchscher's *Transition Shock* and Kramer's *Reality Shock* by applying emotions described by Duchscher into each phase of reality shock. For example, Kramer's Recovery Phase is described as exhibiting the emotions of reduced anxiety and increased coping ability.

CAUSES OF SHOCK IN NOVICE NURSES

Many nurses are familiar with the term culture shock. Culture shock occurs when people are immersed into a culture different from their own with norms that are

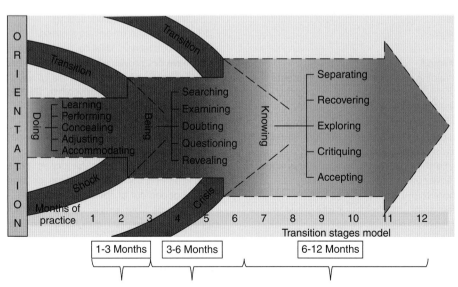

Fig. 25.2 New grad transition stages. (From Duchscher, J. B. [2012]. *From surviving to thriving: Navigating the first year of professional nursing practice.* Saskatoon Fastprint.)

unfamiliar and uncomfortable. Kramer described reality shock as exactly that. Duchscher (2012) described the transition phase as "back pedaling" as the novice nurse focuses more on doing than knowing. Entry into practice in acute care areas, where patients have high acuity but with fewer care resources, is one contributing factor. Because health care delivery still focuses on illness or disease models rather than primary health care, there is a gap between nursing education and nursing practice. When this disparity is paired with lack of experience in delegation and working with teams, the novice nurse may feel unprepared for such a demanding role. Patient-centered nursing is prioritized in nursing school, whereas in the workforce the priority is often the management of tasks and timelines. This disconnect may lead the novice nurse to feelings of failure because of the inability to provide holistic care. First, one should consider how students were taught to think in nursing school. When they prepared a care plan that took hours to complete, how were they to view the patient? The Quality and Safety Education for Nurses (QSEN) competency for patient-centered care is based on the premise of diversity and individual values of the patient, also requiring a more holistic view.

However, in the workforce nurses may function with a partial-person or functional approach, in which different members of the health care team divide the patient care into parts. Although functional nursing is effective and highly productive, it does not deliver holistic care (Indeed, 2022). The American Nurses Association (n.d.) released their definition of appropriate nurse staffing as "Appropriate staffing is a dynamic process that aligns the number of nurses, their workload, expertise, and resources with patient needs in order to achieve quality patient outcomes within a healthy work environment." The Executive Summary describes the five imperatives: (1) reform the work environment, (2) innovate the models for care delivery, (3) establish staffing standards that ensure quality care, (4) improve regulatory efficiency, and (5) value the unique contributions of nurses.

Partial-Task Vs Whole-Task System

The *partial-task system* of health care, in which different members of the health care team divide the patient care into parts, requires only partial knowledge (Kramer, 1974). For instance, one nurse may be assigned to administer all medications, whereas another may be assigned to dressing changes. The nursing assistant aids

with personal hygiene and grooming, the physical therapist provides range-of-motion exercises, and the respiratory therapist teaches pulmonary hygiene techniques. There are many other nursing care delivery models in which the role of the RN varies considerably. The partial-task system described is also congruent with the model known as "functional nursing," which places a high emphasis on completion of tasks. It is an efficient method for working with large numbers of patients, but the nurse cannot provide holistic care within such a system (Indeed, 2022). With functional nursing and the partial-task system the nurse is seen as only part of the care picture, but the RN is the central organizer who is responsible for follow-through on all the care given by other team members. This type of system is popular because fewer professional staff members are required, and it is frequently used on the evening and night shifts, when staffing is considerably lower. This type of system also encourages loyalty to the organization because it forces the nurse to focus on task completion and productivity. The nurse ensures that all tasks are carried out but is not the sole provider of care. A checkmark is often the only quality assessment, with initials being placed next to completed tasks (Box 25.2).

Most novice nurses are more comfortable with the *whole-task system* because it is more consistent with what they were taught in school. The whole-task system requires complete knowledge and encourages loyalty to the profession. The nurse provides total patient care, incorporating physical, emotional, spiritual, and cultural components. The model of nursing care consistent with the whole-task system is total patient care or primary nursing, in which the nurse is responsible for all the needs of the patient (Indeed, 2022). This model provides greater satisfaction for the patient and the nurse. However, because of the need to use an increasing number of lower-salaried employees and the shortage of RNs, few institutions continue to use this model. Nursing moved to a teams-based model during COVID-19 and with the current nursing shortage (Prentice et al., 2022). With this model of care delivery intraprofessional sharing of the workload is promoted and seen as supporting new nursing graduates.

Evaluation Methods

Another inconsistency between school and work environments is the means of evaluation (Kramer, 1974). The school environment evaluates care from the "correct

BOX 25.2   Whole-Task and Partial-Task Checklists

Whole-Task Checklist (Completed by the Same Nurse)		Partial-Task Checklist (Completed by Different Members of the Health Care Team)	
Initials	Task	Initials	Task
TN	✓ Nursing history	SJ	✓ Nursing history
TN	✓ Nursing assessment	TN	✓ Nursing assessment
TN	✓ Patient education	BC	✓ Patient education
TN	✓ Medication teaching	CS	✓ Medication teaching
TN	✓ Bed made	CS	✓ Bed made
TN	✓ Intake and output recorded	SJ	✓ Intake and output recorded
TN	✓ Dressing changed	SJ	✓ Dressing changed
TN	✓ IV fluids hung	CS	✓ IV fluids hung
TN	✓ Patient turned	BC	✓ Patient turned

step" aspect, whereas the evaluation phase in the work environment is based on whether components of care were completed according to established policies and procedures. Were all the steps carried out in a logical, correct, and efficient way? This approach is exemplified in Case Study 25.2.

CASE STUDY 25.2

A graduate nurse was involved in a resuscitation effort. After the incident she exclaimed, "I remembered to keep the time recorded and even had all the needed equipment on hand. I did everything right." But what about the patient? This nurse may have enacted all the steps correctly but may not have completed the components of care according to policies and procedures.

Think back to your first days in the nursing skills course. Can you remember the hours of practice you spent in learning the six "rights" of medication administration and technique of parenteral medication administration? Remember the stress you felt when the instructor observed you drawing up and administering your first intravenous (IV) push medication? How much error did the instructor allow? Probably not much. This is not to say that you should become lax in your tolerance for error. For example, it is never acceptable to have errors in the six "rights" of medication administration. You must and will develop your own system and quality check for performing nursing care. Nursing texts often list supplies followed by a flow diagram for procedures in which each step is listed. For instance, in the resuscitation scenario in Case Study 25.2, even basic

and advanced life support courses focus on algorithms that direct the care of the patient step by step. Always remember that patient safety comes first.

The transition from student to professional nurse is difficult, and changes in the health care environment have only added to the strain. Socialization and a caring relationship with preceptors are key to a nurse's ability to transition throughout the first year (Sherman, 2023). Often new nurses are the target of bullying because of a lack of confidence and professional relationships (Angelis, 2023). According to Angelis (2023), workplace relationships can negatively influence transition. A welcoming environment reduces stress and bullying. Nursing administrators should prevent bullying by nurturing an environment of safety and support reporting of bullying behavior (*Nurse Journal*, 2023)

FROM NOVICE TO EXPERT

Benner (1984) described the following five stages through which novice nurses proceed to become clinically competent:

- *Stage 1:* The nurse has few experiences with clinical expectations and skills are learned by rote; this stage usually occurs while the nurse is completing nursing educational requirements.
- *Stage 2:* Exemplifies the situation of advanced beginners who are able to perform adequately and make some judgment calls on the basis of experience; most novice nurses enter the workforce during this stage.
- *Stage 3:* Describes competent nurses who are able to foresee long-range goals and are mastering skills.

- *Stage 4:* Proficient nurses who view whole situations rather than parts and are able to develop a solution are in stage 4.
- *Stage 5:* Describes expert nurses for whom intuition and decision-making are instantaneous.

The greatest stressors common during transition include workload and time allotment (Fang et al., 2022)

SPECIAL NEEDS OF NOVICE NURSES

The following skills have been identified as needing further refinement in novice nurses. However, it is important to remember that a novice nurse's "need for support" does not end with orientation.

- Collaboration and communication skills (Leonard et al., 2022)
- Critical thinking, clinical skills/judgment/problem solving (Leonard et al., 2022)
- Organizational skills (Kelly (2023)
- Delegation skills (Huber, 2017; Zerwekh & Garneau, 2018)
- Priority-setting skills (Kelly, 2023)
- Assertiveness skills (Mayo Clinic Staff, 2020)
- Dealing with horizontal violence (Germann & Moore, 2017)
- Intuition, connecting the dots, or knowing something needs to be done (Leonard et al., 2022))

According to a survey by Wolters Kluwer (2020), having clinical judgment skills is a primary gap in practice readiness. Only 20% of new nurses feel strong in their general nursing knowledge, with lack of confidence being evident. Discussion of each of these areas follows.

Interpersonal Skills

Most physicians, administrators, and nurse managers expect the novice nurse to immediately develop interpersonal skills that they take for granted. These feelings probably are rooted in the past, when nurses in training spent most of their time on units caring for patients and received little theoretic information or content in the classroom setting. They had time to get to know the members of the health care team and felt comfortable interacting with them. It is difficult for many people, including novice nurses, to be comfortable with interpersonal skills at work when they feel incompetent and inadequate as members of the interprofessional health care team. They are often uncomfortable making rounds, clarifying orders, and participating in interprofessional team conferences. However, effective communication is critical. Development of communication and interpersonal skills is a key success factor for new nurses (Leonard, 2022). These skills are especially important for nurses, who must be able to communicate with other members of the health care team, patients, and coworkers in a fast-paced environment (Kelly, 2023). For example, consider the following scenario:

A novice nurse receives the this order from the patient's physician: "Give Tylenol as needed for pain."

The unit secretary transcribes the order and hands the chart to the new nurse, stating, "You will need to clarify this order: I can't take the new order."

Feelings of fear and uncertainty invade the novice nurse as they practice what to say to the physician. This fear and sense of insecurity can make the novice nurse avoid future contact with the physician, thus compromising patient safety. The nurse must find some way to communicate and may consider the following suggestions: "Can you clarify the Tylenol order on your patient?" or, possibly, "How much Tylenol did you want your patient to have?" or maybe even "Hey stupid, can't you write your orders using the six 'rights'?"

Perhaps the nervous nurse speaks as follows: "Dr. Jones, this is the student nurse. I mean the nurse taking care of your patient. I don't understand your order. I mean can you clarify how much Tylenol you want me to take? I mean how much Tylenol do you want the patient to have?" Then the inexperienced nurse hangs up, feeling ineffective, and the physician questions the nursing care the patient is being given.

Before asking a physician to clarify an order, it is a good idea for the novice nurse to practice what to say and even write it down so as not to forget. Then, when face to face with the person, they can state the facts simply and allow the physician time to consider the correct answer. A smile during the exchange in conversation might provide the receiver with a little more patience.

Gaps in communication may also occur between the novice nurse and the experienced staff because staff are so familiar with the routines that they may leave out information, unintentionally making the novice nurse unable to complete the task.

Novice nurses need to develop interpersonal communication skills by building self-confidence (Forbes & Evans (2022). Kelly (2023) suggests making sure you have investigated the situation before contacting the provider to prevent a negative interaction and use the SBAR format.

Nursing communications skills can be improved by practicing active listening, being aware of nonverbal cues, being sure to offer an open front, and communicating clearly. The ability to accurately pass information between the medical team is vital and the responsibility often falls on the nurse (University of St. Augustine for Health Sciences, 2023).

Clinical Skills

Novice nurses report being caught unaware of the complexity of problem-solving in the clinical environment or "thinking like a nurse." Students are taught skills in terms of objective attributes without situational experience. As an example, the instructor asks the student to listen to heart sounds; as a student you simply follow the pattern of assessment (Zerwekh & Garneau, 2023). Practice increases the effectiveness, efficiency, and correctness of performing skills. However, until the novice nurse has actual experience, there are actions they can take. For example, it is wise to be familiar with the procedure manual on the unit. Also, during the orientation phase the novice nurse should ask for a mentor to observe or assist with procedures for which they have a lower comfort level or a lesser degree of experience, to role-model excellent communication skills, and to answer the mentee's questions. It is important to remember that "practice does make perfect," or at least competency. Every new nurse needs a mentor for support and professional relationships (Zerwekh & Garneau, 2023). Clinical practice in the final semesters of nursing programs also supports the transition shock in which students reported a difference in what was learned in the classroom to actually applying nursing care in the clinical setting, fear of moving from student to nurse, low self-esteem and disenchantment with their how their contributions were not valued, and a struggle with coping in the real practice environment (Yeong-Ju & Soo-Yeon, 2022).

Remember, no one was born with a Foley catheter in one hand and the set of directions engraved in memory.

Organizational Skills

The novice nurse may lack organizational skills. This lack of proficiency may be exaggerated by feelings of being "overwhelmed" by the new environment. Typically, student nurses are responsible for a limited number of patients, and although they must answer for their care the nurses typically are not responsible for as many patients as they will be assigned as new nurses. Someone is usually with students to offer suggestions on how to organize their time. The instructor might question, "Now, what do you plan to do, and what supplies will you need to accomplish the task?" New nurses might consider asking these same questions of themselves. If unsure, the procedure book lists not only the steps to follow but also the supplies that will be needed. List specific time-limited tasks. Avoid scheduling time so tightly that a slight delay causes chaos. Prioritization skills are seen as areas of concern of newly graduated nurses, most likely due to deficits in clinical reasoning. According to the National Council of State Boards of Nursing (2019), nurses should begin practice with the ability to make correct clinical decisions through clinical judgment (NCSBN, 2019). Making lists helps the new nurse, who is predictably task-oriented, to not forget tasks (Kelly, 2023). Chapter 26 offers valuable tips on getting organized, setting priorities, and managing time.

Delegation Skills

Most students have limited exposure to delegation. Uncertainty about or feeling uncomfortable with delegation may be a result of the characteristics of the personnel to whom one is delegating. Consider the licensed practical nurse (LPN), the nursing assistant, and other unlicensed staff. Often these personnel are older and more experienced; therefore the new nurse might feel intimidated when delegating to them. Novice nurses should familiarize themselves with policies concerning which tasks can be performed by which category or level of health care provider. The question "Who can perform this task other than me?" should be considered. Teamwork not only can increase job satisfaction but it has also been found to improve patient outcomes. As you learn to delegate within the team you learn collaboration skills and trust and deliver safe care (American Nurses Association, n.d.). Delegation relies on trust and leadership skills, both of which may be deficient in the novice nurse. Chapter 20 presents a comprehensive overview of delegation.

There are also times when the novice nurse should decline to accept a delegated responsibility because they may not be competent to perform the task even though it is within their scope of practice. Remember that patient safety is always the priority. Show your willingness to learn, and ask someone to demonstrate the task by stating simply, "I would appreciate you demonstrating the procedure and allowing me to observe, and when the next opportunity arises I would like for you to observe me completing the procedure."

Priority-Setting Skills

Priority setting is a skill that all nursing students must demonstrate. The difference between nursing school and the workplace is that serious consequences occur if prioritizing is not done effectively in the workplace. Joswick (2021) suggests adopting the "Do First Things First" philosophy to maintain safety and perform those activities essential to the plan of care.

- Life-threatening or possibly life-threatening conditions
- Activities essential to safety
- Comfort, healing, and teaching

Many novice nurses need help in organizational skills. Novice nurses may derive more satisfaction from performing technical skills, such as starting an IV drip, than from cognitive skills, such as developing a plan of care. Once they are comfortable with basic skills they move on to critical thinking skills. How many people make to-do lists? Many make grocery lists, lists of bills to be paid, or lists of important dates. The same should be done for work—tasks are crossed off as they are completed. At the end of the day consider what time was spent in unproductive ways, what caused interruptions, and what could have been done to save time. The same list may cue the novice nurse to a "forgotten" task or intervention. Kelly (2021) also suggests determining the importance and urgency of the problem.

Assertiveness Skills

When novice nurses are placed in a situation that could possibly jeopardize patient safety and cause distress, it is critical they use assertiveness skills to negotiate the expected orientation time allowing them to effectively care for their patients. Assertive communication allows the novice nurse to say "no" in a respectful way without feeling guilty. Assertive communication shows respect for the other person while acting in ways that boost self-respect. Demonstrating appropriate assertive communication skills can have benefits for one's physical and emotional well-being while preserving relationships. Assertive communication can boost self-esteem and earn respect from others (Zerwekh & Garneau, 2023). Students are often naive when they are told by recruiters,

"Come work for us; we offer a 6-month orientation, and you can ask for an extension if you feel uncomfortable. You will not be placed in charge, and only after a full year's experience will you be allowed to independently care for patients requiring advanced technology, such as ventricular assist devices." Students may be misled into feeling that they are "advanced" in their learning and moving ahead of all the others if they agree to shorten their orientation or if, after only 6 months, they take on the responsibility of caring for patients with special equipment. Assertive communication can help when one tends to have a hard time saying "no."

However, after 6 months, even though novice nurses are becoming more competent and confident, they lack the experience to make instantaneous decisions based on intuition. Unfortunately, novice nurses are often employed on the night shift working with nurses with the same or less experience. As newer novice nurses (those who graduated the following previous semester) are hired, the more experienced novice nurses may even be expected to serve as preceptors. Nursing faculty should invite recent graduates to speak to classes concerning expectations after employment. Faculty should also inform students that they will move through many stages during the next year, and that they should take full advantage of this learning opportunity.

VIOLENCE AT WORK

When one recalls the 1872 children's mantra, "Sticks and stones may break my bones but words will never harm me" by Stephen Fry, we realize lateral violence is not a new occurrence. This mantra is a misnomer—it is well known that the pain inflicted by criticism and insults may last longer than physical pain because we feel emotional pain. It is important to remember that violence is not part of the job (American Nurses Association, n.d.).

When you think of dangerous occupations, law enforcement and military careers may come to mind. However, nursing is one of the most dangerous professions in America. Nursing can actually be more dangerous than a career in law enforcement. According to the American Nurses Association (n.d.), violence is higher in health care workers than in prison guards or police officers. Nurses are three times more likely than other workers to suffer aggression at work. According to the Press Ganey data, more than 5200 nurses were assaulted in the second quarter of 2022 with an average of two nurses assaulted every hour, equating to 57 assaults daily (American Nurses Association (n.d.). According to the National Safety Council (2023), in 2020 there were more than 20,050 injuries and 392 deaths due to workplace violence. Nurses have been victims of workplace violence each year (OSHA, n.d.), but there are most likely many more because most events go unreported. Workplace violence against nurses has increased, especially after the COVID-19 pandemic. The National Nurses United found that 22% of nurses reported an increase in workplace violence, which was credited to staffing deficiencies, visitor constraints, and a change in patient population. Although workplace violence is underreported, social media and policies against violence have exposed the issue. The Workplace Violence Protection for Health Care and Social Service Workers Act (2021) now requires the Department of Labor to mandate violence prevention in both areas. The American Nurses Association (ANA, n.d.) developed a zero-tolerance policy on workplace violence. Some states have increased penalties for assault on nurses (Gooch, 2023 & Benyon, 2019). Student nurses are also leading recipients of violence during their clinical experiences (Hallett et al., 2023), a situation that perpetuates the cycle of lateral violence that continues in nursing. The ANA's goal to stop workplace violence supports many resources for nurses, including contacting your legislator to end nurse abuse and pledging to report all abuses encountered. Box 25.3 shows four types of workplace violence identified by the Centers for Disease Control and Prevention (2020).

Sanner-Stiehr and Ward-Smith (2017) describe horizontal violence and bullying as being prevalent in the nursing profession, especially in newly qualified nurses (Kiprillis et al., 2022). Horizontal violence includes such acts against coworkers as withholding patient information, exclusion, belittling, refusing to assist, badgering, displaying errors for others to observe, eye-rolling, and scapegoating. These researchers suggest that horizontal violence leads to increased stress and job dissatisfaction, which can result in missed work days. In 1996 The Joint Commission (TJC) issued a sentinel event alert in response to a growing number of crimes in health care settings (22). TJC's Sentinel Event Alert 45, revised Alert 59 in 2021, found violence against health care workers to occur in all settings, with the emergency department and inpatient psychiatric setting having the most incidents, with identified nursing floors to be the hardest to secure (The Joint Commission, 2021). The Sentinel Event Database contains reports of permanent harm death, and temporary harm requiring intervention to sustain life and homicide (which are suspected to be much higher due to underreporting). According to the OSHA (n.d.), a well-written and implemented prevention plan to reduce workplace violence is recommended. A secure, improved Injury Tracking Application allows employers to submit their workplace injury information. Lateral violence has been described as an epidemic and must be confronted as if it were an infectious disease because it threatens the health of nurses. Bullying or horizontal violence creates a toxic environment; the high-pressure work environment accompanied by no time to rest and inadequate salaries are believed to be instigators (Detwiler & Vaughn, 2020). The ANA (2015) states that "the nursing profession will no longer tolerate violence of any kind

BOX 25.3 **Types of Workplace Violence**	
Type 1. Violence by a stranger with criminal intent	These violent acts are not committed by employees; rather criminals are strangers without relationship to organization or employees. Robbery most common motive.
Type 2. Violence by a customer or client	Patients or customers become perpetrators of violent acts.
Type 3. Violence by a coworker (worker to worker)	Employee or prior or disgruntled employees threaten or commit violence against current employees and/or management. This is referred to as vertical or horizontal violence.
Type 4. Violence by someone in a personal relationship	Individuals who have a relationship with a current employee commit a violent act in the health care environment.

From Wild Iris Medical Education. (2023). *Workplace violence and safety.* https://wildirismedicaleducation.com/courses/workplace-violence

from any source." You can text PLEDGE to 52886 to #EndNurseAbuse (ANA, n.d.).

The Center for American Nurses (2016) offers a "tip card" on workplace bullying with eight tips before you quit and five behaviors that show respect. The Centers for Disease Control (2022) offers a free course on Workplace Violence Prevention for Nurses, including postevent response.

INTUITION

A nurse walks into a patient's room and senses something is wrong, and even though the data show nothing has changed, the patient confirms feeling anxious. The nurse stops to use all her senses to observe and assess the situation. She is using intuition. Wilding (2022) describes intuition as "that gut feeling." Intuition is not guessing but a nonconscious pattern of recognition and experience based on experience (Nurse Beth, 2021). Benner (1984) described intuition as the function of an expert nurse—implying that intuition develops over time as nurses move from novice to expert. Nursing intuition should be used in combination with knowledge and skills but nurses may have an underlying sense that allows them to suspect changes are occurring in the patient (White, 2022)

STRATEGIES TO EASE TRANSITION

When interviewing for their first positions, novice nurses should determine the philosophies of the agencies and how the various orientation programs assist new nurses to enter the profession. There are many opinions on the best way to accomplish a smooth transition, and each nurse should evaluate the orientation options available. Chapter 27 provides tips for job interviews and ways to learn more about prospective unit culture. Take the time to ask specific questions about retention, length of residency program, assignment of mentor, and patient ratios.

The NCSBN developed an evidence-based model for transitioning novice nurses to practice. The care of patients with complex health needs and a gap in practice readiness were the stimulus for the Transition to Practice Model the NCSBN developed. This model prescribed that a graduate will have the same preceptor for 6 months. In some settings, a team of preceptors is used for ongoing support for an additional 6 months. The

QSEN competencies constitute the five modules used in this model: patient-centered care, teamwork and collaboration, evidence-based practice, quality improvement, safety, and informatics. Feedback and reflection are elicited from the novice nurses throughout the 6-month period.

Biculturalism

Biculturalism is the joining of two contradictory value systems—in this context, those of school values with those of the workplace. Biculturalism is designed to enhance a positive self-image and help novice nurses set realistic goals for practice. This strategy, if accepted in the workplace, allows the new nurse to introduce ideas or values brought from nursing school and integrate them into the work environment. Kramer (1974) recommends that the novice nurse appraise both sides of an issue, determine how their behavior will affect other members of the interprofessional health care team, and single out accessible objectives. Have you ever heard, "We have always done it this way and it works"? Duchscher (2012) acknowledges that tradition is not easily changed but suggests that you "catch more flies with honey than vinegar" (p. 45). Ask yourself, "What is the process for change?" and remember that the solution is not just yours but ours.

Mentors and Preceptors

Mentoring and precepting are often considered to be the same but in fact they are different. Mentoring is a personal relationship with a more experienced person willing to guide a novice or inexperienced person. It is voluntary, ongoing over time, and contributes to lifelong learning (American Nurses Association Massachusetts, n.d.). The socialization achieved through a mentoring relationship can provide the support needed while feeling most vulnerable.

Mentors can help the new nurse experience a sense of safety and improve coping skills. The first year of nursing is "tough" but having a mentor to ask questions and talk to about concerns related to the new role can positively affect the new nurse's overall career trajectory. Mentoring has been shown to be a key strategy for increasing the diversity of the nursing workforce when novice faculty are mentored by culturally competent faculty, thus retaining more diverse students. In comparison, preceptors is a much more defined role for a shorter time. The preceptor guides and supervises the new nurse while evaluating progress (American Nurses Association Massachusetts, n.d.). Foster-Smith (2023) remark that choosing the correct mentor is one of the most important tasks for the novice nurse.

Mentors are experienced nurses who must be willing to commit to a relationship with novice nurses to help them recognize their weaknesses and strengths. Mentors help novice nurses set and reach realistic goals by reinforcing and recommending appropriate courses of action and providing emotional support. Mentors help novice nurses to develop confidence and learn the work culture (Box 25.4).

Some mentoring programs are aimed specifically at male students. Just as women face special challenges when entering a predominantly male profession, so do men entering the predominantly female profession of nursing. Mentors can reduce anxiety and loneliness felt by male students (Eagerton et al., 2019).

Preceptorships

Another popular orientation program is the use of preceptors during the nursing student's final semester of nursing school through their entering the workforce. Preceptor programs have gained popularity as a means to socialize the novice nurse into the profession and to ease the tension of transition from student to nurse.

BOX 25.4	Characteristics of Mentor and Protégé
Mentor	**Protégé**
Empathic and nonjudgmental	Intelligent
Has advanced personal, social, and professional skills	Self-starter
	Curious
Ethical and has moral integrity	Hard worker
Welcomes change	Risk taker
Excellent at communication (both listening and feedback)	Has a sense of humor
	Open to new ideas
Has commitment to excellence in nursing practice	Has a vision both personally and professionally
Sensitive to others' needs	
Has a positive outlook	Embraces challenges
Uses situations to teach	
Is a living example of the values, ethics, and practices of the nursing profession	Possesses interpersonal and communication skills

Adapted from Smith-Trudeau, P. (2014). Will you be my nurse mentor? *Vermont Nurse Connection, 17,* 3.

Preceptor programs often are incorporated into the senior nursing student's final practicum, but they also may be used as part of the orientation program in the first work experience. Preceptors orient novice nurses to the specific nursing area, aid in socialization, and teach skills that are deemed necessary. Preceptor programs lower economic costs by reducing turnover of new graduates and helping novice nurses meet the expectations of their employers and peers. A nurse preceptor encourages independence and confidence by helping develop communication skills, improve organizational skills, improve psychomotor skills including learning the hospital policies and procedures, improve knowledge of medical conditions, develop leadership skills to work with the interdisciplinary team, strengthen critical thinking and make informed decisions, assist with patient education methods, model assertive communication, be a role model by following policies and being a team player, and participate in organized learning experiences such as seminars (Indeed, 2023).

Self-Mentoring

Ultimately no one is as responsible for the transition into the nursing profession as the novice nurses themselves. Mentors and preceptors can ease the transition but novice nurses can also help by using self-mentoring when preceptors or mentors are not available. Novice nurses must be willing to learn appropriate resources, develop problem-solving skills, and ask questions. Novices should reflect back over times when they were self-reliant and believed in themselves. Box 25.5 offers some coping skills that new nurses can use for the transition.

Residency Programs

Residency programs are one innovative way to ease the transition from academia to practice and may also be incentives for graduates selecting that first job. Residency programs often provide didactic or program activities as well as one-to-one preceptor experiences for an extended time, with 12 months being typical. Although residency programs differ, they all focus on retention and increased satisfaction of new nurses with the added bonus of improved patient outcomes and safety. Not all residency programs are the same. It is important for the new graduate to invest the time to research what a particular residency program has to offer. The Vizient/American Association of Colleges of Nursing (AACN) Nurse Residency Program is a 1-year

BOX 25.5   Coping Skills for New Nurses

1. Don't be shy—just introduce yourself to coworkers. Avoid being a wallflower.
2. Have a confidant or mentor—find a nurse or team member who is willing to guide you. Have a "go-to crew" (Wolters Kluwer, 2022).
3. Ask questions—always ask and know where to find the policy and procedure manual.
4. Cheat—yes, you can now look up all those medications. You can also use a calculator the calculate IV fluid rates and verify medication dosages (American Nurse, 2023).
5. Self-care—sleep, eat, follow precautions. Ask your family and friends to support your schedule.
6. Nurse communication—SBAR and use a language your patients understand. Listen to your patient (American Nurse, 2023).
7. Poker face—you are privileged to information and strange things.
8. Don't take things personal—frustration may seem to be all around you but never tolerate bullying. Resolve conflicts (American Nurse, 2023).
9. Time management—adjust to your unit, ask for help, and remember time management is a skill you will learn (Kelly, 2021).
10. You did it—you graduated, enjoy your achievements and rewards. Enjoy your paychecks, cute scrubs, and vacation days.
11. Decision-making—use the nursing process to gather data, prioritize care, and react to dynamic changes confidently (American Nurse, 2023) and "connect the dots" to have a holistic approach (Wolters Kluwer, 2022).
12. Team work—provide shared support and be aware of how personal values affect interactions with coworkers (*American Nurse*, 2023). Be open to different points of view (Wolters Kluwer, 2022).

Data from (Hamstra 2021). *10 tips for new nurses to make you feel better at work.* https://nurse.org/articles/new-nurses-feel-better-at-work/. Wolters Kluwers (2022) include many of the same skills for nursing students.

residency with evidence-based curriculum requiring an academic partner. This program serves as the link for new nurses to transition to practice. Read about other new nurse's success while participating in the nurse residency program (Vizient, 2023).

Preprofessional and Professional Organizations

Students who join preprofessional organizations, such as the National Student Nurses Association (NSNA), gain leadership opportunities and meet not only other students from across the nation and internationally but also leaders in nursing they thought they would only read about. Students participating in the NSNA leadership university network learn how to run for office, problem solve, and disseminate ideas (NSNA, 2020). The NSNA Foundation provides scholarships and mentors future RNs into the profession. The NSNA publishes a magazine with information on job opportunities and legislative issues that affect nursing practice. Participation in preprofessional organizations develops leadership skills that are useful in professional organizations and for potential employers after graduation.

The ANA and some state specialty organizations offer reduced rates for new graduates and student nurses and continue with the previously mentioned benefits after graduation. In addition to lobbying efforts, benefits of involvement in the ANA include access to current information on standards of practice, certification, and networking opportunities.

Self-Confidence and Self-Esteem

Imposter syndrome is a feeling experienced by new nurses that they are not good enough in their new career or their success was not earned on their own (Pate, 2023). To address imposter syndrome don't compare yourself to others, seek a mentor, recognize your achievements, be patient with yourself, celebrate success, don't be a perfectionist, focus on your mental health—a therapist can help, share your feelings, accept positive feedback, and remember how much you have grown as a nurse (Pate, 2023). The Clance Impostor Phenomenon Scale can be used to identify the presence of the impostor phenomenon in new graduates. Take a moment and rate yourself to determine whether you are an impostor (http://paulineroseclance.com/pdf/IPTestandscoring.pdf). Imposter syndrome is not unusual for new graduates, even after completing a rigorous program of study and the licensure exam. A relationship woven with encouragement can inspire self-esteem and self-confidence. It is easy to become discouraged and disillusioned when reality does not quite match our dreams and fantasies. Self-esteem, or belief in oneself, comes as the novice nurse passes through the stages of reality shock and into a career in nursing:

Self-esteem = Self-confidence + Self-respect

Individuals with high self-esteem can problem-solve critically, tackle obstacles, take sensible risks, believe in themselves, and take care of themselves (Positive Way, 1996-2020). Nurses with good self-esteem are effective and respond to themselves and others in healthy ways. They can accomplish more because they feel comfortable with themselves. Take the self-esteem questionnaire in Box 25.6 or https://positive-way.net/self-esteem-questionnaire, then visit the Create Positive Relationships website. If your score is low visit the Positive Way website to learn how to stop your inner critic (http://positive-way.com/stopping%20your%20inner%20critic.htm) (Fig. 25.3).

So far we have discussed ways that the employer and novice nurse can use to ease the transition period—implementing biculturalism, preceptorships, mentoring, and self-mentoring. However, each new nurse must begin by evaluating their own self-esteem. In addition, the novice nurse must realize their uniqueness and rely on instinct and past experiences when maturing and

---

BOX 25.6   Self-Esteem Questionnaire

Answer yes or no to the following questions:
- _____ Do you have a hard time nurturing yourself?
- _____ Have you ever turned down an invitation to a party or function because of the way you felt about yourself?
- _____ Do you get your sense of self-worth from the approval of others?
- _____ Are you supportive of others who berate you?
- _____ When things go wrong in life do you blame yourself?
- _____ Do you react to disappointment by blaming others?
- _____ Do you begin each day with a negative attitude?
- _____ Do you feel undeserving?
- _____ Do you ever feel like an impostor and that soon your deficiencies will be exposed?
- _____ Do you have an inner critic who is disparaging or demeaning?
- _____ Do you believe that being hard on yourself is the best motivation for change?

- _____ Do your good points seem ordinary and your failings all-important?
- _____ Do you feel unattractive?
- _____ Have you ever felt that your accomplishments are due to luck but that your failures are due to incompetence or inadequacy?
- _____ Have you ever felt that if you are not a total success then you are a failure and that there is no middle ground and there are no points for effort?
- _____ Do you feel unappreciated?
- _____ Do you feel lonely?
- _____ Do you struggle with feelings of inferiority?
- _____ Do other people's opinions count more to you than your own?
- _____ Do you criticize yourself often?
- _____ Do others criticize you often?
- _____ Do you hesitate to do things because of what others might think?

The more yes answers you have, the greater the opportunity exists for improving your self-esteem.

From The Positive Way. (2020). *Self-esteem questionnaire*. https://positive-way.net/self-esteem-questionnaire/

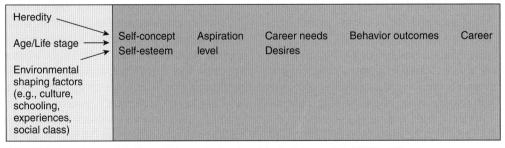

Fig. 25.3 Behavior model. (From Schutz, C., Decker, P.J., & Sullivan, E.J. [1992]. *Effective management in nursing: An-experiential/skill building workbook*. Addison-Wesley.)

moving to a higher level of responsibility. The new nurse should remember to seek a role model or mentor for guidance through the transition. It is important to remember that it is difficult to be successful if one's personal and social life are not kept in balance (e.g., in high school it was great to solve all the chemistry equations on an examination, but if "personal chemistry" was neglected a void was felt that could plague future attempts at maturing).

Violence Prevention

Because new graduates are frequent victims of horizontal violence in their first year of practice, preceptors with zero tolerance for such activities are invaluable. It is also suggested to have nurses remember when they were a new nurse. Unit culture is impacted by high levels of fatigue creating a "toxic environment." Lateral violence was reported as both the cause and effect of this emotional and mental fatigue negatively impacting patient care and personal/professional lives (Bloom, 2019; Wolf et al., 2017). Experienced RNs should consider the following to help ease the transition of the novice nurse to the profession of nursing: The novice nurse should not be expected to enter the work environment and be as productive as experienced staff members. It is important for experienced nurses serving on agency committees to serve as advocates for novice nurses by reminding nurse managers and administrators that it is not possible for nursing students to learn everything necessary for professional practice during school. Also remind other members of the nursing unit about this fact. If a novice nurse develops an initiative, autonomy, and a desire to become a team member they will succeed. Newly graduated nurses are at high risk for lateral violence. Strategies that educators can use to prepare students prior to graduation to handle such situations include: identify and discuss occurrences of lateral violence when in clinical rotations; allow students to rehearse strategies when confronted with lateral violence; role-model professionalism; and develop a Code of Conduct that is consistently enforced (Chisholm, 2019; Sanner-Stiehr & Ward-Smith, 2017). Novice nurses entering the workforce will find the OSHA book *Guidelines for Preventing Workplace Violence for Health Care and Social Service Workers* (n.d.) helpful (https://www.osha.gov/Publications/osha3148.pdf). Novice nurses can also access the ANA website for continuing education resources on conflict competence for help with conflict management and should review the ANA position statement for recommended strategies to help eliminate lateral violence.

KEYS TO SURVIVAL DURING TRANSITION

Morris (2023) shared that learning how to manage stress as a nursing student or nurse can protect both your physical and mental health (Box 25.7). Haskins (2020) shared six tips for new nurses to avoid anxiety. Remember you are not alone; the feelings of being anxious and overwhelmed are normal and the sense of "being on your own" occur when you transition from nursing school to a new nurse. Haskins suggests taking advantage of your orientation time and preceptor to become more confident. She offers these tips to reduce anxiety: rest at least 6 to 8 hours so your mind and body can reset; plan your day in advance, giving you a sense of what is coming; ask to keep the same assignment when possible to improve your familiarity; talk to your mentor, preceptor, or colleague before a situation becomes unbearable; take a deep breath and learn how to regulate your breathing to control your heart rate and be calm; and lastly take care of yourself—stretch, meditate, and perhaps have a spa day. Haskins also recommends you understand your triggers that cause anxiety. Journaling to include the best case scenario to be optimistic can help.

Be dedicated and demonstrate enthusiasm for your career. Passion for nursing allows you to make informed decisions and grow as a professional (American Nurse, 2021). When you are wondering if nurses are even

---

BOX 25.7 Nurse's Transition Strategy

Be a team player

Take the initiative to help a coworker. Be an advocate. A nurse's voice can advocate for a patient when they can't speak for themselves. Be prepared for the unexpected. Stay mentally prepared so you can adapt to the unexpected event. Make sure your off-work hours are fulfilling.

Try new activities where you can use your training as a nurse but in a new environment—volunteer in medical missions or disasters to get a new perspective. Console your coworkers when they need it. Offering emotional support can build camaraderie on the nursing unit.

From Salinas, A. (2018). *My first year as a nurse was a roller coaster ride*. https://www.nurse.com/blog/2018/05/21/my-first-year-as-a-real-nurse-was-a-rollercoaster-ride/ My first year as a nurse was a rollercoaster ride | Nurse.com

appreciated listen to the song by Brown & Gray "You Didn't Have To."

Morris (2023) list ways to manage stress as a nurse to protect yourself. From Morris, 2023, "How to Manage Stress as a Nurse":

1. Eat healthy to support your mental and physical health
2. Keep a routine; it really does decrease anxiety
3. Exercise regularly to improve mood and sleep quality while reducing stress
4. Get better sleep by not watching television and using room-darkening shades or a mask
5. Enjoy nature—just 20 minutes outside can lower your stress hormones
6. Have a social support system and check in with friends and family; being around loved ones releases oxytocin, which helps you relax
7. Set healthy boundaries; "say no" to overtime if you are exhausted
8. Practice mindfulness, which can include yoga, meditation, and body recognition
9. Visit a therapist to identify stressors and learn how to lower your stress level
10. Pet your dog or volunteer at a shelter
11. Journal to release emotional stress
12. Practice deep breathing, which lowers your heart rate and blood pressure while reducing stress
13. Laugh—watch a funny movie, listen to a podcast; laughter improves your immune system
14. Take part in self-care to improve health

Williams (2021) suggests taking time to consider these important issues before accepting your first nursing job: know the nursing job market, talk with past professors, network with nurses you know from your clinical experiences, and visit some online chat rooms with other new nursing graduates.

MEETING SPECIAL NEEDS OF THE NOVICE NURSE

It is important to review some common problems perceived by novice nurses and to offer suggestions to ease the transition period.

Organizational Skills

Lack of organization is common when the novice nurse's assignment becomes much heavier than that of a student nurse. The use of a report sheet can enable the novice nurse to note important information received during the shift report and from other members of the interprofessional health care team as the day progresses. The report sheet can also be used to document occurrences during the shift. Another suggestion for the novice nurse is to contact a former nursing instructor. Most students have developed a special rapport with one or two instructors. Novice nurses might telephone one of their former instructors to discuss the challenges they face during transition so that the instructor can help with problem-solving. Real-time charting to prevent mistakes not only saves time but can help the novice nurse realize when an assessment was skipped, allowing them to complete on time (Kelly, 2021). Kelly (2021) and Morris (2022) suggests a checklist to mitigate stress and provide structure to the day. The checklist constitutes the following questions:

- Why is the patient admitted?
- How do vital signs trend?
- Does the patient have an IV; if so, where?
- What are the patient's active orders for activity, diet, and even code status?

The basic report sheet (Box 25.8) also can be transformed into a unit-specific sheet. For instance, if the novice nurse is on a telemetry floor, there might be a section for "rhythms." The orthopedic nurse could include "traction." This form also can be used to establish and set priorities. Once the care has been prioritized, the nurse can begin these critical interventions. However, it also may be possible to delegate tasks to ancillary staff if the tasks are within their scope of practice. This possibility requires the novice nurse to become familiar with the job descriptions of other nursing personnel, such as licensed professional nurses, nursing assistants, and unlicensed personnel, so delegation will be within their defined roles. Remember that the RN cannot do everything. Kelly (2021) offers free patient care organization sheets for the bedside nurse.

Supply Pockets

Your nursing pockets can be your best friend. They prevent having to revisit the supply room, saving time, and allowing you to feel better prepared to care for the patient. Just think, you have the tourniquet on the patient's arm to start an IV when you realize you forgot the flush and transparent cover. Kelly suggests having the following in your pockets: saline flushes, gauze, alcohol wipes, nursing shears, medical tape, penlight, and your stethoscope (2021).

BOX 25.8 Basic Report Sheet for New Nurses

Patient's Name _____
Room # _____
Diagnosis _____
Diet _____
Activity status _____
Lab ordered/time _____
IV fluids _____

Intake/Output _____
Urine _____ Stools _____
Other _____
IV primary _____
IV secondary _____
Other _____

Patient's Name _____
Room # _____
Diagnosis _____
Diet _____
Activity status _____
Lab ordered/time _____
IV fluids _____

Intake/Output _____
Urine _____ Stools _____
Other _____
IV primary _____
IV secondary _____
Other _____

Patient's Name _____
Room # _____
Diagnosis _____
Diet _____
Activity status _____
Lab ordered/time _____
IV fluids _____

Intake/Output _____
Urine _____ Stools _____
Other _____
IV primary _____
IV secondary _____
Other _____

Patient's Name _____
Room # _____
Diagnosis _____
Diet _____
Activity status _____
Lab ordered/time _____
IV fluids _____

Intake/Output _____
Urine _____ Stools _____
Other _____
IV primary _____
IV secondary _____
Other _____

Clinical Skills

According to Benner's model (1984), the graduate nurse must be allowed to develop clinical skills on the basis of experiences. The novice nurse can develop competence with clinical skills during the orientation phase by asking to observe an experienced nurse perform those skills with which the novice nurse is less familiar. The novice nurse also can provide the nurse manager and mentor with a list of their skills that need further practice. The unit's policy and procedure book is a valuable asset. It should describe in detail the steps to follow for performing a particular procedure. Spend time reviewing the manual before observing the procedure being performed, and then ask questions. Take into consideration that there is more than one correct way to perform a skill; remember, though, that it is not acceptable to take shortcuts that jeopardize the safety of the patient.

Interpersonal Skills

Developing interpersonal skills may be achieved by attending unit meetings, volunteering to serve on committees on the unit or within the agency, and taking an active interest in the nursing unit. These activities aid in the new nurse's socialization into the unit and profession. It is important for all nurses, regardless of their experience, to take part in professional organizations at the local, regional, state, or national level. Specialty organizations often provide valuable information and continuing education pertinent to the nurse's area of practice.

As the nurse becomes more confident in their nursing abilities and is less stressed by performing tasks, they can develop positive relationships with physicians and other members of the interprofessional team. Various methods that may be used to develop professional relationships should be emphasized during the orientation period.

Nurses in staff development positions can be key players in assisting the novice nurse to develop professional communication skills. Making rounds with physicians and helping them with procedures open the door for communication. Asking pertinent and relevant questions ensures that the door remains open.

Delegation Skills

Another important skill that novice nurses need to learn is delegating. First, nurses should consider how others have delegated to them. Body language is important when delegating. Look at the person, be pleasant, and leave room for suggestions from the delegatee; however, do not allow the delegatee to resist or intimidate you so that you end up completing the task yourself. After communicating face to face, give a list of tasks in writing, or post it at the nurses' station; this leaves little room for misunderstanding. Be willing to change the assignment if there are changes in a patient's condition, new patients are admitted, or you realize that the time needed to perform a task was underestimated. If time allows, it is always good to help those to whom you have delegated tasks. For example, if a nurse passes by a door and the attendant is trying to turn a very large patient, the nurse should enter the room and ask, "How can I best help you turn the patient?" Always take time to give sincere positive reinforcement and say "Thank you."

Priority-Setting Skills

Now consider the best way to prioritize. How did you prioritize in nursing school? What worked then will probably work now with a few modifications. Remember: If it is not written down, it will probably be forgotten. Keep a notepad and pen in your pocket. Jot down reminders of things to be done, and place a number next to each indicating its importance. For example, assume that you have already written the following list:

- _____ Start the IV for Mr. B. in room 211
- _____ Check the IV site for Mrs. C. in room 300
- _____ Check the blood sugar for Mrs. M. in room 215

Now you receive a call from the LPN that Mr. T.'s IV line is not dripping in room 212. Next the dietary worker calls to say that when she took the food tray to the patient in room 217, the patient vomited. Then the emergency light goes off in the bathroom of an older, confused patient. Now prioritize. What needs to be done first? First, answer the emergency light; do not even take time to write this one down. Now it is time to reprioritize. The new tasks have been added to the bottom of your previous list. Look over your new list (below). How would you prioritize these tasks?

- _____ Start the IV for Mr. B. in room 211
- _____ Check the IV site for Mrs. C. in room 300
- _____ Check the blood sugar for Mrs. M. in room 215
- _____ Check Mr. T.'s IV line that is not dripping
- _____ Assist the patient in room 217 who is vomiting

Now try out your delegating skills. Place a D next to any tasks that can be delegated in the list below.

- _____ Start the IV for Mr. B. in room 211
- _____ Check the IV site for Mrs. C. in room 300
- _____ Check the blood sugar for Mrs. M. in room 215
- _____ Check Mr. T.'s IV in room 212 that is not dripping
- _____ Assist the patient in room 217 who is vomiting

What had to be considered when you prioritized the tasks? First you needed to consider how much time was required for each task. It usually takes longer to start a new IV line than to check an existing IV site. It also requires less time to determine why an IV is not dripping. However, this fact is insignificant if the patient for whom the IV line must be started is in critical condition and needs the medication to reduce their blood pressure. Delegation may be needed. What tasks can other members perform? The unit secretary can pull reports to check on lab results, and an LPN or nursing assistant can assist the patient who is vomiting, provided that you follow up very soon to assess the patient's condition. A nurse must know how to prioritize. Think through each situation. Change the priority as needed or as situations change throughout the shift.

Now that you know ways to develop organizational skills, refine clinical and interpersonal skills, delegate tasks, and set priorities, take time to remember other important areas of your life. Remember the people you may have neglected during school, and make it a priority to reestablish special relationships with friends, family, and loved ones.

SUMMARY

The period of transition from novice to competent practitioner is critical. New skills must be learned and refined, professional relationships established, and autonomy gained in nursing practice. Knowledge and skills must be refined over time. The transition from student to RN can be compared with that of butterflies as they emerge from their cocoons. It is unfair to judge them while still nymphs; therefore the nursing profession must withhold scrutiny until novice nurses fly with their beautiful wings spread.

REFERENCES

(Note: The American Nurses Association [n.d.] is in the order in which it appears in text)

American Association of Post-Acute Care Nursing (AAPACN). (2020). *Overcoming burnout and compassion fatigue with self-care.* https://www.aapacn.org/blog/overcoming-burnout-and-compassion-fatigue-with-self-care/

American Nurse. (2023). *Nursing Skills Checklist.* https://www.myamericannurse.com/essential-nursing-skills-checklist/

American Nurses Association. (n.d.). *Nurse Staffing Task Force.* https://www.nursingworld.org/~49df79/contentassets/568122c62ddc44bea03b11a71f240a50/nurse-staffing-task-force—-executive-summary-table-1.pdf

American Nurses Association. (n.d.). *Workplace violence.* https://nursesvote.org/issue/workplace-violence/

American Nurses Association. (n.d.). *Workplace violence/#EndNurseAbuse.* https://www.nursingworld.org/practice-policy/work-environment/end-nurse-abuse/

American Nurses Association. (2015). *Incivility, bullying, and workplace violence.* https://www.nursingworld.org/~49d6e3/globalassets/practiceandpolicy/nursing-excellence/incivility-bullying-and-workplace-violence—ana-position-statement.pdf

American Nurses Association. (n.d.). *Text Pledge to 52886 support report share.* https://www.myamericannurse.com/take-pledge-end-nurse-abuse/

American Nurses Association Massachusetts. (n.d.). *Mentoring definitions.* https://www.anamass.org/page/61

American Association of Colleges of Nursing. (n.d.). *Nurse residency program.* https://www.aacnnursing.org/our-initiatives/education-practice/nurse-residency-program

Angelis, N. (2023). *Bullying: Real-life strategies to reduce the frequency and impact of bullying in healthcare.* https://ceufast.com/course/bullying-real-life-strategies-to-reduce-the-frequency-and-impact-of-bullying-in-healthcarenew-graduate-professional-socialization/

Babapour, A.R., Gahassab-Mozaffari, N., & Fathnezhad-Kazemi, A. (2022). Nurses' job stress and its impact on quality of life and caring behaviors: A cross-sectional study. *BMC Nursing, 21,*75. https://doi.org/10.1186/s12912-022-00852-y

Benner, P. (1984). *From novice to expert: Addison-Wesley.*

Benyon, B. (2019). *Violence against nurses: A major issue in healthcare.* https://www.oncnursingnews.com/view/violence-against-nurses-a-major-issue-in-healthcare

Bloom, E.M. (2019). Horizontal violence among nurses: Experiences, responses, and job performance. *Nursing Forum, 54,* 77–83. https://doi.org/10.1002/nuf.12300

Casey K., Oja K.J., & Makic, M.B.F. (2021). The lived experiences of graduate nurses transitioning to professional practice during a pandemic. *Nursing Outlook, 69*(6): 1072–1080. doi: 10.1016/j.outlook.2021.06.006. Epub 2021 J

Centers for Disease Control and Prevention. (2020). *Types of workplace violence.* https://wwwn.cdc.gov/WPVHC/Nurses/Course/Slide/Unit1_5

Centers for Disease Control and Prevention. (2022). *Workplace violence prevention for nurses.* https://www.cdc.gov/niosh/topics/violence/training_nurses.html

Chisholm, J. (2019). Addressing workplace incivility: Facilitating nursing students' transition to the health-care setting. *Creative Nursing, 25*(4), 311–315. https://doi:10.1891/1078-4535.25.4.311

Detwiler, K., & Vaughn, N. (2020). *What is lateral violence in nursing.* Relias. https://www.relias.com/blog/what-is-lateral-violence-in-nursing

Duchscher, J.E. (2009). Transition shock: The initial stage of role adaptation for newly graduated registered nurses. *Journal of Advanced Nursing, 65*(5), 1103–1113. https://doi.org/10.1111/j.1365-2648.2008.04898.x.

Duchscher, J.E.B. (2012). *From surviving to thriving: Navigating the first year of professional nursing practice.* Saskatoon Fastprint.

Duchscher, J., & Windey, M. (2018). Stages of Transition and Transition Shock. *Journal for Nurses in Professional Development, 34,* 228–232. 10.1097/NND.0000000000000461

Eagerton, G. et al. (2019). *Men in nursing: Building diversity in healthcare.* https://www.nbna.org/files/NBNA%20FALL%202019%20REVJAN07.pdf

Fang, Y., Yang, J., Zhang, M., Song, J., & Lin, R.A . (2022). Longitudinal study of stress in new nurses in their first year of employment. *Int J Clin Pract, 21,*2022,6932850. doi: 10.1155/2022/6932850. PMID: 36567777; PMCID: PMC9705110

Forbes, T.H. 3rd, & Evans, S. (2022). From anticipation to confidence: A descriptive qualitative study of new graduate nurse communication with physicians. *Journal of Nursing Management, 30*(6),2039–2045. doi: 10.1111/jonm.13656. Epub 2022 May 19. PMID: 35506538; PMCID: PMC9790247

Foster-Smith, R. (2023). Choosing the right mentor. *Nursing Management,* 54(9), 56, September 2023. DOI: 10.1097/ nmg.0000000000000047

Germann, S., & Moore, S. (2017). Lateral violence, a nursing epidemic? *Reflections on Nursing Leadership, 43*(1), 39–43.

Glynn, C. (2022). *Nurses eat their young.* https://nursingcen-tral.com/lateral-violence-in-nursing.

Gooch, K. (2023). *The states increasing penalties for violence against hospital workers.* https://www.beckershospitalre-view.com/workforce/the-states-increasing-penalties-for-violence-against-hospital-workers.html

Hallett, N., Gayton, A., Dickenson, R., Franckel, M., & Dickens, G.L. (2023). Student nurses' experiences of workplace violence: A mixed methods systematic review and meta-analysis. *Nurse Education Today, 128,* 105845. https://doi.org/10.1016/j.nedt.2023.105845

Hamstra, B. (2021). *10 tips for new nurses to make you feel better at work.* https://nurse.org/articles/new-nurses-feel-better-at-work/

Haskins, A. (2020). *6 tips for new nurse who feel anxiety.* https://nurse.org/articles/new-nurse-anxiety

Huber, D. (2017). *Leadership and nursing care management* (6th ed). Saunders.

Indeed. (2022). *Functional nursing: Definition, advantages, and disadvantages.* https://www.indeed.com/career-advice/career-development/functional-nursing

Indeed. (2023). *What is a nurse preceptor? (And how to become one.).* https://ca.indeed.com/career-advice/finding-a-job/nurse-preceptor

Joswick, P.J. (2021). Time management and setting patient care priorities. In Kelly Vana's Nursing Leadership and Management (1st ed., p 490–510). John Wiley & Sons.

Kelly, L.A., Gee, P.M., & Butler, R.J. (2021). Impact of nurse burnout on organizational and position turnover. *Nursing Outlook, 69*(1), 96–102. doi:10.1016/j.outlook.2020.06.008.

Kelly, W. (2023). *How to stay organized as a new nurse.* https://healthandwillness.org/how-to-stay-organized-as-a-new-nurse/

Kiprillis, N., Gray, R., Robinson, E., & McKenna, L. (2022). Prevalence of horizontal violence of nurses in their first year of practice: A systematic review. *Collegian 29*(2), 236–244.

Kleber, K. (2022). *For the overwhelmed new graduate nurse.* https://www.freshrn.com/for-the-overwhelmed-new-graduate-nurse/

Kramer, M. (1974). *Reality shock: Why nurses leave nursing.* Mosby.

Laskowski-Jones, L., & Castner, J. (2022). The great resigna-tion, newly licensed nurse transition shock and emergency nursing. *Journal of Emergency Nursing 48*(3), 236–242. https://doi.org/10.1016/j.jen.2022.03.010

Leonard, J.C., Whiteman, K., Stephens, K., Henry, C., & Swanson-Biearman, B. (May 31, 2022) "Improving com-munication and collaboration skills in graduate nurses: An evidence-based approach" *OJIN: The Online Journal of Issues in Nursing Vol. 27, No. 2, Manuscript 3.*

MasterClass. (2022). *Compassion fatigue vs burnout: What's the difference?* https://www.masterclass.com/articles/compassion-fatigue-vs-burnout

Mayo Clinic Staff. (2020). *Being assertive: Reduce stress, communicate better.* https://www.mayoclinic.org/healthy-lifestyle/stress-management/in-depth/assertive/art-20044644

Mcleod, C. (2019). *Nursing burnout: We are not doing enough.* https://www.canadian-nurse-.com/en/articles/issues/2019/october-2019/nursing-burnout-we-are-not-doing-enough

Meriam-Webster Dictionary. (2020). https://www.merriam-webster.com/dictionary/transition

Minnesota.gov Handout 6: ABCs of addressing compassion fatigue. https://education.mn.gov/mdeprod/idcplg?IdcService=GET_FILE&dDocName=PROD04622 0&RevisionSelectionMethod=latestReleased&Rendition= primary

Morris, G. (2022). *How to manage stress as a nurse.* Nurse Journal. https://nursejournal.org/articles/how-to-manage-stress/

Morris, G. (2023). *How to manage stress as a nurse.* https://nursejournal.org/articles/how-to-manage-stress/

Najafi, B., & Nasiri, A. (2023). Explaining novice nurses' experience of weak professional confidence: A qualitative study. *SAGE Open Nurs 20,*9:23779608231153457. doi: 10.1177/23779608231153457. PMID: 36969365; PMCID: PMC10031601.

National Council of State Boards of Nursing. (NCSBN). (2018). *Transition to practice.* http://www..ncsbn.org/transition-to-practice.htm

National Council of State Boards of Nursing. (2019). *Clinical judgment measurement model in next generation NCLEX news winter 2019* (pp. 1-6).

National Council of State Boards of Nursing. (2023). *Transition to Practice.* https://www.ncsbn.org/nursing-regulation/practice/transition-to-practice.page

National Council of State Boards of Nursing. (2023). *2023 NCSBN Symposium: Solutions addressing nursing workforce crisis/report.*

National Safety Council. (2023). *Assault fifth leading cause of workplace deaths.* https://www.nsc.org/workplace/safety-topics/workplace-violence

National Student Nurses Association (NSNA). (2020). *Lead-ership conference.* http://www.nsna.org/meetings.html

National Solutions, Inc. (2023). *2023 NSI National Health Care Retention & RN Staffing Report.* https://www.nsinursingsolutions.com/Documents/Library/NSI_National_Health_Care_Retention_Report.pdf

Nursing Solutions Inc. (2023). *2023 NSI National health care retention & RN staffing report.* https://www.wpchange.org/resources/2023-nsi-national-health-care-retention-rn-staffing-report

Nurse Beth. (2021). *Nursing intuition—what is it, and do you have it?* https://allnurses.com/nursing-intuition-what-is-it-t734342/

Nurse Journal. (2023). *Ask A Nurse: How to Combat Nurse Bullying in the Workplace.* https://nursejournal.org/ask-a-nurse/how-to-combat-bullying-in-nursing/

Occupational Safety and Health Administration (OSHA). (n.d.). *Guidelines for preventing workplace violence for healthcare and social service workers.* https://www.osha.gov/Publications/osha3148.pdf

Pate, K. (2023). *Imposter syndrome in nursing: A barrier to personal growth.* https://www.aacn.org/blog/imposter-syndrome-in-nursing-a-barrier-to-personal-growth

Prentice, D., Moore, J., Fernandes, B., & Larabie, E. (2022). Nursing care delivery models and intraprofessional collaborative care: Canadian nurse leaders' perspectives. *SAGE Open Nursing, 8.* doi:10.1177/23779608221133648

Sanner-Stiehr, E., & Ward-Smith, P. (2017). Lateral violence in nursing: Implications and strategies for nurse educators. *Journal of Professional Nursing: Official Journal of the American Association of Colleges of Nursing, 33*(2), 113–118. https://doi.org/10.1016/j.profnurs.2016.08.007

Sherman, R.O. (2023). *Ensuring new graduate professional socialization.* EmergingRNLeader. https://emergingrnleader.com/ensuring-new-graduate-professional-socialization/

The American Institute of Stress. (2023). Compassion Fatigue: Coping with secondary traumatic stress disorder in those who treat the traumatized. https://www.stress.org/military/for-practitionersleaders/compassion-fatigue from Figley, 2001.

The Center for American Nurses (2016). *New information for nurses.* https://centerforamericannurses.org/

The Joint Commission. (2021). *Sentinel Event Alert.* https://www.jointcommission.org/-/media/tjc/documents/resources/patient-safety-topics/sentinel-event/sea-59-workplace-violence-final2.pdf

University of St. Augustine for Health Sciences. (2023). *The importance of effective communication in Nursing.* https://www.usa.edu/blog/communication-in-nursing/

Vizient (2023). *Nurse Residency Program News for Nurse Residents.* https://www.aacnnursing.org/Portals/0/PDFs/NRP/Nurse-Residency-Newsletter-July-2023.pdf

White, A. (2022). *The importance of nursing intuition.* https://nursingcecentral.com/the-importance-of-nursing-intuition/

Wilding, M. (2022). *How to tell the difference between fear and intuition.* https://www.forbes.com/sites/melodywilding/2022/06/07/how-to-tell-the-difference-between-fear-and-intuition/?sh=360e87e75dd0

Williams, E. (2021). *Ensure you love your first nursing job—choose wisely!.* https://www.nurse.com/blog/love-first-nursing-job-choose-wisely/

Wolf, L. A. et al. (2017). Workplace aggression as cause and effect: Emergency nurses' experiences of working fatigued. *International Emergency Nursing, 33*, 48–52. https://doi.org/10.1016/j.ienj.2016.10.006

Wolf, L.A., Perhats, C., Clark, P.R., Moon, M.D., & Zavotsky, K.E. (2018). Workplace bullying in emergency nursing: Development of a grounded theory using situational analysis. *International Emergency Nursing, 39*, 33–39. https://doi.org/10.1016/j.ienj.2017.09.002

Wolters Kluwer (2022). *Top 10 skills nursing students need to succeed.* https://www.wolterskluwer.com/en/expert-insights/top-10-skills-nursing-students-need-to-succeed-today

Workplace Violence Prevention for Health Care and Social Service Workers Act, 2021 Workplace Violence Prevention for Health Care and Social Service Workers Act, H.R. 1195, 117 Cong. (2021). https://www.congress.gov/bill/117th-congress/house-bill/1195?r=1

Yeong-Ju, K., & Soo-Yeon, K. (2022). Transition shock experience of nursing students in clinical practice: A phenomenological approach. *Healthcare, 10*(4), 613.

Zerwekh, J., & Garneau, A.Z. (2018). Role transitions. In J. Zerwekh & A.Z. Garneau (Eds.), *Nursing today: Transition and trends* (9th ed.). Elsevier.

Zerwekh, J., & Garneau, A.Z. (2023). *Nursing today: Transition and trends* (11th ed). Elsevier

Zhou, L., Kachie Tetgoum, A.D., Quansah, P.E., & Owusu-Marfo, J. (2022). Assessing the effect of nursing stress factors on turnover intention among newly recruited nurses in hospitals in China. *Nursing Open, 9*(6), 2697–2709. doi: 10.1002/nop2.969. Epub 2021 Jun 30. PMID: 34190432; PMCID: PMC9584492

26

Managing Time: The Path to High Self-Performance

Barbara Cherry, DNSc, MBA, RN, NEA-BC*

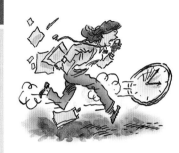

Our lives revolve around time; use it as a way ensure high performance, positive energy, focus in all aspects of your life.

ⓔ Additional resources are available online at: http://evolve.elsevier.com/Cherry/

LEARNING OUTCOMES

After studying this chapter, the reader will be able to:

1. Understand the unique demands of complex health care environments in today's fast-paced world of high technology and communication transfer and its effects on personal time management.
2. Articulate one's own time-management preferences and style.
3. Create an action plan to manage procrastination and distraction.
4. Adopt a time-management plan unique to one's own style to ensure high-level personal performance in work and home life.
5. Articulate the impact of personal time-related choices made by individuals on the risk to patients and the organization.

KEY TERMS

Energy management Ensuring that the right amount of effort matches the right task to optimize an outcome.

Goal A tangible, measurable, and attainable act in a specific time. It has broad-term results, experiences, or achievements toward which someone is willing to work.

Objective An identifiable, measurable act that implements one's goal and is typically short-term.

Prioritizing The act of deciding what should be done first and what activities should follow sequentially; establishing an ordered list or ranked items based on importance or urgency; method used to determine what actions need to be accomplished ahead of others.

Procrastination The act of intentionally and/or habitually putting off doing something that should be done.

Technology management Application of information systems and equipment to enhance work and life activities to maximal benefit.

Time management The development of processes and tools that increase efficiency and productivity within a set standard of time.

---

*We would like to acknowledge and thank Genevieve J. Conlin, DNP, MEd, MS/MBA, RN, NEA-BC, and Patricia Reid Ponte, DNSc, RN, FAAN, NEA-BC, for their contributions to this chapter in editions 1–8.

474

PROFESSIONAL/ETHICAL ISSUE

Karen is a busy staff nurse working on a medical-surgical unit at the local community hospital. She has returned to work from her vacation and is getting report for her patient assignment. While she was away some significant updates were made to the clinical documentation system. Karen wasn't able to attend the training session to review the changes and is not familiar with the changes. Her manager had told Karen that she needed to attend the training before she could return to practice. She hadn't been concerned, as she feels she has strong computer skills, and assumed she'd figure it out upon her return. "I mean, really, how hard can it be?" Karen had said. One of her colleagues offers to take a few minutes to show her some of the new workflows in the system but Karen brushes her off, stating, "I don't have time to review this; I need to get my meds passed so I can go to the uniform sale in the café before it closes."

Karen soon discovers there are some big differences in how to document medications, as well as some of the procedures. She quickly falls behind in her documentation and starts writing things on a piece of paper.

Karen has plans after work to meet friends for dinner. She's eager to finish her shift and get on with her evening. She has missed some important pieces of documentation, although she does give a thorough handoff to the next nurse at shift change report. The oncoming nurse asks about a patient's response to a pain medication given. Karen replies, "I need to remember to note that; I'll just deal with it next time I work .... Hopefully I'll remember everything I did!" She laughs it off as she leaves the unit at the end of her shift.

You are the nurse receiving report from Karen, and you realize her documentation is not complete. What do you do? What systems could have been put in place to ensure that Karen did not return to work before completing the new documentation system training? What could Karen have done when she realized the enormity of the gap in her knowledge and skills in using the new documentation system? What are the ethical considerations involved in this situation for both the individual and the organization?

VIGNETTE

Approximately 4 months ago, Ashley Jade transferred to a position as a staff registered nurse (RN) at an ambulatory cancer treatment center. Today Ashley arrived at the chemotherapy infusion room 15 minutes before the start of her shift. She knew it was going to be a busy day and, given her lack of experience in this work setting, she thought she should get a head start on her assignment. She was heading toward the workstation when one of her colleagues stopped her to discuss a holiday party, and they both spoke fervently about how much fun it would be.

Ten minutes later, Ashley resumed her trek to the workstation. As she arrived the phone rang, and Ashley answered it. A patient was seeking information about her appointment time. It took Ashley quite a while to open up the computer screen, log in, and find the information, which she communicated to the patient. By now many of her colleagues were on site, already starting to work on their assignments. Ashley looked at her assignment and realized that in addition to her other assigned patients, one of her patients would be receiving the first treatment of a new chemotherapy protocol. She knew that given the time necessary to work with the patient and family, triple-check orders with her physician and pharmacist colleagues, and administer the premedication and chemotherapy, all while monitoring this very ill patient, she would be very busy all day.

While she was reviewing the new chemotherapy protocol one of Ashley's primary patients came in unexpectedly with a fever and low blood pressure, needing hydration and platelets. The physician gave Ashley orders to stabilize the patient and arrange for transfer to the inpatient unit. The hospital was full, so the transfer would take some time. Ashley began to get very anxious about being able to complete all of her assigned duties while giving her patients the specialized care and attention they needed. Unfortunately, this anxious feeling was becoming a common occurrence in Ashley's workday.

Meanwhile, Bella Callahan, a staff RN who had been working on the inpatient oncology floor for slightly less than a year, was passing out 10:00 a.m. medications. She received a call from Ashley to take report before accepting the patient later in the day when a room became available. Bella was already behind in passing medications because of the barcoding system now in use for medication administration. Despite the fact that this system would be safer and more efficient, using the new application took more time in the first few weeks. The training was great, but medication administration took longer. Bella asked the charge nurse whether she could take report for her, but the charge nurse said she was in the midst of transferring another patient to the medical intensive care unit.

Bella took the report from Ashley and agreed to accept the patient at 1:00 p.m., when another patient's discharge would be completed and the room cleaned. Bella wondered, "How will I ever get finished in time to pick up my daughter from daycare by 4:00 p.m.?" Her day was lining up like so many before, with her not finishing her work before the end of the shift. Bella would have to call her mother to help out again by picking up her daughter.

Both Ashley and Bella were working frantically to ensure that patients' needs were met in a timely way, but it seemed impossible to both of them before they decided to call their respective managers and seek assistance.

Questions to Consider While Reading This Chapter:

1. When Ashley arrived on duty, what are some strategies she could have used to be sure she made the most of her early arrival?
2. What factors should Ashley and Bella consider when deciding how to prioritize their patient care assignment?
3. What are some strategies that Bella and Ashley can use to ensure balance between their work and personal lives?

CHAPTER OVERVIEW

The previous scenarios are typical of what happens daily in the lives of busy professionals. Managing multiple priorities during a particular workday and integrating personal and work-related demands is the constant dilemma of so many men and women today. Additionally, performing well in both arenas is not only a goal of most working professionals but more importantly also an obligation to ensure quality and safety in care delivery. To accomplish the important goals in life, it is necessary to understand your own preferred style of managing priorities, recognize your typical distractions, identify a personal performance approach, and consistently use strategies and tools to make the most of every minute. This chapter is designed to assist students, new nurses, and busy professionals in implementing self-management strategies to better use their time and energy to ensure a highly productive, focused life.

HEALTH CARE TODAY

Health care environments are fraught with incredible complexities: high-acuity patients, vigilant and knowledgeable family members, ever-growing information technology geared toward supporting staff in their work, often tight quarters in which to deliver high-tech and high-risk care, and little time to interact with patients on an interpersonal therapeutic level. Interprofessional practice models demand collaborative teamwork, when in reality disciplines often function in parallel work processes. The need to move patients quickly from one site of care to another on a constantly growing continuum that reaches into patients' homes is the norm in today's health care environment. Fast-paced clinics, high-tech ambulatory care practice settings, and quaternary care in high-intensity critical care units and operating rooms are typical. The nature of the intimate human element inherent in the delivery of health care makes it like no other work.

As health care continues to evolve with a focus on improving quality and reducing costs, managing time and organizing care efficiently have become critical components of health care delivery. The Covid-19 Pandemic of 2020 made health care professionals realize the vital need to address their personal mental and physical health and work–life balance. Therefore it becomes critical for each professional working in these dynamic settings to receive education and coaching in managing time, energy, balance, and focus to ensure high performance. Florence Nightingale's words resonate: "Knowing how you manage when you are there [at work] ... impacts how your work should be done when you are not there" (1969).

PERSPECTIVES ON TIME

Each person has a specific perspective of time, which is based on their own experiences, values, education, socioeconomic factors, age, personality, culture, and genetic makeup. To understand one's own perspective on time and the resulting behaviors, it is necessary to create opportunities to think introspectively and examine personal preferences, traits, habits, and tendencies. This is the critical first step in achieving an individualized time-management strategy and plan.

Review the following 10 psychologic obstacles that influence how you create and sustain focused and productivity work habits (Morgenstern, 2004). Then carefully consider how one or more of these might affect your ability to develop productive, energetic work habits:

1. *Unclear goals and priorities:* Within a particular work shift or within your life as a whole, if you lack clarity about purpose and expected outcomes the ability to manage time to meet your desires becomes a futile task.

2. *Conquistador of chaos:* If you are constantly overburdened with tasks, events, urgent requests, and last-minute cancellations, you are a better crisis manager than a manager of time.

3. *Fear of downtime:* Some individuals fear the possibility of standing still too long. They feel guilty with time-outs or time off. Staying too busy to think keeps long-term planning and personal introspection at bay.

4. *Need to be a caretaker:* In professions such as nursing the need to be a caretaker is a common devotion and can be very gratifying. However, when this need becomes unbalanced it can cause you to feel resentful, unappreciated, and overwhelmed.

5. *Fear of failure:* If you are unable to get to the things that are important to you and are unable to meet your personal goals, you may be afraid of failure. It can be very upsetting to go after your dreams and find out you cannot reach them. Sometimes it is easier to avoid making the effort. Take time to understand what your fears are and to openly address them.

6. *Fear of success:* You may have been given a message somewhere in your life that you do not deserve to be a success. Therefore it can be anxiety provoking to garner success and stand apart from others, who may distance themselves from you. Take time to think through whether or not this issue is playing out in your life.

7. *Fear of disrupting the status quo:* Not pursuing your goals for fear of the reactions of those around you is very common. Your family, coworkers, or supervisors may be critical of what you want to pursue. Gradually approaching changes gives you and those around you time to acclimate.

8. *Fear of Completion:* If you are afraid of completing a project that is creative and fun because you are fearful that another similar project will not find its way to you or the project may no longer be important to you, take the time to understand why you are not completing a routine task or a major project that has been with you for some time.

9. *Need for perfection:* If you are a perfectionist and feel that everything should be completed with the same level of excellence, you are not keeping things in perspective. If you demand extremely high standards for every single task you undertake, you simply will not get everything done.

10. *Fear of losing creativity:* Many creative people think that creating an organized time-management structure or approach to life will squelch their creative natures or tendencies. However, creating a framework to manage priorities will allow more freedom and time to enhance your creative juices.

Why Is Your Personal Time Perspective Important?

Following are some of the benefits that will result if you take the time to uncover your own tendencies, fears, strengths, and weaknesses and become more mindful in your nursing practice (Ponte & Koppel, 2015):

- Improved patient outcomes through implementation of productive work habits and processes
- Increased satisfaction with your work accomplishments as a result of applying something new in your setting
- Improved interpersonal relations because of your ability to be fully present and engaged to do your best work
- Better future direction because there is more attentiveness to proactively managing and engaging in the environment
- Improved personal health because of decreased anxiety and a restoration of emotional balance

It is more crucial than ever that you strive to understand what you value, recognize your purpose in life, and determine strategies to ensure that your focus and energy are geared toward your major goals in life. Whether you are trying to organize how to approach a particular workday or trying to balance your personal and work life, the strategies that you will learn and integrate into your daily activities now will play out the rest of your life. To help you get a perspective on your current time-management skills, take the following free assessment from MindTools: https://www.mindtools.com/aavjrgg/how-good-is-your-time-management. Then we will move to a discussion on the full engagement in managing your time and performance though the management of your physical, mental, spiritual, and emotional energy.

ENERGY MANAGEMENT

In their classic work on full engagement in the workplace, Loehr and Schwartz (2005) note that "Energy, not time, is the fundamental currency of high performance."

Striving to be more efficient and more organized, or to manage time and priorities better, is all in the interest of becoming a better performer in one's work or personal life. Only when we are fully engaged do we perform our best. Full engagement requires drawing on four separate but related sources of energy: (1) physical, (2) mental, (3) spiritual, and (4) emotional. Just as we build physical capacity through disciplined exercise and strengthening routines, we can also strengthen our emotional, spiritual, and mental capacities.

Consider Ashley from our earlier Vignette. Her decision to transfer to the chemotherapy infusion center, her third transfer in 18 months, came only after the sheer frustration of not feeling in control of her work life and home life. At work Ashley felt overwhelmed, underappreciated, and unprepared physically for the daily challenges of 12-hour shifts. She was exhausted every morning, and she fell into bed as soon as she got home. Her energy level was poor. She felt dissatisfied with her inability to spend more time with friends on her days off. Ashley could not bear the thought of getting out of bed early another day, even if it was for something fun. Because of this she gained weight over the past 6 months, and the only thing that seemed to make her happy was to visit her sister on Sunday afternoons. Getting to work the next day often proved difficult because her motivation was low and her energy level even lower. With this new job Ashley was attempting to get back on track. "It's going to be different this time," she said to herself. With a focus on physical, mental, spiritual, and emotional energy Ashley may really have a different—and much better—life and work experience!

Physical Energy

Key components of physical energy for a productive and highly energizing life include paying attention to a routine of:

- eating properly
- getting adequate sleep and exercise
- taking appropriate breaks during long shifts
- drinking plenty of water
- focusing on one activity while collecting thoughts about what to prioritize next

Once the physical capacity of your holistic self is working well, you can pay attention to your mental, spiritual, and emotional capacities.

Mental Energy

The mental energy that is most potent to ensure full engagement and high performance is that of realistic optimism. *Realistic optimism* is seeing the world as it is but always working toward an optimal solution or goal. *Mental energy* is the ability to maintain sustained concentration on a task and move flexibly between issues. Mental energy includes:

- preparation
- visualization
- positive self-talk
- effective time management
- creativity

Ashley has begun to identify this mental energy in her desire to get back on track. She realizes that change is necessary. To move in this direction Ashley needs to spend some time reflecting on the following questions: (1) What are my major goals in life? and (2) What is my purpose?

Spiritual Energy

Often we do not take the time to reflect about what is important to us. Being in a quiet place helps us identify our vision of life—our purpose and direction in life. Ashley from the Vignette has yet to determine her life vision, resulting in frequent job changes and her lack of clarity about how she wants to spend her downtime. Having direction and purpose is the key factor in one's spiritual capacity.

Emotional Energy

Physical, mental, and spiritual energy provide fuel for building our emotional capacity. Managing emotions skillfully in the service of high positive energy and full engagement is called *emotional intelligence* (Goleman, 2006). Striving to increase one's emotional capacity—which includes improving one's self-confidence, self-control, self-regulation, social skills, interpersonal effectiveness, empathy, patience, openness, trust, and enjoyment—will result in a more positive, invigorating work experience and personal life (Box 26.1 How to Improve Your Emotional Intelligence).

Practicing Mindfulness

There is growing interest in and evidence of the positive impact of adopting a mindful attitude and incorporating mindfulness practices into one's personal and professional life. Mindfulness practices help you stay focused on the present and be attentive to what is happening in the moment, so that distractions are held at bay while the mind continuously brings you back to the present moment. One mindfulness practice is to use focused breathing for 1 to 2 minutes to stay calm and reflect on the priority at hand, allowing yourself the opportunity to remember the importance of what is happening in the moment. This practice results in less rumination about the future or extraneous phenomena and allows you to be clear-minded, focused, and attentive to the situation at hand, whether it be the need to administer a medication, to calm an upset family member, or to document in the medical record.

Incorporating a mindful attitude and mindful practices into your way of life can result in a more balanced and effective focus to carry out activities of everyday life and nursing practice (Penque, 2019; Ponte & Koppel, 2015). Mindfulness practices can also have an impact on your greater well-being and perceived health. Mindfulness-based practices, in addition to focused breathing, include meditation, yoga, reflective journaling, and incorporating music, art, and nature into your daily life and into nursing practice. There are many excellent online resources to learn more about mindfulness including one from Mayo Clinic: https://www.mayoclinic.org/healthy-lifestyle/consumer-health/in-depth/mindfulness-exercises/art-20046356.

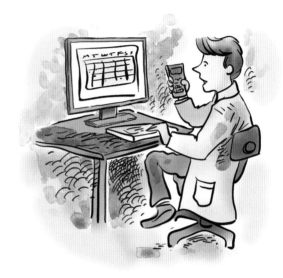

Nurses who adopt a mindful attitude and practices are more apt to be better at time and energy management in all aspects of their work and personal lives.

Becoming Resilient

Resiliency is an important concept that can help nurses manage stressful work environments and not become overwhelmed by challenging situations. Traits of a resilient nurse are (1) being psychologically strong and able to maintain self-control and optimism in the face of complex work conditions; (2) proactively adopting problem-solving methods to cope with stress; (3) addressing negative emotions in a respectful way and not carrying those emotions personally; (4) having an optimal work–life balance; (5) maintaining a high degree of confidence in the face of difficulties; and (6) owning a sense of achievement and positive professional values for the work done as nurses (Han et al., 2023). Resiliency takes time and experience to develop but new nurses are strongly encouraged to work toward becoming more resilient. Following are some keys for developing and enhancing your resiliency (Han et al., 2023):

- Work on improving and growing in your nursing skills and knowledge to build your confidence
- Take an active approach to solving problems in the workplace by offering solutions and working proactively with your team
- Contribute to building a collaborative team spirit and having colleagues to support you
- Seek out at least one trusted colleague or nurse leader who you can talk to and who can provide support when needed
- Seek out mental health support when needed
- Be proud of your personal sense of achievement as a nurse and seek to continue to learn and grow
- Establish supportive relationships outside of the work environment and nurture your home life
- Take care of your personal health

TIME AND ENERGY DISTRACTIONS

We are all subject to distractions in our work and personal lives that may influence our propensity to procrastinate or not reach our goals. Nurses experience stress and distraction when they assume unplanned responsibilities while simultaneously conducting their planned work. It is important to recognize and understand the distractions or complexities that inhibit our ability to complete tasks and to meet our objectives and goals in a planned way. Box 26.2 lists some common internal and external time and energy distractions that each of us may experience in a typical day. The reader is encouraged to be aware of these time distractions and consider actions to address those that are affecting you. The following sections in the chapter provides examples of how to strategically avoid these common time distractions.

TIME-MANAGEMENT STRATEGIES

It is easy to apply the perspectives-on-time concept to nurses because many nurses have type A personalities, meaning that they are oriented toward high achievement. As high achievers nurses go above and beyond for their patients, colleagues, and families and are often attracted to activities that are challenging, difficult, and even risky. When high achievers mismanage themselves in relation to time they experience frustration and stress. To assist nurses in improving their self-management and

BOX 26.2 **Time and Energy Distractions**	
External Distractions	**Internal Distractions**
Interruptions	Failure to set goals and
Socializing or visitors	priorities/inadequate
Meetings (unnecessary)	planning
Understaffing	Procrastination
Lack of information/	Ineffective delegation
ineffective communi-	Personal disorganization
cation	Inability to say no
Lack of feedback	Lack of self-discipline or
Inadequate information	indecisiveness
about policies and	Leaving tasks unfinished
procedures	Not setting time limits
Personnel or coworkers	Attempting too much at
with problems	once
Lack of teamwork/	Overinvolvement in
duplicating efforts	routine detail
Confusing lines of author-	Making numerous errors
ity, responsibility, and	
communication	

time management, various strategies to help overcome time and energy distractors and improve time management are outlined in the following sections. While planning, organizing, and implementing are essential to control the use of time, it is important to note that *planning* is the most important step in time management.

Planning for Control

Planning is the most important step in time management. Unfortunately, few people expend as much energy planning as they should. Some shy away from planning because they believe it is too time-consuming and never leads to closure. In reality planning allows people to better use their time and can lead to completion of goals. For example, 1 minute of planning can transfer to at least 10 minutes of productivity, proving to be a great return on the investment of taking the time to review and plan for the day. If you arrive 10 to 15 minutes early for your scheduled shift and map out the day's priorities, your likelihood of executing those priorities is far greater than had you not taken the time to plan up front.

Having a priority-planning list as you work is useful in keeping you on track to accomplish tasks by the end of the shift or day. Those who plan well also tend to encounter fewer problems when Murphy's Law—*If anything can go wrong it will*—becomes a reality. Thus it is important to plan before beginning any task, project, or day's activities. Planning involves (1) setting goals and establishing priorities, (2) scheduling activities, and (3) making to-do lists.

Setting Priorities. Prioritizing is about making choices about what to do and what not to do. To prioritize effectively you need to be able to recognize what is important as well as to see the difference between urgent (must be done immediately) and important (must be done, but there may be flexibility as to when the task can be accomplished). A major component of prioritization is deciding what should be done first and what activities should follow sequentially. The factors that influence how to establish priorities include:

- urgency of a situation
- demands of others
- closeness of deadlines
- existing time frame
- your level of familiarity with the task
- ease of the task
- amount of enjoyment involved
- consequences involved
- size of the task
- congruence with personal goals

Unfortunately, not all of these factors carry the same weight in the consideration of the use of time. Several processes have been proposed to assist people in setting priorities, including the ABCD approach, the Pareto principle, and the continuum approach:

1. The *ABCD approach* requires making a list for every task that needs to be done (Hackett & Bigott, 2021). An A is assigned to the items that must get done right away, the B is assigned to items that should get done sooner rather than later, the C is assigned to items that can wait till later, and the D is assigned to items that should be delegated. The A items should stand out from the others because of their priority for patient care and their worth to the person making the list. Also the A items are likely to require more energy and time, but they should be completed before any of the B or C items. This system or prioritizing allows for reflection and change while maintaining focus.

2. The *Pareto principle* is another process that is suggested for setting priorities. This principle is also referred to as the "80/20 rule," suggesting that 80% of the time expended produces 20% of the results, and

20% of the time expended produces 80% of the results (Koch, 2014). The essence is in determining the "vital few" activities that should be done and eliminating the "trivial many." This principle emphasizes selecting the most productive activities, eliminating trivial ones, and learning to say "no."

3. The *continuum approach* to setting priorities encourages a person to select priorities by categorizing or ranking items according to four continuums. As you read about the four continuums think about Ashley's assignment in the opening Vignette and consider which of her tasks would have been high priorities according to this approach.

   - *Intrinsic importance:* Very important and must be done; important and should be done; not so important and may not be necessary, but may be useful; or unimportant and can be eliminated entirely.
   - *Urgency:* Very urgent and must be done now; urgent and should be done soon; not urgent and can wait; time is not a factor.
   - *Delegation:* Must be done by me because I am the only one who can do it; can be delegated; can be dumped because the task does not need to be done or delegated.
   - *Visitations and conferences:* People I must see each day; people to see frequently but not daily; people to see regularly but not frequently; people to see only infrequently.

   Obviously these continuums have varying usefulness, depending on the activity being scrutinized.

   Overall it does not matter which method is used to establish priorities as long as priorities are established using a sound rationale. Fortunately, setting priorities becomes easier with practice. If Ashley had established her priorities for the day, it is unlikely that talking about the holiday party or calling the inpatient unit to give a report on a patient that would not transfer for several hours would have taken precedence over reviewing the new chemotherapy regimen protocol she would be administering to a patient. Setting priorities would have allowed Ashley to better use her time and decreased her anxiety about not managing her assignment appropriately.

Establishing a To-Do List. Writing something on paper often is the first step to accomplishing it. A to-do list tends to keep people on track and focused on specific activities. Thus the list should be reflective of your priorities and goals. To-do lists should be made and revised daily to be the most useful in managing your time. Sometimes they require revision more frequently, even hourly, when priorities shift for valid reasons. The list should be legible and easily accessible to review throughout the day. It is helpful to review the list at the end of the shift or day to assess how you achieved or did not achieve your goals. This is an opportunity to reflect on the distractions you experienced so that you can make note of what not to do when the next situation arises. The list will give you the opportunity to reevaluate your tasks to see what needs to be carried over to the next day. Different people find it useful to construct their lists on note cards, in day-planner calendars, on pocket calendars, in electronic recall devices, on computers, and myriad other ways. There is no right or wrong way to make a to-do list, but it should always be available to you.

Scheduling Activities. Scheduling activities is an important component of planning. It is one way to control Parkinson's Law, which states that work will expand to fill the time that is available. By scheduling activities a person determines how much time is spent on a specific activity. Such time delineations tend to focus attention and activity so that the task gets completed more efficiently and effectively. A schedule of activities can be constructed using a variety of different methods, including hourly time schedules. Everyone has used an hourly schedule for appointments, classes, or leisure activities. In addition, nurses become adept at using hourly time schedules to administer medications appropriately. Unfortunately, most people, including nurses, do not use time schedules frequently or consistently enough.

The process of scheduling activities is an important part of planning to use your time more efficiently. However, scheduling needs to be done appropriately to ensure adherence. Remember to schedule activities so that they coincide with your internal "prime time," when you concentrate best, and your external "prime time," when you deal best with other people. As a general rule 15 minutes of focused time and energy toward a project equates to 1 hour of productivity. Be sure to include some flexible time just for yourself.

Another support for scheduling activities is to use technology wisely. Technology continues to advance at a feverish pace and these systems can support a nurse's workflow and assist with prioritizing patient care activities through alerts and clinical decision support systems.

Organizing for Control

Organizing yourself and your environment is an important component of time management. Such organization requires that you be able to deal effectively with:

- The cluttered-mind syndrome
- The art of "no detourism"
- The art of "wastebasketry"
- E-mail mania

The Cluttered-Mind Syndrome. The clutter-mind syndrome is exactly what the label implies—a mind cluttered with many thoughts and ideas, which can be distractions to accomplishing your goals and divert your attention sufficiently that you do not know where to begin. When you lose your concentration you will again become distracted by the clutter. To stay focused keep your to-do list organized and stick with accomplishing your priorities, plan ahead and set deadlines for completing tasks, avoid procrastination, take short breaks and drink plenty of water, and engage in positive self-talk about what you can accomplish. You can do this!

The Art of "No Detourism." To effectively organize, or clear the mind, you must practice the art of "no detourism." This requires complete concentration on one activity or task until—with no detours—it is completed. It mandates that only one activity at a time be undertaken and that it be completed before you move to a different task. This method also implies that the task should be completed correctly the first time so that you do not waste time redoing it. Inherent in the concept of "no detourism" is the fact that the tasks undertaken are directly related to personal goals and objectives, thus completing them will result in internal satisfaction.

The Art of "Wastebasketry." Perfecting the art of "wastebasketry" is mandatory for better use of time. The art of physical wastebasketry involves "circular filing" (in the trash can or with the delete key on the computer) of any documents, including e-mails and other paperwork, that has limited use or needs no response. The goal is to handle a paper (or e-mail) only once, then either act on it (do it), send it along to another appropriate person (delegate it), or throw it away (dump it). This art involves being sufficiently knowledgeable and skilled to ascertain which documents, e-mails, and paperwork are appropriate candidates for the "circular file" and then daring to follow through. The art of mental wastebasketry also involves organizing your mind to deal with the established priorities. It requires using selective perception to attend only to those tasks at hand. It also assists in discarding useless information. Mental wastebasketry is a valuable skill to perfect in relation to achieving a better use of time.

E-Mail Mania. E-mail has become the primary method of communication for the majority of individuals in professional, health care, and academic settings. It is an expedient route to contact people, regardless of their location. It is also a useful way to conduct business with a group of people concurrently, when appropriate, because of the ability to share information with many parties at once. Keep in mind, however, that e-mail is a professional channel of communication; messages should contain a greeting, a clear body of text, specific and clear requests for information, and an acceptable closing. Messages should be free of grammatical and typographic errors. Also keep in mind that a telephone call may be a sufficient and more efficient means of response and often is more appropriate.

Effective communication in health care is critical and it is important for a health care organization to recognize the diversity of its staff, noting that many nurses are steeped in technology. This technologic adeptness continues to evolve, and organizations are actively working to accommodate their staff by using multiple medias to communicate. Chapter 19 provides additional information about how to use e-mail effectively.

Implementing for Control

Implementing for control refers to carrying out activities that assist people in managing time use. Further exploring these activities in the following sections clarifies how they can be implemented easily in daily life.

Attacking the Priorities. It is important to attack your priorities early to gain control of your time. Delay in beginning tasks will only result in crises when deadlines or personal goals are not met. One of the most cited reasons for delaying this process is fear—a very real

symptom of procrastination. Regardless, it is important to analyze your inability to attack your priorities to be able to identify how to better manage your time to achieve the results you established. If the priority is a big project or large task, it can be successfully approached by examining how the project can be divided up into smaller, more manageable tasks.

Avoiding Procrastination. Procrastination is a bad habit that ranks high on the list of time wasters. It has been referred to as an obstacle to success and can wear many disguises, including fear, laziness, indifference, overwork, and forgetfulness. Procrastination is most frequently evident when a person is faced with an unpleasant task, a difficult task, or a difficult decision. Usually procrastination is recognizable easily because it involves doing low-priority rather than high-priority tasks, and it always welcomes interruptions. Procrastination is the art of "never doing today what can be put off until tomorrow." The result is less productivity, less internal satisfaction, and more stress.

To overcome procrastination you should (1) recognize when it is occurring and (2) admit that what is occurring is procrastination. Once those two steps are accomplished, the work of overcoming procrastination can begin. Following are mechanisms for overcoming procrastination (Emmett, 2009):

- Identify the tasks that are being put off.
- Ask why the task is being avoided.
- Determine whether the task could or should be done by someone else.
- Identify consequences of the procrastination.
- Set priorities in relation to the task.
- Establish deadlines and adhere to them.
- Focus on one aspect at a time.
- Do not strive for perfection if 95% or 98% will be just as effective.

The last item is clearly one in which good clinical discernment must be exercised because there are clearly instances in which providing nursing care that is anything less than 100% could cause harm. It also helps if you can eliminate those tasks that make up the procrastination. For example, if rearranging the desk or the medication cart is part of how a person procrastinates, then eliminate that activity as unnecessary. Most important, emphasize the benefits that are to be gained by completing the task and accomplishing the goals that will provide internal satisfaction.

Engaging a Mentor. Observe nurses in your work setting who exhibit excellent time-management skills; they are organized, able to complete their assignments on time, and even available to help others. These individuals would be excellent mentors on time management. Reach out to a time-management mentor for advice and suggestions to create a more manageable and enjoyable workday for yourself.

Delegating Appropriately. Most simplistically, *delegation* is the art of giving other people tasks to accomplish. In reality, however, there is nothing simple about delegation. It usually requires considerable time and energy to delegate, but the rewards are greater in the overall context of accomplishing goals. Following are some important benefits of delegation (Mancini, 2003):

- Extends the results that can be accomplished from what one person can do alone to what they can manage through others.
- Frees time for more important tasks.
- Assists in developing the initiative, skills, knowledge, and competence of others.
- Maintains the responsibility and decision level.
- Provides for more cost effectiveness.

With these potential benefits, it would seem that everyone would want to use delegation. Unfortunately this is not the case. Many barriers, internal and external, can hinder the delegation process.

A brief exploration of those barriers may clarify why delegation is such a problem for some people. The internal barriers to delegating include: preferring that tasks are accomplished in a certain way; demanding that everyone know all the details; believing that no one else can complete the task as well; lacking experience in delegating; feeling insecure; fearing being disliked; lacking confidence in others; striving for perfectionism, resulting in over-control; lacking organizational skills; failing to delegate authority commensurate with the responsibility delegated; fostering indecision; possessing poor communication skills; and lacking commitment to the development of others.

The external barriers to delegating are inherent either in the situation or in the person to whom something is being delegated. External barriers within the situation may include understaffing, stringent policies that mandate who can do what, low tolerance of mistakes, the critical nature of the work, and confusion regarding responsibilities and authority. External

barriers to delegation that reside within the person to whom tasks are being delegated include lack of experience, lack of competence, avoidance of responsibility, overdependence on others, disorganization, procrastination, work overload, and immersion in trivia and clutter (Mancini, 2003). When the barriers are identified and overcome the delegation process can proceed. Implementing the following steps will facilitate appropriate delegation (also see Chapter 20 for a complete discussion of legal and effective delegation in the clinical setting):

1. Identify exactly what is to be delegated and why.
2. Select the person who is qualified, able, and willing to perform the task.
3. Communicate the assignment in detail, perhaps even including written instructions.
4. Involve the delegatee in establishing the objectives and deadlines for the task.
5. Have the delegatee repeat the details of the task.
6. Give the delegatee the authority for accomplishing the task.
7. Provide adequate resources and support as needed.
8. Follow up regularly for progress reports.
9. Establish controls and monitor the results.
10. Evaluate the process and progress of the delegatee.
11. Let the delegatee do the job.

It is not prudent to take shortcuts when delegating tasks because the results might be different from what was originally intended. Avoiding delegation shortcuts is an important consideration because the nurse who does the delegating also retains accountability for the task and the patient care.

Delegation would have been useful to Ashley in the opening Vignette. It could have helped her meet her patient care goals and decrease her anxiety. Unfortunately Ashley was overwhelmed, and she could not identify those things that needed to be done or direct someone else to do them. In addition, Ashley had not established any priorities so it was difficult for her to plan for appropriate delegation.

Controlling Interruptions. To focus on your priorities it is important to establish uninterrupted blocks of time. Frequent causes of interruptions are telephone calls, meetings, and visitors. Learning how to control such interruptions helps you accomplish more in less time. One of the easiest ways to manage incoming calls is to not answer them during time that is scheduled for other activities. Use voicemail to manage calls that come at inconvenient times. The same goes for e-mails. Establish a set time for reading and responding to e-mails. Take advantage of the auto responder function to let others know that you will be responding to their e-mail at a set time. A good example of controlling interruptions in the opening Vignette would have been for Ashley to ask the unit secretary to help the patient requesting information about an appointment.

Meetings can become a major time waster if they are poorly managed and unproductive. This includes virtual meetings, which may also take additional time when there are technology glitches. The first step in controlling the interruption of a meeting is deciding whether to attend. For virtual meetings, consider if it is the type that will be recorded so that you may watch it later at a more convenient time. Such a decision should be based on an evaluation of the potential productivity of the meeting. For example, ask such questions as: Is the meeting absolutely necessary? Does the agenda contain items that you should be informed about? Is it necessary for you to contribute to the discussion? Will decisions be made that will affect you and your functioning? Are you conducting the meeting? These questions should guide your decision (Mancini, 2003). Once a person is committed to attending a meeting, they are responsible for helping ensure that the meeting remains focused and productive. The person conducting the meeting not only shares these same responsibilities but also has a more direct role in affecting the outcome.

Learning the Art of Saying "No."

"No" is such a small word but it is sometimes more difficult to say than any 14-syllable word. The first step in learning to say "no" is determining when to say it. The cost–benefit ratio of each opportunity must be evaluated in relation to the overall goals. If the activity will be a benefit overall, obviously it must be given careful consideration. If it will not be a significant benefit you should decline gracefully but emphatically. There is no need to provide an elaborate qualifier to your "no" response; a clear, succinct reply is acceptable. For example, when asked to review a clinical guideline do not refuse on the basis of the fact that you are overworked and do not have a free minute for 3 weeks. The person requesting the review is likely to agree on the later time frame, in which case you will find yourself committed to doing something that has low benefit unless you create another excuse. Instead be polite and gracious in the refusal, but do not allow leeway so you are manipulated into saying "yes." Always consider the opportunity that "no" offers in terms of your overall goals.

Using Technology.

Many of today's technologic advances can be used to improve time management by improving technology management. Most health care settings have adopted more uses of technologic resources to better improve the use of time and enhance patient care. Examples include electronic order entry systems that allow clinicians to enter and activate orders that are then transmitted to the pharmacy to fill medication requests and patient acuity rating systems that are completed online and used by admitting departments to send patients to the appropriate units for care.

Just about every workplace has a professional office system that supports e-mail and scheduling activities. The scheduling features available can be very useful for staff in the planning phase of time management. Many people use smartphones to synchronize their personal and professional calendars. These devices also become valuable resources in the clinical setting if programmed with drug information and lab value databases, which allow a nurse to have a wealth of information at their fingertips without having to carry or look for resource manuals. However, when you are considering the many technologic devices available keep in mind that the tools and devices should improve workflow and processes, not hinder them or create cumbersome ones. Also remember that taking time to learn to use new technology correctly will pay off in the long run by increasing your effective use of time.

Rewarding Yourself.

All people function more productively when they are motivated. The sources of motivation vary from person to person. A person needs to identify their motivators and use them as rewards for accomplishing goals. It is important to identify long- and short-term rewards so that they can be implemented appropriately. Most people are familiar with rewarding themselves in exchange for doing something, and they do it frequently. For some it is a way of life. It usually amounts to bargaining with yourself to facilitate the completion of a task. For example, "If I finish reading these two work-related articles then I can read my novel for 30 minutes," or "If I complete this paper I will treat myself to ice cream." You should know which rewards work best and use them appropriately to accomplish long-term goals.

Using Clinically Focused Time-Management Strategies

Time-management strategies specific to the clinical setting are recommended for nurses to use for a more productive and balanced workday (Box 26.3). While situations in each nursing unit will vary widely, it is imperative for the new nurse to consider time-management strategies appropriate to their work setting and learn and use other strategies as recommended by experienced nurses and nurse leaders.

CONTINUING TO SUCCEED

Improving time management to enhance self-performance and accomplish goals is a lifelong process. The process becomes easier the longer you engage in it, but time management still requires continual attention and energy. Obviously time management does not just happen—it requires a strong personal commitment. For continued success use the following strategies (Lakein, 1989):

- When feeling overwhelmed always stop and plan activities.
- Keep focused on priorities and act accordingly.
- Avoid procrastination.
- Maintain a positive attitude about the established goals or revise them so that they coincide with your value system.
- Do something for yourself every day.
- Continue to work on overcoming your fears.
- Resist doing the easy but unimportant tasks.

In addition, delete the words "if only" from your vocabulary. Regret is a luxury and a great time waster. You can spend significant time rehashing mistakes or determining how to make something perfect when it was a one-time occurrence that is now over. It is more productive to accept responsibility for mistakes, identify how to prevent such mistakes in the future, and move on. The reader is encouraged to review the tips for continuing success in managing time presented in Box 26.4.

BOX 26.3 Specific Clinically Focused Time-Management Strategies

1. Make a "to-do" list and use a technique such as the *ABCD* approach (previously discussed) to prioritize your activities. Be aware about how you are progressing on your duties and be prepared to reprioritize as situations in the clinical setting change.
2. Take opportunities to be proactive with use of your time. If you have some downtime, complete a low-priority task to create a time buffer if unexpected or unanticipated events occur. For example, prepare discharge instructions for a patient and family earlier in the day when you have some downtime even though you do not need them right away.
3. Use bedside reports at shift change to improve communication between the caregivers and the patient and significant others; the plan of care can be prioritized during this shared report.
4. Learn to "cluster care," which means to be prepared to perform as many tasks as possible when you are in a patient's room, including performing the physical assessment, answering questions, and providing education.
5. Use critical thinking to determine what tasks can be delegated to another team member (see Chapter 20 for a detailed discussion on safe and effective delegation).
6. Use purposeful hourly rounding to proactively address any patient needs.
7. Become familiar with key team members who can be a resource for you when you need help.

Data from Hackett, R., & Bigott, V. (2021). New graduate nurse time management. *American Nursing Journal, 16*(5), 30–32.

BOX 26.4 Tips for Successful Time Management

1. Clarify objectives, make a to-do list, and establish priorities on the list to work from.
2. Make sure the first hour of every workday is productive.
3. Do the task right the first time so that time will not be wasted doing it over.
4. Develop the habit of finishing whatever task is started.
5. Conquer procrastination and learn to do tasks now.
6. Make better time management a daily habit.
7. Take time for yourself—time to relax, time to live, time to just be.
8. Develop a personal philosophy of time that is consistent with your values.
9. Do tomorrow's planning tonight.
10. Ask yourself often, "Why am I doing what I am doing right now?"

From Skillpath Seminars. (2011). Managing multiple projects, objectives and deadlines. Skillpath.

SUMMARY

This chapter has focused on how to better manage your energy to control one of our most precious and seemingly scarce resources—time. Regardless of your work location, time management is important to achieving any personal or professional goals, and it helps decrease frustration and anxiety in high achievers. Without time management most professionals could never achieve their established goals, and for nurses many patient care activities would never be completed, perhaps resulting in poor patient outcomes. Ashley's and Bella's experiences in the opening Vignette are an example of what your life could be like in nursing unless you implement strategies for better self-management. Let's address the questions posed in the opening Vignette.

1. When Ashley arrived on duty, what are some strategies she could have used to be sure she made the most of her early arrival?

    In keeping with the idea of controlling interruptions and distractions Ashley should have had a quick, 1-minute friendly conversation with the colleague she met in the hall and planned a time later to visit about the holiday party. When she got to the unit, using her delegation strategies, she should have asked the unit secretary to take the call from the patient about her scheduled appointment. In setting her plan and priorities for the day she needed to focus on the reviewing the new chemotherapy protocol and managing the care for her ill primary care patient that came to the unit unexpectedly.

2. What factors should Ashley and Bella consider when deciding how to prioritize their patient care assignment? *Planning* and *prioritization* are the key to completing a successful workday. By reviewing and understanding their assignments early in their workday nurses can quickly establish their priorities, create

"to-do" lists as needed, and use all of the strategies noted in this chapter to focus on their priorities, understand internal and external time distractors, control interruptions, delegate appropriately, avoid procrastination, use technology to support time management, and engage in brief mindfulness activities when feeling overwhelmed. Another key to successful time management is to get a mentor who has demonstrated excellence in time management and ask them for advice and suggestions to create a more manageable and enjoyable workday.

3. What are some strategies that Bella and Ashley can use to ensure balance between their work and personal lives?

    Learning to manage physical, mental, spiritual, and emotional energy and build resiliency will provide nurses with the competencies they need for a successful professional career and a happy, uplifting personal life. The first key is managing one's health, followed by developing one's mental and spiritual energy, and then becoming more emotionally intelligent and resilient (ideas for each of these areas are discussed in the chapter).

Remember, it is essential for success in your professional career to initiate habits related to time management that will continue throughout the years. Frequently throughout the day ask yourself, "What is the best use of my time right now?" (Lakein, 1989). You may be surprised to learn that the answer does not coincide with your current activity. When that occurs stop and implement the strategies for self-management to better control your time. You will become more productive and gain internal satisfaction as a result.

CLINICAL JUDGMENT AND NEXT-GENERATION NCLEX® EXAMINATION-STYLE QUESTIONS

Consider Ashley from the opening chapter Vignette who had recently transferred to a new job in the outpatient chemotherapy infusion center. As noted in the chapter, Ashley's decision to transfer to the chemotherapy infusion center, her third transfer in 18 months, came only

after the sheer frustration of not feeling in control of her work life and home life. As Ashley reflects on her new job she is determined to have a better experience in her professional life and her home life. She vows to be more in control of her workday, both physically and mentally, and to have more energy when she is off work for the things she enjoys! What time-management and self-performance improvement actions recommended in this chapter can Ashley take to ensure success in her new job and more enjoyment in her home life?

For each action step, use an X to indicate if it was Effective (helped to meet expected outcomes), Ineffective (did not help meet expected outcomes), or Unrelated (not related to the expected outcomes).

Action	Effective	Ineffective	Unrelated
Create a plan to improve physical health and energy.			
Reflect and clarify career goals.			
Rely on help every day from coworkers who seem to be able to get their work done more quickly and easily.			
Identify distractions that affect time management and how to better manage them.			
Plan to eat lunch in the cafeteria every day.			
Plan the workday in advance to ensure that priority tasks are accomplished.			
Follow chemotherapy protocols exactly and triple-check orders with her physician and pharmacist colleagues.			
Ask the nursing supervisor for several new projects and committee assignments.			
Learn how to manage emotions if the workday gets overwhelming.			
Improve motivation for staying focused at work by planning rewards.			
Seek out a mentor to provide guidance about time management			

REFERENCES

Emmett, R. (2009). *Manage your time to reduce your stress: A handbook for the overworked, overscheduled, and overwhelmed.* Walker and Company.

Goleman, D. (2006). *Emotional intelligence: Why it can matter more than IQ.* Bantam Books.

Hackett, R., & Bigott, V. (2021). New graduate nurse time management. *American Nursing Journal, 16(5)*, 30–32.

Han, P., Duan, X., Jiang, J., Zeng, L., Zhang, P., & Zhao, S. (2023). Experience in the development of nurses' personal resilience: A meta-synthesis. *NursingOpen, 10(5)*, 2697–3436. https://doi.org/10.1002/nop2.1556

Koch, R. (2014). *Living the 80/20 way: Work less, worry less, succeed more, enjoy more.* Nicholas Brealey.

Lakein, A. (1989). *How to get control of your time and your life.* Signet.

Loehr, J., & Schwartz, T. (2005). *The power of full engagement.* Free Press.

Mancini, M. (2003). *Time management.* McGraw-Hill.

Morgenstern, J. (2004). *Time management from the inside out.* Henry Holt.

Nightingale, F. (1969). *Notes on nursing: What it is, and what it is not.* Dover.

Penque, S. (2019). Mindfulness to promote nurses' well-being. *Nursing Management, 50(5)*, 38–44. doi.org/10.1097/01.NUMA.0000557621.42684.c4

Ponte, P.R., & Koppel, P. (2015). Cultivating mindfulness to enhance nursing practice. *American Journal of Nursing, 115(6)*, 48–55. doi.org/10.1097/01.NAJ.0000466321.46439.17.

Skillpath Seminars. (2011). *Managing multiple projects, objective and deadlines.* Skillpath

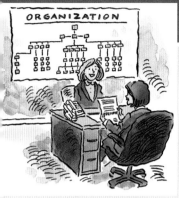

27

ORGANIZATION

Finding the right match can be exciting.

Job Search: Finding Your Match

Susan R. Jacob, PhD, MS, RN*

ⓔ Additional resources are available online at: http://evolve.elsevier.com/Cherry/

LEARNING OUTCOMES

After studying this chapter, the reader will be able to:
1. Use the interview process to evaluate potential employment opportunities.
2. Prepare an effective résumé and nursing portfolio.

3. Compare and contrast various professional nursing employment opportunities.
4. Summarize the employment process.

KEY TERMS

Orientation Activities that enhance adaptation to a new environment.
Portfolio A collection of evidence demonstrating acquisition of skills, knowledge, and achievements related to a professional career.

Professional objective Occupational position for which one aims.
Résumé Summary of a job applicant's previous work experience and education.

PROFESSIONAL/ETHICAL ISSUE

Alice and Renardo had just finished their senior seminar class, in which the nursing recruiters from the local hospital held a session on job interviewing. The recruiters told the class about potential job opportunities at their hospital and described their intensive 3-month orientation process for new graduates. The recruiters discussed the high cost of orienting one new nurse and told the class that it was well worth the investment to have the

assurance that the new graduates would be skilled and comfortable in their new positions. The recruiters added that once the hospital made an investment in a new nurse, they expected a commitment of at least 2 years.

Alice told Renardo she planned to apply at this hospital because it was likely there would be positions available, but she also planned to apply at the other local hospital closer to her home, where she really wanted to work, even though there were currently no openings for new graduates.

Renardo said, "I may hold out for the hospital I really want because I would hate to take a position and start orientation, and then find out there were openings in the hospital that is my first choice."

*We thank Kathryn S. Skinner, MS, RN, CS, and Laura H. Day, MS, BSN, RN, for their contributions to this chapter in the fourth edition.

Alice responded, "Not me! I will take the first position I am offered because I can always quit if I get a better offer."

"Even if you have already started orientation?" asked Renardo.

"Yes, sir," Alice said. "I need to do what is best for me and my family."

What are the professional and ethical issues involved in Alice's plans to take a job and quit if a better offer comes along? What are the implications for the hospital and for other new graduates if Alice quits a job at the hospital after only a few weeks or months?

VIGNETTE

"For 2 years I've struggled to meet deadlines for term papers, nursing care plans, and examinations," sighed Leslie. "Now that graduation is almost here, I'm scared that I don't know enough to be a 'real nurse.' And I'm confused about where to begin and what kind of nursing position I should seek. This first job seems so important."

Questions to Consider While Reading This Chapter:

1. How should the new graduate in the scenario decide where to apply for that first position?
2. What kinds of questions should the applicant ask about a prospective position?
3. How can the applicant demonstrate knowledge, skills, and experience to the recruiter?

CHAPTER OVERVIEW

This chapter helps student nurses prepare to successfully negotiate their first employment as professional nurses. It discusses the importance of networking, researching available opportunities, and examining their personal aptitudes, interests, lifestyle priorities, and long-term goals to find the best job fit.

Readers are shown how to create and use cover letters and résumés to market themselves in written introductions and how to prepare for and actively participate in a recruitment interview. The chapter describes what can be expected from a recruiter and how to obtain the information needed to make thoughtful and rewarding job choices. Putting these recommendations into practice will ensure the new graduate of the best chance for finding a good job match as an entry-level nurse practicing in a suitable work environment.

EXPLORING OPTIONS

The job market for graduate nurses is extensive. There are many opportunities in urban as well as rural areas. Health care economics ride a roller coaster from robust to lean times, but the high demand for the skills of professional registered nurses (RNs) remains constant, and the potential for finding suitable employment is good. Trends in health care delivery direct today's health care providers to change their orientation from disease to health and from inpatient to outpatient services, leading to a growing need for professional nurses in nonacute community-based care settings, such as primary care clinics; ambulatory surgery centers; and home, school, and work environments. However, although rapid changes in health care delivery systems continue to create new and varied opportunities outside the acute care settings where nurses have traditionally practiced, hospitals remain the most likely starting place for new graduates to acquire general experience that will be helpful in opening career path doors. In fact, with a nursing shortage there is an increased demand for nurses to work in acute care settings.

Numerous marketing strategies have been tried in an effort to aggressively attract bright, energetic new graduates in times of demand and short supply. For some institutions in selected areas of the country cost seems irrelevant. Sign-on bonuses, promises of tuition reimbursement for continued education, and student loan repayment, just to name a few, have been offered as enticements. However, in other areas of the country, for the first time in several years, it is taking graduates longer to find employment than in the past, when it was common for new graduates to have promises of employment prior to graduation. Ultimately, being aware of one's own qualities and taking advantage of networking opportunities are more important keys to finding just the right match in today's job market.

Knowing Oneself

The choice of a first nursing position deserves careful study. For some, the opportunities seem to be a smorgasbord of possibilities, all of them attractive. The neophyte nurse should carefully explore any job under consideration and its responsibilities in light of their own personal qualities. Some students find it helpful to consult an instructor or a trusted nursing mentor for objective input and perspective. An experienced nurse can see the pros and cons that may not be visible to a new nurse. A thoughtful review of one's general interests, abilities, and strengths (especially those pointed out by clinical instructors) and awareness of the types of patients who have provided the greatest emotional reward are essential.

Other important considerations are one's physical and emotional stamina, energy level, and responsibilities to others—spouse, children, and other family members; volunteer commitments; and social activities—all of which make legitimate demands on one's schedule. Long-term goals must be factored into the first job choice as well. Is the first job a stepping-stone to an advanced degree, to a narrowly specialized area of nursing, to a traveling nurse position, or to a management role? Selection of a position that fits one's abilities, lifestyle, and career aspirations will affect job satisfaction, career advancement, and overall sense of success and happiness.

Be aware that many acute care settings offer transition to practice programs or nurse residency programs that can impact the job search. Some organizations require new graduates to apply for a position in their nurse residency or transition to practice program rather than an open RN position. Once accepted into the residency program, the new graduate is matched to a unit or service line based on their interest, interview, demonstrated ability, and organizational need. Other organizations may require participation in a nurse residency or transition to practice program for new graduates once applicants have accepted a position with the organization in question (C. Crook Clancy, personal communication, September 1, January 24, 2023).

- Finding the right practice environment is essential to long-term success and job satisfaction. The American Association of Colleges of Nursing (AACN, n.d.a) developed a white paper titled *Hallmarks of the Professional Practice Environment*. On the basis of this paper a brochure for nursing school graduates was developed titled "What Every Nursing Student Should Know When Seeking Employment" (AACN, n.d.b). This brochure, which can be downloaded from the website, identifies eight key characteristics, or hallmarks, of the professional practice setting, and suggests that applicants ask the following questions about the employer they are considering. Does the potential employer:

- Manifest a philosophy of clinical care emphasizing quality, safety, interdisciplinary collaboration, continuity of care, and professional accountability?
- Recognize the value of nurses' expertise on clinical care quality and patient outcomes?
- Promote executive-level nursing leadership?
- Empower nurses' participation in clinical decision-making and organization of clinical care systems?
- Demonstrate professional development support for nurses?
- Maintain clinical advancement programs based on education, certification, and advanced preparation?
- Create collaborative relationships among members of the health care team?
- Use technologic advances in clinical care and information systems?

Box 27.1 provides other statistics and information to request from a potential employer. The numbers of hospitals seeking and receiving Magnet hospital credentialing are growing, and where these work environments are available the nurse may wish to consider these organizations. Generally hospitals with Magnet status have demonstrated excellence in areas such as low RN turnover rates, adherence to standards of nursing care as defined by the American Nurses Association (ANA), and mechanisms in place for staff participation in decision-making. Dierkes et al. (2021) found that Magnet hospitals had a more positive nurse work environment and outcomes and

---

BOX 27.1 Statistics and Information That Applicants May Request From a Potential Employer

RN vacancy rate and turnover rate
Patient satisfaction scores (preferably a percentile ranking)
Employee satisfaction scores
Average tenure of nursing staff
Education mix of nursing staff
Percentage of registry or travelers used
Key human resources policies (e.g., reduction in workforce; tenure vs performance criteria)
Copy of the most recent The Joint Commission report on the institution, and the number of contingencies cited
Information about whether the nurses are unionized
Copy of the contract

From American Association of Colleges of Nursing. (2002). *What every nursing school graduate should consider when seeking employment.* American Association of Colleges of Nursing.

were more likely to have specialty-certified nurses and a higher percentage of baccalaureate-prepared nurses. The American Nurses Credentialing Center (ANCC) lists all Magnet hospitals on its website (https://www.clinicalman-agementconsultants.com/ancc-list-of-magnet-recog-nized-hospitals–cid-4457.html).

Many graduate nurses have discovered that working in an environment that did not match well with their personal attributes and long-term goals not only made them unhappy but also damaged their future employment options. Poor job fits lead to frequent job changes, which could lead to poor references and the attachment of the label "job hopper."

Appropriate job choice is critically important and can be costly to the new graduate. Accordingly, an ineffective hiring decision can also be expensive for the employer. Hospitals routinely pay for drug testing and criminal background checks. The preemployment costs alone can tally close to $2000 before the person even steps in the hospital door to begin employment. Classroom and hospital orientation includes the salary of the graduate nurse (GN) and the nursing educators. Additionally, various other paid employees teach mandatory classes, such as infection control and fire safety, and the GN gets an official welcome from the organization's chief nursing officer.

Following the classroom orientation is approximately 4 weeks of classroom and clinical instruction before the nurse arrives on the patient care unit. This time period of one-on-one instruction to review basic nursing skills incurs the cost of not only the GN's salary but the salaries of nursing educators.

Subsequently, assignments are made for the GN to follow a preceptor for the next 8 to 12 weeks, depending on how quickly the nurse achieves competency in each area. This phase of the training process costs the hospital the GN's salary and the preceptor's salary.

The clinical nursing educator, who follows the nurse through completion of orientation to eventual competency, is also paid for the duration of the process. The additional time it takes to teach is another consideration in adding up the cost, a cost to which it is difficult to assign a dollar value. Nurse residency and transition to practice programs may occur concurrently with and extend beyond the orientation period or begin following completion of unit orientation. The nurse residency program coordinator or director, facilitators, and content experts are a considerable organizational investment

in successful transition to practice of newly licensed RNs. Other nonspecific cost considerations include the cost of provision of space required for the education of new staff. Included in this category would be building utilities, engineering staff that support the operation, housekeeping costs, and general administration costs associated with the procurement of new GNs.

- In general the cost of an RN turnover ranges between $33,900 and $58,300, with an overall average of $46,100 in 2021. In comparison, the average cost of an RN turnover was $40,038 in 2020. https://www.advi-sory.com/daily-briefing/2022/10/17/nurse-turnover

Critical to effective selection is high-level nurse leader competency in resource management processes and attention to creation of an effective, healthful practice environment. A great decision on the part of the new graduate and the nurse leader will have better outcomes for the individual nurse in areas of job satisfaction and retention and for overall organizational outcomes in terms of employee engagement and retention and patient outcomes.

Networking

The investigative process of researching potential employers begins with networking at school, in the community, and within student nurse organizations. One may question other nurses, employees, and former employees, especially alumni of one's own school, who have worked in various settings. Faculty will have pertinent observations based on their experiences with clinical sites in the community. It is also valuable to listen to neighbors, friends, and family members who have been patients.

Some employers now offer "phone-a-thons," in which they invite nurses to speak directly with recruiters or nursing department supervisors. Websites, open houses, health care job fairs, and virtual online career events are great places to pick up information about institutions. Recruitment materials and brochures often contain interesting facts about the organization, such as the mission, vision, values statements and goals, available services, and information about associate benefits.

The Internet offers links to actual jobs and information on career planning. Most hospital and large health care systems maintain websites to post their employment needs and invite applications online. The Internet is a cost-effective recruiting method, and larger health care systems expect early communications to take place by fax and e-mail. Applicants who use this method to follow up on a job posting should pay particular attention to the application and résumé that is sent electronically, being sure to follow the online prompts correctly and ensuring there are no errors before submitting materials online. To make sure one's online information is secure one should never share the username or password with anyone. If there is no response to Internet inquiries within a week applicants should follow up with a phone call.

Internet sites are helpful for exploring job opportunities, writing résumés, and preparing for employment interviews. If a new graduate is seeking a position in a large community with multiple job choices available, this informal research will help narrow the list to the best place to begin the job application process. Later in the interview, the applicant may wish to describe to the recruiter how their search resulted in this employer's being the number-one choice over others for the graduate's first job. This process of researching potential employers will continue through the interview process. Assessing the climate of the work environment is a valuable tool in "finding a match" and is discussed more thoroughly later in this chapter.

WRITTEN INTRODUCTIONS

Three of the most important steps in a job search are writing a cover letter, preparing a professional résumé, and assembling a professional portfolio. These tools introduce the applicant to a prospective employer. The first impression should be persuasive; there may not be a second chance. Presenting oneself on paper can make a difference, perhaps the difference between getting a desired interview and being passed over in favor of someone else. These written introductions should present a conscientious, mature, competent, committed professional who would be an asset to an agency that prides itself on its nursing services.

How to Write a Cover Letter

The cover letter is a chance for an applicant to sell themself and make the recruiter look forward to meeting an attractive candidate (Box 27.2). A convincing cover letter will show how this candidate is different and convey to the recruiter why they are the best fit for the position. The letter should also address why this institution is the applicant's first choice.

A cover letter should reflect the nurse's own style of writing, should never appear to have been copied from

---

BOX 27.2   Cover Letter

Bonnie McCray Pino
416 Melody Avenue
Bristol, TN 37620
555-912-3120 (Home)

April 8, 2024

Ms. Donna Henderson, MS, RN
Director of Nurse Recruitment
Charleston Memorial Hospital
1600 Beckley Avenue
Memphis, TN 38104

Dear Ms. Henderson:

I would like to apply for a new graduate position on a cardiology nursing unit at Charleston Memorial Hospital. After graduating from Smith College with a BSN on June 6, I will be ready to start work immediately. I plan to take the RN licensing examination in early July.

Through reading about your hospital and my own personal experience in a recent clinical rotation at Charleston Memorial, I have learned that your institution is a modern, professional one with an emphasis on quality patient care. For this and many other reasons I am convinced that Charleston Memorial is where I want to work as a nurse.

I will be in Memphis from April 20 to April 25 and will call to schedule an appointment to see you then. My home phone number is 555-912-3120; my cell phone number is 555-200-9999.

I look forward to meeting you and discussing how I can contribute to Charleston Memorial Hospital.

Sincerely,
(Name signed here in pen)

Bonnie McCray Pino
Enclosure: Résumé

---

a book, and should be tailored to the particular job. Like any business document it should be clean, direct, and letter perfect. It should be attractive and effortless to read. There must be no typing errors and no grammar or spelling mistakes. Everything should fit on a single page of 8.5" by 11" white heavyweight bond paper with ample margins on the top, bottom, and sides.

The letter should follow a business format with the applicant's name and address at the top in case the cover letter gets separated from the résumé. The letter should be addressed to a specific person. If the person's name or title is unknown, the applicant should refer to a marketing brochure or call the recruitment office to ask for correct title and spelling of the appropriate person's first and last names.

If spelling is not one's strength one should use the spell-check tool on the computer, but should not depend on its accuracy. Using a dictionary and asking a competent friend to proofread the final copy is also a good idea. Poor typists would be well served to pay someone to type for them. A sloppy letter will cast doubt on one's abilities to practice as a professional.

The body of the letter should be single-spaced, three or four block paragraphs long, with blank lines between paragraphs, and organized as follows:

- Paragraph 1 should be a statement of purpose that tells the recruiter what kind of position is being sought, the writer's expected date of graduation, state licensing status, and the date the writer will be ready to begin work.
- Paragraph 2 should emphasize the writer's suitability. The implied message should be "I'm just the person for the job" without going into all the details that will be included in the résumé. A sentence should describe past work or educational experiences that relate to the agency's particular needs and philosophy. The more homework the nurse has done in learning about the institution the more persuaded the recruiter will be. The final sentence should refer to the enclosed résumé.
- Paragraph 3 should request an interview appointment and give a range of dates of availability. It is a good idea for the writer to promise a phone call "next week" or "soon" to schedule a meeting time and to provide a phone number by which the writer can be reached if the number is different from the permanent phone number listed on the résumé.
- The letter can end with a "written handshake" such as, "I look forward to meeting with you to discuss available nursing positions in your institution"—a cautiously optimistic note.
- The letter closes with "Sincerely," and after four lines of space for a signature, the writer's name is typed. A line is skipped and "Enclosure" is typed on the left margin to indicate that a résumé is enclosed.

The letter should be proofread carefully, signed, and copied, and the copy filed. If the nurse has chosen to use different approaches with different institutions, it would be wise to review the appropriate cover letter before each interview.

One week later the writer should follow up by phone to be sure the letter was received. This attention to detail and follow-through will impress the recruiter or personnel office and improve chances of getting an interview soon. These phone calls usually become mini-interviews, and the applicant should be extra courteous, aware that it usually is the secretary who controls the interview schedule. By keeping a written list of all contacts made the new graduate will be able to add the flattering personal touch of acknowledging previous phone contacts when meeting them for the first time during the interview process.

The cover letter serves as the foundation on which all other follow-up is built: résumé, call for appointment, and interview. What is presented in the letter should prompt the person responsible for hiring to take a close look at the enclosed résumé.

How to Prepare a Résumé

A résumé is a short compilation of one's education, work experience, credentials, and accomplishments. In many cases the résumé is the first document a hiring manager will look at when reviewing the application and therefore is a true "first impression." Accordingly, it is important to put time and effort into developing and maintaining an updated, accurate résumé (Box 27.3). The résumé is different from a curriculum vitae (CV), which is a chronologic account of one's entire educational and professional work experience, usually required by academic institutions for educator positions. The résumé is the most appropriate format for the new graduate and will complement the cover letter by filling in important details about educational and work experiences. It is important to provide accurate information because inaccurate information on a résumé or application can lead to dismissal later. An effective résumé should compress education and employment history into an attractive, easy-to-read one-page summary. A wealth of valuable information can be communicated simply and straightforwardly by saying more with less. The key is writing concisely. For example, "BSN with high honors" speaks for itself. Citing exact grade point average or "dean's list" standing adds little. Succinct ways to convey a message can be found by experimenting with phrases and word choices. The writer should avoid pompous language and use of the passive voice, instead using active verbs such as *improved*, *established*, *trained*, *administered*, *prepared*, *wrote*, and *evaluated*.

A basic résumé contains three essential sections: (1) identifying information, (2) education, and (3) work

BOX 27.3 Résumé

Bonnie McCray Pino
416 Melody Avenue
Bristol, TN 37620
555-912-3120 (Home)
555-200-9999 (Cell)
E-mail: bpino@xyz.com

Professional Objective:	**Staff Nurse Position (Cardiology)**
Licensure:	Eligible to take NCLEX examination after June 6, 2021. Anticipated date of NCLEX: July 2021
Education:	
2020 to 2024	Smith College School of Nursing, Bristol, TN BSN, June 4, 2024
2017 to 2020	Oakview High School, Nashville, TN, Diploma, June 2020
Experience:	
June 2018 to August 2018	Drs. Smith and Jones OB/GYN office, Bristol, TN, Office Assistant: Accompanied patients to treatment area, weighed patients, and recorded vital signs
May 2017 to August 2017	St. Mary's Hospital, Knoxville, TN. Patient Care Assistant: Assisted RNs in providing basic nursing care including feeding, bathing, assisting with ADLs, and patient teaching in a pediatric setting
Professional Organizations:	Tennessee Student Nurses Association, 2022–2024
References:	Provided on request

experience. In addition, optional information may include professional objectives, honors, achievements, and memberships in professional organizations. A well-designed résumé marks the writer as a career-minded professional, just what recruiters are seeking. A succinct, well-organized résumé indicates that the applicant is focused and organized in other areas as well.

The first section of the résumé, the identifying information, contains the applicant's name, address, and home and work phone numbers, followed by licensure information. The states of licensure and license numbers are listed. Graduating students should indicate when and where they have taken or will take the National Council of Licensing Examination (NCLEX).

If the résumé writer opts to include a professional objective it should come next. Some interviewers like to see this because it shows that the nurse has put some thought into career planning. The writer should keep in mind, though, that it is limiting to put forth a singular objective that ties the nurse to only one particular clinical area. If there is no such opening available in that department the recruiter will consider the applicant an unlikely candidate to pursue. It is better to have an objective statement that is broad and general.

The second section should include details about education, including degrees and diplomas awarded, names and locations of schools, and graduation dates, starting with the most recent graduation and degree and going in reverse chronologic order.

The third section presents the information apt to be the greatest help in obtaining a job: work experience and employment history. Many recruiters are nurses themselves so a detailed description of what a routine job entails is not needed. Instead efforts should be directed toward illustrating any special knowledge or contributions. The new graduate's résumé might reflect student accomplishments or elaborate on jobs in which they have demonstrated skills also applicable to nursing responsibilities, such as organization of tasks, time management, delegation to subordinates, and ability to work well with others. The summary should start with the current or most-recent position and work chronologically backward, including places of employment, job titles, dates worked, and responsibilities. Accomplishments during employment should be listed, including number and type of patients cared for, any special techniques used, or any participation in the development of programs, policies, or forms pertinent to the position.

This section closes with optional information, such as seminars attended, honors received, and memberships in professional organizations. It is not advisable to list community activities or activities from more than 5 years ago unless it can be clearly shown that they are pertinent to a nursing career. Similarly, personal information—such as marital and health status, age, number of children, and hobbies—should be excluded. This information is not job related and should not be used by the employer to screen applicants.

References do not need to be included in the résumé but should be ready for presentation in a neatly typed list when requested from any future employer. The résumé should conclude with the simple statement "References provided on request" or "References available." When someone agrees to be listed as a reference the applicant should take time to discuss with them what prospective employers may want to know. Former instructors or former employers may require written permission before releasing information. As the job search continues the nurse should keep references informed of the names of employers who may be inquiring.

The résumé should be produced neatly and inexpensively on a computer because a good résumé will be used repeatedly with revisions, and the nurse will want to be able to produce an up-to-date version without completely rewriting it. Production methods should be kept as simple as possible. Many tools and templates are available in most word processing software programs for résumé building and formatting. It is not necessary to go to the added trouble and expense of having the résumé professionally typeset and printed. Having it neatly typed and reproduced using good-quality photocopying services suffices. These resources as well as laser/color printers are available at public or university libraries. To make the text easy to read one style of serif font should be used throughout, in 11- or 12-point size. Again the applicant should have someone review the final copy for typing errors, then use a photocopying service for "quick copying" onto good-quality white or ivory paper. It is important to remember that when it comes to résumés appearances do count. A well-formatted résumé that is properly organized and neatly typed makes a great first impression.

How to Prepare a Portfolio

The nursing portfolio contains more information than a résumé and provides documentation to support the résumé. As health professionals nurses are responsible for staying abreast of current professional knowledge and managing their own careers and professional growth and development. Ideally practices to support these activities should start during their student years. Professional development is a lifelong and continuous process, which is essential to the maintenance of clinical skills and knowledge required in today's ever-changing health care environment. By creating a professional portfolio a professional may showcase personal and professional development, practice excellence, and clinical leadership. Portfolio compilation gives one an opportunity to assess abilities, identify learning goals, and devise a plan for further personal and professional development. In addition to validating accomplishments and highlighting milestones, this tool may illustrate a professional's progression along the continuum from novice to expert.

The portfolio introduces the professional nurse to recruiters, employers, admissions committees, and potential supervisors in a visual and tangible way. It includes traditional documents, such as a résumé, license to practice and certifications, educational documents (e.g., diplomas, transcripts), and examples of significant professional, community, and student activities (Box 27.4).

The simplest way to build a portfolio is to start with an attractive three-ring binder. A table of contents gives interviewers a map to guide their review of the information. Dividers can separate sections, each with its own

---

BOX 27.4 Documents for a Professional Portfolio

Professional Credentials
Résumé
Licenses
Certifications
Specialty practice certifications
Basic cardiac life support (BCLS)
Advanced cardiac life support (ACLS)

Educational Credentials
Diplomas
Transcripts
Continuing education certificates
Honors and awards (including program from awards ceremony, letters regarding awards, newspaper articles)

Research and Scholarly Activity
Publications
Evidence-based Practice Project or Quality Improvement Project Title
Teaching materials for patients, staff, handouts
Case studies
Photo of poster sessions, classroom presentations
PowerPoint outline of presentation
Student papers and projects

Professional Activities
Membership cards
Evidence of service as an officer or leader in student organizations
Community involvement and volunteer activities
Performance evaluations
Letters of recommendation

cover page, and plastic sleeves or pocketed pages work well to hold loose items. Appropriate documents are assigned to each section. Copies should be made of important originals, such as diplomas, certifications, and licenses that would be difficult to replace. Samples of letters from grateful patients, congratulations from peers, and complimentary notes from supervisors should be included. Sentences in longer letters or performance appraisals that address the information considered to be most important for the reader to note should be highlighted. The GN may want to include supervisor evaluations from nonnursing positions to demonstrate leadership qualities, dependability, and attention to detail, characteristics also relevant to the nursing work setting.

Interest in electronic portfolios, or e-portfolios, is gathering momentum as a strategy for fostering lifelong learning and enhancing ongoing personal and professional development. The e-portfolio can represent an authentic means of assessing cognitive, reflective, and affective skills. Furthermore, e-portfolios provide a means through which nurses can record and provide evidence of skills, achievements, experience, professional development, and ongoing learning, not only for themselves but also for the informing and scrutiny of registration boards, employers, managers, and peers (Holtzman et al., 2022).

Graduation is the perfect time to create a career portfolio, one that will be easy to build on and update as one's nursing career evolves. If documents are created on the computer, updates and revisions will be easy when the nurse pursues new and different professional roles and responsibilities. Many baccalaureate educational programs require students to create such a portfolio as part of their preparation for graduation and entry into the first job. Nurses who present portfolios to the recruiter may have a competitive edge over nurses who do not; increasingly, boards of nursing and many specialty organizations are making portfolios (or other methods of documenting evidence of competency) mandatory for relicensure and recertification. Continuing education and testing provide a limited picture of an individual's knowledge and/or skill acquisition in a limited area at one point in time. However, portfolios promote critical thinking, self-assessment, and individual accountability. A portfolio is a portable mechanism for evaluating competencies that may otherwise be difficult to assess.

HOW TO INTERVIEW EFFECTIVELY

No matter how qualified and self-confident a person may feel, sitting across the desk from an interviewer can be intimidating. One's conduct in the recruiter's office may determine whether a job offer is made. Being a little anxious is normal but panic is not. When the applicant has made a good first impression in the cover letter and résumé they can expect to be called for an interview. The graduate's task then becomes to enter the interview prepared to answer and ask questions that will help determine whether this organization, with its available job opportunities, is a good match.

Every agency has its own hiring and interviewing policies. Generally the smaller the organization and the more decentralized the nursing department, the more involved the lower-level manager is in the recruitment and hiring process. The same person who interviews nurse applicants also may be the manager, staff development instructor, quality assurance director, employee health nurse, or chair of the product standards committee. A large organization with many employees may have a separate human resources department with a nurse recruiter on staff. Within such large organizations the hiring process becomes more complicated and more formal; applicants are more tightly screened, and the hiring decisions are further removed from the actual work position.

Increasingly, hospitals are conducting panel interviews. A panel interview can be more efficient because several people can be in the room together and all have the same experience. The interviewers learn from the responses to one another's questions. Some organizations find this approach to be the easiest way to reach consensus on job candidates. If the applicant knows a panel interview is a possibility, they should learn as much as possible about the panel members and the departments they represent (C. Crook Clancy, personal communication, 2021).

Some "nurse recruiters" are not nurses themselves, a situation that may make a difference in the kind of information exchanged in the interview. A nonnurse is not likely to be able to fully discuss questions that pertain directly to a nurse's job description, patient care workload, and nursing responsibilities. Also, the applicant does not have to answer questions that are not job related. In fact some questions are not legally allowed to be asked (Box 27.5). After a job offer is made the prospective employer may ask certain non–job-related questions but not

BOX 27.5 Legal and Illegal Areas of Questioning

Some questions are inappropriate to be asked of an applicant before a job offer is made.

Legal	Illegal
Educational preparation	Race
Licensure preparation	Creed
Licensure status	Color
Work experience	Age
Reasons for leaving previous jobs	Nationality
	Marital status
Reasons for applying to this institution	Sexual preference
	Religious beliefs
Qualifications for this job	Number of children or dependents
Strengths and weaknesses	
Criminal convictions	Financial or credit status

before. They should not be a part of deciding whether the applicant is offered a position.

How to Prepare: Planning Ahead

It is recommended that interview appointments be made as early as possible and that senior students not wait until graduation day. Ideally interviews should be scheduled at least 2 months prior to graduation. Job hunting takes time, and appointments are not easily scheduled near nursing school graduation dates, times that tend to be busy weeks for recruiters.

How to Prepare: Self-Talk

As the day approached Mary obsessed about the interview, thinking to herself, "What if they ask me something I cannot answer, and I go blank like I used to do in clinicals when the instructor quizzed me about my patient's medicines? I will look like an idiot, and maybe even start to cry." The night before the appointment Mary could not sleep.

One's thoughts dictate one's reality. Nurses, especially new nurses, should be aware of what they are saying to themselves. The applicant who thinks "Why would anyone want to hire a GN like me with no practical experience?" will project a lack of self-trust that may be interpreted by the recruiter as a lack of enthusiasm or even incompetence. However, a confident graduate's self-talk may be something like this: "I have successfully completed a difficult nursing course of study. I am now ready to take on the responsibilities of a professional. With orientation, on-the-job training, and the support of experienced nurses I can succeed as an RN. I have everything I need to begin practice." This reality-based self-talk is an important internal dialogue for establishing feelings of confidence before the job interview.

The reality is that all graduates have met the criteria for graduation from a nursing education program and have been deemed ready by that credentialing body for entry-level positions as RNs. The final test of competence to practice, the NCLEX examination, will provide further proof. GNs who fear failure of this final test must remind themselves of those now successfully practicing who preceded them from the same educational program with the same preparation.

How to Prepare: Rehearse

A simple visualization of how the graduate wants to appear to the recruiter can bring about the self-assurance needed to create an attractive candidate. It is helpful to mentally review and to be prepared to describe pride in any past work experiences, especially the parts of any job that relate to what is required of a nurse. Even babysitting jobs can validate a worker as a responsible adult if that person worked consistently for the same family and showed stability and good judgment as a trusted caretaker for children. Applicants tend to discount minimum-wage, part-time, adolescent, or summer employment, but these experiences often reveal a great deal about the applicant: Would attendance records attest to the worker's dependability? Was the worker given greater responsibility over time? Was the worker allowed to open or close the business? Handle the cash receipts? Consider Case Study 27.1.

Remember that it is not only the graduate's academic standing or honors and awards that measure success as a student. Perhaps the student was not in the top 10% of the class but was active in student affairs. Perhaps the student was chair of a student government committee or a contributor to the campus newspaper. The graduate should be prepared to describe other areas of student accomplishments.

Unfortunately many nurses are not accustomed to selling themselves and are uncomfortable in situations in which they need to discuss their best attributes and market their qualifications. Therefore after rehearsing in one's own mind how to present these qualifications to interviewers it would be wise to rehearse with another person, role-playing the expected interview dialogue.

CASE STUDY 27.1

The only job Sam had before nursing school had been working at the customer service desk at a large children's toy store, where he scheduled and supervised the cashiers. His title was "designated key carrier," which he listed on his résumé. The interviewer reasonably interpreted this to be a position that demonstrated the employer's trust in Sam.

BOX 27.6 Applicants' Rights

Applicants have the right to:

- Be informed of available positions at an institution and the minimal qualifications required.
- Apply for any available position for which they are qualified.
- Be seriously and fairly considered for any available position for which they are qualified.
- Be interviewed, be shown a job description, and be made aware of the requirements and expectations of the job.
- Have the work schedule discussed.
- Be informed of the benefits package.
- See the nursing unit and meet the manager if they are being considered seriously.
- Be made aware of the orientation program.
- Be given an expected time by which a decision will be made.

The nurse should role-play with another student or an experienced nurse (even better), rehearsing answers to questions the interviewer is expected to ask, and practicing descriptions of the key points of past employment. A few minutes spent in rehearsing with another person will contribute to composure and self-confidence in the actual situation.

Finally, it is important for the graduate to remember that the job interview is not an examination to pass or fail nor is it an interrogation. It is an exchange of information—the recruiter hoping to find a potential employee to fill a staff vacancy, and the applicant hoping to find employment as a nurse in this organization. Each has responsibilities for informing the other, and each has rights to obtain information from the other (Box 27.6).

The Phone Interview

Phone interviews are becoming a standard first step to narrowing down the applicant pool, and they minimize travel expenses for out-of-town applicants. The purpose of the phone interview is to screen applicants and determine which ones to invite for a face-to-face interview. The applicant should be prepared for the interview just as if it were an in-person interview. Use a quiet, comfortable, and private space with no distractions so you can focus on the interview.

If you'll be using your cell phone make sure it's fully charged and you are in a spot with good reception for the call. You may also find that standing during an interview helps you sound more energetic during the call.

Review these guidelines for appropriate phone interview etiquette so you make the best impression on your interviewer.

Answer the Phone Yourself. First, be sure to let family members and/or roommates know you are expecting a call. When you answer the phone respond with your name. You can say, "This is Jane Doe" or "John Smith speaking!" That way the interviewer will know they've reached the right person. Make sure to use an upbeat tone of voice (try smiling as you speak).

Follow the Interviewer's Lead. Some interviewers may wish to engage in a few minutes of small talk. Others may want to get right into the interview. Let the interviewer steer the start to the conversation but be prepared to talk about the weather or make other small talk.

Listen carefully to the interviewer and don't start speaking until the interviewer finishes the question. If you have something you want to say jot it down on your notepad and mention it when it's your turn to talk. It can also be helpful to jot down the question (or at least some keywords).

Don't worry if you need a few seconds to think of a response, but don't leave too much dead air. If you need the interviewer to repeat the question, ask.

Many job applicants have found it helpful to dress in business attire for the interview because it makes them feel and act more professionally. The applicant should control the surroundings by eliminating distracting background noise. Whether the interviewer is calling the applicant or vice versa, the applicant should be ready before the appointed time, anticipate any time zone differences, and respect the employer's time constraints. The applicant should also eliminate any possible distractions from the phone room by (1) making sure children and pets are quiet; (2) putting a "do not ring or knock" sign on the door; and (3) turning off call waiting, cell phones, music, and television sets. The résumé should be printed out, a pen and paper should be ready for note-taking, and a glass of water should be nearby in case of a dry throat. The applicant should have a list of thoughtful questions available to ask the interviewer(s). Standing may make the applicant sound more confident, and smiling can be heard in the voice (Doyle, 2020a).

In preparation for a phone interview or a call from a potential employer it is wise to make sure one's voice-mail message sounds professional. Although friends may enjoy listening to a favorite band or sarcastic message, the potential employer might find it unprofessional (Doyle, 2020a). The same caution goes for social media. It is important to remember that the messages and pictures posted on YouTube, MySpace, Facebook, Twitter, or other Internet websites are generally not private. Potential employers often research applicants' social media presence during the screening phase of the employment process (Doyle, 2020a).

How to Prepare: The Interview Itself

Dress Appropriately. Business-appropriate clothing, such as a neat dress, suit, or pantsuit, projects a professional attitude. Casual attire projects a casual attitude. Jeans are not acceptable, nor are shorts, tennis shoes, flip-flops, or any clothes that are too short, too tight, too revealing, or too trendy. Conservative and simple are always best. When people are dressed to look their best their attitudes improve and levels of self-confidence increase. Makeup should be light, and the use of perfume or cologne should be avoided. Most institutions are fragrance free because of patients' and employees' allergic reactions to perfumes. Large, distracting jewelry should be avoided. Applicants who have lots of piercings should wear only earrings; tattoos should be covered. Smartphones should be muted or put on vibrate during the interview. Applicants should also avoid distracting behavior such as chewing gum and drinking coffee or other beverages.

Arrive on Time. Arriving late for a job interview creates a poor first impression. The applicant should be considerate of the interviewer's time and agenda. If delayed they should call to reschedule. Arriving too early can make the interviewer feel rushed or the applicant appear overanxious; however, 10 to 15 minutes early is a reasonable target.

Bring a Résumé. Even if a résumé has already been submitted the applicant should bring extra copies. The recruiter may have routed the mailed copy to a manager for review. Applicants probably will be asked to complete an employment application, and the résumé is a ready reference for past employers and dates of employment. A Social Security card, driver's license, and nursing license, if available, also will be requested as necessary parts of the identification process. Some agencies request that a current cardiopulmonary resuscitation card be made available to photocopy. These documents will be easy to produce if the applicant has also brought a professional portfolio folder.

Video Interviewing

Skype and Zoom, online phone and video Internet services, are being used to conduct long-distance initial interviews. Advance preparations should include (Doyle, 2020b):

- Downloading software.
- Conducting a quick test the morning of the interview to make sure the camera and the microphone are working.
- Considering your appearance: It is important to choose colors that look good on video, such as blue, rather than colors that may look too bright, like red. Patterns can be less attractive than solids, so think about a pattern that will not be distracting to your viewer. During the video interview it is important to remember to smile and focus direct eye contact.
- Remembering the background that the viewer will see and hear. Are you sitting so that a blank wall is behind you or is there a cluttered bookshelf behind you? Set up the webcam accordingly. Is the space quiet and unlikely to have distracting background noise?
- Having a few notes written down about what you would like to talk about and a pen handy to jot down thoughts for additional comments you think of to add during the conversation is important.

The Face-to-Face Interview

The in-person interview is the most time-consuming and subjective part of the employment process. For professionals it is appropriate for interviews to be unstructured, using open-ended questions (see Box 27.7); both recruiter and applicant will have questions. Many organizations conduct panel interviews including as many as

BOX 27.7   Open-Ended Interview Questions

Applicants may expect to be asked a series of open-ended questions such as:

- How do you evaluate success?
- How would you describe yourself?
- Tell me about yourself.
- Tell me about something that's not on your résumé.
- What is your greatest strength?
- How will your greatest strength help you perform?
- What challenges are you looking for in a position?
- What are your goals for the future?
- How do you handle conflict?
- What is your greatest weakness?
- Why are you leaving your job?
- How do you handle stress and pressure?
- What motivates you?
- What do you find are the most difficult decisions to make?
- What are you passionate about?
- Why are you the best person for the job?

From Doyle, A. (2019). *Open-ended job interview questions and answers.* The Balance: Careers. https://www.thebalancecareers.com/open-ended-interview-questions-and-answers-2061635

6 to 8 interviewers and subsequent interviews with a clinical manger on the unit. Other organizations may schedule individual interviews with the nurse recruiter, nurse manager, and a staff RN. Hospital tours are often part of the interview process. The interview process can be expected to last as long as 4 hours. It is important to maintain professional communication with direct eye contact and to avoid casual chatter about things that are unrelated to the job. Being prepared is key and planning answers to the questions most likely to be asked is the best way to prepare. Nine of the most frequently asked questions follow. Mentally reviewing practiced responses to these questions will give the applicant confidence.

1. What Positions Interest You? The interviewer needs to know whether there are positions available in the applicant's area of interest and whether the applicant has the required qualifications to fit the vacant positions. If there is no fit in interest or qualifications with jobs available, neither applicant nor recruiter needs to waste more time in the interview.

Because titles and position names vary from organization to organization, it is better to answer the question with favorite clinical experiences. Applicants might share short- and long-term goals and how they visualize laying the groundwork today for tomorrow's professional roles. A good response might be, "I'm interested in a position that will help me grow as a professional and give me opportunities to develop greater competency as a nurse. Ultimately I would like to work as a critical care clinical nurse specialist." If interest, qualifications, and the available positions match, the interviewer will want to start planning secondary interviews and tours.

2. Tell Me About Your Work History. Even if previous jobs were not nursing related, the applicant can highlight the responsibilities carried out, the skills acquired, and how these skills can transfer to the professional nursing role. This is the point at which the interviewer will get an idea of motivation, drive, energy level, and reliability. No new graduate will be expected to have all the knowledge and skills of an experienced RN; however, when answering the graduate may stress other aptitudes, such as verbal skills or interpersonal skills. It is best to start with the current or most recent job and proceed backward. A new graduate might discuss student clinical experiences, which clinical areas were favored, and why.

3. How Did You Choose to Apply for a Job Here? Any previous investigative homework done on the institution is useful and helps form honest responses. For example, an applicant might say, "This hospital has a reputation for its quality care, and I like that," or "I am interested in research and have heard you have a nursing research committee for staff nurses."

4. Do You Want a Full-Time or Part-Time Position, and Which Shift Do You Prefer? If there is a need or desire for a particular schedule the nurse should be honest and ask for that schedule. If the recruiter does not have that schedule available ask what is available so that a decision can be made. Can the nurse be flexible to accept an undesirable shift until a preferred one becomes available? Part of one's investigation of an institution should include looking at a current list of posted positions. Particularly with smaller agencies, if what the nurse desires is not posted it may be beneficial to ask for a particular schedule but, if willing, express an interest in working a schedule that is posted. For example, "I'm willing to work the evening shift posted for the medical-surgical unit; however, I'm most interested in moving into a day position in labor and delivery."

5. and 6. What Are Your Strengths/Weaknesses? Sometimes these questions may be asked in less direct ways, such as, "What are some of the areas you know you need to improve?" or "How have your skills developed in your advanced nursing courses?" Honesty always is best. In asking this question the interviewer may only be trying to pinpoint the special skills and preferences of the nurse. For example, with which kind of patients has the nurse been most effective, and which ones proved most difficult? The clearer the applicant can be in articulating specific talents and deficiencies, the more closely the recruiter will be able to match the candidate to a position suited to their abilities. The closer these match, the more likely the employee will flourish and be able to use special talents.

It is not advisable to avoid the issue of weaknesses. Everyone has them. It is better to admit them but to present them in a positive way. In addition, it may be helpful to tell the interviewer what is being done to correct weaknesses. For example, "Sometimes I tend to see the big picture and have to remind myself to pay more attention to the details. I've started keeping lists, and they seem helpful." Another suggestion might be, "I have limited bedside nursing experience, but I am excited about building on the clinical skills I have learned in school."

7. What Would You Do If ...? The recruiter probably will ask some situational questions related to decision-making and critical thinking skills. The nurse will be asked to explain how to assess a particular situation, set priorities, decide what should be implemented first for a patient, and what can be delegated. Rather than fabricate an answer about unfamiliar circumstances, one can honestly say, "I've never been in that situation, but I think I would ..." or "I was in a similar situation in which ... occurred, and this is what I did in that circumstance."

When an interviewer says, "Tell me about a time when ..." or "Give me a specific example of ...," they are conducting a behavioral interview. The applicant must be prepared to respond to these questions because many employers use a behavioral interview as part of the hiring process for nursing positions (LaMaster & Larsen, 2010). This type of job interview is based on the logic that past behavior predicts future behavior and seeks previous experience of required job-related behaviors. If the job requires the ability to analyze and find solutions to problems, then the candidate may be asked to provide an example of when they previously found solutions to a difficult problem. The question might be: "Tell me about a time when you faced a difficult problem. What steps did you take to solve that problem?" Examples may be taken from any context as long as they include the required behavior. The applicant should remember that there are no right or wrong answers to this question.

8. Why Should We Hire You? This question gives the applicant an opportunity to share their special assets that the applicant would bring to the employer's institution. Without embellishment or selling oneself short, it is important to convey pride in being a nurse and conviction that one has something special to offer.

9. What Questions Do You Have? Usually the interview ends with the interviewer asking whether the applicant has any questions. This is an opportunity for the applicant to demonstrate initiative, and they should take advantage of it, although not to excess. In an effective interview with an experienced interviewer most questions regarding salary, benefits, and human resource policies will have been addressed (Box 27.8). If they have not been addressed this is the time they should be asked about. Should a tour of the nursing unit and a meeting with the supervisor be arranged many such concerns will be answered then.

Further Questions. Box 27.7 presents an additional list of open-ended interview questions that the applicant may be asked, and Box 27.9 lists questions appropriate for the applicant to ask. The more information gathered, the easier it will be to make a decision, and the more likely it is that the nurse will be happy in the long term.

Simulation or Circuit Interviewing

Simulation or circuit interviews are a newer form of interviewing. Applicants are asked to participate in brief simulations and/or interviews with a variety of organization leaders and educators. This style of interviewing can vary among organizations based on facility space and accommodations. An advantage to this type of interview is the applicant can demonstrate abilities in addition to answering behavioral-based questions (C. Crook Clancy, personal communication, January 24, 2021).

BOX 27.8 What to Expect a Recruiter to Communicate

Recruiters should inform applicants of basic human resource policies regarding job descriptions, compensation, benefits, and staff development, including:

- Conditional period
- Job descriptions
- Shift rotation
- Weekend rotation
- Salary
- Staff development
- Parking
- Security
- Health insurance and other insurance benefits
- Preemployment physical examinations
- Credit union
- Overtime
- Scheduled paydays
- Paid time off
- Leaves of absence
- Employee discounts
- Transfer and promotion policies
- Resignation policies
- Preemployment policies
- Pay increases

BOX 27.9 Appropriate Questions for the Applicant to Ask

1. May I see the job description for the position we are discussing?
2. What is the nurse-to-patient ratio?
3. What support staff are available on the unit to assist nurses?
4. What about clerical help and support services? What nursing care delivery systems or models are practiced here (e.g., team nursing, primary nursing, centralized, decentralized)?
5. How available are physicians? Admitting physicians and house staff?
6. How often are nursing care conferences held on this unit?
7. What type of nursing documentation is used?
8. How long is the orientation program? What does the program include? What continuing education programs are available after my initial orientation?
9. How will my performance be evaluated? How often and by whom?
10. What exact schedule or shift will I be working in this position?
11. What will my salary be? Is there a shift differential?
12. Are there differentiated practice levels or roles and differentiated pay scales for nursing congruent with differences in educational preparation, certification, and other advanced nursing preparation?
13. How are pay increases decided?
14. What other benefits are there (e.g., health, life insurance, vacation time, tuition reimbursement, retirement plan)?
15. What input do staff nurses have in decision-making about nursing practice?
16. What is the work culture?

THE APPLICANT'S TASKS

Assess the Climate of the Work Environment

As mentioned in the discussion of researching potential employers, there are ways other than direct questioning to learn a lot about the institution. Every organization has its own personality and atmosphere. The first impression probably came from the secretary who answered the phone when the applicant called for an appointment with the recruiter, followed by the greeting on arrival at the recruiter's office. A tone of respect and pride in being associated with the organization may have been communicated in the first encounter. Every subsequent encounter builds on the first.

In the hallways of the agency how do people acknowledge each other? A visit to the employee cafeteria to buy a cup of coffee or a sandwich at mealtime can be enlightening. Are nurses eating there? Does it seem that the staff members are enjoying themselves? The applicant should pick up for later reading any available in-house publications, such as employee newsletters or bulletins.

Ask for a Tour

If the interviewer does not automatically offer a tour of the unit the applicant can request to see it and will certainly want to meet with the person who would be the immediate supervisor. Some employers arrange for the recruit to actually shadow a staff nurse for part of a shift. To get an accurate feel for the unit the applicant should pay close attention to the pace, the tone of the staff interaction, and the morale. Is this a group the prospective employee would like to join? Are the manager's philosophy and management style similar to the applicant's own?

The astute applicant can get an accurate feel for the nursing unit's culture and personality by observing the manager's interactions with staff. Is the manager accessible to the staff and supportive in response to them? How are phone calls and other interruptions handled? How well do people seem to be getting along? The applicant should pay attention to the way people on the unit relate to each other—nurses to physicians, nurses to families, nurses to nurses. How are the patients responded to on the intercommunication system? The efficiency with which staff work should be noted. How rushed are they? Also, bulletin boards and any public displays of staff recognition (e.g., "employee of the month" plaques or brag boards) should be examined. Even a second visit to the unit might be requested before a final decision is made. The more information gathered the easier it will be to make a decision (DeLuca & DeLuca, 2010).

Some managers offer opportunities for the applicant to meet with staff, and formal interviews with staff nurses may be scheduled as a routine part of the hiring process. It is important for the applicant to realize that even the informal peer interview is important because the peer is assessing the applicant and will provide a recommendation regarding hiring. Such experiences give the applicant a closer view of the actual work organization and enable representative staff members a chance to have a voice in selecting new coworkers. Staff nurses provide bedside care to patients and best understand the qualities appreciated in a good team member. Whether the introduction to staff is a formal interview or a casual conference room encounter, the applicant can be made to feel welcome and wanted while learning about the real work and the real workers of the agency. Once firsthand knowledge has been obtained, if the applicant confers again with these employees and former employees before applying, they can ask more informed questions.

Follow-Up

Thank-You Letter. A follow-up letter thanking the recruiter is a courtesy and a reminder of the nurse's interest in receiving a timely response. It is also a final chance for the applicant to make the case for being chosen for the role and to inquire about when a hiring decision will be made (Box 27.10). If the nurse does not hear from the employer within a reasonable length of time (1 to 2 weeks) after the interview, it is appropriate to inquire by phone about the status of a hiring decision.

BOX 27.10 **Interview Follow-up Letter**

May 18, 2024
Ms. Donna Henderson, MS, RN
Director of Nurse Recruitment
Charleston Memorial Hospital
1600 Beckley Avenue
Memphis, TN 38104

Dear Ms. Henderson:

It was a pleasure meeting with you on Monday. I now have a clear picture of what I might expect as a new graduate nurse in your hospital. Everyone on the units I visited was very friendly.

I look forward to hearing from you with good news about a position at Charleston Memorial. I can be reached in the afternoons at 555-912-3120 or on my cell, 555-200-9999.

Thank you again for your time and interest.

Sincerely,
(Name signed here in pen)

Bonnie McCray Pino

Avoid Impulse Decisions. If offered a position and time is needed to make a decision the applicant should postpone a decision and should not feel pressured into acceptance while still unsure. An offer to phone the recruiter with an answer within an agreed-on time is appropriate.

If there are other job opportunities, certainly comparisons need to be made by weighing the pros and cons of each position and each organization. How do benefits compare? What are the possibilities for lateral and vertical movement within the systems? How available are continuing education opportunities to staff nurses? How do observations of the work culture fit with the nurse's ideas of what is needed to support professional success? Does the schedule that is offered fit the applicant's lifestyle? When a decision has been reached a phone call should be made promptly to the recruiter, whether the answer is yes or no.

Weighing Options. Applicants should take time to weigh options, especially if they have applied to several different organizations. It is not professional to accept a position while knowing one would resign if a more appealing offer came along. Employers invest significant resources in orienting a new nurse and should expect a commitment rather than the casual attitude of "I'll keep this job until the job I really want becomes available." What questions might one ask oneself while weighing the merits of one position against others? Remembering that no job is perfect, the following four questions should be considered. Box 27.11 further helps applicants evaluate potential employment opportunities.

Does the position match the nurse's qualifications? Although it is flattering to receive a job offer for a position for which a nurse has little or no preparation, one should not be influenced by such a compliment. When there is a nursing shortage a position that is beyond an applicant's present skills and experience may sound wonderfully challenging, but in actuality it may be overwhelming and a disastrous beginning for a new graduate. Being overzealous, overconfident, and overeager to please can only lead to feelings of guilt and inadequacy if the job is not appropriate. It is wiser to accept a position in which adequate orientation and clinical support exist, which would allow the graduate to gain the experience and preparation necessary to accept a position requiring more skills at a later time.

What are the actual responsibilities of the job? The newly hired nurse has the right to completely understand what will be expected in the position offered, including the overall and daily responsibilities and the length and nature of on-the-job training that will be provided. What will be the supervisory responsibilities? How many and what skill level of employees will be under the RN's leadership? What orientation is planned to prepare the RN for practicing independently? Are there arrangements for a preceptor to guide the graduate through the difficult transition of entering a first nursing job? Reality shock can be anticipated, and the more assistance a new graduate receives in adjusting to the new role of the nurse the more likely the beginner is to be successful and satisfied.

Does this position lead the nurse in the direction of projected career goals? Is the offered job a step toward meeting long-term career objectives? For example, a graduate who wants to be a nurse-midwife would be wiser to accept a position in postpartum if labor and delivery is not available rather than a position in neurosurgery just because it offers a slightly higher salary or a few more weekends. No position or job change should be accidental or the result of a snap decision. Wise career moves result from deliberate planning and purposeful preparation.

How will the work be compensated? Experienced nurses often advise novices that money, although important, is not the only reward associated with a job. However, money does matter, especially to a new graduate who may have subsisted on a limited income while in school. It is common for loans to have accumulated, along with unpaid bills. Inadequate salary can be a real source of job dissatisfaction, of course, but because of the 24-hour responsibilities in health care nurses traditionally have basic salaries that include other income-contributing factors, such as shift differentials, weekend differentials, holiday pay, paid vacation days, and expected salary increases over time. Compensation comes in other packages besides paychecks. There are policies that allow for maternity leaves, medical leaves, tuition reimbursement, sick days, discounts on prescriptions and health insurance, retirement benefits, and malpractice insurance coverage, all of which affect income in indirect but important ways. As is true in other areas of consideration, the better the total compensation package fits one's needs, the greater the likelihood that one will remain satisfied with the job.

Well-prepared job applicants will have listed those benefits they consider essential, and these vary with individual circumstances. For example, the essentials for someone who is the sole family breadwinner probably include health insurance, paid time off, and an employer-provided retirement plan. Available child care would be especially important for parents of preschool children.

THE EMPLOYER'S TASKS

In any agency providing nursing services its nurses are the indispensable employees. The selection of new nurse employees is a critically important responsibility, and it is the recruiter's duty to make sure the best selection is made.

First the nurse must meet the minimal requirements for the position desired. For example, 1 year of experience might be required for a nurse to work a weekender program or in a critical care area. Operating room (OR) experience may be required for OR nursing positions, and perinatal nursing experience may be required for labor and delivery positions. A secondary consideration is the nurse's suitability for contributing to the mission of the health care delivery system. The recruiter is selling the organization to the applicant and measuring the skills and aptitudes the applicant would bring to the organization.

The bottom line for any employer who provides health care services to the public is to ensure that its nursing staff practice safely. Recruiters are looking to uncover anything that would impair a nurse applicant's ability to provide safe nursing care, such as incompetence, unprofessional conduct, unreliability in attendance, chemical dependency, or record of criminal activity. For screening recruiters have four primary sources of information: the application, interview impressions, test results, and references.

Applications are validated. Work history and references are checked to ensure accuracy. Many employers are checking credit history because they may assume that an individual who has good credit is reliable and accountable and will likely be a dependable nurse. Previous supervisors are asked about attendance, dependability, performance, attitude, ability to get along with others, integrity, and eligibility for rehire. The applicant's stated reason for termination is compared with information obtained from work references. The employer has a right to obtain reasonable information about the people who are hired. Most employment applications ask whether the applicant has ever been convicted of a crime other than a minor traffic violation. The question is about convictions, not arrests, and the response is verified by a background or criminal record check. Response to this or any other question in the application process must be honest and truthful. Each institution has its own policies regarding convictions, but most are vitally concerned about their responsibilities regarding negligent hiring. The applicant is rejected if they committed a crime that, if repeated while in the employ of the institution, would cause harm to patients, families, other employees, or the institution.

A physical examination is often required. It usually is performed on-site and at the employer's expense. It may involve obtaining the applicant's full medical history and vital signs, routine blood tests, a urine drug screen, and sometimes a chest radiograph. The purpose of the examination is to provide protection for patients and to ensure that the caregiver can carry out the necessary physical responsibilities of the job. For example, are illegal mood-altering substances evident that would impair the nurse's abilities and judgment? Are there physical limitations the institution should know about to determine whether any special accommodations are necessary to allow the candidate to perform the usual duties associated with the position? Employers may do job function matching, a process to determine whether the applicant has the physical capability to perform functions such as bending or stooping required by a specific job. Psychological testing is also frequently part of the preemployment screening process.

Even with a job offer made and a date for employment set, actual start dates are contingent on receipt of documentation of these final screenings, plus a reference check to verify the résumé; these items establish the practitioner's safety and reliability. Other parts of screening for safety might include paper-and-pencil testing, such as skills tests, pharmacology tests, and, in some cases, personality testing and psychologic testing for specialty areas. Some screening assessments such as personality testing may be completed prior to the interview.

Although a preemployment pharmacology test is becoming less common, many institutions still give such a quiz to determine basic knowledge of routinely administered medications, their purposes, and their side effects. Simple dosage questions and calculation methods may be asked. Some questions may be situational ones, such as, "What would you do in this case?" or "The first nursing action in this scenario should be ..."

A few larger institutions also may administer a clinical skills test. Such a test might be conducted in a simulated laboratory setting, where frequently used patient care equipment is set up. Usually a staff development instructor accompanies the nurse through a series of stations where the nurse is asked to plan and perform the appropriate nursing actions. Examples might be starting cardiopulmonary resuscitation on a simulated patient, demonstrating the proper procedure for starting an intravenous line, and talking through the assessment of a patient.

It is far better to be prepared and even better to be proactive and to offer to produce some of the documentation required. For instance, the nurse may be able to get a written reference from a former employer or a statement from a physician sooner than the institution can. The employment start date depends on the receipt of all necessary information, so it will expedite the process if the candidate volunteers to initiate some of the documentation gathering or even has references in hand with other documentation at the time of interview.

Once an applicant is selected the agency has committed itself to costly training, orientation, and additional benefits that may cost as much as 30% to 40% of the employee's salary. A major element of control, which any organization possesses, is its ability to choose its employees. A thorough selection process is a sign to the committed professional that this is a reputable employer.

SUMMARY

To summarize the chapter let's review the questions posed at the beginning of the chapter and see what you have learned.

1. How should the new graduate in the scenario decide where to apply for that first position?

    The neophyte nurse should carefully explore any job under consideration and its responsibilities in light of their own personal qualities. Some students find it helpful to consult an instructor or a trusted nursing mentor for objective input and perspective. An experienced nurse can see the pros and cons that may not be visible to a new nurse. A thoughtful review of one's general interests, abilities, and strengths (especially those pointed out by clinical instructors) and awareness of the types of patients who have provided the greatest emotional reward are essential.

    Other important considerations are one's physical and emotional stamina, energy level, and responsibilities to others—spouse, children, and other family members; volunteer commitments; and social activities—all of which make legitimate demands on one's schedule. Long-term goals must be factored into the first job choice as well. Is the first job a stepping-stone to an advanced degree, to a narrowly specialized area of nursing, to a traveling nurse position, or to a management role?

2. What kinds of questions should the applicant ask about a prospective position?

    RN vacancy rate and turnover rate

    Patient satisfaction scores (preferably a percentile ranking)

    Employee satisfaction scores

    Average tenure of nursing staff

    Education mix of nursing staff

    Percentage of registry or travelers used

    Key human resources policies (e.g., reduction in workforce; tenure vs performance criteria)

    Information about whether the nurses are unionized

    Job responsibilities of the position

3. How can the applicant demonstrate knowledge, skills, and experience to the recruiter?

    The applicant can create a portfolio as part of their preparation for graduation and entry into the first job. Nurses who present portfolios to the recruiter may have a competitive edge over nurses who do not. Including specific hours and skills obtained in clinical experiences on the résumé will assist the recruiter in assessing knowledge, skills, and experience of the applicant.

REFERENCES

Advisory Board. *Daily briefing: Nurse turnover.* https://www.advisory.com/daily-briefing/2022/10/17/nurse-turnover Accessed August 31, 2023.

American Association of Colleges of Nursing Task Force on Hallmarks of the Professional Practice Setting. (n.d.a). *Hallmarks of the professional practice environment.* https://www.aacnnursing.org/news-data/position-statements-white-papers/hallmarks-of-the-professional-nursing-practice-environment

American Association of Colleges of Nursing. (n.d.b). *What every nursing student should know when seeking employment.* https://www.aacnnursing.org/students

Holtzman, D., Kraft, E., & Small, E. (2022). Use of ePortfolios for making hiring decisions: A comparison of the results from representatives of large and small businesses. *Journal of Work Applied Management, 14(1),*18–34.

DeLuca, M., & DeLuca, N. (2010). *Stand out and get hired: Best answers to the 201 most frequently asked interview questions* (2nd ed.) The McGraw Hill Companies, Inc.

Doyle, A. (2020a). *Phone interview tips that will get you hired.* https://www.thebalancecareers.com/how-to-ace-a-phone-interview-2058579

Doyle, A. (2020b). *Tips on using skype for video job interviews.* https://www.thebalance.com/video-interviewing-with-skype-2061627

Dierkes, A.M., Riman, K., Daus, M., Germack, H.D., Lasater, K.B. (2021). The Association of Hospital Magnet° Status and Pay-for-Performance Penalties. *Policy, Politics & Nursing Practice, 22*(4):245–252. doi: 10.1177/15271544211053854. Epub 2021 Oct 22. PMID: 34678085; PMCID: PMC9394674

LaMaster, M.A., & Larsen, R.A. (2010). Prepare for a behavioral interview, then ace it!. *American Journal of Nursing, 40*(1), 8–10. https://doi.org/10.1097/01.NAJ.0000366152.10576.00

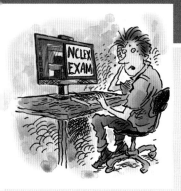

28

The NCLEX-RN® Examination

Trina Barrett, DNP, RN, CNE, CCRN-K

...dequate preparation for the NCLEX-RN exami-
...ation can reduce panic and ensure success.

ⓔ Additional resources are available online at: http://evolve.elsevier.com/Cherry/

LEARNING OUTCOMES

After studying this chapter, the reader will be able to:

1. Explain the purpose of the Next Generation NCLEX-RN (NGN-RN) examination.
2. Describe changes in the NGN-RN examination.
3. Create a personal plan for preparing for the NGN-RN examination.
4. Analyze the relationship between the client needs' categories/subcategories and the integrated processes as they relate to NGN-RN test items.
5. Use the NGN-RN Test Plan to plan review and remediation strategies.
6. Recognize the National Council of State Boards of Nursing Clinical Judgment Measurement Model (NCJMM).

KEY TERMS

Clinical judgment Defined by the National Council of State Boards of Nursing (NCSBN) as the observed outcome of critical thinking and decision-making. It is an iterative process with multiple steps that uses nursing knowledge to observe and assess presenting situations, identify a prioritized client concern, and generate the best possible evidence-based solutions to deliver safe client care (NCSBN, 2022).

Clinical judgment Measurement Model (CJMM) A framework for the valid measurement of clinical judgment and decision-making (NCSBN, 2019).

Computer adaptive testing (CAT) A type of testing taken on a computer, in which the computer reestimates a candidate's ability based on all the previous answers and the difficulty of those items. The CAT is able to produce results that are more precise and

efficient, using fewer items by targeting items to the candidate's ability (NCSBN, 2023a).

National Council of State Boards of Nursing An independent not-for-profit organization that supports state boards of nursing by monitoring trends in nursing practice and develops the licensing examination for both registered and practical nursing.

NCLEX-RN NCLEX stands for National Council Licensure Examination for Registered Nurses, an examination taken by qualified graduates of approved schools of nursing. Graduates who pass the NCLEX-RN are granted licenses to practice as RNs.

Next Generation NCLEX-RN (NGN-RN) An extension of the current NCLEX to focus on the assessment of clinical judgment as this skill has evolved as a vital aspect of entry-level nursing practice.

PROFESSIONAL/ETHICAL ISSUE

Jamie Wilcox, senior nursing student, just left a meeting with the director of her Bachelor of Science in Nursing (BSN) program. Jamie was devastated. She learned that she would not graduate in a few weeks as planned because her score on the final standardized exam was not high enough and, according to the program director, was a predictor that she might not pass the NGN-RN. Jamie did not realize there was so much at stake when she took the standardized exam, and she admitted to herself that she really did not prepare or take the exam seriously. After all, she had passed every course in the nursing program; her grades were not outstanding, but they were passing. She wondered: "Can this be fair? Was this high-stakes testing even ethical?"

Over the next week Jamie learned more about standardized exams. She learned they were used at various points throughout the nursing school curriculum to provide students and faculty with insight into how a student's performance compares with other students' at other schools. These exams also provide individual assessment by noting a student's strengths and weaknesses, and they are used to develop remediation plans. Standardized exams are often used by nursing schools to predict the chance for being successful on the NGN-RN and to determine whether a student will graduate, so they are considered "high stakes." However, Jamie also learned that standardized exams are just "predictors" or, at best, estimates of future performance. Although Jamie was determined to be successful in completing her remediation plan and performing well on the next standardized exam, she still had many questions about such "high-stakes" testing.

- What responsibility belongs with the nursing program that progressed a student through the program but then deemed a student ineligible to graduate because of their performance on a standardized exam?
- What responsibility lies with the student who had poor performance on a standardized exam?
- Should standardized exams become the "standard" that determines whether a student should graduate from nursing school? Why or why not?

VIGNETTE

Consider for a moment how nursing and licensure examinations have changed as society has changed. Nursing is a reflection of society's values, knowledge, and needs.

Test items or questions found on the NGN-RN examination today have little resemblance to questions asked on state board examinations administered during the early part of the 20th century. The examinations of that era dealt with practical issues and consisted mainly of knowledge-based questions that had little to do with assessment, application, evaluation, or need. Consider, for instance, the following questions taken from the 1919 state board questions and answers for nurses (Foote, 1919):

- What are the advantages of fireplaces?
- How would you sterilize silkworm-gut and silk sutures?
- What care regarding nourishment would you give a gynecological patient to prevent a common discomfort?
- Give some general rules for preparing meats.
- Give three common complaints that the public makes about graduate nurses.

Questions to Consider While Reading This Chapter:

1. What is the purpose of the NGN-RN examination?
2. What type of questions can I expect on the NGN-RN examination?
3. What is the best way to prepare for the NGN-RN examination?

CHAPTER OVERVIEW

This chapter helps student nurses prepare to successfully pass the Next Generation NCLEX (NGN-RN) examination. The purpose of the NGN-RN is discussed, an overview of the format and content is given, and reasons why the NCLEX-RN was updated to the NGN-RN and what to expect are presented. Various strategies for preparing for the examination are given, and students are encouraged to develop a personal plan of study.

ARE YOU PREPARED FOR THE NGN-RN EXAMINATION?

You are pursuing a degree in nursing and plan to take the Next Generation NCLEX-RN (NGN-RN) licensure examination after graduation. Do you know what to expect on the examination itself? Do you feel you have the knowledge necessary for NGN-RN examination success? If not you should be interested in this chapter, which offers an overview of the format and content you can expect on the test and strategies for success.

THE NGN-RN EXAMINATION

The NGN-RN examination and licensure to practice nursing go hand in hand. To receive a license to practice as a registered nurse (RN) in the United States and its territories, candidates must furnish evidence of competency to provide safe and effective nursing care by successfully completing the NGN-RN examination (NCSBN, 2023b). Graduates from all RN programs in all states take the same NGN-RN examination. The examination content common to all of these programs reflects current entry-level nursing practice (NCSBN, 2022). Individuals taking the examination must have graduated from approved schools of nursing.

Purpose of the NGN-RN Examination

The purpose of the NGN-RN examination is to:
1. Safeguard the public from unsafe practitioners.
2. Assist state boards of nursing in determining candidates' capabilities for performing entry-level RN positions.

To keep the NGN-RN examination current the National Council of State Boards of Nursing (NCSBN) conducts a practice analysis on a 3-year cycle by investigating current practice that entry-level nurses are performing in various health care settings in the United States. The practice analysis provides data to support the NCLEX as a reliable, valid measure of competent, entry-level nursing practice. The practice analysis is conducted every 3 years. In addition to the practice analysis NCSBN conducts a knowledge, skills, and abilities (KSA) survey. In 2021 this comprehensive survey included questions regarding the frequency and importance of entry-level nursing activities as well as the relevancy of using clinical judgment in performing the activities. Because clinical judgment is important in the delivery of safe and effective nursing care at the entry level, NCSBN added clinical judgment to the NCLEX Practice Analyses and the subsequent NCLEX Test Plans (NCSBN, 2022).

In the most current practice analysis completed in 2021 entry-level registered nurses ($n = 4758$) were asked to rank various activity statements from highest to lowest. The panel of 13 subject matter experts (SME) developed a survey of 146 nursing activity statements. The survey activity topics related to *frequency performed*, *importance*, and *clinical judgment relevancy*. The panel used the current test plan category structure describing the types of activities performed by newly licensed RNs and developed a list of activities performed within each category of the structure (NCSBN, 2022).

General Characteristics of the NGN-RN Examination.

The NCLEX-RN examination is a pass–fail examination and has been computerized since 1994. Before that time it was a paper-and-pencil examination requiring 2 days to complete. Today the examination is offered at Pearson Professional Centers throughout the United States and international test centers (NCSBN, 2023c). The NGN-RN can have anywhere from 85 to 150 items. Regardless of the number of items the time limit for examination is 5 hours, which includes examination instructions and breaks. All breaks (restroom, stretching, etc.) are optional. The official results of the examination are sent to candidates within 6 weeks after they have taken the examination. Unofficial results are available on the NCLEX website (NCSBN, 2023d).

Computer Adaptive Testing. The NCLEX-RN examination uses computer adaptive testing (CAT), a test-administering technique that uses computer technology and measurement theory. As a candidate answers questions on the examination, CAT adapts to the level of the candidate's knowledge, skills, and ability. After a candidate answers a question at a particular level of difficulty the computer selects the next item that the candidate should have a 50% chance of answering correctly. All examinations are consistent with the NGN-RN examination Test Plan, which controls inclusion of nursing content. Candidates have ample opportunity to demonstrate their competence because the examination does not end until stability of the pass or fail result is certain, or time runs out (NCSBN, 2023a).

Candidates taking the examination answer a minimum of 85 questions to a maximum of 150 questions, of which 15 are pretest and not scored. The NCSBN advises that the length of an NGN-RN examination be based on the performance of the candidate on the examination, and it has established a goal to be *95% sure of pass–fail decisions*. The computer determines whether a candidate passes or fails according to the following three rules:
1. *95% confidence interval rule:* 95% certainty that the candidate's ability is obviously above or below the passing standard.
2. *Maximum-length examination rule:* When the candidate is very close to the passing standard, the computer continues to give test items until the maximum number of items is reached; at this point, the computer disregards the 95% confidence rule and considers only the final ability estimate.

3. *Run-out-of-time rule:* If the candidate runs out of time before reaching the maximum number of items, the computer has not been able to decide whether the candidate passed or failed with 95% certainty, an alternate rule will be implemented:
   - If the candidate has not answered the minimum number of required items, the candidate automatically fails.
   - If at least the minimum number of required items were answered, then the final ability estimate will be based on all responses given before the exam time expired. If the score is at or above the passing standard the candidate will pass; otherwise the candidate will fail
   - It is important for students to understand that the goal of CAT is to determine competency based on the difficulty of questions answered correctly rather than on the number of questions answered correctly. The CAT is individualized, and two people taking the examination at the same time will not have the same questions (NCSBN, 2023a).

Question Formats

The NGN-RN will have test items in a variety of question formats to include **Traditional:** multiple choice, multiple response, ordered response, fill-in-the-blank calculations, and/or hot spots, charts, graphics, sound, video, tables, and multimedia; and **Next Generation**: matrix multiple choice, multiple response, case study, and stand-alone items that reflect the clinical judgment measurement model. The NCSBN website (www.ncsbn.org) has detailed information about the NCLEX-RN examination, including information on the *Next Generation NCLEX, CAT methodology,* the *candidate bulletin,* downloadable *Sample Pack,* and *Exam Preview* for candidates to view. Students are encouraged to visit the NCSBN website for multiple resources that will help them understand and prepare for taking the NGN-RN.

Traditional Format: Multiple Choice, One Option.

With this type of format, the candidate is presented with a question followed by four possible responses. The candidate is asked to select the one option that best answers the question. Multiple-choice, one-option format is the style most commonly used on the examination. See the following example.

> *The nurse has received the following information about assigned clients. The nurse should assess which client **first**?*

A. A 64-year-old client who had a total knee replacement 3 hours ago and has 15 mL of serosanguineous drainage in the collection device.

B. A 32-year-old client who had closed reduction of a fractured right malleolus 5 hours ago and has swelling of the right toes.

C. A 56-year-old Type 1 diabetic who has a left below-the-knee amputation and is complaining of left foot pain.

D. A 69-year-old client who was admitted 6 hours ago with congestive heart failure and is becoming increasingly more restless.
(Answer: D)

Alternate Item Formats. Because of the nature of CAT, the type of item presented to the candidate will depend on the content area. Following are examples of the alternate item formats.

- *Hot spot (questions based on illustrations and charts):* With the hot spot item, the candidate is asked to identify one or more area(s) on a picture or graphic and answer using the mouse button when the cursor is over the area identified. See the following example:

> *The nurse palpates the point of maximum impulse as part of the assessment exam. Where would the nurse locate the point of maximal impulse (PMI)?*
> 1. A
> 2. B
> 3. C
> 4. D
> *(Answer: D)*

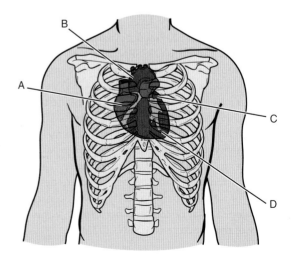

- *Multiple-response:* The candidate is presented with a question followed by five or more responses. The candidate is asked to check all responses that are correct; partial credit is not given. See the following example:

  *A nurse is caring for a 47-year-old female client who has been diagnosed with hypothyroidism. Which manifestations might the nurse expect the client to report? (**Select all that apply**.)*
  - ☐ Intolerance to heat
  - ☐ Periorbital edema
  - ☐ Weight loss
  - ☐ Menorrhagia
  - ☐ Constipation
  - ☐ Fatigue

    (Answer: periorbital edema, menorrhagia, constipation, and fatigue)

- *Fill-in-the-blank:* The candidate is presented with a dosage calculation question to which the answer must be typed, instead of selecting from among a set of options. A drop-down calculator is available for the candidate to use. Type only a number including a decimal point if indicated. Do not enter unit of measurement such as milligrams. The question tells you to round your answer. See the following example:

  The patient weighs 80 kg and the order is to infuse 500 mg dobutamine in 500 mL of LR at 5 mcg/kg/min. How many milligrams of dobutamine should be infused per hour?
  Answer: 24 mg/hour
  Calculations:
  5 mcg/min × 80 kg = 400 mcg/min
  400 mcg × 60 = 24,000 mcg/hr
  24,000 divided by 1000 = 24 mg/hr
  (1000 mcg = 1 mg)

- *Ordered response "Drag-and-drop":* The candidate is presented with a set of responses to a question and asked to place them in logical order to prioritize them. The unordered items appear on the left side of the screen and the candidate must drag each box to the right side of the screen in the correct order. See the following example:

  A nurse is preparing to perform a sterile dressing change. In what order would the following steps be performed?
  1. Gather supplies. ☐
  2. Set up the sterile field. ☐
  3. Assess the wound. ☐
  4. Explain the procedure to the patient. ☐
  5. Remove the soiled dressing. ☐
  6. Document the dressing change. ☐

     Candidates will be asked to click on the steps and drag items in the correct order.
     (Answer: 1 4 5 3 2 6)

- *Exhibit:* The candidate is provided with a problem and exhibit. To view the exhibit, the candidate must click on the "exhibit" button and read information found behind the tabs. See the following example, in which the candidate must look in the chart to find pertinent information to report:

  A patient is ordered Lanoxin 0.25 mg daily. The nurse assesses the patient's heart rate as 48 beats per minute. Prior to calling the physician, what additional information is needed?

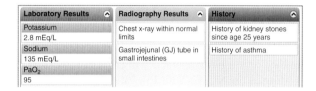

  A. Laboratory results: Potassium 2.8 mEq/L
  B. Laboratory results: Arterial blood gases (PaO₂) 95
  C. History: Kidney stones since age 25 years
  D. Radiography: Chest x-ray within normal limits
     (Answer: A)

- *Audio:* Each candidate is furnished with earphones and listens to an audio clip. The candidate is asked to identify specific assessment findings. See the following example:

  Candidate listens to an adventitious breath sound such as crackles.
  Candidate is asked to identify the abnormal finding.

- *Graphic:* The candidate is presented with options that are either pictures or graphic images rather than text. Options are preceded by circles and the candidate can only select one answer.

COGNITIVE DOMAINS AND THE NCLEX-RN EXAMINATION

The cognitive levels may be viewed as consecutive steps, with *remembering* being the lowest, most fundamental step and *creating* being the highest, most highly evolved of the steps. Table 28.1 shows the Bloom's cognitive levels

TABLE 28.1 Bloom's Taxonomy
Creating (highest level)
Evaluating
Analyzing
Applying
Understanding
Remembering (lowest level)

from the lowest level to the highest level. Because nursing requires application of knowledge, skills, and abilities, the majority of NGN-RN examination questions are written at the application or higher cognitive levels and reflect clinical judgment (Anderson & Krathwohl, 2001; Bloom et al, 1956; Dickison et al., 2019).

COMPONENTS OF THE NCLEX-RN TEST PLAN

The Test Plan for the NCLEX-RN examination is based on the current nursing practice of entry-level RNs. According to the NCSBN (2023b), "The NCLEX® assesses the knowledge, skills, abilities and clinical judgment that are essential for the entry-level nurse to use to meet the needs of clients requiring the pro-motion, maintenance or restoration of health" (p. 2). The NCLEX-RN Test Plan is framed by four major categories of *client needs*, which are further subdivided into a total of six subcategories, as follows (NCSBN, 2023b):

1. Safe, effective care environment
   - Management of care
   - Safety and infection control
2. Health promotion and maintenance
3. Psychosocial integrity
4. Physiologic integrity
   - Basic care and comfort
   - Pharmacologic and parenteral therapies
   - Reduction of risk potential
   - Physiologic adaptation

Each of these will be examined individually here, followed by a discussion of several processes that are fundamental to nursing and integrated throughout the client needs' categories and subcategories.

Client Needs

"The goal of nursing for client care in any setting is preventing illnesses and potential complications; alleviating suffering; protecting, promoting, restoring, and facilitating comfort and health; and dignity in dying" (NCSBN, 2023b, p. 3). *According to the NCSBN (2023b), the profession of nursing contributes in helping clients achieve an optimal level of health in a variety of settings. For the purposes of the NCLEX, a client is defined as the 'individual, family, or group, which includes significant others and population'."*

(NCSBN, 2023b, p. 3).

Safe and Effective Care Environment. The category safe and effective care environment pertains to the provision and direction of nursing care delivery to safeguard clients, their families or significant others, and health care providers. It is further divided into two subcategories, management of care, from which 15% to 21% of the Test Plan is constructed, and safety and infection control, from which 10% to 16% of the Test Plan is constructed (NCSBN, 2023b). Within this section, the nurse should have the knowledge, skills, and ability to meet the client's needs for a safe and effective environment.

Health Promotion and Maintenance. The health promotion and maintenance category pertains to the provision and direction of nursing care that takes into consideration projected growth and development principles, early detection and prevention of health problems, and techniques of physical assessment to achieve optimal health outcomes. Six percent to 12% of NCLEX-RN examination questions are related to this category (NCSBN, 2023b).

Psychosocial Integrity. In the psychosocial integrity category, "The nurse provides and directs nursing care that promotes and supports the emotional, mental, and social well-being of the client experiencing stressful events, as well as clients with acute or chronic mental illness" (NCSBN, 2023b, p. 11). Psychosocial integrity is addressed in 6% to 12% of NCLEX-RN examination questions (NCSBN, 2023b).

Physiologic Integrity

The physical aspects of health and wellness are the focus of physiologic integrity. This category is further divided into four subcategories (NCSBN, 2023b):

- Basic care and comfort, accounting for 6% to 12% of examination questions, is directed at the provision of comfort and assistance in performing activities of daily living.

- The pharmacologic and parenteral therapies subcategory, to which 13% to 19% of NCLEX questions are devoted, is concerned with administration of medications and parenteral therapies.
- Reduction of risk potential, addressed in 9% to 15% of the questions, correlates with reducing the risk of development of complications related to clients' current conditions or treatments.
- Physiologic adaptation, accounting for 11% to 17% of examination questions, is the management or coordination of care for clients with acute or chronic and life-threatening disease processes.

Integrated Processes

Processes that are fundamental to nursing are integrated throughout the previously noted client needs' categories and subcategories (NCSBN, 2023b). The integrated processes are:

- Caring: defined as "the interaction of the nurse and client in an atmosphere of mutual respect and trust. In this collaborative environment, the nurse provides encouragement, hope, support and compassion to help achieve desired outcomes" (NCSBN, 2023b, p.4).
- Clinical Judgment: defined as the observed outcome of critical thinking and decision-making; an iterative process with multiple steps that uses nursing knowledge to observe and assess presenting situations, identify a prioritized client concern, and generate the best possible evidence-based solutions to deliver safe client care.
- Communication and documentation: defined as the "verbal and nonverbal interactions between the nurse and the client, the client's significant others and the other members of the health care team. Events and activities associated with client care are validated in written and/or electronic records that reflect standards of practice and accountability in the provision of care" (NCSBN, 2023b. p. 4).
- Culture and Spirituality: defined as regard for the unique and personal preferences for care, the applicable standard of care, and legal requirements (NCSBN, 2023b).
- Nursing Process: defined as "a scientific, clinical reasoning approach to client care that includes assessment, analysis, planning, implementation and evaluation (NCSBN, 2023b, p. 4).
- Teaching/Learning: defined as "facilitation of the acquisition of knowledge, skills and abilities promoting a change in behavior" (NCSBN, 2023b, p 4).

Such examples can include a health promotion and maintenance question also involves teaching/learning or a psychosocial integrity question that also addresses communication and documentation. All questions relate to some activity in which an entry-level nurse may engage when caring for or managing a patient. A more complete overview of these integrated processes follows.

Nursing Process. The nursing process, defined previously as one of the integrated processes on the NGN-RN, is applicable to all situations in which the nurse and patient interact and may be used with any theoretic framework. The nursing process involves the following five steps:

1. Assessment: Establishes a database for the client and consists of gathering information or data about an identified client. Depending on the nurse's focus, the client may be a person, a family, a group of people, or a community. Assessment information comes from a variety of sources, including the client, the family and significant others, laboratory or radiographic reports, physician records, hospital or clinic records, and other caregivers. Assessment also includes verification and communication of data.
2. Analysis: Client-related data gathered during assessment provide the basis for analysis. During this step, the nurse classifies or groups assessment data and identifies actual or potential client problems. During classification data also are validated and interpreted, and additional data may be required.
3. Planning: Consists of setting realistic and measurable mutual goals, developing interventions to meet or resolve identified patient needs or problems, and modifying goals as necessary. Goal setting should include the collaboration of members of the interdisciplinary health care team, the client, their family, and significant others as indicated. As with the previous steps of the nursing process, the plan must be communicated to other members of the health care team to ensure continuity of care.
4. Implementation: Includes initiating and carrying out nursing interventions or actions to achieve the goals set in the planning stage. The nurse implements interventions that will allow the patient to achieve goals and outcomes to support or improve the patient's health status.
5. Evaluation: Data is collected to document the progress the patient has made, or not made, in relation to

the stated goal. Once data have been collected and analyzed the nurse must decide what action to take or what modification to make regarding the goal. Using evidence the nurse makes a judgment to determine whether the established outcome has met the actual response.

Clinical Judgment Measurement Model (CJMM)

The movement to the CJMM for the NGN-RN was based on the recognition that entry-level nursing practice relies upon a strong foundation of clinical judgment and effective decision-making to ensure patient safety. Chapter 24 gives a detailed description of Clinical Judgment. The CJMM is a framework designed for testing and does not replace evidence-based theories of nursing, nor does it replace the nursing process. Rather, it provides an evidence-based framework for measuring whether candidates can demonstrate clinical judgment and decision-making. Unfolding scenarios with new test item types and stand-alone items are designed to test critical thinking, clinical judgment, and decision-making. The six steps of the CJMM include (NCSBN, 2023b):

1. **Recognize cues**—identify relevant and important information from different sources (e.g., medical history, vital signs).
2. **Analyze cues**—organize and connect the recognized cues to the client's clinical presentation.
3. **Prioritize hypotheses**—evaluate and prioritize hypotheses (urgency, likelihood, risk, difficulty, time constraints, etc.).
4. **Generate solutions**—identify expected outcomes and use hypotheses to define a set of interventions for the expected outcomes.
5. **Take actions**—implement the solution(s) that address the highest priority.
6. **Evaluate outcomes**—compare observed outcomes to expected outcomes.

The following section describes the structure of NGN-RN test items designed to test critical thinking, clinical judgment, and decision-making.

NGN-RN Test Items. NGN-RN *case study items* are item sets composed of six items that are presented as part of an unfolding case scenario that are displayed with exhibit tabs such as Nurses' Notes, Vital Signs, and Diagnostic Results. NGN *stand-alone* items are items administered independent of other items. Both items

measure the clinical judgment steps of *Recognize Cues, Analyze Cues, Prioritize Hypothesis, Generate Solutions, Take Actions, and Evaluate Outcomes*.

A common feature of NGN-RN test items is that components of the item are displayed on a split screen with the left side stating the scenario and data and the right side presenting the question to be answered. The question to be answered will be in the form of the new NGN item types such as stand-alone, bowtie, trend, drag-and-drop, drop-down, highlight, matrix multiple, and multiple response. Students are encouraged to visit the NCSBN website to review sample questions and previews at https://www.nclex.com/prepare.page. Students are also encouraged to visit the following website for an explanation about how the NGN-RN text items are scored: https://www.ncsbn.org/public-files/NGN_Summer21_ENG.pdf.

PREPARING FOR THE NCLEX-RN EXAMINATION

The NCLEX-RN is considered to be a "high-stakes" examination to evaluate nursing competence and protect the public. There is no one best method for preparing to take the NCLEX-RN. Success depends on a candidate's nursing knowledge and ability to use that knowledge, test-taking skills, and confidence level. The best preparation any candidate can have is what the candidate brings from their nursing program.

Some measure of preparation for the NCLEX-RN examination after graduation from nursing school is a must for all candidates seeking success on the examination. Candidates should NOT convince themselves that they do not need to review because they made average or above-average grades in their academic and nursing coursework, nor should they decide that review will serve no purpose because they made average or below-average grades in their coursework.

In preparation for the NCLEX-RN examination, it is important to remember that review is a personal undertaking. What works for one candidate may not work for another, and vice versa. Each candidate should use the study and review methods that have proved successful in their nursing program. To allow ample time to review content successful candidates usually start studying about 5 or 6 months prior to taking the test, but depending on your end-of-program predictor exam results or practice exam results you may need longer.

Build Your NCLEX Study Plan

Use the following tips and strategies to build your own study plan and increase the likelihood of passing the NCLEX-RN examination:

- *Review the most current NCLEX-RN Candidate Bulletin* found on the NCSBN website (www.ncsbn.org).
- *Become familiar with the test plan* (find the most current Test Plan at www.ncsbn.org).
- *Locate your test site early.* Be sure to obtain an Authorization to Test (ATT). Remember, you must apply to your board of nursing or regulatory body before registering with Pearson Vue (http://www.pearson-vue.com) to take the examination. Be certain you have acceptable identification as stated on the NCSBN website. You may need to order replacement identification before testing. If you have changed your name, the only identification documents accepted are a marriage license, divorce decree, or legal court name change documents.
- *Perform a needs assessment.* Determine content areas of strengths and weaknesses. Look at previous academic and nursing coursework, class notes and handouts, examination grades, and grades made on nursing care plans or process papers. If your school uses nationally normed assessment examinations use their report to determine areas of strengths and weaknesses. The rationale provided when reviewing these exams provides a wealth of information and validates the correct answers. Talk with faculty in courses in which you had weakness or difficulty. Determine where the greatest amount of review is needed. Be honest in performing the needs assessment. The foundation for success or failure on the NCLEX-RN examination may be determined here.
- *Analyze standardized examinations.* If your school uses standardized examinations to compare you with your peers and the national population of test takers, look at where you rank in comparison with both groups. Again, do not be overconfident if you scored higher than either group. This fact should give you positive affirmation that you have a high chance of passing the NCLEX—not that you can delete your NCLEX-RN study plans. Even when students score at the highest level, many miss some questions. The "focused review" provided by the standardized examination describes the area of the nursing process, and the specific content area should be used to remediate. Remember, these exams cannot test all content

matter so always consider that you received only what is highly tested on the NCLEX-RN.

- *Determine the number of days or weeks necessary for review.* Candidates with a strong nursing knowledge base may need less time than candidates with weaknesses. As with the needs assessment, you should be realistic in planning the amount of review time you need.
- *Decide which method of review will be used.* Both individual and group study methods have strong and weak points. Strong points of individual study include having total control over content and time spent in review. Weak points include having no immediate resources to explain or assist with understanding difficult concepts. Candidates with weakness in disciplining themselves may have problems sticking to review schedules and focusing on specific content with individual study. Strong points of group study include the support that members can give one another and learning from others in the group. Also, many minds working together are stronger than one working alone. Weak points of group study include lack of preparation by some group members, the group being held back by weaker members, and a tendency of the group to focus on socialization rather than review. If you use a study group, get the others to agree that all members coming to sessions must be prepared to work.
- *Decide what materials or resources will be used during review.* Textbooks and class notes from nursing or nursing-related courses, such as anatomy and physiology, psychology, and nutrition, are helpful. It has been suggested that rereading your nursing school notes may not be the best use of time. Computer-assisted instructions used during the nursing program may be available. Numerous NCLEX-RN examination review books are available. Many review books include online resources to be used during review.
- *Structure review time.* Schedule review during your times of peak performance. Learning is enhanced when reviewing for short blocks of time, around 50 minutes, instead of for several unbroken hours at a time. Remember that you are reviewing for an examination, not cramming for one.
- *Control the review environment.* Keep noise and distraction at a minimum. Have adequate space and lighting for review. Control the room temperature when possible; if not possible, dress for the environment. Have all materials needed for review, including

drinks and snacks, close at hand so as not to waste time gathering these items during review time. Make sure that friends and family know not to interrupt you during review time.

- *Have a game plan for each review session.* Develop a review schedule complete with subject matter to be considered and specific tasks to be completed during each session. Stick to the schedule.
- *Learn concepts and principles, not isolated facts.* The NCLEX-RN examination tests a candidate's ability to apply, analyze, and evaluate nursing knowledge and does not focus on isolated events. Candidates whose past test-taking success has been based on memorization rather than actual learning have an increased risk for failure on this examination.
- *Use learning techniques that have proved successful in the past.* People have different learning styles and therefore benefit from different learning techniques. You might choose to use flash cards, underscore key points, take notes or outline material, or record pertinent information for later playback. Quiz yourself or ask others to pose questions. Many people find downloading application software (i.e., an "app") to practice NCLEX-style questions is helpful.
- *Seek qualified help when reviewing information that is particularly difficult.* Faculty members are an excellent resource. If you invest in an external course review, ask for help during the question and answer sessions or determine whether an open forum to ask questions extends beyond the actual review class. Some review courses offer individual coaches to address these difficult topics.
- *Practice taking NCLEX-RN–type examinations, paying particular attention to the rationales or reasons provided for correct and incorrect answers.* Successful test takers know why a specific option is correct or incorrect. Even though candidates may spend as much time as they want on a question when actually taking the examination, you should get into the habit of taking about 1 minute for each question. Poor time management may cause a candidate to not have enough time to complete the test and therefore to be unsuccessful on the NCLEX-RN examination. Practice also will help reduce test anxiety. NCLEX-RN–type examinations are commonly found in NCLEX-RN review books.
- *Use the Internet.* It provides numerous sources that may aid in preparation for the NCLEX-RN examination.

- *Avoid excessive stimulants* (e.g., caffeine) *to increase review time.* The best learning takes place when your head is clear.
- *Maintain a healthy, positive attitude toward reviewing and taking the NCLEX-RN examination.* Have confidence in your abilities to be successful on the examination. Remember that even practicing nurses with years of experience do not know everything there is to know about every aspect of nursing and that your goal on the NCLEX-RN examination is to demonstrate minimal competency for an entry-level RN position, not competency required for an advanced RN position.
- *Remember to use the NCSBN website* (www.ncsbn.org), which offers tips related to how to prepare for the NCLEX-RN exam, the registration process, what to expect on exam day and how to get your results.

Consider an NCLEX-RN Review Course: Food for Thought

Just as there is no one best method for preparing to take the NCLEX-RN examination, there is no one best review course for a candidate to take in preparation for the examination. The most important thing to remember is that a review course is exactly what it says it is—a review course. Such courses are designed to reconsider or reexamine content common to the three types of nursing programs and to improve test-taking strategies.

The purpose of a review course is to enhance or polish what candidates already know from their nursing programs. Review courses are not intended to teach totally new concepts. For a candidate who has an extreme weakness in one or more content areas the review course may not provide enough content to bring them up to speed on the topic.

Numerous companies and people offer review courses. Each review offering has strong and weak points, and what appeals to one candidate may not appeal to another. Some companies offer financial discounts or other incentives if more than one candidate from a school of nursing registers for their course. Review courses can be expensive and may last from 1 or 2 days to a complete week. Some courses provide books or other written or online materials. Others may offer additional materials for a fee. Some companies will refund a part or all of the cost of the review course if a candidate who takes it does not pass the NCLEX-RN.

Investigate who is teaching the review course you are considering. Are the credentials and nursing background of those teaching the course available? And do they appear to be competent to teach the course? A review course is no better than the person or people teaching it. The decision to take a review course in preparation for the NCLEX-RN examination is a personal one. Some candidates find the structure and schedule of a review course helpful in preparation. Other candidates may find the structure and schedule restrictive and overly time-consuming.

Candidates seriously interested in taking an NCLEX-RN examination review course should look to the faculty at their school of nursing for guidance. Many faculty have had experience with review courses or may teach them. Candidates should also talk to peers who have recently graduated about recommendations for review courses. Serious candidates also should obtain written information from several different offerings and compare and contrast them. Selection of a review course should be based on more than the cost—it should meet the candidate's unique needs.

SUMMARY

Success on the NCLEX-RN examination is needed to obtain a license and practice as an RN. Entry-level nurses are required to make complex decisions while delivering client care. These increasingly complex decisions often require the use of clinical judgment to support client safety. Research studies analyzed items and documented the validity of these items to measure clinical judgment. The NGN-RN exam is designed to capture entry-level CJ understanding more directly. The NGN-RN should be viewed as an extension of the current NCLEX rather than radically different. The key to success on the NCLEX-RN examination is sound preparation from the nursing program, adequate preparation for the examination, and confidence in oneself.

REFERENCES

Anderson, L.W., & Krathwohl, D.R. (Eds.). (2001). *A taxonomy for learning, teaching, and assessing: A revision of Bloom's taxonomy of educational objectives.* Addison-Wesley.

Bloom, B.S., et al. (1956). *Taxonomy of educational objectives: The classification of educational goals. Handbook I. Cognitive domain.* David McKay.

Dickison, P., Haerling, K.A., & Lasater, K. (2019). Integrating the national council of state boards of nursing clinical judgment model into nursing educational frameworks. *Journal of Nursing Education, 58*(2), 72–78.

Foote, J. (1919). *State board questions and answers for nurses.* Lippincott.

National Council of State Boards of Nursing. (2019). *Next generation NCLEX news: The NGN clinical judgment measurement model and action model.* https://www.ncsbn.org/publications/ngn-news-spring2019

National Council of State Boards of Nursing. (2022). *RN practice analysis: Linking the NCLEX-RN examination to practice, U.S. and Canada.* https://www.ncsbn.org/public-files/21_NCLEX_RN_PA.pdf

National Council of State Boards of Nursing. (2023a). *The NCLEX uses computer adaptive testing.* https://www.nclex.com/the-ngn-uses-cat.page

National Council of State Boards of Nursing. (2023b). *2023 Next generation NCLEX-RN test plan.* https://www.nclex.com/test-plans.page

National Council of State Boards of Nursing. (2023c). *NCLEX test center.* https://www.nclex.com/testing-locations.page

National Council of State Boards of Nursing. (2023d). *Quick results: How to access your unofficial NCLEX results. National Council of State Boards of Nursing.* https://www.nclex.com/quick-results.page

INDEX

Note: Page numbers followed by *b* indicate boxes, *f* indicate figures, and *t* indicate tables.

A

AACN. *See* American Association of Colleges of Nursing
AANA. *See* American Association of Nurse Anesthetists
ABCD approach, time management and, 481
Abstract, 97
ACA. *See* Affordable Care Act
Accommodation, conflict resolution and, 369
Accountability, 132, 135, 179, 187
    challenge of, 195
    definition of, 374
Accreditation, 69, 80
    patient safety improved with, 416–417
    quality improvement through, 409–410
    staffing affected by, 393
Accuracy, in communication, 360
Active listening, 351, 359
Active shooter, 302, 313–314, 314t
Activities, scheduling of, time management and, 482
Act, purpose of, 73
Acuity, patient
    definition of, 391
    level of, 392
Acupuncture, 223–224, 224f
Acute care setting, nursing care delivery model for, 399–400
Adaptation model, 93
Ad hominen abusive, 359t
Advance care plan, 245, 251–252
    definition of, 239
Advance directives, 132, 166, 167, 240, 250
    definition of, 239
Advanced practice nurse (APN), 69, 73
Advanced practice registered nurse (APRN) regulation, 80
Affordable Care Act (ACA), 18, 123, 435
    components, 124b
Agency for Healthcare Research and Quality (AHRQ), 101–102
Aggressive communication, 363–364
AHRQ. *See* Agency for Healthcare Research and Quality
Alexander technique, 220, 231b
Algorithm, health care protocols described with, 414, 415f
All-hazards approach, 305
    definition of, 302
Alternate item format, 512–513
AMA. *See* American Medical Association
Ambulatory care, nursing care delivery model, 400
American Academy of Nursing (AAN), 62b
American Assembly for Men in Nursing (AAMN), 32–33
American Association of Colleges of Nursing (AACN), 62b, 419, 464–465, 491
American Association of Nurse Anesthetists (AANA), 32
American Association of Occupational Health Nurses, 270
American Indians, poverty rate of, 202
American Medical Association (AMA), 425
American Nurses Association (ANA), 34, 69, 72, 433, 491–492
    Code of Ethics for Nurses, 242

American Nurses Association (ANA) *(Continued)*
    Code of Ethics for Nurses with Interpretive Statements, 258
    collective bargaining and, 278
    Crisis Standard of Care: COVID-19 Pandemic, 258
    health policy development of, 426–429
    Nursing: Scope and Standards of Practice, 328
    workplace advocacy by, 258
American Nurses Association code of ethics, 182b
American Nurses Credentialing Center (ANCC), 34, 69, 78–79, 261, 270
American Organization for Nurse Leadership (AONL) COVID Impact Longitudinal Study, 19–20
Americans with Disabilities Act, 137, 138–139
ANA. *See* American Nurses Association
Analysis
    of health policy issues, 433–434
    as stage of nursing process, 331
ANCC. *See* American Nurses Credentialing Center
Antiestablishment, 22, 27–28
APN. *See* Advanced practice nurse
Appropriate staffing, 457
Arbitration, 280
    definition of, 275
Art, 22, 23
Art and literature, nursing in, 26–31
    1980s to 1990s, 28
    as Angel of Mercy, 27
    antiestablishment era, 27–28
    antiquity's image, 26
    early 20th-century, 27
    as heroine, 27
    media campaigns, 30–31
    millennial media, 29
    nursing's response, 30
    sexual revolution, 28
    social media, 29–30
    Victorian image, 26–27
Artificial intelligence (AI), 103, 296
Assertive communication, 363, 461
Assertiveness skills, novice nurse development of, 461
Assessment
    function of, delegation of nursing tasks and, 25
    of health policy issues, 433–434
    NCLEX-RN® examination and, 515
Assessment tool, for decision-making, 505b
Assignment, definition of, 374
Assistive personnel (AP), 374, 376, 389
Associate degree programs, 57
Association of Perioperative Registered Nurses, 270
Attitudes
    culturally diverse groups, 203–204, 203f
    verbal communication affected by, 354
Audio, as alternate item format, 513
Augmented reality (AR), 297